FOURTH EDITION

INTRODUCTION TO
GLOBAL HEALTH

Kathryn H. Jacobsen, PhD, MPH
Professor of Health Studies
William E. Cooper Distinguished University Chair
University of Richmond

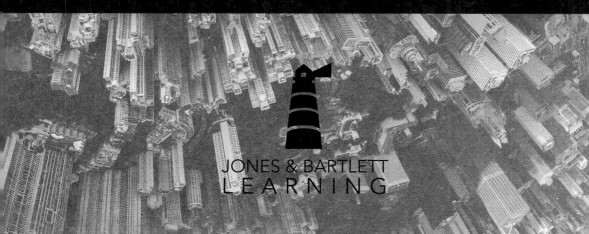

JONES & BARTLETT
LEARNING

World Headquarters
Jones & Bartlett Learning
25 Mall Road
Burlington, MA 01803
978-443-5000
info@jblearning.com
www.jblearning.com

Jones & Bartlett Learning books and products are available through most bookstores and online booksellers. To contact Jones & Bartlett Learning directly, call 800-832-0034, fax 978-443-8000, or visit our website, www.jblearning.com.

Substantial discounts on bulk quantities of Jones & Bartlett Learning publications are available to corporations, professional associations, and other qualified organizations. For details and specific discount information, contact the special sales department at Jones & Bartlett Learning via the above contact information or send an email to specialsales@jblearning.com.

40335-0

Production Credits

Vice President, Product Management: Marisa R. Urbano
Vice President, Product Operations: Christine Emerton
Director, Product Management: Matthew Kane
Product Manager: Sophie Fleck Teague
Director, Content Management: Donna Gridley
Manager, Content Strategy: Carolyn Pershouse
Content Strategists: Sara Bempkins, Tess Sackmann
Director, Project Management and Content Services: Karen Scott
Manager, Project Management: Jackie Reynen
Project Manager: Jennifer Risden
Senior Digital Project Specialist: Angela Dooley
Senior Marketing Manager: Susanne Walker

Content Services Manager: Colleen Lamy
Vice President, Manufacturing and Inventory Control:
    Therese Connell
Product Fulfillment Manager: Wendy Kilborn
Composition: Straive
Cover Design: Michael O'Donnell
Media Development Editor: Faith Brosnan
Rights & Permissions Manager: John Rusk
Rights Specialist: Liz Kincaid
Cover Image (Title Page, Part Opener, Chapter Opener):
    © Tavarius/Shutterstock
Printing and Binding: LSC Communications

Library of Congress Cataloging-in-Publication Data

Names: Jacobsen, Kathryn H., author.
Title: Introduction to global health / Kathryn H. Jacobsen.
Other titles: Global health
Description: Fourth edition. | Burlington, Massachusetts : Jones & Bartlett
    Learning, [2024] | Includes bibliographical references and index. |
Identifiers: LCCN 2022006405 | ISBN 9781284234930 (paperback)
Subjects: LCSH: World health. | Public health. | Globalization–Health
    aspects. | MESH: World Health. | Communicable Disease Control. | Health
    Transition. | Internationality. | BISAC: MEDICAL / Public Health
Classification: LCC RA441 .J33 2022 | DDC 362.1–dc23/eng/20220225
LC record available at https://lccn.loc.gov/2022006405

6048

Printed in the United States of America
26 25 24 23 22   10 9 8 7 6 5 4 3 2 1

Brief Contents

Preface   xi

New to This Edition   xiii

About the Author   xv

CHAPTER 1   Global Health Transitions......................1

CHAPTER 2   Global Health Priorities.......................21

CHAPTER 3   Socioeconomic Determinants
              of Health......................................55

CHAPTER 4   Environmental Determinants
              of Health......................................75

CHAPTER 5   Health and Human Rights.......................107

CHAPTER 6   Global Health Financing.......................133

CHAPTER 7   Global Health Implementation..................155

CHAPTER 8   HIV/AIDS and Tuberculosis.....................177

CHAPTER 9   Diarrheal, Respiratory, and
              Other Infections..............................213

CHAPTER 10   Malaria and Neglected Tropical
              Diseases......................................253

CHAPTER 11   Reproductive Health...........................297

CHAPTER 12   Nutrition.....................................331

CHAPTER 13   Cardiovascular Diseases.......................361

CHAPTER 14   Cancer..391

CHAPTER 15 **Diabetes, Chronic Respiratory Diseases, and Other Noncommunicable Diseases** ... 419

CHAPTER 16 **Mental Health Promotion**................... 457

CHAPTER 17 **Injury Prevention** 481

CHAPTER 18 **Promoting Neonatal, Infant, Child, and Adolescent Health** 507

CHAPTER 19 **Promoting Healthy Adulthood and Aging** 529

CHAPTER 20 **Interprofessionalism in Global Health** 547

Glossary **555**
Index **591**

Contents

Preface.........................xi

New to This Edition............xiii

About the Author xv

CHAPTER 1 Global Health Transitions 1

1.1 Defining Global Health 1

1.2 Population Health 3

1.3 Prevention and Intervention
Science 4

1.4 Risk Factors 8

1.5 Health Transitions 12

1.6 Global Health History and
Functions 15

1.7 Global Health Achievements..... 17

References 18

CHAPTER 2 Global Health Priorities 21

2.1 Globalization and Health 21

2.2 Global Health Security.......... 22

2.3 Prioritization Strategies 24

2.4 Millennium Development Goals .. 28

2.5 Sustainable Development Goals.. 30

2.6 Vital Statistics................. 34

2.7 Mortality 36

2.8 Morbidity..................... 40

2.9 Burden of Disease Metrics 41

2.10 Sources of Health Information ... 44

2.11 Country Income Level and Health 46

2.12 Featured Countries 50

References 52

CHAPTER 3 Socioeconomic Determinants of Health........ 55

3.1 Health Equity and the Sustainable
Development Goals............. 55

3.2 Economics 56

3.3 Education 59

3.4 Gender 61

3.5 Employment................... 63

3.6 Culture, Discrimination,
and Health 65

3.7 Migrant and Refugee Health..... 67

3.8 Governance and Politics 70

References 72

CHAPTER 4 Environmental Determinants of Health........ 75

4.1 Environmental Health and the
Sustainable Development Goals...75

4.2 Water, Sanitation, and Hygiene ... 79

4.3 Energy and Air Quality.......... 84

4.4 Occupational and Industrial
Health.......................88

4.5 Urbanization................... 92

4.6 Sustainability 96

4.7 Ecosystem Health 99

4.8 Climate Change and Health 100

References 103

CHAPTER 5 Health and Human Rights 107

5.1 Health and Human Rights...... 107

5.2 Access to Health Services...... 110

5.3 Access to Essential Medicines . . 111

5.4 People with Disabilities 114

5.5 Health in Prisons 117

5.6 Health Workforce 119

5.7 Access to Basic Human Needs . . 121

5.8 Emergency Management 123

5.9 International Health Regulations . . 126

References 129

CHAPTER 6 **Global Health Financing** **133**

6.1 Medicine and Public Health 133

6.2 Global Health Financing 135

6.3 Health Systems 137

6.4 Paying for Personal Health 141

6.5 Health Insurance 143

6.6 Paying for Global Health Interventions 145

6.7 Official Development Assistance . . 146

6.8 Foundations and Corporate Donations 149

6.9 Personal Donations 150

References 152

CHAPTER 7 **Global Health Implementation** **155**

7.1 Global Health Channels and Implementers 155

7.2 Global Health Interventions 157

7.3 International Cooperation 159

7.4 The United Nations 160

7.5 Development Banks 163

7.6 Global Partnerships 165

7.7 Local and National Governments . . 166

7.8 The Nonprofit Sector 168

7.9 The Corporate Sector 170

7.10 Research and the Academic Sector 171

7.11 Measuring Impact 171

References 174

CHAPTER 8 **HIV/AIDS and Tuberculosis** **177**

8.1 HIV/AIDS, Tuberculosis, and Global Health 177

8.2 Viruses, Bacteria, and Fungi 179

8.3 HIV and AIDS 181

8.4 HIV/AIDS Epidemiology 184

8.5 HIV Interventions 189

8.6 Sexually Transmitted Infections . 195

8.7 Tuberculosis 197

8.8 TB Epidemiology 199

8.9 TB Interventions 202

8.10 Antimicrobial Resistance 205

References 207

CHAPTER 9 **Diarrheal, Respiratory, and Other Infections** **213**

9.1 Infectious Diseases and Global Health 213

9.2 Diarrheal Diseases 217

9.3 Diarrhea Interventions 221

9.4 Acute Respiratory Infections 224

9.5 Pneumonia Interventions 228

9.6 Influenza 230

9.7 Coronaviruses 234

9.8 Immunization 235

9.9 Vaccine-Preventable Infections . . 238

9.10 Viral Hepatitis 242

9.11 Meningitis 245

References 245

CHAPTER 10 **Malaria and Neglected Tropical Diseases** . . **253**

10.1 Malaria, NTDs, and Global Health 253

10.2   Protozoa and Helminths 255

10.3   Malaria 257

10.4   Malaria Epidemiology 259

10.5   Malaria Interventions. 260

10.6   Dengue 265

10.7   Other Arboviruses 266

10.8   Lymphatic Filariasis. 269

10.9   Onchocerciasis. 270

10.10 Schistosomiasis 272

10.11 Soil-Transmitted
       Helminths. 273

10.12 Chagas Disease and
       Trypanosomiasis 274

10.13 Leishmaniasis 276

10.14 Leprosy, Buruli Ulcer,
       and Trachoma 276

10.15 Skin NTDs. 278

10.16 Foodborne NTDs 279

10.17 Rabies and Snakebite
       Envenoming 282

10.18 Eradication 283

10.19 Guinea Worm Disease 285

10.20 Polio 287

10.21 Emerging Infectious
       Diseases. 288

References 291

**CHAPTER 11 Reproductive
Health** . . . . **.297**

11.1   Reproductive Health
       and Global Health 297

11.2   The Fertility Transition. 299

11.3   Population Planning. 302

11.4   Family Planning 306

11.5   Contraception. 308

11.6   Healthy Pregnancy. 311

11.7   Maternal Mortality 313

11.8   Stillbirths and Neonatal
       Mortality 317

11.9   Infertility 322

11.10 Gynecological Health. 323

11.11 Men's Reproductive Health 324

11.12 Sexual Minority Health 324

References 325

CHAPTER 12 Nutrition **331**

12.1   Nutrition and Global Health 331

12.2   Macronutrients. 332

12.3   Breastfeeding and
       Infant Nutrition. 335

12.4   Child Growth. 337

12.5   Severe Acute Malnutrition. 341

12.6   Food Security and
       Food Systems. 343

12.7   Micronutrients 345

12.8   Iron Deficiency Anemia 346

12.9   Iodine Deficiency Disorders. 348

12.10 Other Mineral Deficiencies 348

12.11 Vitamin A Deficiency 349

12.12 Other Vitamin Deficiencies 350

12.13 Overweight and Obesity. 350

12.14 Obesity Interventions. 353

12.15 Food Safety. 355

References 357

**CHAPTER 13 Cardiovascular
Diseases** **361**

13.1   Cardiovascular Disease and
       Global Health 361

13.2   The Epidemiologic Transition . . 363

13.3   CVD Epidemiology 365

13.4   CVD Prevention. 367

13.5   Health Behavior Change 371

13.6   Physical Inactivity and
       Sedentariness 373

13.7   Ischemic Heart Disease. 375

13.8   Stroke 379

13.9 Hypertension 381

13.10 Other Cardiovascular
      Diseases .384

References 387

CHAPTER 14 Cancer 391

14.1 Cancer and Global Health 391

14.2 Cancer Biology 392

14.3 Cancer Epidemiology 394

14.4 Cancer Prevention 398

14.5 Cancer Screening 401

14.6 Cancer Treatment 402

14.7 Lung Cancer 406

14.8 Breast Cancer 407

14.9 Cervical Cancer 409

14.10 Prostate Cancer 410

14.11 Liver Cancer 412

14.12 Esophageal, Stomach, and
      Colorectal Cancers 413

14.13 Other Cancers 414

References 416

**CHAPTER 15 Diabetes,
Chronic Respiratory Diseases,
and Other Noncommunicable
Diseases 419**

15.1 Noncommunicable Diseases and
      Global Health 419

15.2 Diabetes 425

15.3 Chronic Respiratory Diseases . . 429

15.4 Tobacco Control 433

15.5 Chronic Kidney Disease 436

15.6 Liver Diseases 437

15.7 Digestive Diseases 440

15.8 Neurological Disorders 442

15.9 Genetic Blood Disorders 443

15.10 Musculoskeletal Disorders 445

15.11 Vision Impairment 446

15.12 Hearing Loss 449

15.13 Skin Diseases 451

15.14 Dental and Oral Health 451

References 452

**CHAPTER 16 Mental Health
Promotion 457**

16.1 Mental Health and
      Global Health 457

16.2 Depressive Disorders 459

16.3 Anxiety Disorders 460

16.4 Schizophrenia 461

16.5 Bipolar Disorder 463

16.6 Drug Use Disorders 463

16.7 Alcohol Use Disorders 464

16.8 Other Mental Health Disorders . .468

16.9 Suicide 469

16.10 Autism and Neurodevelopmental
      Disorders 471

16.11 Dementia and Neurocognitive
      Disorders 472

16.12 Mental Health Care 473

References 475

CHAPTER 17 Injury Prevention . . 481

17.1 Injuries and Global Health 481

17.2 Transport Injuries 484

17.3 Falls 488

17.4 Drowning 490

17.5 Burns 492

17.6 Other Unintentional Injuries . . . 492

17.7 Intentional Injuries 494

17.8 Interpersonal Violence 494

17.9 Gender-Based Violence 497

17.10 Conflict and War 498

17.11 Bioterrorism 501

References 503

CHAPTER 18 **Promoting Neonatal, Infant, Child, and Adolescent Health 507**

18.1   Global Child Health 507

18.2   Improving Neonatal Survival 510

18.3   Supporting Infant Health and Development. 514

18.4   Health Interventions in Early Childhood 516

18.5   Children with Special Needs . . . 520

18.6   Promoting Health in Middle Childhood 521

18.7   Promoting Adolescent Health . . 522

References 525

CHAPTER 19 **Promoting Healthy Adulthood and Aging 529**

19.1   Healthy Adulthood 529

19.2   Promoting Health in Early Adulthood 531

19.3   Promoting Health in Middle Adulthood 534

19.4   The Aging Transition 537

19.5   Aging and Global Health 539

19.6   Supporting Health in Older Adulthood 543

References 544

CHAPTER 20 **Interprofessionalism in Global Health. 547**

20.1   Core Knowledge in Global Health 547

20.2   Multidisciplinary Learning in Global Health 547

20.3   Interprofessional Skills for Global Health Practice. 550

20.4   Intercultural Communication and Global Health Practice 551

20.5   Experiential Learning in Global Health 551

20.6   Professional Development in Global Health 552

20.7   Global Health Matters 553

References 554

Glossary. 555

Index 591

Preface

The first and second editions of *Introduction to Global Health* were written during the era of the Millennium Development Goals (MDGs). The MDGs spelled out an ambitious plan for significantly reducing global poverty between 2000 and 2015. Thanks to the support of partners around the world, many of the MDG targets were achieved. The number of people living in extreme poverty dropped substantially during the first 15 years of the 21st century, and significant progress was made toward alleviating hunger, preventing maternal and child mortality, and controlling HIV/AIDS and malaria.

The Sustainable Development Goals (SDGs), which were launched at the end of 2015 as the follow-up to the MDGs, were used as an organizing framework for the third edition of *Introduction to Global Health*. The SDGs consist of 17 goals for enhancing human flourishing by 2030 by promoting prosperity while upholding human rights, protecting the planet, and fostering peace and security. Improvements in any of the 17 areas will yield benefits for population health, and improvements in global public health will enable other SDGs to be achieved. While the MDGs focused on health problems that primarily burden low-income countries, the SDGs include targets that apply to every country worldwide, including containing the spread of infectious diseases, improving management of noncommunicable diseases, promoting mental health, and preventing injuries. The priorities spelled out in the SDGs continue to guide funding and policy decisions in global health, and they remain a core theme in the revised edition of the textbook (**Table 1**).

The major updates for this new fourth edition of *Introduction to Global Health* feature emerging themes related to what might come to be known as the pandemic era. New and expanded content about global health security, health equity, health metrics, and other areas of global health that have grown in importance as a result of the COVID-19 pandemic are integrated into chapters throughout the text. The sections of the text that feature the SDGs and various other health targets established by the World Health Organization and global partnerships acknowledge the setbacks that have been caused by the COVID-19 pandemic, and a series of new tables summarizes the many types of interventions that can be used to resume progress toward achieving improved world health. Global health has never been more visible than it is today. This text provides a forward-looking perspective on the numerous actions that are helping promote the physical, mental, and social health of people across the life span and across the globe.

Table 1 The SDGs and *Introduction to Global Health*

SDG	Goal	Target		Chapter/Section
1	No poverty			3.2
2	Zero hunger			12
3	Good health and well-being	3.1	Maternal mortality	11
		3.2	Infant and child mortality	18
		3.3	HIV/AIDS and tuberculosis	8
		3.3	Hepatitis, waterborne diseases, and other communicable diseases	9
		3.3	Malaria and neglected tropical diseases	10
		3.4	Noncommunicable diseases	13, 14, 15
		3.4	Mental health and well-being	16
		3.5	Substance abuse	16.6, 16.7
		3.6	Road traffic injuries	17.2
		3.7	Sexual and reproductive health	11
		3.8	Universal health coverage	6
		3.9	Hazardous chemicals; air, water, and soil pollution; and contamination	4
		3.a	Framework Convention on Tobacco Control	15.4
		3.b	Access to vaccines and medicines	5.3
		3.c	Health workforce	5.6
		3.d	Emergency management	5.8
4	Quality education			3.3
5	Gender equality			3.4
6	Clean water and sanitation			4.2
7	Affordable and clean energy			4.3
8	Decent work and economic growth			3.5
9	Industry, innovation, and infrastructure			4.4
10	Reduced inequalities			3.6, 3.7
11	Sustainable cities and communities			4.5
12	Responsible consumption and production			4.6
13, 14, 15	Climate action and biodiversity			4.7, 4.8
16	Peace, justice, and strong institutions			3.8
17	Partnerships			7

New to This Edition

The fourth edition of *Introduction to Global Health* has been updated to integrate content about the COVID-19 pandemic and to include more comprehensive coverage of the full spectrum of topics that are now included on the global health agenda.

The first seven chapters present the core theories, principles, and purposes of global health:

- Chapter 1 has been rewritten to emphasize the history, values, and functions of global health. The chapter explains how populations, action, cooperation, equity, and security express the values of global health; introduces new content about foundational concepts such as health equity, population health, prevention science, intervention science, and health transitions theory; and adds a new section about the history of international health and global health.
- Chapter 2 has been rewritten to have a greater emphasis on how travel, trade, and other aspects of globalization affect health, disease, and health disparities. Global health security is presented as a growing global health priority due to the COVID-19 pandemic. The chapter introduces the Sustainable Development Goals (SDGs), which will guide many international cooperation efforts through 2030, then presents several new sections that explain how global health metrics are used to track progress toward achieving global health targets.
- Chapters 3 and 4 continue to use the SDGs as a framework for exploring the socioeconomic and environmental determinants of health. Chapter 3 has a new emphasis on the cultural and political contributors to health that are embedded

in sections on health and economics, education, sex/gender, employment, race/ethnicity, migration, and governance. Chapter 4 examines the links between health and water, sanitation, energy, air quality, occupational and industrial health, and urbanization. New sections on sustainability, ecosystem health, and climate change engage with these critical themes.

- Chapter 5 continues to use the SDGs and the Universal Declaration of Human Rights to highlight some of the major ethical issues in global health, including questions about the right to access healthcare services, essential medicines and vaccines, and basic human needs such as drinking water; emergency management and humanitarian responsibilities after natural disasters; and the rights of people in prison, people with disabilities, and other special populations.
- Chapter 6 focuses on the financing and delivery of medical care and public health services in countries with different types of health systems and different income levels. The chapter opens with a new section comparing medicine and public health that provides a foundation for understanding the funding mechanisms for both personal and public health interventions.
- Chapter 7 continues to describe the roles, responsibilities, and relationships of the agencies and organizations involved in financing and implementing public health interventions locally and internationally. The revised chapter has a stronger emphasis on the roles of channels (first-level

recipients) and implementers (second-level recipients) of funding from major donors.

Chapters 8 through 17 systematically describe the global health interventions being used to reduce the population health burden from the major causes of disease, disability, and early death worldwide. Each chapter begins with a section that explains why the featured topic is considered to be a global health issue, then presents the basic pathophysiology of selected conditions, relevant health metrics, and information about the financing and implementation of interventions for the conditions. All of these chapters have been significantly updated to feature new scientific, epidemiological, policy, and practice developments.

- Chapter 8 examines the progress that has been made toward eliminating HIV/AIDS and tuberculosis as global public health problems.
- Chapter 9 discusses the heavy toll that child mortality from diarrheal diseases and pneumonia continues to take on lower-income countries and describes the tools that are available to contain outbreaks of influenza and other vaccine-preventable infections. A new section describes the emergence of SARS, MERS, and COVID, complementing content about coronaviruses that has been integrated into other chapters.
- Chapter 10, which focuses on malaria and neglected tropical diseases (NTDs), has a much stronger focus on interventions for disease prevention and control. Emerging NTD priorities such as chikungunya, strongyloidiasis, scabies, and snakebite envenoming have been added to the chapter.
- Chapter 11 highlights a diversity of reproductive and sexual health issues, including family planning, infertility, pregnancy, maternal mortality, neonatal health, gynecological and urological health, and sexual minority health.
- Chapter 12 is now organized to align with nutrition across the life course. New

sections on infant nutrition and child growth complement revised sections on the nutrition transition, macronutrient and micronutrient undernutrition, overweight and obesity, and food safety.
- Chapter 13 focuses on cardiovascular diseases. This is now the first of the three chapters on noncommunicable diseases (NCDs), and it introduces the epidemiological transition and health behavior theories. Chapter 14 focuses on cancer, and Chapter 15 focuses on diabetes, chronic respiratory diseases, chronic kidney disease, cirrhosis, and other NCDs.
- Chapter 16 describes the diversity of mental health disorders that contribute to disability worldwide and emphasizes the need for greater access to mental health services.
- Chapter 17 discusses injury prevention interventions across the life span.

The final chapters synthesize the core messages of the text by examining evidence-based, cost-effective, sustainable interventions for promoting health and preventing illness across the life span. Chapter 18 presents the major improvements in neonatal, infant, child, and adolescent health that have been achieved in recent decades and the opportunities for continued progress. Chapter 19 describes the emerging challenges associated with aging populations and the opportunities for promoting healthy adulthood and aging. Chapter 20 has been rewritten to emphasize the multidisciplinary and interprofessional nature of global health and to describe the various educational pathways and experiential learning activities that can serve as preparation for a career in global health.

More than 330 figures and tables highlight key material, and nearly all of these illustrations are new for the fourth edition. All of the statistics in the text have been updated. An updated and expanded glossary provides definitions for more than 900 key terms in global health, and all of the terms in the glossary are embedded in sentence form within the main text.

About the Author

Kathryn H. Jacobsen, PhD, MPH, is a professor of health studies and holds the William E. Cooper Distinguished University Chair at the University of Richmond, where she teaches courses on global health, epidemiology, research methods, and disease prevention and control. She was previously a professor of epidemiology and global health at George Mason University.

Dr. Jacobsen's research focuses on the population health transitions that occur with globalization, socioeconomic development, and environmental change. Her research portfolio includes analyses of the global epidemiology of hepatitis A virus, emerging infectious and noncommunicable diseases, adolescent risk behaviors, and other global public health concerns. She has authored more than 200 peer-reviewed scientific articles.

Dr. Jacobsen has served as a technical expert for the World Health Organization and other public health agencies, global health partnerships, and international health groups. She is an active Global Burden of Diseases, Injuries, and Risk Factors (GBD) Study collaborator, serves on several editorial boards, and has chaired the undergraduate and master's education committee for the Consortium of Universities for Global Health.

In addition to being the author of *Introduction to Global Health*, Dr. Jacobsen is also the author of *Introduction to Health Research Methods: A Practical Guide* (Jones & Bartlett Learning).

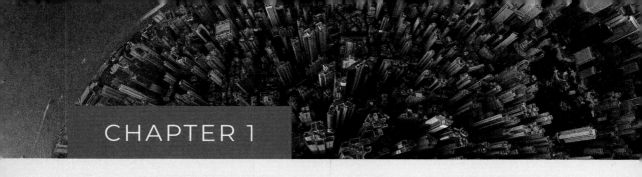

CHAPTER 1

Global Health Transitions

Global health brings together partners from around the world to solve shared population and environmental health concerns. Investments in global health are motivated by a desire to improve millions of lives, prevent avoidable illnesses and deaths, mitigate transnational threats like pandemics and climate change, promote health equity, and protect international trade and security.

1.1 Defining Global Health

Global health is a field of academic study, research, and applied practice that seeks to improve population health worldwide. The word "global" conveys two meanings: worldwide and comprehensive. Some global health initiatives focus on health concerns that primarily affect people who live in low-income countries, but most seek to address complex transnational problems that affect or have the potential to affect people in every country. Global health researchers take a holistic approach to examining the many socioeconomic, environmental, political, and other contributors to health and well-being, and global health practitioners apply tools from public health, medicine, environmental science, the social sciences, engineering, law, and other professions toward the improvement of population and environmental health in countries and communities across the globe.

Some of the core values that guide global health can be summarized by the acronym PACES: population, action, cooperation, equity, and security (**Figure 1.1**). The **P**opulation dimension of global health emphasizes that global health interventions typically target health issues that adversely affect large numbers of people across multiple world regions. Some global health initiatives focus on the diseases that cause the most deaths, disability, and lost productivity worldwide. Some target emerging threats to population health that have the potential to affect every country in the world in the future, such as pandemic influenza and global warming. Some aim to improve the socioeconomic and environmental conditions that cause millions or even billions of people worldwide to have suboptimal health status.

The **A**ction lens accentuates the value of global health principles and theories leading to improved health in the real world. Global health researchers use scientific studies to identify the most effective and economical

Populations	Global health prioritizes the exposures and diseases that cause a considerable proportion of preventable deaths and/or disabilities in multiple world regions.
Action	Global health uses evidence-based, cost-effective, sustainable interventions to prevent illness and injury, treat existing diseases, and alleviate suffering.
Cooperation	Global health uses international, multisectoral partnerships to solve complex health concerns.
Equity	Global health reduces health disparities by prioritizing the needs of low-income countries and other disadvantaged populations.
Security	Global health tackles the health issues that are most likely to contribute to political and economic instability and conflict.

Figure 1.1 PACES: Global health values.

interventions for prioritized health issues, then practitioners use those research findings to design and implement policies and practices that will prevent new population health problems and solve existing concerns. Many global health initiatives seek to increase access to health literacy, safe drinking water, essential medicines, nutritious foods, and other fundamental tools for preventing, diagnosing, and treating health problems, because these have been identified as some of the "best buys" that yield the greatest benefits for population health per dollar spent.

The Cooperation aspect of global health recognizes that there are many cross-border threats to population health and well-being that can only be solved through international partnerships. Pollution generated in one country may adversely affect the air and water quality of many neighboring lands. A drug-resistant strain of tuberculosis or another infection that emerges in one nation may quickly spread around the globe. One country acting alone cannot contain these hazards to health. Solving these global challenges will require governments and representatives from business and other sectors in many countries to work together to identify priorities, generate action plans, and follow through on achieving shared goals.

An Equity lens brings attention to health issues that predominantly affect low-income countries and other disadvantaged populations

and marginalized groups. **Health equity** is present when everyone has an equal opportunity to be as healthy as possible.[1] High-income countries have experienced significant improvements in population health status over the past century as they have become wealthier, built infrastructure that supports healthy living, and expanded access to medication, surgery, vaccines, and other health technologies. Health status in low-income countries is improving, but life expectancy and other health metrics are still less favorable in these areas than in higher-income places. Besides these between-country gaps in health status, there are also within-country health inequalities. For example, people with mental health disorders in any country may encounter systematic challenges to accessing health care and social services. Many global health campaigns are guided by social justice principles and seek to ensure that the voices of individuals who represent marginalized groups are heard so that the needs of their communities can be acknowledged and acted on.

The Security aspect of global health underscores health as a foundation for safe and peaceful societies. Places that are burdened by infectious disease outbreaks, chronic hunger, or high rates of preventable disability and early death due to lack of access to routine medical, surgical, and psychological care may experience economic turmoil and political unrest. Instability may lead to violent conflict, and conflict in one place may lead to disruptions and violence in other locations. Investments in global health can support economic growth, political stability, and national and international security.

Many diseases, environmental hazards, and other population health issues are classified as global health priorities based on the PACES criteria. Pandemics are one obvious example of a global health priority. Within a few months after COVID-19 was first identified in late 2019, the coronavirus had spread to dozens of countries and met all five of the PACES criteria:

- Population: Billions of people were at risk of SARS-CoV-2 infection, millions became infected, and hundreds of thousands of people died from the infection.
- Action: Control measures, such as testing, contact tracing, and isolation and treatment of infected individuals, were widely deployed to slow the spread of the virus while researchers worked to develop and test medications and vaccines.
- Cooperation: National efforts to respond to the pandemic relied on global sharing of information about the most effective protocols for diagnosing SARS-CoV-2 infection and treating COVID-19 patients, and decisions related to international travel and trade were dependent on reliable access to up-to-date statistics about case counts and locations.
- Equity: The pandemic affected some populations disproportionately, with healthcare, food service, and other essential workers at high risk of on-the-job exposure to SARS-CoV-2 and older adults and people with chronic diseases especially vulnerable to severe illness and death after contracting the virus.
- Security: The emergence of COVID-19 caused major social and economic disruptions due to school and workplace closures, travel bans, supply chain interruptions, and other hardships.

The PACES criteria can similarly be used to justify investment in interventions for a diversity of other health issues, such as HIV/AIDS, maternal mortality, child hunger, hypertension, lower back pain, and depression. All these health concerns, and many more, can become global health foci when groups of people representing diverse cultures and nationalities work together to raise awareness about health issues and then solve them.

1.2 Population Health

The goal of global health is to improve the health of the world's people. Health is often defined as the absence of disease or injury, but that is an incomplete explanation because the focus is on what health is not, rather than on what health is. Some definitions of health emphasize the ability to conduct normal daily activities, but that construct is inadequate because the definition of "normal" varies from person to person. For example, many people assume that it is normal for an older adult to have limited mobility and forgetfulness, but that is not an inevitability. Many older people are very active and mentally sharp, and therapy and assistive technologies could improve the quality of life of many seniors who have joint pain and memory loss. Similarly, parents in many parts of the world assume that it is normal for children to have intestinal worms. Even though a cheap medication can kill these parasites, millions of children are currently living with untreated intestinal worms that can significantly impair their health, growth, and school performance.

A more comprehensive definition of health encompasses both physical and mental health as well as the presence of social connections that facilitate health. The Constitution of the World Health Organization (WHO), written in 1948, defines **health** as "a state of complete physical, mental, and social well-being and not merely the absence of disease or infirmity."[2] This definition recognizes that health is about more than just biology; it is also about psychology, sociology, and a host of other factors. Although there is almost no one in the world today who would be classified as having "complete" health according to the WHO statement,[3] this definition provides a target for medical and public health professionals and organizations as they work together to improve the health status of individuals and communities.

Global health initiatives aim to improve health at the population level. A **population** is a group of individuals, communities, nations, or other entities. Some global health interventions seek to improve the well-being of large regions or the entire world population. For example, strengthening early warning systems for emerging infectious diseases that could cause pandemics is an action that protects all humans, not just a few selected individuals or countries. Some global health interventions provide services directly to individuals because healthier individuals collectively will form healthier populations. Health is improved when infectious diseases (such as HIV, tuberculosis, cholera, influenza, measles, and malaria) and noncommunicable diseases (such as cardiovascular disease, cancer, and diabetes) are prevented, managed, or cured. Health is improved when nutritional deficiencies like protein-energy malnutrition and iron deficiency anemia are remediated. Health is improved when women do not die in childbirth, when people who have depression and anxiety have access to counseling and medications, and when people who are injured in a traffic collision or an act of violence have access to surgery and rehabilitation that restore function.

Population health encompasses health outcomes and the determinants of health in groups of humans at the community, regional, national, and/or worldwide level.[4] The **determinants of health** are the biological, behavioral, social, environmental, political, and other factors that influence the health status of individuals and populations. Individual

behaviors like handwashing often, eating several portions of fruits and vegetables daily, and using sidewalks rather than walking in traffic contribute to reducing the risk of infections, managing chronic diseases, and preventing injuries at the individual level, but the ability of individuals to engage in these activities is a function of both individual willpower and community resources. If someone lives in a community that does not have public washrooms, affordable fresh foods, and pedestrian walkways, these actions may be impossible. Community-wide interventions related to these determinants of health will enable individuals to adopt healthier behaviors that improve their own health outcomes. When the health outcomes for individuals improve, the overall health status of their community also improves. A similar pattern exists for the health of nations. Worldwide efforts related to the determinants of health can improve health outcomes in all the participating countries.

1.3 Prevention and Intervention Science

Global health is an action-oriented field that works to improve health status for every age group and extend healthy life expectancy. For an individual, an ideal health trajectory begins with a consenting adult becoming pregnant and that pregnancy leading to an uneventful full-term delivery of a healthy newborn. After birth, the ideal health trajectory continues with that healthy infant growing into adulthood without experiencing serious infections, illnesses, or injuries and that adult remaining healthy and active for many decades. Because everyone eventually dies, the ideal health trajectory ends in very old age with a gentle death that is not preceded by months or years of disability and pain. However, few people achieve this ideal pathway (**Figure 1.2A**).

In very low-income communities, a large proportion of children are born with low birthweight and struggle with repeated bouts

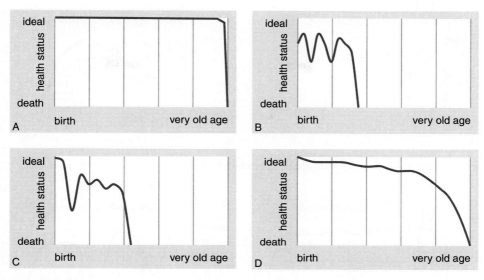

Figure 1.2 Examples of health trajectories.

of infectious diseases like pneumonia and malaria, and it is not uncommon for young women to die in childbirth (**Figure 1.2B**). A healthy child may develop permanent physical impairments due to a catastrophic car crash in adolescence, have reduced health status from alcohol abuse or misuse of prescription painkillers in middle adulthood, and then die from a heart attack before reaching retirement age (**Figure 1.2C**). Even when people live to be very old, they usually experience a gradual decline in function and loss of independence prior to dying (**Figure 1.2D**). Actions implemented at the individual, community, and higher levels can prevent many of these events that decrease health status and can lessen the level of reduced health associated with them.

In global health, an **intervention** is a strategic action intended to improve individual and population health status. A variety of medical, behavioral, social, economic, environmental, and other interventions and changes can help individuals and their communities make progress toward having longer, healthier life trajectories.[5] For example, nutrition support programs for pregnant and breastfeeding women can reduce the risk of low birthweight and malnutrition in infants; the use of antibiotics to treat childhood pneumonia soon after the onset of a cough can prevent life-threatening illness; the availability of skilled birth attendants can prevent women from dying during childbirth; and numerous other interventions during adulthood, such as injury prevention technology, mental health care, and lifestyle changes that reduce the risk of heart attacks, can improve both quality of life and the number of years lived (**Figure 1.3**). Together, these interventions can have a strong positive impact on an individual's health, allowing a person who might otherwise have experienced poor health in childhood and died young to instead have a healthy childhood and live to old age. When these interventions reach millions of people, they make a huge difference in population health, happiness, and productivity.

The adage that prevention is better than a cure expresses one of the foundational principles of global health. It is usually cheaper to spend relatively small amounts of money on interventions that keep people healthy across the life span than it is to spend relatively large amounts of money helping people recover from

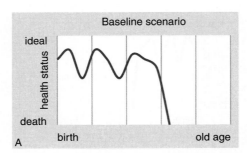
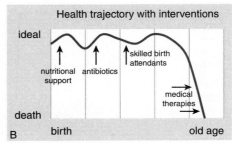

Figure 1.3 Examples of interventions that improve health trajectories across the life span.

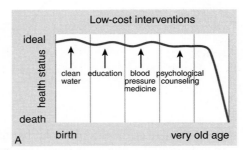
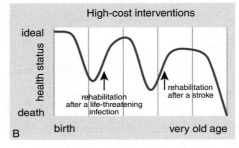

Figure 1.4 Maintaining good health status through preventive interventions is less costly than paying for rehabilitation after health crises.

health crises (**Figure 1.4**). Lengthy hospitalizations, long-term disabilities, and untimely deaths are expensive and exhausting for the affected individuals and their families and caregivers. They are also costly for the communities and nations that lose the economic, social, and other contributions the affected individuals would have made through work productivity, tax revenue, and service if they had lived longer, healthier lives. **Systems thinking** is the process of identifying the underlying causes of complex problems so that sustainable solutions can be developed and implemented. **Prevention science** is the process of determining which preventive health interventions are effective at improving health status, how successful those interventions are in various populations, and how readily they can be scaled up for widespread implementation.[6] **Implementation science** is the scientific study of how to increase uptake of evidence-based practices

and policies after effective interventions have been identified.

There are three levels of prevention that together capture the full range of health interventions (**Figure 1.5**). **Primary prevention** consists of protective actions that help keep an adverse health event from ever occurring. Some primary prevention interventions promote healthy behaviors, such as vaccinating children to reduce their risk of contracting measles and polio infections, keeping mosquitoes out of homes to reduce the risk of malaria and other vector-borne diseases, and using a seat belt to reduce the risk of severe injuries during a motor vehicle collision. Some primary prevention programs work to modify the health environment by increasing access to improved sanitation facilities to prevent diarrheal infections, spraying insecticides to kill the mosquitoes that spread dengue virus, implementing clean delivery room practices

Level	Goal	Target Population	Key Interventions	Examples
Primordial prevention	Prevent risk factors for disease	People without disease	Prevention	■ Healthy lifestyles ■ Healthy environments
Primary prevention	Prevent disease from ever occurring	People without disease	Prevention	■ Vaccinating children to protect them from paralytic polio ■ Giving vitamin A capsules to at-risk children to prevent blindness
Secondary prevention	Reduce the severity of disease and prevent disability and death	People with early, nonsymptomatic disease	Early diagnosis	■ Checking blood pressure routinely to detect the onset of hypertension ■ Screening with mammography to detect early stage breast cancer
Tertiary prevention	Reduce impairment and minimize suffering	People with symptomatic disease	Treatment and rehabilitation	■ Extracting teeth with severe decay to alleviate pain ■ Providing physical therapy to people who have been injured in a vehicle collision to restore function

Figure 1.5 Levels of prevention.

to prevent infections of newborns and their mothers, and building roads that are safe for bicyclists and pedestrians. Others use policy changes to improve access to healthcare services, essential medications, and nutritious foods. Primary prevention interventions are often the most cost-effective interventions, but there are many adverse health conditions for which the risk factors remain poorly understood and the options for primary prevention therefore remain limited.

Secondary prevention is the detection of health problems in asymptomatic individuals at an early stage when the conditions have not yet caused significant damage to the body and can be treated more easily. (**Asymptomatic** means not symptomatic.) Cancer screening tests, such as mammography for breast cancer, Pap smears for cervical cancer, and colonoscopies that look for the polyps that

are precursors to colorectal cancer, are forms of secondary prevention. Similarly, routine HIV tests, blood pressure checks in adults, and sports physicals for student athletes are intended to detect health issues in people who might otherwise have remained unaware of the presence of manageable but potentially serious health conditions for many years.

Tertiary prevention consists of interventions that reduce impairment, minimize pain and suffering, and restore function in people with symptomatic health problems. Examples of tertiary prevention include managing chronic diseases with medication, alleviating the pain that can be caused by advanced cancer, and providing physical therapy and occupational therapy to people recovering from strokes or serious injuries.

Given the three levels of prevention, there is almost always some intervention that could improve the health of individuals who are vulnerable to various adverse health conditions or are already sick. Primary prevention is the preferred option, especially when a cost-effective intervention is available. When primary prevention is not possible with current technologies and when health problems are already present, secondary prevention and tertiary prevention can improve longevity and quality of life.

1.4 Risk Factors

The ability of individuals, nations, international partnerships, and other groups to make informed decisions about what interventions to invest in and collaborate on is dependent on understanding the risk factors for adverse health outcomes. **Etiology** is the cause of a disease or another adverse condition. The **proximal cause** is the most immediate cause of an adverse event. For diseases, the proximal etiological agents may be intrinsic (internal) causes, such as genetics and psychological factors, or extrinsic (external) causes, such as infections and environmental hazards. Beyond proximal causes, there are many other factors that contribute to creating the situations in which illnesses and diseases occur.[7] A **distal cause** is a social, environmental, or other factor that is not an immediate cause but contributes to the causal pathway for an adverse event. Epidemiologists and prevention scientists are often able to identify a variety of immediate exposures that are associated with increased risk of illness, but it is harder to quantify the ways that social, economic, political, historic, and other distal factors that are parts of causal webs have created and perpetuated public health problems.[8] Research by anthropologists, sociologists, and other social scientists and humanities scholars provides insights about the ways that political structures (like colonialism and capitalism), prejudices (like racism and sexism), and other contextual factors have shaped and continue to shape health.[9]

For most adverse health conditions, there are many different combinations of events that might lead to the onset and progression of the disease or disorder. **Multicausality** describes a causal pathway in which many different risk factors contribute to an adverse event occurring.[10] The terms *necessary* and *sufficient* are often used to describe the various sets of exposures that can lead to adverse outcomes. A risk factor is said to be a necessary part of the disease pathway if it must be present for a person to develop a disease. For example, an individual can have a genetic disorder only if he or she carries the gene for that disorder. The gene is necessary. A risk factor is sufficient if that exposure or characteristic by itself can cause disease. Being exposed to a high dose of radiation could be sufficient to cause some types of cancer, but most of those cancers could also develop in someone who was never exposed to radiation. Radiation is sufficient but not necessary to cause cancer. Some exposures are necessary but not sufficient on their own to cause disease. Many adverse health outcomes result from dozens or even hundreds of exposures that are neither sufficient nor necessary on their own but in the aggregate can lead to a situation in which an infection, illness, or injury occurs.

Consider the example of child pneumonia, which is a more frequent cause of pediatric mortality than diarrheal diseases, malaria, HIV, or injuries.[11] Nearly 1 million children die from pneumonia each year, and almost all these deaths occur in lower-income countries.[12] A variety of pathogens can cause child pneumonia, and there are countless sets of distal and proximal causes that may lead to a child contracting a respiratory infection. Medical interventions tend to focus on the proximal causes of pneumonia cases and deaths, emphasizing primary prevention methods like vaccination and tertiary prevention methods like access to antibiotics. A more comprehensive prevention package will include interventions related to distal causes as well as proximal ones.

An **exposure** is a personal characteristic, behavior, environmental encounter, or intervention that might change the likelihood of developing a health condition. Individuals may have different risks of infection, disease, and complications from disease as a result of age, genetics, immunology, comorbidities, nutritional status, health behaviors, psychological factors, environmental hazards, and many other characteristics. A **risk factor** is an exposure that increases the likelihood of experiencing a particular health outcome. Some risk factors are specific to one disease, but many biological, behavioral, environmental, and other risk factors are associated with a diversity of adverse health outcomes (**Figure 1.6**).[13] For child pneumonia, some of the risk factors are biological. Infants and young children may have underdeveloped immune systems that leave them vulnerable to certain types of pathogens, or they may have poor immune response due to being chronically undernourished. Some risk factors are environmental. Children who are exposed to indoor air pollution from cooking fires and children exposed to outdoor air pollution because they live near dirty industrial areas are more susceptible to respiratory infections. Some risk factors are social, economic, or behavioral. Parents who have never attended school or had the opportunity to learn how to read may not have the education to recognize when a child requires medical assistance. Parents who are subsistence farmers or work for very low wages might not have the money to pay for transportation to a hospital when a child is critically ill.

In prevention science, the term **primordial prevention** is sometimes used to describe the general lifestyle habits and environmental conditions that prevent risk factors for adverse health events from developing. In that framework, primordial prevention is about general conditions that protect health—such as eating a nutritious diet, exercising, avoiding tobacco and other harmful substances, and getting adequate sleep each night—and primary prevention is about specific actions that mitigate the risk of developing specific diseases. A person who eats a low-fat diet to keep blood lipid levels low is practicing primordial prevention; a person with elevated blood lipid levels who takes cholesterol-lowering medication to reduce the risk of cardiovascular disease later on is practicing primary prevention. A person who chooses not to start smoking is engaging in primordial prevention; a tobacco-using person who works to quit smoking to reduce the risk of developing lung cancer later on is engaging in primary prevention. For child pneumonia, primordial prevention includes conditions such as adequate nutrition and clean air.

Health-Related Behaviors	Nutritional Exposures	Environmental Exposures	Untreated Medical Conditions
▪ Tobacco use ▪ Physical inactivity ▪ Unsafe sex ▪ Alcohol abuse ▪ Injecting drug use	▪ Obesity and overweight ▪ Child underweight ▪ Low fruit and vegetable intake ▪ Suboptimal breastfeeding ▪ Vitamin A deficiency ▪ Zinc deficiency ▪ Iron deficiency	▪ Indoor smoke from solid fuels ▪ Unsafe water, sanitation, and hygiene ▪ Urban outdoor air pollution ▪ Occupational risks ▪ Lead exposure	▪ High blood pressure ▪ High blood glucose ▪ High cholesterol ▪ Unmet contraceptive need

Figure 1.6 Examples of modifiable risk factors for adverse health outcomes.

Data from *Global Health Risks: Mortality and Burden of Disease Attributable to Selected Major Risks.* Geneva: World Health Organization; 2009.

The links between hundreds of exposures and child pneumonia have been confirmed by health researchers. **Causation** is a relationship in which an exposure directly causes an outcome. A **causal factor** is an exposure that has been scientifically tested and shown to occur before the disease outcome and contribute directly to its occurrence. An **association** is a statistical relationship between two variables, but tests of association are not enough to prove that a relationship is or is not causal. The presence of causality is typically determined by using both quantitative analysis, such as laboratory testing and statistics, and a qualitative consideration of causal theory. The **Bradford Hill criteria** are a set of conditions that provide support for the existence of a causal relationship between an exposure and an outcome, such as the strength of the association, the presence of a dose–response relationship between the exposure and outcome, and the consistency of the risk across numerous studies (**Figure 1.7**).[14] There

is no expectation that all of the Bradford Hill criteria have to be met for an exposure to be considered causal, but the evidence for causality is stronger when more criteria are met.[15] When many different exposures contribute to the onset and progression of a disease, many different interventions can be effective at preventing adverse outcomes.

An individual's health status at any age is a function of his or her experiences throughout the life course.[16] Some of the circumstances that lead to adverse health outcomes are ones that cannot be altered. A **nonmodifiable risk factor** is a risk factor that cannot be changed through health interventions. We do not have the ability to change a person's age or the technology to change a person's inherited genes, and we cannot erase past behaviors and previous medical events that have damaged the body. However, there are many actions that support improved health today and reduce the risk of health problems in the future. A **modifiable risk factor** is

Criterion	Key Question
Temporality	Did the exposure happen before the onset of disease?
Strength of association	Is the statistical association between the exposure and outcome strong?
Dose–response relationship/ biological gradient	Do people with a higher level of exposure have a higher risk of the outcome than people with a lower level of exposure?
Cessation	Does stopping the exposure reduce the risk of the outcome?
Specificity	Are the exposure and outcome both narrowly defined rather than general concepts?
Theoretical plausibility	Is there a reasonable biological explanation for why the exposure might cause the outcome?
Consistency	Has a potentially causal relationship between the exposure and outcome been observed in other studies and other populations?
Coherence	Is a causal relationship between the exposure and outcome congruent with other knowledge about the variables?
Consideration of alternate explanations	Are there reasons why what appears to be a causal relationship might not actually be causal?

Figure 1.7 Criteria for evaluating whether an exposure causes a disease or other health outcome.

a risk factor that can be avoided or mitigated. For example, a **behavioral risk factor** is a behavior that can be adopted, stopped, or changed in order to reduce the risk of disease. Behavior change interventions may encourage the reduction of hazardous behaviors or may promote the adoption of healthier behaviors.

Some modifiable risk factors can be mitigated with behavior change at the individual or household level. For child pneumonia, health education programs can encourage parents not to cook indoors without adequate ventilation and can teach parents the importance of seeking medical care for children with moderate breathing difficulties rather than waiting until the onset of severe respiratory distress. However, many risk factors can only be mitigated at the community level or higher levels. One family cannot force a factory to stop releasing toxins into the air. Reducing outdoor air pollution might require a national clean air law to be enacted and enforced. One small rural community will not have the resources to build and staff a hospital that provides affordable, high-quality health services. Rural communities could pool their funds to establish a network of clinics, but they would probably need to coordinate their efforts with an urban referral hospital and with a national organization that trains and certifies rural health workers and other clinical care providers. One county or parish will not be able to develop and manufacture all the medications and vaccines its residents need. Pharmaceutical products are typically developed by international research teams, and few factories have the technical capacity to produce chemically complex substances that are reliably safe and effective. One nation cannot prevent antibiotic-resistant bacterial strains from emerging and spreading across the globe. If all countries do not work together to promote antimicrobial stewardship and combat drug resistance, respiratory infections that are currently curable may cause widespread death in the future. Reducing child deaths from pneumonia requires a mix of individual- and household-level, community-level, national-level, and global interventions.

It can be comforting to assume that individuals have the power to control their own health destiny, but that is a false assumption. Health is a complex function of individual (intrapersonal) factors plus interpersonal factors (relationships), institutional and organizational factors, community factors, and public policy.[17] Many people do not have the ability to choose to eat healthy meals, exercise daily, breathe fresh air, get enough sleep, access routine medical screenings, and manage mild health conditions so that they do not become severe. Low-income individuals and households may not have the money to buy adequate amounts of nutritious food, time to do much of anything other than work, or the resources to access health services. Even the world's richest people do not have full control over their personal health trajectories. Some people who apply the best available science to every aspect of their lives will still become seriously ill long before they reach old age. The factors that cause their health status to diminish may be ones that they cannot control. Even billionaires do not have the ability on their own to ensure that the influenza vaccine they get annually will protect against the strains that end up circulating in a particular year, that the air they breathe outside their homes is clean, or that the other motorists they encounter on public roads will not be driving recklessly.

Individuals can and should accept responsibility for their own health decisions, but there are some threats to health that can only be solved at the population level. The health of individuals is a function of their own biology and behaviors, and it is also a function of a broad set of economic, social, cultural, political, environmental, occupational, and other factors.[18] For many adverse health outcomes, the distal causes of the health problem are ones that cannot be solved by individuals or even by states, provinces, or nations acting alone. Many threats to health can only be resolved with global cooperation.

1.5 Health Transitions

A **health transition** is a shift in the health status of a population that usually occurs in conjunction with socioeconomic development (**Figure 1.8**). One hundred years ago, most populations across the globe had similar health profiles: high birth rates, high child mortality rates, short life expectancies, and a considerable proportion of illnesses and deaths due to infections and undernutrition. During the 20th century, high-income nations transitioned to having longer life expectancies and lower rates of infection and chronic hunger. Low-income countries did not experience such dramatic improvements in population health status. Because low-income countries did not undergo the health transitions observed in high-income countries, gaps in health equity between the highest- and lowest-income countries increased.

Population health status is related to socioeconomic and environmental factors. Places with more poverty and pollution tend to have limited access to health services and less favorable health profiles (**Figure 1.9**). Economic growth, infrastructure development, and new health technologies in high-income countries in the 20th century enabled high-income countries to improve population health in all age groups. In the United States, for example, the leading causes of death in both 1800 and 1900 were pneumonia (including pneumonia caused by influenza), tuberculosis, and diarrhea, all of which are infectious diseases.[19] Many of these deaths occurred in children and young adults. By 1950, the risk of dying in childhood or early

Type of Transition	Pre-transition Populations	Post-transition Populations
Fertility transition	The typical woman gives birth to several children.	The typical woman gives birth to only one child or two children.
Demographic transition	The total population size may be increasing due to high birth rates.	The total population size may be shrinking because birth rates are so low.
Obstetric transition	Pregnancy-related conditions are a major cause of death in women of reproductive age.	The maternal mortality rate is very low.
Nutrition transition	Underweight is a major population health concern.	Obesity is a major population health concern.
Risk transition	Environmental exposures like unsafe drinking water and polluted indoor air are major contributors to disease.	Lifestyle factors like physical inactivity and tobacco use are major contributors to disease.
Epidemiologic transition	Infectious diseases in children are a significant burden to the population.	Chronic diseases in adults are the dominant health concern in the population.
Mortality transition	High death rates in children and reproductive-age adults mean that few people live to very old age.	Low mortality rates for children and reproductive-age adults allow many people to live to old age.
Aging transition	Children comprise the majority of the total population.	Older adults are a growing proportion of the population.

Figure 1.8 Examples of health transitions.

Today, in Very LOW-Income Populations...	Today, in Very HIGH-Income Populations...
■ There are high rates of poverty, illiteracy, and unemployment, which can have negative effects on personal, family, and community health.	■ Most people have access to the basic tools for health, although there are still health disparities based on socioeconomic status.
■ Many people do not have access to an outhouse or other type of toilet, and many do not have reliable access to safe drinking water.	■ Almost everyone has indoor plumbing and safe drinking water.
■ Many infants and young children die from diarrhea, pneumonia, malaria, and other infections.	■ Almost every baby will survive to adulthood.
■ The typical woman gives birth to many children, and it is not uncommon for women to die in childbirth.	■ The typical woman gives birth to one or two children, and very few women die due to pregnancy-related conditions.
■ The median (average) age of the population is 15 to 20 years.	■ The median (average) age of the population is 40 to 45 years.
■ The typical adult dies at around 65 years of age.	■ The typical adult dies at around 85 years of age.
■ Visits to hospitals and clinics are usually because of infections (such as malaria or tuberculosis) or serious injuries.	■ Visits to hospitals and clinics are usually due to chronic noncommunicable diseases (such as arthritis, back pain, hypertension, and diabetes).
■ Access to effective management of chronic diseases (such as hypertension and diabetes) is very limited.	■ Screening tests often detect emerging health problems early, so they can be treated or managed before they cause severe disease.
■ Undernutrition (including protein energy and micronutrient deficiencies) remains a significant public health concern.	■ Overweight and obesity are major public health concerns, and many people have diets that are high in fat and calories.
■ Very few people with mental health disorders receive clinical care because there are so few psychiatrists and psychologists.	■ Clinical mental health services are usually available, but they are often underused.
■ Serious injuries often lead to death because no surgical services are available.	■ Serious injuries can often be treated with surgery and rehabilitation.

Figure 1.9 Examples of significant differences in health status and access to the tools for health in low-income and high-income countries.

adulthood had decreased considerably and the most frequent causes of death had shifted to heart disease, cancer, and stroke, the same aging-associated diseases that remain the most frequent causes of death in the United States today.[20] These changes in population health status were attributed in part to vaccines, antibiotics, contraceptives, and other medical advances, but they were also the result of improved sanitation, better nutrition, increased education, and economic growth.[21]

The **risk transition** is a health transition characterized by a shift from exposures like undernutrition, unsafe water, and indoor air pollution that increase the risk of childhood infectious diseases causing most preventable morbidity and mortality in a population to exposures like obesity, physical inactivity, and tobacco use that increase the risk of chronic diseases being the most prominent risk factors.[13] As the risk transition occurs (**Figure 1.10**),[22] the major causes of illness and death change (**Figure 1.11**).[23] Comparing high-, middle-, and low-income countries provides insights into how these health transitions occur. Middle-income countries tend to have health and risk profiles that are somewhere between those of low-income and high-income countries. Middle-income countries usually continue to have some populations burdened by undernutrition and infectious diseases while other populations within the same country experience the challenges associated with obesity and chronic noncommunicable conditions. This need for health systems in middle-income countries to be responsive to both pre-transition and post-transition health problems is sometimes called the dual or double burden of disease.

Some health and risk transitions are not wholly favorable ones. Global health interventions seek to postpone death and prevent disability. People who live in high-income

	Low-Income Countries	Middle-Income Countries	High-Income Countries
#1	Child and maternal malnutrition	High blood pressure	Tobacco
#2	Air pollution	Tobacco	High body mass index (overweight and obesity)
#3	Unsafe water, sanitation, and handwashing	Dietary risks (such as a diet that is high in sodium and low in whole grains and fruits)	High fasting plasma glucose (blood sugar)

Figure 1.10 Major risk factors for reduced health status and early death in countries with low-, middle-, and high-sociodemographic status.

Data from GBD 2019 Risk Factors Collaborators. Global burden of 87 risk factors in 204 countries and territories, 1990–2019: a systematic analysis for the Global Burden of Disease Study 2019. *Lancet*. 2020;396:1223-1249.

		Low-Income Countries	Middle-Income Countries	High-Income Countries
Leading causes of death	#1	Cardiovascular diseases	Cardiovascular diseases	Cardiovascular diseases
	#2	Respiratory infections (such as tuberculosis and pneumonia)	Cancer	Cancer
	#3	Maternal and neonatal disorders (such as preterm birth)	Chronic respiratory diseases	Neurological disorders (such as Alzheimer's disease)
	#4	Enteric infections (diarrheal diseases)	Diabetes and chronic kidney disease	Chronic respiratory diseases
	#5	Cancer	Respiratory infections	Diabetes and chronic kidney disease

Figure 1.11 Leading causes of death in countries with low-, middle-, and high-sociodemographic status.

Data from GBD 2019 Diseases and Injuries Collaborators. Global burden of 369 diseases and injuries in 204 countries and territories, 1990–2019: a systematic analysis for the Global Burden of Disease Study 2019. *Lancet*. 2020;396:1204-1222.

countries often live to old age, but many older adults are disabled by chronic diseases and experience a lot of pain. Increasing rates of obesity and sedentary lifestyles among younger adults are likely to exacerbate the burden from noncommunicable diseases in post-transition countries in the coming decades. However, transitions that shift the burden of death and disease from children and young adults to older adults are considered to be population health successes. Everyone will eventually die of something, but a population is healthier when the typical age at death is 85 years rather than 65 years. Since hunger and infectious diseases tend to disproportionately burden children, a shift toward obesity and chronic diseases that usually affect older adults is a relative improvement in population health.

A **health disparity** (also called a health inequality) is an avoidable difference in health status between population groups. Health disparities can be observed between countries and within countries. One of the key goals of global public health is to reduce health disparities by increasing the health status of disadvantaged populations through interventions that target proximal or distal causes of suboptimal health.[24] Minimizing health disparities by reducing the health status of advantaged populations would not be a global health gain. Health equity is only achieved when progress toward greater health occurs in all populations.

1.6 Global Health History and Functions

Long before bacteria were first viewed through a microscope, people were aware that travel and trade could bring deadly diseases into vulnerable populations. Thousands of years ago, people with skin lesions and other signs of disease were ostracized and forced to live away from healthy-looking people. Hundreds of years ago, port authorities started requiring incoming ships to stay in harbor for several weeks before they could dock and allow crew members to disembark and goods to be offloaded.[25] Modern transportation has accelerated the speed at which pathogens can spread to new locations through international travel and trade, but the population health threats associated with globalization are long-established concerns.

One of the primary goals of early international health pacts was to limit the spread of dangerous infections. For example, a series of International Sanitary Conferences held in various European cities starting in 1851 assembled representatives from several countries to discuss concerns about the shipping industry spreading cholera to new ports.[26] The delegates sought to identify policies and practices that would protect population health while allowing international supply chains to flow uninterrupted.[27] The signatories of the resulting agreements committed to notifying other countries about outbreaks of cholera, plague, yellow fever, and other epidemic diseases, and they pledged to monitor health at ports and impose quarantines on disease-carrying ships.[28] By the early 1900s, international regulations also incorporated several other cross-border health issues, including ones related to water pollution; alcohol, opium, and other drugs; and occupational health and safety.[29] These treaties set the stage for the International Sanitary Regulations, later renamed the International Health Regulations, which were approved by the World Health Organization 100 years later in 1951 and are still in force today.

Economic and political interests were central to early investments in international health.[30] By around 1870, the industrial revolution had transformed manufacturing and rail networks enabled mass movement of people and goods across land. European countries that had colonized the Americas and parts of Asia and the Pacific in previous centuries began laying imperial claim to more of Africa's natural resources. The United States, Russia, and Japan also acquired overseas territories so

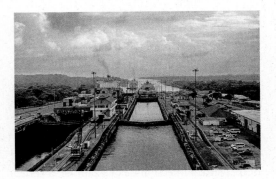

The Panama Canal.

Courtesy of Pixabay

that they could access raw materials, take advantage of cheap labor, expand the market base for the goods they produced, and control strategic military positions. Many of these colonies and territories were located in tropical climates where mosquito-borne infections like malaria and yellow fever were constant threats. The field of tropical medicine was established in the late 1800s and early 1900s as more European (and American) businessmen, military personnel, and their families relocated to tropical areas to oversee commercial and defense activities.[31] Tropical medicine specialists aimed to protect settlers and visitors from parasitic and infectious diseases and to ensure that the workforce in these areas was healthy enough to be productive.[32]

Today, some of the functions of tropical medicine are performed by travel medicine specialists. Tropical medicine was also the precursor for the field of **international health**,[33] a term that in current usage usually describes efforts to alleviate poverty-related health conditions in lower-income areas, not just the tropics.[34] International health interventions typically involve cooperative efforts between a high-income country sponsor and one or more lower-income country recipients who work together to improve a health issue that is a public health priority in the lower-income country.[35] Many international health programs have humanitarian origins and aims that overlap with commercial and diplomatic motivations.[36] Charitable projects that improve the health

of adults and children in recipient countries enable more workers and consumers in those countries to participate in the global economy. That outcome can generate economic and other benefits for all the collaborating countries.

One of the criticisms of some traditional ways of doing international health is that partnerships between high-income donor countries and lower-income recipient countries perpetuate power hierarchies rather than promoting true equity among partners.[36] Calls to "decolonize" global health push for wider recognition of how colonialism and settler-colonialism (which occurred when European immigrants to the United States, Canada, Australia, and other places participated in a systematic process that displaced Indigenous populations and took possession of their lands) have harmed and continue to harm individual, public, and global health.[9] Decolonizing global health requires rethinking global health concepts and practices as well as improving diversity, equity, and inclusion within the global health workforce.[37]

The distinction between international health and global health is still under debate, but global health interventions are more likely to include partners from many countries across the income spectrum (rather than being sponsored by one high-income country), emphasize how globalization processes affect the health of all people (rather than focusing exclusively on the most disadvantaged populations), and apply interprofessional and multisectoral lenses to the development and implementation of public health interventions.[35] International health efforts often have an intergovernmental focus, whereas global health initiatives typically welcome partners from governments, nonprofit foundations, and corporations.[38]

The global HIV epidemic of the late 1990s demanded new models for how countries from all world regions and all income levels can work together to respond to shared threats to population health. The success of the broad-based collaborations that were formed to accelerate scientific discoveries related to HIV/AIDS and to increase access to HIV medications showed that global partnerships can achieve their goals.[39] Over the past 20 years, many large global partnerships have been formed to address numerous population health issues. Some focus on security threats that require commitments from every country in the world, such as antimicrobial resistance, food safety, emerging infectious diseases, global climate change, and geopolitical violence. Some focus on the traditional foci of international health investments: infectious disease prevention and control, including support for vaccination and eradication campaigns; responses to famines, natural disasters, and humanitarian crises; and promotion of maternal and child health and survival through literacy programs, micro-loans, and other community development activities as well as directly health-related ones. Some partnerships have goals related to noncommunicable diseases, mental health promotion, injury prevention, and healthy aging. A century ago, international health was a recognized tool for promoting economic and political stability, a component of diplomatic efforts, and a foundation for economic and infrastructural development. Today, global health continues to serve an important role in enabling international trade and travel, fostering safety and security, and promoting sustainable development.

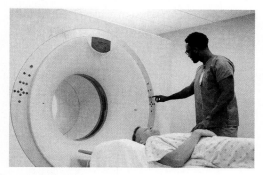

© Cavan Images/Getty Images

1.7 Global Health Achievements

Innovations in health technology over the past 100 years have created an incredible set of tools for global health work. New antibiotics were discovered along with a host of medications for managing and treating noncommunicable diseases like heart disease, cancer, and diabetes. Life-saving vaccines were developed. Smallpox was eradicated. Oral contraceptives transformed family planning, and assisted reproductive technologies enabled many couples with infertility to have biological offspring. Electrocardiographs, magnetic resonance imaging, and other new diagnostic tools improved the quality of medical care. New therapies like dialysis for kidney disease and contact lenses for vision impairments enhanced quality of life. Modern surgical techniques made joint replacements, open heart surgery, and organ transplants routine in some parts of the world. These technological advances enabled many of the top 10 public health achievements of the 20th century that were highlighted by the U.S. Centers for Disease Control and Prevention (CDC) at the start of the new millennium (**Figure 1.12**)[40] as well as many

1	Vaccination
2	Motor-vehicle safety
3	Safer workplaces
4	Control of infectious diseases
5	Decline in deaths from ischemic heart disease and stroke
6	Safer and healthier foods
7	Healthier mothers and babies
8	Family planning
9	Fluoridation of drinking water
10	Recognition of tobacco as a health hazard

Figure 1.12 The U.S. CDC's top 10 public health achievements of the 20th century (1900–1999).

Centers for Disease Control and Prevention. Ten great public health achievements: United States, 1990–1999. *MMWR Morb Mort Wkly Rep.* 1999;48:241–243.

of the leading global health achievements during the first years of the 21st century (**Figure 1.13**).[41]

While these health technologies are indisputably beneficial, the uneven distribution of access to them generated a massive intensification of health disparities during the 20th

1	Reductions in child mortality
2	Vaccine-preventable diseases
3	Access to safe water and sanitation
4	Malaria prevention and control
5	Prevention and control of HIV/AIDS
6	Tuberculosis control
7	Control of neglected tropical diseases
8	Tobacco control
9	Increased awareness and response for improving global road safety
10	Improved preparedness and response to global health threats

Figure 1.13 The U.S. CDC's top 10 global health achievements in the first decade of the 21st century (2001–2010).

Centers for Disease Control and Prevention. Ten great public health achievements: worldwide, 2001–2010. *MMWR Morb Mort Wkly Rep.* 2011;60:814–818.

century. People living in the world's richest countries now have access to an array of tools for health that would have been unimaginable 100 years ago, while children living in the world's poorest areas continue to succumb to easily preventable conditions like starvation and vaccine-preventable and antibiotic-treatable infectious diseases. Global health aims to end these disparities by using a holistic, comprehensive approach to improving population and planetary health worldwide. Thanks to coordinated global health and development initiatives, the 21st century has already seen improvements in health equity. Life expectancies and other health metrics are improving in low- and middle-income countries even as these measures hold steady or continue to improve in high-income countries.[42] The goals of global health in the 21st century include continuing to create innovative solutions to public health problems; increasing access to health, healthcare services, and health technologies around the world; and expanding global communication and action about shared health concerns. Population health is not a "zero sum game" in which one country can "win" only when another country "loses." Everyone gains when world health increases.

References

1. Braveman P, Gruskin S. Defining equity in health. *J Epidemiol Community Health.* 2003;57:254–258.
2. *Constitution of the World Health Organization.* New York: United Nations; 1946.
3. Huber M, Knottnerus JA, Green L, et al. How should we define health? *BMJ.* 2011;343:d4163.
4. Kindig D, Stoddart G. What is population health? *Am J Public Health.* 2003;93:380–383.
5. Keller LO, Strohschein S, Lia-Hoagberg B, Schaffer MA. Population-based public health interventions: practice-based and evidence-supported. *Public Health Nurs.* 2004;21:453–468.
6. Flay BR, Biglan A, Boruch RF, et al. Standards of evidence: criteria for efficacy, effectiveness and dissemination. *Prev Sci.* 2005;6:151–175.
7. Krieger N. Epidemiology and the web of causation: has anyone seen the spider? *Soc Sci Med.* 1994;39:887–903.
8. Richardson ET. *Epidemic Illusions: On the Coloniality of Global Public Health.* Cambridge MA: MIT Press; 2020.
9. Büyüm AM, Kenney C, Koris A, Mkumba L, Raveendran Y. Decolonising global health: if not now, when? *BMJ Glob Health.* 2020;5:e003394.
10. Rothman KJ, Greenland S. Causation and causal inference in epidemiology. *Am J Public Health.* 2005;95(Suppl 1):S144–S150.
11. UNICEF, WHO, World Bank, UN-DESA Population Division. *Levels and Trends in Child Mortality Report 2019: Estimates Developed by the UN Inter-agency*

Group for Child Mortality Estimation. New York: UNICEF; 2019.

12. McAllister DA, Liu L, Shi T, et al. Global, regional, and national estimates of pneumonia morbidity and mortality in children younger than 5 years between 2000 and 2015: a systematic analysis. *Lancet Glob Health.* 2019;7:e47-e57.

13. *Global Health Risks: Mortality and Burden of Disease Attributable to Selected Major Risks.* Geneva: World Health Organization; 2009.

14. Howick J, Glasziou P, Aronson JK. The evolution of evidence hierarchies: what can Bradford Hill's 'guidelines for causation' contribute? *J Roy Soc Med.* 2009;102:186–194.

15. Susser M. What is a cause and how do we know one? A grammar for pragmatic epidemiology. *Am J Epidemiol.* 1991;133:635–648.

16. Kuh D, Ben-Shlomo Y, Lynch J, Hallqvist J, Power C. Life course epidemiology. *J Epidemiol Community Health.* 2003;57:778–783.

17. McLeroy KR, Bibeau D, Steckler A, Glanz K. An ecological perspective on health promotion programs. *Health Educ Q.* 1988;15:351–377.

18. *Committee on Assuring the Health of the Public in the 21st Century. The Future of the Public's Health in the 21st Century.* Washington DC: National Academies Press; 2002.

19. Jones DS, Podolsky SH, Greene JA. The burden of disease and the changing task of medicine. *New Engl J Med.* 2012;366:2333–2338.

20. Guyer B, Freedman MA, Strobino DM, Sondik EJ. Annual summary of vital statistics: trends in the health of Americans during the 20th century. *Pediatrics.* 2000;106:1307–1317.

21. Martens P. Health transitions in a globalising world: towards more disease or sustained health? *Futures.* 2002;34:635–648.

22. GBD 2019 Risk Factors Collaborators. Global burden of 87 risk factors in 204 countries and territories, 1990–2019: a systematic analysis for the Global Burden of Disease Study 2019. *Lancet.* 2020;396:1223–1249.

23. GBD 2019 Diseases and Injuries Collaborators. Global burden of 369 diseases and injuries in 204 countries and territories, 1990–2019: a systematic analysis for the Global Burden of Disease Study 2019. *Lancet.* 2020;396:1204–1222.

24. *Innov8 Approach for Reviewing National Health Programmes to Leave No One Behind: Technical Handbook.* Geneva: World Health Organization; 2016.

25. Gensini GF, Yacoub MH, Conti AA. The concept of quarantine in history: from plague to SARS. *J Infect.* 2004;49:257–261.

26. Huber V. The unification of the globe by disease? The International Sanitary Conferences on cholera, 1851–1894. *Historical J.* 2006;49:453–476.

27. Harrison M. Disease, diplomacy, and international commerce: the origins of international sanitary regulation in the nineteenth century. *J Global History.* 2006;1:197–217.

28. Fidler DP. From International Sanitary Conventions to global health security: the new International Health Regulations. *Chinese J Int Law.* 2005;4:325–392.

29. Fidler DP. The globalization of public health: the first 100 years of international health diplomacy. *Bull World Health Organ.* 2001;79:842–849.

30. Birn AE. The stages of international (global) health: histories of success or successes of history? *Glob Public Health.* 2009;4:50–68.

31. Gibson AD. Miasma revisited: the intellectual history of tropical medicine. *Aust Fam Physician.* 2009;38:57–59.

32. Brown ER. Public health in imperialism: early Rockefeller programs at home and abroad. *Am J Public Health.* 1976;66:897–903.

33. Packard RM. *A History of Global Health: Interventions Into the Lives Other Peoples.* Baltimore MD: Johns Hopkins University Press; 2016.

34. Koplan JP, Bond TC, Merson MH, et al. Towards a common definition of global health. *Lancet.* 2009;373:1993–1995.

35. Holst J. Global health: emergence, hegemonic trends and biomedical reductionism. *Global Health.* 2020;16:42.

36. Abimbola S, Pai M. Will global health survive its decolonisation? *Lancet.* 2020;396:1627–1628.

37. Affun-Adegbulu C, Adegbulu O. Decolonising global (public) health: from western universalism to global pluriversalities. *BMJ Glob Health.* 2020;5:e002947.

38. Brown TM, Cueto M, Fee E. The World Health Organization and the transition from "international" to "global" public health. *Am J Public Health.* 2006;96:62–72.

39. Brandt AM. How AIDS invented global health. *N Engl J Med.* 2013;368:2149–2152.

40. Centers for Disease Control and Prevention. Ten great public health achievements: United States, 1990–1999. *MMWR Morb Mort Wkly Rep.* 1999; 48:241–243.

41. Centers for Disease Control and Prevention. Ten great public health achievements: worldwide, 2001–2010. *MMWR Morb Mort Wkly Rep.* 2011;60:814–818.

42. Goli S, Moradhvaj A, Chakravorty S, Rammohan A. World health status 1950–2015: converging or diverging. *PLoS One.* 2019;14:e0213139.

CHAPTER 2

Global Health Priorities

Globalization processes have helped improve global population health in recent decades, but international travel and trade also increase the risk of pandemics and other threats to human security. Global partnerships and agendas like the Sustainable Development Goals shape global health priorities and establish frameworks for evaluating progress toward achieving shared targets.

2.1 Globalization and Health

Globalization is the process of countries around the world becoming more integrated and interdependent across economic, political, cultural, and other domains. Globalization can be observed in the proliferation of multilateral trade agreements and the rising complexity of global supply chains; the growing number of multinational corporations and international nonprofit organizations; and increases in population mobility, cross-border communication, data sharing, and cultural diffusion. Globalization contributes to the favorable and unfavorable health transitions that are occurring in many parts of the world by increasing access to health technologies, encouraging urbanization, changing social and cultural practices, and accelerating environmental changes.[1]

One of the most obvious examples of the links between globalization and health is the threat from contagious diseases. A **pathogen** is a bacterium, virus, or other microorganism that can cause disease. Pathogens have never stopped at international borders. Infectious diseases like plague and smallpox spread across Asia and Europe more than 1,000 years ago when sea and land trade routes like the Silk Road linked China, India, and the Mediterranean. The pathogens carried by the Europeans who explored the Americas in the 15th century caused the decimation of many Indigenous American populations, while some infections that originated in the Western hemisphere, such as syphilis, made their way back to Europe and sparked widespread epidemics.[2] Today, modern transportation allows for a new infectious disease that emerges in any part of the world to be transported by aircraft to any other part of the world within hours rather than weeks or months. Concerns about globalization and health also encompass a diversity of other emerging health issues, such as bioterrorism, drug resistance, food safety, and the health effects of climate change.

Globalization is not a uniformly good or bad process but one that yields a mix of positive and negative outcomes.[3] For example, globalization processes have shifted a lot of manufacturing from high-income countries to middle-income countries, where lower salaries for workers allow products to be made more cheaply. In high-income areas, globalized supply chains have reduced the cost of consumer products but also caused the loss of many manufacturing jobs. In middle-income countries, the growth of the manufacturing sector has created jobs, but it has also demanded increased worker productivity even when that compromises worker safety and causes environmental damage. In low-income areas, some residents benefit from being able to buy consumer products manufactured in middle-income countries, but countries that do not have educational systems geared toward producing a technologically skilled workforce are unable to reap the most valuable benefits of the global economy. Globalization tends to create greater income inequalities between and within countries.

In many countries, concerns about the adverse impacts of globalization have led to the rise of nationalistic political movements that call for greater self-reliance and less engagement with other nations. However, even if countries implement isolationist policies, it is not possible to eliminate the need for involvement in global health activities. The threat from emerging infectious diseases is an ancient one that will continue to exist for future generations, and environmental hazards can easily cross international borders when they are carried by air, water, or animals.[4] Whether a country has pro- or anti-globalization policies, every country benefits from active communication about transnational health concerns, collaboration on scientific research that enables populations to fortify themselves against threats to health, and cooperation on health interventions that promote prosperity, peace, and security.

Due in part to globalization processes, today's population health and risk profiles are different than the patterns observed 100 years ago. The general trend toward improved global health that has been observed in recent decades is expected to continue, but new and sometimes unpredictable health transitions will occur. The coronavirus pandemic that began in early 2020 was a rapid health transition that quickly shifted health behaviors and caused periodic spikes in the mortality rate from infectious disease in high-income countries. Economic- and climate-related shocks may also adversely affect population health at unexpected times.

Countries that proactively engage in global health dialogues and actions are able to use prevention strategies and other interventions to shape a healthier, safer future for their own citizens as well as the world at large.[5] All participating countries benefit from collaboratively working to prevent and respond to outbreaks, achieve shared health and development goals, promote goodwill and humanitarian values, and protect economic and political interests at home and abroad.[6]

2.2 Global Health Security

Human security was defined in the United Nations Development Programme's 1994 *Human Development Report* as the freedom from fear and freedom from want that results from having the following types of security:

- Economic security (freedom from extreme poverty)
- Food security (freedom from hunger)
- Health security
- Environmental security (freedom from preventable environmental vulnerabilities)
- Personal security (freedom from violence)
- Community security (freedom from discrimination)
- Political security (freedom from human rights violations)[7]

Ideally, the protection and empowerment that facilitate human security for one generation should not compromise the ability of future generations to enjoy similar freedoms.[8]

Human security focuses on individual and community well-being, while national security focuses on the protection of the collective interests of people living within a country's borders. For many countries, support for health security and other aspects of human security is a core component of national security plans.[9] For example, the National Academies of Sciences, Engineering, and Medicine, which has been chartered as an advisory board by the U.S. Congress since 1863, has recommended that the United States invest in global health activities as part of its overall strategy for protecting Americans from emerging and continuing threats to health, enhancing economic growth and productivity, and enabling Americans to remain leaders in innovation (**Figure 2.1**).[10] The investment in global health activities by high-income countries generates major returns through fortified homeland security, expanded

Priority Area		Recommendation
Secure against global threats	Achieve global health security	Improve international emergency response coordination
		Combat antimicrobial resistance
		Build public health capacity in low- and middle-income countries
	Address continuous threats	Envision the next generation of the President's Emergency Plan for AIDS Relief (PEPFAR)
		Confront the threat of tuberculosis
		Sustain progress toward malaria elimination
Enhance productivity and economic growth	Invest in women's and children's health	Improve survival in women and children
		Ensure healthy and productive lives for women and children
	Promote cardiovascular health and prevent cancer	Promote cardiovascular health and prevent cancer
Maximize returns on investments	Catalyze innovation	Accelerate the development of medical products
		Improve digital health infrastructure
	Smart financing strategies	Transition investments toward global public goods
		Optimize resources through smart financing
	Global health leadership	Commit to continued global health leadership

Figure 2.1 Recommended actions from the National Academies of Sciences, Engineering, and Medicine's Committee on Global Health and the Future of the United States.

Data from National Academies of Sciences, Engineering, and Medicine. *Global Health and the Future Role of the United States.* Washington DC: National Academies Press; 2017.

markets for international trade, and strengthened diplomatic relationships.[11]

Global health security describes public health interventions implemented by governmental and military personnel in collaboration with other stakeholders in order to protect populations from threats to health and safety.[12] The current concept of global health security is an extension of the historic international health policies and practices that aimed to slow the spread of epidemics as international travel and trade intensified.[13] Communities and countries suffering from widespread health problems are more likely to have economic and political instability, and poverty and unrest can further exacerbate public health problems that might spill over into other parts of the world. International and global health initiatives can help break this cycle, facilitating productivity and peace. Global health security recognizes that countries participating in global health activities reap the benefits of self-protection in addition to the humanitarian gains and goodwill that these actions may generate.[14]

One of the major foci of global health security is pandemic preparedness and response. For example, the Global Health Security Agenda (GHSA), launched by the United States in collaboration with the World Health Organization (WHO) in 2014, aims to strengthen the ability of dozens of partner countries to prevent epidemics when possible, to detect emerging threats early, and to respond quickly and effectively to outbreaks.[15] Progress toward achieving these GHSA goals is made by supporting laboratory capabilities, surveillance systems, workforce development, and sustainable financing mechanisms in less-resourced countries as well as with specific programs focused on themes such as antimicrobial resistance, zoonotic diseases, and vaccination.

However, global health security is not just focused on pandemics and other infectious disease threats, such as HIV/AIDS and drug-resistant tuberculosis. Any health issues

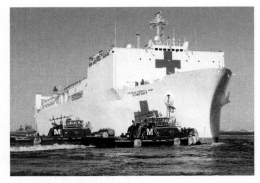

© MC2 Justin Yarborough/U.S. Navy

that reduce human security can be part of a global health security strategy, including maternal and child health, malnutrition, noncommunicable diseases such as cardiovascular disease and cancer, mental health issues, and violence. Investments in improving any area of public health in other countries and world regions can fortify the national security of partner nations.

2.3 Prioritization Strategies

In an ideal world, there would be enough resources for all worthy global health goals to receive the funding they need to be achieved. In the real world, the amount of funding available for health interventions is limited. Advocates for various health problems and solutions must compete for attention and support, and only the proposals that garner buy-in from well-resourced groups are able to move forward. The gap between commendable ideas and the resources to implement them has created a demand for prioritization strategies that allow funders to make informed decisions about where and how to invest in global health. When future generations compile lists celebrating the major global health accomplishments of the 21st century, those lists will reflect the decisions today's global health leaders make about which projects to prioritize.

Each funding agency and planning committee applies its own criteria for the types of activities that it will support.[16] For example, some focus specifically on health and nutrition interventions, while others support broader educational and economic development activities. Some give priority to preventive interventions, and some prioritize treatment of existing health issues. Some prepare primary health facilities to diagnose and treat a diversity of health issues, and some focus on increasing access to advanced disease-specific care at tertiary hospitals. Additionally, each group may prioritize one or more of the global health values summarized by the acronym PACES: populations, action, cooperation, equity, and security (**Figure 2.2**).

For example, one approach is to establish priorities based on the health concerns that affect the greatest number of people (**Figure 2.3**). The WHO's five-year plan for 2019–2023 was built around a "triple billion" target: 1 billion more people enjoying improved health, 1 billion more people protected from health emergencies, and 1 billion more people accessing universal health coverage.[17] The term **burden of disease** describes the adverse impact of a particular health condition (or group of conditions) on a population. Groups that prioritize global health investments based on a population lens make their decisions after looking at statistics about the conditions that cause the greatest burden of disease in the populations they support. Disease burden can be measured using health metrics, such as the number of annual hospitalizations and deaths from a particular disease, or using economic indicators, such as the total direct costs of medical care for a disease and the indirect costs of absences from work or school due to the condition. As part of the strategic planning for achieving the triple billion target, the WHO identified 10 global health issues that already affect billions of humans or have the potential to do so in the near future. The list included air pollution and climate change, noncommunicable diseases (such as heart disease,

Lens	Key Questions
Populations	■ What are the health issues that cause the greatest number of deaths, illnesses, and disability worldwide? ■ Which populations have the greatest need?
Action	■ What are the "best buys" among the available interventions? ■ How do we allocate resources to do the greatest good for the greatest number of people?
Cooperation	■ Who are the partners, and what are their shared goals? ■ What problem is the partnership best equipped to solve?
Equity	■ What actions will do the most to improve the health status of vulnerable populations? ■ How will the intervention improve health equity?
Security	■ What are the greatest threats to peace? ■ How will the intervention help to achieve the national interests of sponsoring governments?

Figure 2.2 PACES: Strategies for prioritizing global health issues.

Lens	Sample Priority		Sample Priority	
Populations	Cardiovascular disease (CVD)	CVD is the leading cause of adult mortality worldwide.	Drinking water	Unsafe drinking water causes billions of cases of severe diarrhea annually.
Action	Hunger	Adequate nutrition in early childhood is critical for healthy development, and many low-cost interventions can improve child nutritional status.	HIV	HIV medications can extend the lives of infected individuals by many years or even decades, but millions of people who would benefit from these drugs do not have access to them.
Cooperation	Environmental health	Pollution generated by one country can cause adverse health effects in neighboring lands; international collaborations can mitigate threats to environmental health.	Drug-resistant infections	One country with poor regulations for antibiotic use can put the whole world at risk; global partnerships can slow the emergence and spread of drug-resistant pathogens.
Equity	Neglected tropical diseases	The world's poorest children are disabled and disfigured by parasitic diseases that do not affect children who happen to have been born in higher-income places.	Mental health	In every country, people with mental health disorders encounter stigma that may exclude them from full participation in society.
Security	Violence	The violence in conflict areas can spill over into new locations and create migration crises.	Emerging infectious diseases	Outbreaks of deadly infectious diseases threaten public safety and can cause social, economic, and political instability.

Figure 2.3 PACES: Examples of global health priorities.

cancer, and diabetes), global influenza pandemics, fragile and vulnerable settings, antimicrobial resistance, Ebola and other high-threat pathogens, weak primary health care, vaccine hesitancy, dengue, and HIV.[18] Work on these widespread areas of concern will contribute significantly to improving health for more than 1 billion of the world's people.

Prioritization based on an action orientation often awards the highest rankings to interventions that have been identified as "best buys" because they help many people make meaningful gains in health status at a low cost per person or at a low cost per adverse event averted by the intervention.[19] In general, low-cost primary prevention activities are the most cost-effective interventions.[20] For example, the interventions that the Disease Control Priorities (DCP) project has identified as having good "value for money" in low- and middle-income countries include improving the basic care of newborns; vaccinating children against infections such as measles, pneumococcus, rotavirus, and *Haemophilus influenzae* type b (Hib); preventing malaria and HIV infections; treating tuberculosis and other communicable diseases to prevent them from spreading to other people; and expanding the use of medications to manage cardiovascular diseases.[21] DCP also identifies basic surgical interventions for issues such as emergency obstetric complications, appendicitis, hernias, and traumatic injuries as good values in population health.[22]

Some groups make decisions based on the special interests and capabilities of the collaborators. For example, in 2003 the Bill & Melinda Gates Foundation introduced a set of Grand Challenges in Global Health that could be solved with new technologies, such as creating new and improved vaccines, controlling insects that transmit pathogens, improving nutrition through the creation of nutrient-rich staple plant species, improving treatment of infectious diseases by limiting drug resistance, curing chronic infections, and measuring health status with new diagnostic tools.[23] Research proposals related to these areas of research or to more recently released sets of Grand Challenges are prioritized for funding. Because the Gates Foundation is led by people with expertise in computing and information technology, the foundation is uniquely prepared to support the development and dissemination of new tech products. When funding and implementation agencies have special areas of expertise, they can maximize their impact by applying their knowledge and experience to new projects that build on past achievements.

Groups focused on equity prioritize projects that will confront perceived injustices and reduce health disparities. Many equity-oriented programs focus on the health of infants and children because of the nearly universal belief that no child anywhere should suffer from abuse, hunger, or preventable and treatable diseases.[24] Other equity-focused initiatives seek to improve the health of other vulnerable populations, such as refugees and other migrants, incarcerated people, people with disabilities, older adults, and members of marginalized population groups. Equity-focused global health organizations may also advocate for human rights.

Another approach is to make prioritization decisions based on the security interests of sponsoring governments, including direct and indirect threats to national, regional, and global peace and stability. For example, at the beginning of the 21st century, the U.S. Centers for Disease Control and Prevention (CDC) recognized that the leading public health challenges for the United States included protecting the environment, responding to emerging infectious diseases (including pandemic influenza and drug-resistant pathogens), and reducing the burden from violence (including the physical and psychological traumas sustained by military personnel deployed to conflict areas) (**Figure 2.4**).[25] These types of threats to health and security cannot be alleviated by any one country working in isolation. Once a country has identified its own strategic global health priorities, that country is prepared to advocate for those priorities in conversations with potential partners. Working with partner nations on achieving shared aims will then advance health security at home and abroad.

The priorities identified by groups viewing global health with different lenses provide insight into the health challenges of nations and populations around the world, and they point toward solutions for shared concerns. Because there are so many governmental, nonprofit, corporate, academic, and other initiatives and partnerships with different priorities for global health, a wide range of health issues are active global health priorities.

1	Institute a rational healthcare system (balance equity, cost, and quality).
2	Eliminate health disparities.
3	Focus on children's emotional and intellectual development.
4	Achieve a longer "healthspan" (healthy aging).
5	Integrate physical activity and healthy eating into daily lives.
6	Clean up and protect the environment.
7	Prepare to respond to emerging infectious diseases.
8	Recognize and address the contributions of mental health to overall health and well-being.
9	Reduce the toll of violence in society.
10	Use new scientific knowledge and technological advances wisely.

Figure 2.4 The U.S. CDC's top public health challenges for the early 21st century.

Data from Koplan JP, Fleming DW. Current and future public health challenges. *JAMA*. 2000;284:1696–1698.

2.4 Millennium Development Goals

During the Cold War, which emerged in the aftermath of World War II, Western capitalistic democracies were sometimes classified as "First World" countries; communist bloc countries labeled as "Second World" countries; and the remaining nations, which were home to the majority of the world's people, categorized as "Third World" countries.[26] By the time the Union of Soviet Socialist Republics (USSR) split into independent republics and the Berlin Wall was dismantled in 1991, this hierarchical language had fallen out of favor. The new terminology often divided the world into just two groups, developed countries and developing (or less-developed or underdeveloped) countries. That language still implies a hierarchy of rich and poor nations or donor and recipient countries, and it does not acknowledge that every country is developed in some way and no country ever stops developing. Similar language about the "Global North" and the "Global South" is of limited use because geography has little to do with economic status. Today, quantitative language like high income, middle income, and low income is typically used to describe the relative economic status of countries. Rather than dividing the world into two or three fixed groups, country income levels are visualized as a spectrum.

The changing geopolitical terrain of the late 20th century sparked calls for every country in the world to participate in global governance. A series of United Nations–related conferences in the 1990s, such as the "Earth Summit" held in Rio de Janeiro, Brazil, in 1992 and a World Summit on Social Development held in Copenhagen, Denmark, in 1995, promoted the idea of sustainable, equitable development. The momentum from these events was channeled into a new push to try to eradicate global poverty.[27] The **Millennium Development Goals (MDGs)** were a set of eight goals endorsed by the United Nations and hundreds of partners that aimed to significantly reduce global poverty between 2000 and 2015 (**Figure 2.5**). Many of the eight goals had direct links to health, including ones seeking to eradicate extreme poverty and hunger (MDG 1); reduce child mortality (MDG 4); improve maternal health (MDG 5); combat HIV/AIDS, malaria, and other diseases (MDG 6); and

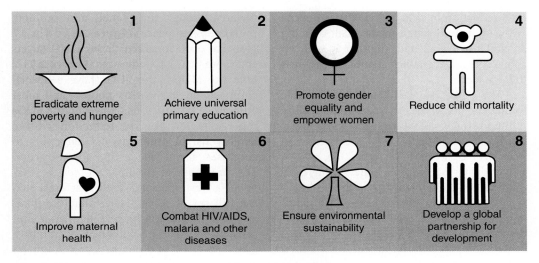

Figure 2.5 Millennium Development Goals (MDGs) (2000–2015).

ensure environmental sustainability (MDG 7). While the MDGs overall were about general socioeconomic development, they were also a major contributor to the global health successes thus far in the 21st century.

One of the reasons the MDGs were so influential is that they provided a clear strategy for evaluation by defining sets of goals, targets, and indicators. A **goal** is a desired future outcome. Some goals are commitments that are easily attainable within a set time frame but still require buy-in from the relevant stakeholders. Some goals are aspirational ones that are intended to encourage incremental progress toward achieving ambitious aims. A **target** is a specific, measurable objective that contributes to achieving a desired future outcome. Targets point toward the actions that should be taken to demonstrate progress toward achieving goals. An **indicator** is a variable used to measure performance, achievement, or change. When the eight MDGs were launched in 2000, they were accompanied by 18 targets and 48 indicators. These were later expanded to 21 targets and 60 indicators. Each goal had at least one target associated with it, and

each target was assessed with one or more measurable indicators. Data about each of the 60 indicators were collected annually from most participating countries as part of evaluating how much progress had been made toward reaching national, regional, and global targets.

For example, MDG 1 aimed to "eradicate extreme poverty and hunger." A 0% rate of poverty was an aspirational goal that no one believed would actually be achieved by 2015. One of the targets associated with MDG 1 was to "halve, between 1990 and 2015, the proportion of people whose income is less than $1 a day" (target 1A). A 50% reduction in extreme poverty over 25 years was an ambitious target, but the MDG partners agreed that it could be achieved within the stated timeline. Three indicators were used to assess progress on this target, including one for the proportion of the population living on less than $1.25 per day (indicator 1.1). The final data collected in 2015 showed a 68% reduction in extreme poverty, as measured by this indicator, between 1990 and 2015.[28] The target of a 50% reduction was met or, more precisely, exceeded. While a

68% reduction in extreme poverty is not the 100% reduction stated in the goal, defining an ambitious goal and aligning it with an achievable target enabled significant progress to be made.

The MDGs facilitated remarkable improvements in health status and quality of life for the world's lowest-income populations. Globally, there was a 44% reduction in hunger between 1990 and 2015, a 53% reduction in the mortality rate among children between birth and their fifth birthdays between 1990 and 2015, a 44% reduction in pregnancy-related deaths during that time period, a 45% reduction in new cases of HIV compared to the rate in 2000, and a 62% reduction in the percentage of people without reliable access to safe drinking water sources.[29] Although not all of the goals and targets were achieved, most lower-income countries had healthier populations in 2015 than they had when the MDGs were launched in 2000.[28]

While some concerns were raised about how well the MDGs promoted equity, sustainability, local ownership of priorities, and holistic development (rather than relatively narrow, single-sector silos of focus), the general consensus was that the MDGs provided a helpful framework for global cooperation toward international development.[30] Each signatory country was committed to working toward these goals, so the MDGs provided a blueprint for national- and international-level priority setting.

2.5 Sustainable Development Goals

The success of the MDGs was the impetus to create a follow-up set of global goals. The **Sustainable Development Goals (SDGs)** are a set of 17 goals endorsed by the member nations of the United Nations at the end of 2015 that aim, by 2030, to end poverty, protect the planet, and promote prosperity and peace (**Figure 2.6**).[31] The 17 goals are operationalized through 169 targets and more than 230 indicators (**Figure 2.7**).[32] Like the MDGs, the SDGs have a special emphasis on the world's poorest and most vulnerable populations. However, the SDGs mix goals for poverty reduction with a lengthy list of other targets that apply to countries across the economic spectrum. The preamble of the *2030 Agenda for Sustainable Development*, which first presented the full set of SDGs, states that the goals are "a plan of action for people, planet, and prosperity" that are intended to improve "the lives of all" and not just some countries and some stakeholders.[31]

Many of the areas of success during the MDG era have been assigned even more ambitious targets in the SDGs. For example, the MDGs aimed to reduce extreme poverty by 50% between 1990 and 2015 (MDG 1.A) and the SDGs aim to eradicate extreme poverty by 2030 (SDG 1.1). The MDG indicator for this target (MDG 1.1) measured the proportion of people living on less than $1.25 per day. The SDG indicator (SDG 1.1.1) measures the proportion of the population below the international poverty line (updated to $1.90 per day) at the total population level and in subgroups defined by sex, age, employment status, and urban and rural geographic locations. Most of the MDG targets that were not achieved have also been retained in the SDGs, and they are accompanied by a host of new targets and indicators covering a broader diversity of socioeconomic, health, and environmental issues.

Like the MDGs, the SDGs treat health as both a necessary prerequisite to and an outcome of economic growth.[33] Two of the 17 SDGs focus specifically on health (SDG 3) and nutrition (SDG 2), but all of the other goals are relevant for health. Several of the SDGs pertain to the socioeconomic determinants of health: economics (SDG 1), education

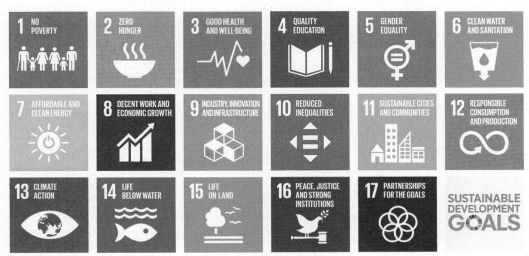

Figure 2.6 Sustainable Development Goals (SDGs) (2016–2030).

(SDG 4), gender equality (SDG 5), employment (SDG 8), equal opportunities for all people (SDG 10), peace (SDG 16), and good governance (SDG 17). The remaining SDGs relate to the environmental determinants of health: water and sanitation (SDG 6), affordable clean energy (SDG 7), safe work environments (SDG 9), healthy urban areas (SDG 11), sustainable consumption and production practices (SDG 12), and healthy climates (SDG 13), including healthy oceans (SDG 14) and land (SDG 15).

The sole SDG that is specifically focused on health (SDG 3) includes a much greater diversity of targets and indicators than were encompassed by the three MDGs that aimed to reduce the burden from child mortality, maternal mortality, and infectious diseases (primarily HIV, malaria, and tuberculosis). The health-focused SDG targets include ambitious aims for further reducing maternal mortality (SDG 3.1) and child mortality (SDG 3.2); alleviating the burden from

a diversity of infectious diseases, including HIV, tuberculosis, malaria, neglected tropical diseases, and hepatitis B virus (SDG 3.3); reducing the number of adults who die before their 70th birthdays from noncommunicable diseases (SDG 3.4); improving treatment of substance use disorders (SDG 3.5); preventing transportation-related deaths (SDG 3.6); increasing the accessibility of health services, medications, and vaccines (SDG 3.7 and 3.8); improving environmental health (SDG 3.9); and reducing tobacco use (SDG 3.a) **(Figure 2.8)**.[34]

A **benchmark** is a standard or point of reference for comparison. Most of the SDG targets have 2015 as the baseline benchmark for evaluating improvements by 2030. Some of the SDG targets use strong verbs like "eliminate," "eradicate," "prohibit," or "end" that call for dramatic improvements during the 15 years that the SDGs will be in force. Some use weaker verbs like "promote," "enhance," "support," or "encourage" that anticipate that only minor

SDG	Theme	Goal
1	No poverty	End poverty in all its forms everywhere
2	Zero hunger	End hunger, achieve food security and improved nutrition, and promote sustainable agriculture
3	Good health and well-being	Ensure healthy lives and promote well-being for all at all ages
4	Quality education	Ensure inclusive and equitable quality education and promote lifelong learning opportunities for all
5	Gender equality	Achieve gender equality and empower all women and girls
6	Clean water and sanitation	Ensure availability and sustainable management of water and sanitation for all
7	Affordable and clean energy	Ensure access to affordable, reliable, sustainable, and modern energy for all
8	Decent work and economic growth	Promote sustained, inclusive, and sustainable economic growth, full and productive employment and decent work for all
9	Industry, innovation, and infrastructure	Build resilient infrastructure, promote inclusive and sustainable industrialization, and foster innovation
10	Reduced inequalities	Reduce inequality within and among countries
11	Sustainable cities and communities	Make cities and human settlements inclusive, safe, resilient, and sustainable
12	Responsible consumption and production	Ensure sustainable consumption and production practices
13	Climate action	Take urgent action to combat climate change and its impacts
14	Life below water	Conserve and sustainably use oceans, seas, and marine resources for sustainable development
15	Life on land	Protect, restore, and promote sustainable use of terrestrial ecosystems, sustainably manage forests, combat desertification, and halt and reverse land degradation and halt biodiversity loss
16	Peace, justice, and strong institutions	Promote peaceful and inclusive societies for sustainable development, provide access to justice for all and build effective, accountable, and inclusive institutions at all levels
17	Partnership for the goals	Strengthen the means of implementation and revitalize the global partnership for sustainable development

Figure 2.7 The 17 Sustainable Development Goals (SDGs).

Goal.Target.Indicator	
2.2.2	Child malnutrition
3.1.1	Maternal mortality
3.2.1	Child mortality
3.3.1	HIV
3.3.2	Tuberculosis
3.3.3	Malaria
3.3.4	Hepatitis B virus
3.3.5	Neglected tropical diseases
3.4.1	Noncommunicable diseases (cardiovascular disease, cancer, diabetes, and chronic respiratory disease)
3.4.2	Suicide
3.5.1	Substance abuse
3.6.1	Road traffic injuries
3.7.1	Sexual and reproductive health
3.8.1	Universal health coverage
3.9.1	Air pollution
3.9.2	Unsafe water and sanitation
3.9.3	Unintentional poisoning
3.a.1	Tobacco use
3.b.1	Access to essential medicines and vaccines
3.c.1	Health workforce
3.d.1	Emergency preparedness
6.1.1	Drinking water
6.2.1	Sanitation
7.1.2	Clean household energy
11.6.2	Air pollution
13.1.1	Natural disasters
16.1.1	Homicide
16.1.2	Conflicts

Figure 2.8 Examples of Sustainable Development Goals targets related to health.

Data from *World Health Statistics 2016: Monitoring Health for the SDGs.* Geneva: World Health Organization; 2016.

signs of progress will be attained before 2030. The indicators for each target provide further evidence about whether bold leaps or merely incremental steps forward are intended to be achieved by 2030. The expectation is that by 2030 the less ambitious targets will have been met and good progress will have been made toward achieving the grander targets.

2.6 Vital Statistics

As more resources have been devoted to global health efforts, it has become increasingly important to quantify population health concerns, identify major modifiable risk factors for diseases and other adverse health conditions, assess the impact of new public health interventions, and monitor changes in the health status of populations over time. The key measures of health and disease in populations include information about population size, birth rates, death rates, the frequency and causes of various illnesses and disabilities, the causes of death, and the rates at which members of the population engage in risky behaviors. All these measures provide an evidence base for making policy and funding decisions.[35]

A **statistic** is a measured characteristic of a sample population. **Vital statistics** are population-level quantifications of births, deaths, and other life events. Most countries maintain vital statistical records on their residents by issuing birth and death certificates, logging marriage and divorce certificates, and compiling data from other sources. A **census** collects demographic data about every individual in a population. Many countries conduct routine censuses because enumerating (counting) the total population in each of its geopolitical units enables resources to be allocated proportionally. Demographers use vital statistics and census records to understand the current population and predict the size and characteristics of the population in future years.

Counts of life events in a population can be translated into proportions and rates. Percentages and rates can then be compared in two or more populations. A **ratio** is a comparison of two numbers. A **proportion** is a ratio in which the numerator (the top number) is a subset of the denominator (the bottom number). When a proportion expresses part of a whole, the value ranges from 0 to 1. A **percentage** expresses a ratio in units of "per 100." When a percentage expresses part of a whole, the value ranges from 0% to 100%. A **rate** is a ratio in which the numerator and denominator have different units. The denominator for a rate often expresses a measure of time. For example, the **birth rate** is the number of births per 1,000 people (or other units) in a population over a one-year period.

Survival analysis is a statistical evaluation of the distribution of the durations of time that individuals in a population experience from an initial time point (such as birth) until some well-defined event (such as death). **Life expectancy** is the average number of additional years of life an individual of a particular age can be expected to survive based on population mortality patterns. **Life expectancy at birth** is the average number of years a newborn in a population can be expected to survive based on population mortality patterns at the time of birth. Life expectancy at birth captures the burden from infant and child deaths in addition to the average age at death of adults. In places with high infant mortality rates, the life expectancy at birth is often in middle adulthood. This does not mean that the typical adult dies at 40 or 50 years of age. Instead, that number represents an age somewhere between a large number of child deaths and a large number of deaths among older adults (**Figure 2.9**). Life expectancies have increased over time in most countries, but they remain much higher in high-income countries than in low-income countries (**Figure 2.10**).[36]

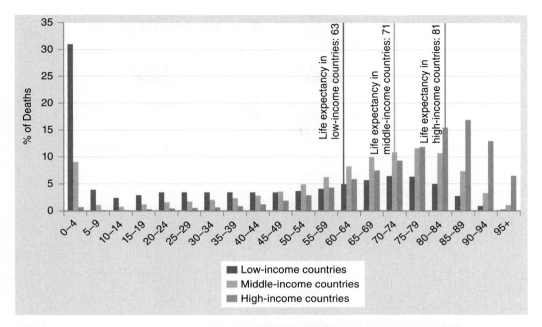

Figure 2.9 Distribution of deaths by age and life expectancy at birth, by country income group.

Data from United Nations Department of Economic and Social Affairs. *World Population Prospects: The 2019 Revision.* New York: United Nations; 2019.

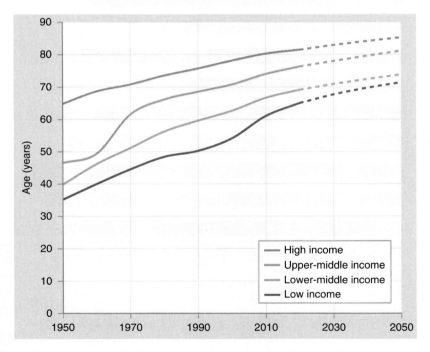

Figure 2.10 Life expectancy at birth has increased over time for all country income groups.

Data from United Nations Department of Economic and Social Affairs. *World Population Prospects: The 2019 Revision.* New York: United Nations; 2019.

Some life expectancy statistics present estimates of **healthy life expectancy** (HALE), the average number of additional years an individual of a particular age in a population can expect to live without disability. The typical adult can expect to experience about 10 years of poor health before dying (**Figure 2.11**).[37] Global health aims to increase life expectancies and increase HALE so that people live to older ages without experiencing extended periods of disability prior to death. Interventions that reduce the likelihood of dying before old age increase life expectancies. Interventions that reduce the likelihood of dying or the likelihood of having a chronic illness or disability increase HALE.

2.7 Mortality

Epidemiology is the study of the distribution and determinants of health and disease in human populations. Epidemiologists quantify health problems in populations, identify the risk factors for developing those conditions, and test the effectiveness of interventions for these concerns. In public health, **biostatistics** is the science of analyzing health data and interpreting the results so that they can be applied to solving public health problems. One of the major roles of epidemiologists and biostatisticians is tracking the causes of illness, disability, and death in communities and nations.

Mortality means death. The **mortality rate**, also called the **death rate**, is the number

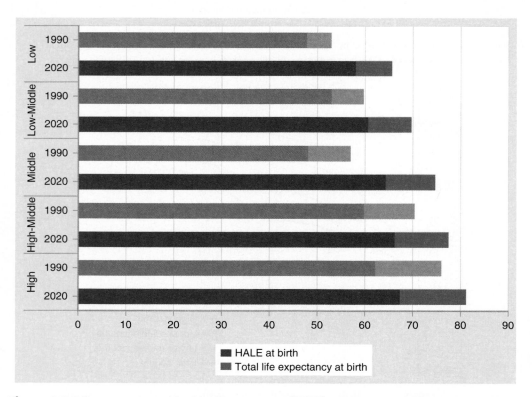

Figure 2.11 Life expectancy and healthy life expectancy (HALE) at birth, by country sociodemographic group.

Data from GBD 2019 Demographics Collaborators. Global age-sex-specific fertility, mortality, healthy life expectancy (HALE), and population estimates in 204 countries and territories, 1950–2019: a comprehensive demographic analysis for the Global Burden of Disease Study 2019. *Lancet.* 2020;396:1160–1203.

of all-cause or cause-specific deaths per 1,000 people (or other units) in a population during a stated period of time. An all-cause mortality rate might describe the rate of death from any cause among all Canadians during one calendar year. A cause-specific mortality rate might quantify the rate of death from lung cancer in Canada that year. An age-specific mortality rate might report the rate of death from any cause among Canadians who were 60 to 69 years old during a selected year. An age- and cause-specific mortality rate could describe the rate of death from lung cancer among Canadians aged 60 to 69 years that year.

Tallying deaths at the population level is challenging in lower-income countries that do not have reliable systems for registering vital statistics. In places where most births and deaths occur in homes instead of in hospitals, government officials may document only a fraction of these events. The most disadvantaged populations, often the ones with the highest mortality rates, are the least likely to have their life events accurately counted. Thus, while very precise mortality statistics are available in high-income countries, death rates in low-income countries often must be estimated based on incomplete registries. Demographers and epidemiologists use advanced computational methods to collate the best available data and make reasonably accurate assessments of the annual number and causes of death by age group and sex in every region of the world.

Higher-income countries usually have older populations than lower-income countries. Because of the age differential, higher-income countries usually have higher all-ages mortality rates than lower-income countries. However, when age-specific mortality rates are compared, the opposite trend is observed. A five-year-old who lives in a low-income country is much more likely to die this year than a five-year-old who lives in a high-income country. A 70-year-old who lives in a low-income country is more likely to die this year than a 70-year-old who lives in a high-income country. The same trend is observed for all ages from birth through older adulthood (**Figure 2.12**).[37] The lower age-specific mortality rates in higher-income countries allow more residents to live to old age, and then the higher proportion of older adults in higher-income countries makes the all-ages mortality rate higher.

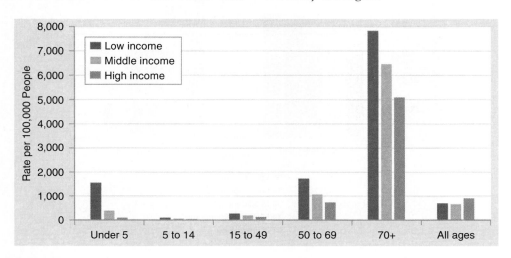

Figure 2.12 Age-specific all-cause mortality rates per 100,000 people, by country sociodemographic group.

Data from GBD 2019 Demographics Collaborators. Global age-sex-specific fertility, mortality, healthy life expectancy (HALE), and population estimates in 204 countries and territories, 1950–2019: a comprehensive demographic analysis for the Global Burden of Disease Study 2019. *Lancet*. 2020;396:1160–1203.

A **crude statistic** is a raw or unadjusted statistical measure. Because of the different age structures in different countries, it can be misleading to compare their crude all-ages health statistics. **Age standardization** is the generation of comparable statistics for populations with different age structures. Summary age-standardized statistics are calculated from age-specific rates that are combined with weights that are proportional to the distribution of people by age worldwide (or in another reference population). While the crude (unadjusted) all-cause mortality rates are highest in high-income countries that have a large proportion of older adults, the age-standardized (adjusted) mortality rates are highest in low-income countries (**Figure 2.13**).[37] When reporting the value of a statistic in one population, the crude (unadjusted) rate is the correct one to report. The crude mortality rate (CMR) truly is higher in high-income countries than in low-income countries. When comparing mortality rates in two or more populations with different

population age structures, age-adjusted mortality rates are the best option for making the comparison a fair one. These values are artificial, but they are directly comparable.

Some mortality statistics look at the distribution of causes of deaths within a selected population and time frame. The **proportionate mortality rate** (PMR) is the percentage of all people who die in a population whose death is the result of a particular cause. The **case fatality rate** (CFR) is the proportion of people with a particular disease who die as a result of that condition. Cause-specific mortality rates, PMRs, and CFRs provide different views about the impact of one selected health issue on deaths in a population. Suppose that the goal is to examine COVID-19 deaths in Australia during the year 2020. For the cause-specific mortality rate, the denominator would be the total number of people living in Australia in 2020 (as of the middle of the year, roughly around July 1) and the numerator would be the total number of deaths from COVID-19 in

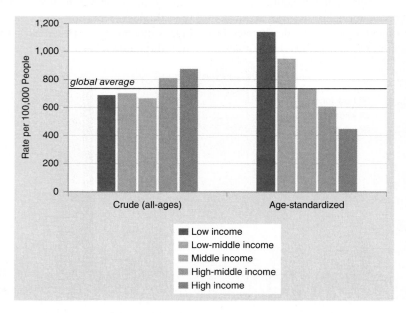

Figure 2.13 Crude and age-standardized all-cause mortality rates per 100,000 people, by country sociodemographic group.

Data from GBD 2019 Demographics Collaborators. Global age-sex-specific fertility, mortality, healthy life expectancy (HALE), and population estimates in 204 countries and territories, 1950–2019: a comprehensive demographic analysis for the Global Burden of Disease Study 2019. *Lancet.* 2020;396:1160–1203.

Australia across all of 2020. For the PMR, the denominator would be all deaths that occurred in Australia in 2020 and the numerator would be the subset of those deaths that were due to COVID-19. For the CFR, the denominator would be all people living in Australia who developed COVID-19 at any point during 2020 and the numerator would be the total deaths from COVID-19 among those individuals.

Looking at a variety of statistics provides a more complete picture of health and risk status than examining just one measure. For example, consider the comparison of deaths from respiratory infections, such as tuberculosis and pneumonia, and deaths from cardiovascular disease (CVD) in countries with different income levels (**Figure 2.14**).[38] In low-income countries, the percentage of deaths due to respiratory infections is about equal to the percentage of deaths due to CVD. In high-income countries, only a small percentage of deaths are due to respiratory infections but nearly one in three deaths is due to CVD. However, while the percentage of deaths from CVD in low-income countries

is about half the crude PMR of CVD in high-income countries, the age-standardized CVD-specific mortality rate in low-income countries is almost twice the rate in high-income countries. Crude PMRs and age-standardized mortality rates show different stories about the burden from infectious diseases and noncommunicable diseases in low-income countries.

One of the challenges when tabulating causes of death in a population is that only one primary cause can be assigned to each deceased individual. Decisions about how to assign causes of death when there are multiple contributing factors can have a significant impact on which diseases appear to be the most frequent causes of mortality in a population. For example, when people with HIV/AIDS die of tuberculosis, their deaths are typically attributed to HIV. That coding pattern may cause the true burden from tuberculosis to be underrepresented in statistical tables. Statistics should only be compared when similar decisions about how to allocate causes of death were applied to all of the populations being examined.

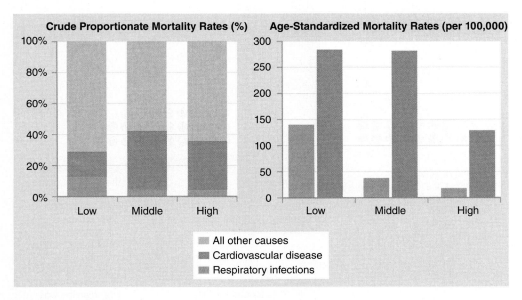

Figure 2.14 Comparing crude proportionate mortality rates and age-standardized mortality rates, by country sociodemographic group.

Data from GBD 2019 Diseases and Injuries Collaborators. Global burden of 369 diseases and injuries in 204 countries and territories, 1990–2019: a systematic analysis for the Global Burden of Disease Study 2019. *Lancet.* 2020;396:1204–1222.

2.8 Morbidity

Morbidity is the presence of nonfatal illness or disease. Morbidity does not describe whether an illness or disease is mild or severe, just that it is present. The two measures that are most often used to quantify the morbidity rate for a particular disease in a population are incidence and prevalence (**Figure 2.15**). **Incidence** is the number of new cases of a disease in a population during a specified period of time. An **incidence rate** is calculated as the number of new cases of a disease in a population during a specified time period divided by the total number of people in the population who were at risk of the disease during that period. Incidence is usually used to quantify infectious diseases, acute diseases (diseases that occur suddenly), and outbreaks. **Prevalence** is the percentage of members of a population who have a given trait at a particular time.

Prevalence is calculated as the number of total existing cases, whether newly diagnosed or long established, divided by the total number of people in the population at the time the prevalence is measured. Prevalence is usually used to describe the frequency of chronic (long-lasting) exposures and diseases in a population, such as the percentage of adults in a country who have diabetes or asthma or smoke tobacco products.

A **case definition** is a list of the inclusion and exclusion criteria that must be met in order for an individual to be classified as having a particular disease or disability. Epidemiologists measuring incidence and prevalence must establish clear case definitions that state exactly which characteristics indicate that a person has (or does not have) conditions of interest. The International Classifications of Diseases (ICD) code is a standard system for recording diagnoses. The 11th major revision of the ICD manual (ICD-11)

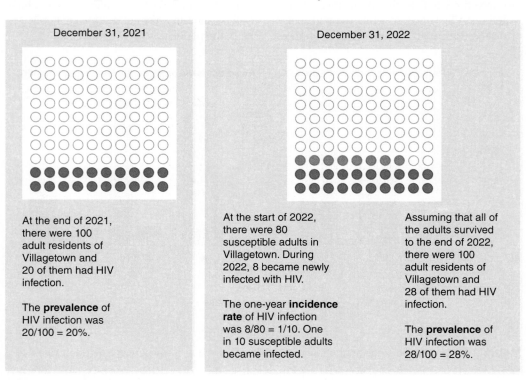

December 31, 2021

December 31, 2022

At the end of 2021, there were 100 adult residents of Villagetown and 20 of them had HIV infection.

The **prevalence** of HIV infection was 20/100 = 20%.

At the start of 2022, there were 80 susceptible adults in Villagetown. During 2022, 8 became newly infected with HIV.

The one-year **incidence rate** of HIV infection was 8/80 = 1/10. One in 10 susceptible adults became infected.

Assuming that all of the adults survived to the end of 2022, there were 100 adult residents of Villagetown and 28 of them had HIV infection.

The **prevalence** of HIV infection was 28/100 = 28%.

Figure 2.15 An example of incidence and prevalence.

was released by the World Health Organization in 2018 and continues to be updated as needed.[39] For example, several codes related to COVID-19 were added in 2020. To calculate rates of disease rather than just counts of cases, epidemiologists must also have a system in place for ascertaining the total number of people in the population being studied, especially if changes in the health status of a population are being tracked over time and the population might be growing or shrinking or aging.

The incidence of an adverse health condition may increase due to behavioral changes (like more people becoming heavy alcohol consumers), nutritional changes (such as vitamin deficiencies increasing during humanitarian crises), environmental changes (like more mosquitoes during rainy seasons accelerating the spread of malaria), and a diversity of other factors. Preventive health interventions may reduce the incidence rates. For example, vaccines may reduce the incidence of infections, smoking cessation support may reduce the incidence of noncommunicable diseases, and enforcement of traffic laws may decrease the frequency of injuries. The prevalence of an adverse health condition may increase when the incidence increases or when new therapies allow people to live with the disease for a longer duration. The prevalence of a chronic disease may decrease if the incidence goes down or a new cure becomes available.

2.9 Burden of Disease Metrics

A **metric** is a composite indicator derived from two or more other measures. A variety of complex health metrics that combine information about epidemiology, demography, and other factors are used to evaluate disease burden at the population level. **Premature mortality** is any death before a selected target survival age. **Years of life lost (YLLs)** is a burden of disease metric used to quantify population-level reductions in health status due to premature mortality. For example, if the goal is for everyone in a population to live at least 75 years, someone who dies on her 70th birthday would contribute five YLLs to the population total. If the target for survival is 80 years, someone who dies on his 60th birthday would contribute 20 YLLs to the population total. The leading causes of YLLs globally include cardiovascular diseases, cancers, injuries, maternal and neonatal disorders, and lower respiratory infections.[38]

Everyone eventually dies, so preventing all deaths is not a population health goal. Instead, the goal is for people to die in old age rather than at younger ages. YLLs are sometimes a better indicator of population health priorities than total deaths. Diseases that kill children, who would have had decades of productive life remaining if they had survived, generate more YLLs per case than diseases that primarily affect older adults. An intervention that keeps one five-year-old from dying will prevent the loss of 75 YLLs in a population that has a target survival age of 80 years, while an intervention that keeps a 75-year-old in that population alive for at least five more years will generate only five averted YLLs. One criticism of YLLs is that they assign limited value to interventions that extend life for older adults, but this weighting aligns with the action orientation of population health.

Many nonfatal conditions cause significant impairment and distress. **Years lived with disability (YLDs)** is a burden of disease metric used to quantify the population-level reductions in health status attributable to nonfatal conditions (**Figure 2.16**). In most burden of disease models, disability refers to any short- or long-term reduction in health status.[40] The total number of YLDs from a selected health problem in a population is a function of how much disability (reduction in function) the condition causes, how often the condition occurs, and how long the condition typically persists.[41] A person who spends a year in a coma would contribute about one full YLD to the population total for the year. Someone who is unable to work or go to school for one week due to a bout of influenza or a severely sprained ankle would contribute a tiny fraction of one

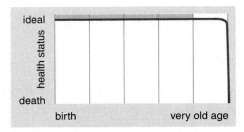 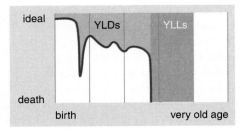

Figure 2.16 Examples of years lived with disability (YLDs) and years of life lost (YLLs) to premature mortality for different health trajectories.

YLD to the tally. The typical person contributes a small portion of one YLD to the population total each year, but those many small contributions from individuals add up to a large number of YLDs across a population. Some of the most frequent causes of YLDs worldwide are musculoskeletal disorders (such as back pain and arthritis), mental health disorders (such as depression and anxiety), sense organ disorders (such as age-related hearing and vision loss), neurological disorders (such as migraines and Alzheimer's disease), and injuries.[38]

The main criticism of YLDs is the need to assign weights to the amount of disability caused by various illnesses and impairments. It will never be possible to assign an accurate weight to the decrease in quality of life caused by blindness, loss of a limb, depression, a brain tumor, or asthma because the experience of disability varies so much based on the individual, access to healthcare services, living conditions, the level of community support, and other factors. For example, the amount of disability caused by an amputated foot would be much higher for a manual laborer in a low-income country where prosthetics are not available than it would be for an office worker in a high-income country who uses a customized prosthesis.

A **disability-adjusted life year (DALY)** is a burden of disease metric that is quantified as the sum of years of life lost (YLLs) to premature death and years lived with disability (YLDs) in a population. The DALY summarizes the total burden of disease in a population from deaths before old age and from nonfatal causes of reduced health status. The leading causes of DALYs include some of the top causes of YLLs and some of the most frequent causes of YLDs (**Figure 2.17**).[38] Economists frequently use health-adjusted life year estimates similar to the DALY as part of cost-effectiveness analyses. A **quality-adjusted life year (QALY)** is a metric used in health economics to represent the additional duration of life and quality of life conferred to populations by effective public health interventions.[42] A DALY is a bad thing to be avoided (the loss of a healthy year of life), while a QALY is a good thing to save.[43]

When looking at the burden of disease within one country, the best option may be to look at the relative percentages from various causes. When comparing the burden of disease in two or more countries, it is usually better to examine the rates of YLLs, YLDs, and DALYs per 100,000 people, especially when the countries have different demographic, socioeconomic, and health profiles. Lower-income countries tend to have higher overall rates of disability than high-income countries. For example, a resident of a low-income country may have reduced health status due to depression, malaria infection, and low vision due to cataracts, while a resident of a high-income country who has depression is unlikely to also have malaria and untreated cataracts. When the rate of DALYs from a particular condition is the same in a low-income country and a high-income country, the relative proportion of DALYs from that condition will be higher in the high-income country because the overall rate of DALYs is lower in the high-income country (**Figure 2.18**).

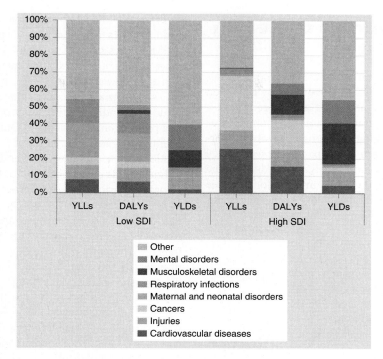

Figure 2.17 Distribution of YLLs, YLDs, and DALYs, by country sociodemographic group.

Data from GBD 2019 Diseases and Injuries Collaborators. Global burden of 369 diseases and injuries in 204 countries and territories, 1990–2019: a systematic analysis for the Global Burden of Disease Study 2019. *Lancet.* 2020;396:1204–1222.

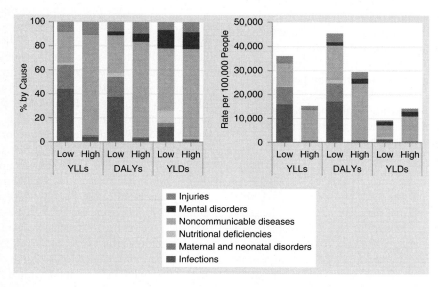

Figure 2.18 YLLs, YLDs, and DALYs by proportion and by rate per 100,000 people in the high- and low-sociodemographic groups.

Data from GBD 2019 Diseases and Injuries Collaborators. Global burden of 369 diseases and injuries in 204 countries and territories, 1990–2019: a systematic analysis for the Global Burden of Disease Study 2019. *Lancet.* 2020;396:1204–1222.

2.10 Sources of Health Information

Data are raw or unprocessed facts, figures, symbols, or signs. **Information** is generated when data are processed and presented in a format that is usable for understanding a situation and making decisions. A **health information system** encompasses the technology used to collect, store, analyze, and disseminate health-related data and information.[44] Some health information systems enable clinicians to access and share relevant information about their patients and some focus on population-level health indicators. The WHO uses the acronym SCORE to describe the major functions of a public health information system[45]:

- **S**urvey populations using tools such as population-based surveys, surveillance of public health threats, censuses, and other tools.
- **C**ount births, deaths, causes of death, and other health-related events.
- **O**ptimize health service data so that it is easy to examine the availability, quality, and effectiveness of healthcare facilities, health financing, and the health workforce.
- **R**eview progress and performance regularly in order to identify and act on opportunities to improve health sector performance.
- **E**nable data use for policy and action because providing information about population health to the public enables individuals, households, businesses, governments, and other entities to make informed decisions and plan for the future.

It can take many months or years to gather and analyze large data sets, and even the most robust data sources typically are incomplete. For example, everyone knew in 2020 that data about the true extent and impact of the coronavirus pandemic during that year would not be available until years later and that the exact number of cases of COVID-19 would never be known. Various statistical and mathematical techniques are used to overcome those logistical barriers and provide timely information for decision making. **Data science** is an interdisciplinary field that uses statistics, machine learning, and other computational tools to generate information and knowledge from various types of data.

An **estimate** is a calculation of the likely value of an indicator, metric, or other variable in a population. Data about a country's overall health status are rarely gathered from 100% of residents. Instead, surveys of random samples of households or patients are used to infer the values of various health, demographic, and socioeconomic statistics at the population level. Global health statistics are often presented as a point estimate with a confidence interval. The point estimate is the value of the number in the sample, and the confidence interval shows the likely range of numbers that might be found to be the true value in the population if everyone were sampled. The point estimate falls halfway between the lower end of the confidence interval and the upper end of the confidence interval. Larger samples generate narrower confidence intervals.

Many types of health statistics are disseminated through the websites and annual reports of major governmental and nongovernmental health organizations. The websites of the WHO, U.S. CDC, U.S. National Institutes of Health (NIH), and other health agencies provide easy-to-read and regularly updated information about hundreds of diseases. For example, the WHO's *Weekly Epidemiological Record* and the CDC's *Morbidity and Mortality Weekly Report* (*MMWR*) provide timely information about emerging health issues, such as new infectious disease outbreaks. For comparative global health statistics, the best sources are often the appendices of the annual reports of United Nations agencies. For disease-specific statistics, the reports of specialty organizations can be helpful references. For example, both the International Agency for Research on Cancer (IARC), which is part of the United Nations system, and the American Cancer Society, which is an independent nonprofit organization, report some global cancer statistics and estimates every year.

Some of the numbers that are used to describe population health status cannot be directly measured. In those situations, models can be used to estimate and visualize population health trends. A mathematical **model** is a set of equations that define relationships among many variables. For example, burden of disease metrics are generated using complex models that incorporate assumptions about the target survival age and the disability weights assigned to various conditions as well as data about demographics, morbidity and mortality, socioeconomic indicators, and other measurable variables. Models can also be used to generate projections and forecasts. A **forecast** describes the most likely estimate of future trends based on past data. A **projection** describes the future outcomes that can be anticipated if various interventions are implemented or other events occur.

Statistical and model-based estimates from different populations can be compared when they are calculated based on similar methods and assumptions. For example, the **Global Burden of Disease (GBD)** project is a massive collaborative effort to quantify the epidemiologic profiles of every country in the world. The GBD project was initiated by the WHO in the 1990s and is now housed at the Institute for Health Metrics and Evaluation (IHME) in Seattle. The GBD collaborators use models to generate regular updates of the estimated rates of disability and death by cause for every country worldwide. The outputs from the models include point estimates and confidence intervals, just like the outputs of other types of statistical analyses. The GBD collaborators also use advanced computational methods to identify the contributing risk factors for adverse health outcomes. The leading modifiable risk factors worldwide include behavioral risks such as malnutrition and tobacco use, environmental and occupational risks such as air pollution and unsafe drinking water, and metabolic risks such as unmanaged high blood pressure and high blood sugar levels (**Figure 2.19**).[46] These numbers inform the development of policy recommendations that

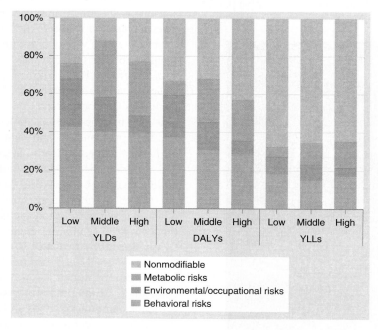

Figure 2.19 Distribution of major risk factors, by country sociodemographic group.

Data from GBD 2019 Risk Factors Collaborators. Global burden of 87 risk factors in 204 countries and territories, 1990–2019: a systematic analysis for the Global Burden of Disease Study 2019. *Lancet.* 2020;396:1223–1249.

can be acted on by governmental bodies and other public health funders and implementers.

The best sources of detailed information about the research methods used to generate estimates of population health statistics and metrics are often academic and professional journal articles. **Peer review** is the process of a scientific manuscript being evaluated by experts who scrutinize the methodology and the reasonableness of the results prior to a report being published. Formal scientific reports and journal articles undergo peer review prior to publication, which means that experts have evaluated the validity of the methods and results. An **abstract** is a one-paragraph summary of the objectives, methods, results, and implications of a scientific investigation. Abstract databases like MEDLINE can be used to search for abstracts summarizing journal articles on selected topics. The full reports can then be found online or in a library. These high-quality resources, along with books and other reports published by trusted organizations, provide an evidence-based foundation for those who seek to create, implement, evaluate, and improve global public health policies and practices.

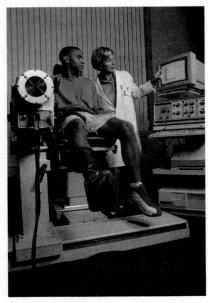

2.11 Country Income Level and Health

Many analyses of global health and health transitions compare population health status in countries with different income levels. The term **low- and middle-income countries (LMICs)** encompasses all low-income, lower-middle-income, and upper-middle-income countries. Health status in LMICs is often compared with health status in high-income countries (HICs) (**Figure 2.20**). Some global health reports compare LMICs to countries that are members of the **OECD (Organisation for Economic Co-operation and Development)**, an intergovernmental organization that represents about three dozen of the world's richest countries.

The threshold for what constitutes low-income or middle-income status can be defined based on a variety of indicators and metrics. For example, **gross national income (GNI)** is the total income from the selling of goods and services produced in one country, including consumer spending, government spending, investments, and exports. The GNI per capita correlates with a variety of health metrics. For example, higher GNI per capita is associated with lower child mortality rates and higher life expectancies (**Figure 2.21**).[47] The World Bank uses GNI per person to divide countries into four income-level categories: low, lower middle, upper middle, and high. Nearly 75% of the world's people live in a country classified as middle income (lower middle or upper middle income) by the World Bank.[36]

Health economists also use a variety of other macroeconomic indicators to measure the amount of economic activity in a country. **Gross domestic product (GDP)** is the total amount of goods and services produced in one country by domestic- and foreign-owned companies. **Gross national product (GNP)** is the total amount of goods and services produced by one country's companies in that country and by companies owned by that

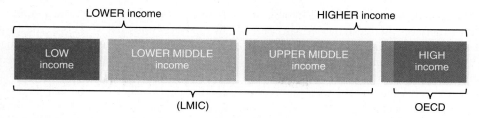

Figure 2.20 Income-level terminology.

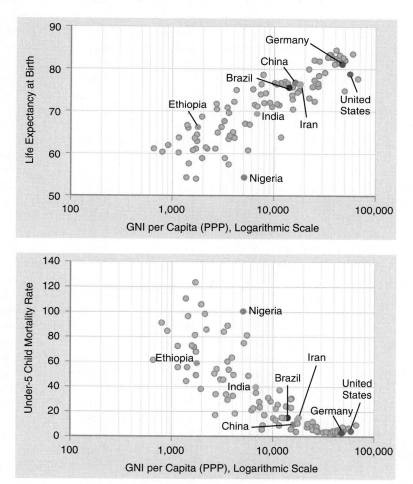

Figure 2.21 Gross national income (GNI) per capita (PPP) versus mortality rate per 100,000 children less than five years old and life expectancy at birth.

Data from World Development Indicators. World Bank. Accessed 2020. https://data.worldbank.org/

country's companies but operating in other countries. That means that Germany's GNI is the total income from the selling of goods and

services produced in Germany, its GDP is the total amount of goods and services produced in Germany by both German and foreign companies, and its GNP is the total amount of goods and services produced by German companies in Germany and by German companies operating in other countries. All three of these metrics can be recorded in per capita (per person) terms by dividing the total monetary value by the population of the country.

It is impossible to accurately measure all economic transactions in a country, so macroeconomic metrics are estimated using the best available data. There are a variety of methods that can be used for the estimation process. The World Bank often uses the Atlas method to estimate the GNI. The **Atlas method** is an estimation method that improves economic comparisons by reducing the impact of market and exchange rate fluctuations on metrics. The Atlas method calculates the GNI by adding together the value of product sales and taxes, minus subsidies, within the country plus salaries and property income from abroad, and then adjusting the total to account for inflation.

Because the amount of goods and services that can be purchased with a given amount of money varies from place to place—for example, it costs fewer U.S. dollars to rent an apartment in Lagos, Nigeria, than to rent an apartment in New York City—it can be helpful for economic indicators to account for cost of living differences. An alternative way of estimating GNI uses **purchasing power parity (PPP)**, an estimation method that improves economic comparisons by adjusting metrics based on how many goods, services, and other products can be purchased in various populations with a fixed amount of money, such as $1,000 U.S. dollars. A clever example of PPP is the "Big Mac Index," which uses the relative price of a McDonald's hamburger in different countries to determine the relative value of other items.[48] If a Big Mac costs $6 in one country and $3 in another, it is likely that the cost of living is about twice as high in the $6-per-hamburger country. Workers in the higher-priced country will have to

earn a much higher salary to stay above the local poverty line than workers in the $3-per-burger country. The PPP GNI is usually higher than the Atlas GNI, especially in lower-income countries (**Figure 2.22**).[49]

Summary values like the GNI have some major limitations as indicators of economic development. They do not count unpaid labor like caring for children and growing food to feed a family, and they ignore important societal issues such as environmental sustainability and wealth inequality. These values show the economic experience of the "average" person living in each country, but the economic mean may be misleading if most people in a country are very poor, a few are extremely rich, and there is almost no middle class. Even when a large proportion of the population experiences something near the average reported for the country, there will still be variability in the experiences of individuals. There are millionaires in every country, even the countries with the poorest per capita economic metrics, and there are people in every country, even the wealthiest ones, who live on almost no income.

Some socioeconomic metrics combine monetary variables with social and health indicators. The **Human Development Index (HDI)** is an estimate of national development calculated from data on income (GNI per capita in purchasing power parity dollars), education (the mean and expected years of schooling), and life expectancy at birth.[47] The United Nations Development Programme (UNDP) uses the HDI to divide countries into four groups: low, medium, high, and very high. Researchers at IHME have developed a **Sociodemographic Index (SDI)** that is calculated from data on income per capita, the average number of years of education, and fertility rates.[50] Both the HDI and SDI are calculated using income per person and statistics about education, but for the SDI the third component is fertility rather than life expectancy. GBD

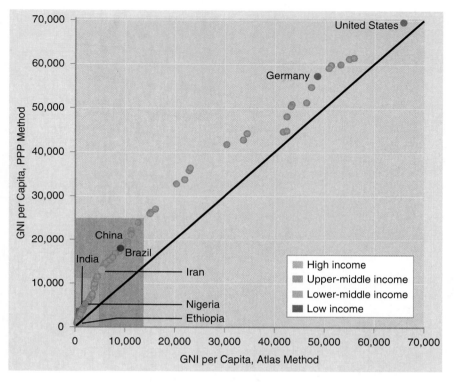

Figure 2.22 Gross national income (GNI) per capita: Atlas method versus purchasing power parity (PPP).

Data from World Development Indicators. World Bank. Accessed 2020. https://data.worldbank.org/

analyses often compare health metrics in five SDI quintiles: low, low-middle, middle, high-middle, and high. The HDI has increased in most countries over the past 25 years as incomes, levels of school enrollment, and life expectancies have risen, but there are still significant gaps between the richest countries and the poorest countries (**Figure 2.23**).[47] Similar trends are observed for the SDI.[37] A variety of more complex indices, such the Social Progress Index[51] and the summary values in the *World Happiness Report*,[52] add additional variables about basic human needs, health, and freedom to their calculations.

The HDI and SDI do not adjust for within-country inequalities. The **Gini coefficient** is a measure of the inequality in the

distribution of incomes within a particular country. A country in which everyone has exactly the same income would have a Gini coefficient of 0 (perfect equality). A country in which one person has all the income and everyone else has zero income would have a Gini coefficient of 100 (perfect inequality). The general trend is that countries with higher development levels have lower Gini coefficients, indicating greater equality (**Figure 2.24**).[47] However, there is a lot of variability in Gini coefficients. For example, the United States has high inequality for a country classified as having very high human development. When two countries have similar economic profiles, the country with greater income inequality tends to have a less favorable health profile.[53]

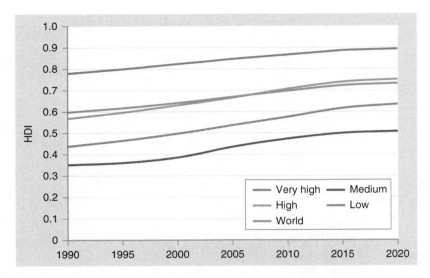

Figure 2.23 Human Development Index (HDI) over time.

Data from *Human Development Report 2020: The Next Frontier.* New York: United Nations Development Programme; 2020.

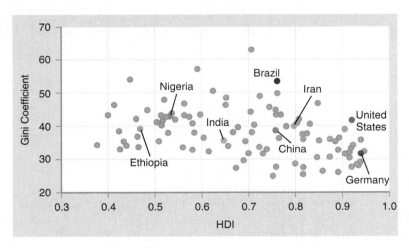

Figure 2.24 HDI versus Gini coefficient.

Data from *Human Development Report 2020: The Next Frontier.* New York: United Nations Development Programme; 2020.

2.12 Featured Countries

Throughout this book, data from eight large countries will be used to represent the diversity of the world's health profiles (**Figure 2.25**). These eight countries include the three with the largest populations—China and India, which each have more than 1.3 billion residents, and the United States, which has more than 330 million inhabitants—as well as five other countries that are among the 19 countries that are each home to more than 80 million people (and are therefore each home to more than 1% of the global population).[49]

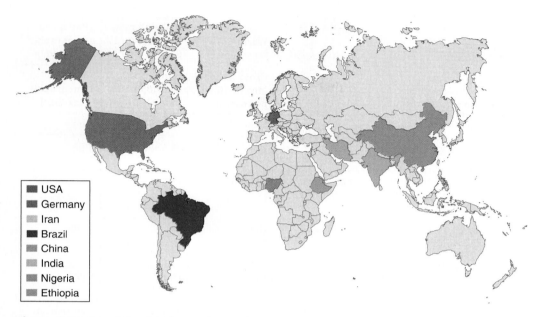

Figure 2.25 Map of the eight featured countries.

Together, these eight countries are home to about half of the world's people (**Figure 2.26**).

The featured countries represent geographic diversity (**Figure 2.27**), including all seven World Bank regions and all six WHO regions. The featured countries also represent a diversity of economic profiles, with six of the eight featured countries being LMICs and two OECD-member HICs. The World Bank classifies one of the eight countries as low income, two as lower-middle income, three as upper-middle income, and two as high income. The eight countries also represent all four UNDP classifications. The UNDP levels generally align with the World Bank groupings, but one of the featured lower-middle-income countries (Nigeria) is classified as having a low rather than a medium human development level. The eight countries also span all five of the SDI groups used by IHME.

There is often considerable diversity in the socioeconomic and health profiles of countries within the same world region. There is also considerable diversity among different states

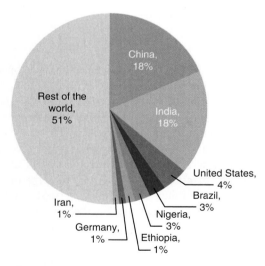

Figure 2.26 The eight featured countries represent nearly half of the world's population.

Data from United Nations Department of Economic and Social Affairs. *World Population Prospects: The 2019 Revision.* New York: United Nations; 2019.

or provinces within countries and between urban and rural areas. These types of within-country differences can be observed in all eight

Country	World Bank Region	WHO Region	World Bank Income Group	UNDP Human Development Level	IHME Socio-demographic Index Group
Basis for classification	Geography	Geography	Gross national income (GNI) per capita	Human Development Index (HDI)	Socio-demographic Index (SDI)
United States	North America	Americas	High	Very high	High
Germany	Europe and Central Asia	Europe	High	Very high	High
Iran	Middle East and North Africa	Eastern Mediterranean	Upper middle	High	High-middle
Brazil	Latin America and the Caribbean	Americas	Upper middle	High	Middle
China	East Asia and Pacific	Western Pacific	Upper middle	High	Middle
India	South Asia	Southeast Asia	Lower middle	Medium	Low-middle
Nigeria	Sub-Saharan Africa	Africa	Lower middle	Low	Low-middle
Ethiopia	Sub-Saharan Africa	Africa	Low	Low	Low

Figure 2.27 Eight featured countries by geographic location and income group.

of the featured countries. For example, parts of southern Nigeria have a middle-income or upper-middle-income economic profile, while some of the northern areas of Nigeria have a very low-income profile and are at risk of famine.[54] National statistical reports present the average values for various metrics, and those averages do not express the wide range of values that may be present within diverse regions of the country. Despite that limitation, general patterns can be observed by comparing statistics from large countries. This can be valuable for understanding past health transitions, current trends in population health status, and projections of future population health profiles.

References

1. McMichael AJ. Globalization, climate change, and human health. *N Engl J Med*. 2013;368:1335–1343.
2. Morens DM, Folkers GK, Fauci AS. Emerging infections: a perpetual challenge. *Lancet Infect Dis*. 2008;8:710–719.
3. Osland JS. Broadening the debate: the pros and cons of globalization. *J Manage Inquiry*. 2003;12:137–154.
4. Labonté R. Reprising the globalization dimensions of international health. *Global Health*. 2018;14:49.

5. Huynen MMTE, Martens P, Hilderink HBM. The health impacts of globalisation: a conceptual framework. *Global Health.* 2005;1:14.

6. *Response, Recovery and Resilience: The Power of U.S. Investments in Global Health.* Washington DC: Global Health Council; 2021.

7. *Human Development Report 1994: New Dimensions of Human Security.* New York: United Nations Development Programme; 1994.

8. Commission on Human Security. *Human Security Now: Protecting and Empowering People.* New York: United Nations; 2003.

9. Oslo Ministerial Declaration: global health: a pressing foreign policy issue of our time. *Lancet.* 2007;369:1373–1378.

10. National Academies of Sciences, Engineering, and Medicine; Health and Medicine Division; Committee on Global Health and the Future of the United States. *Global Health and the Future Role of the United States.* Washington DC: National Academies Press; 2017.

11. *The Case for U.S. Investment in the Global Fund and Global Health.* Washington DC: Friends of the Global Fight against AIDS, Tuberculosis and Malaria; 2017.

12. Aldis W. Health security as a public health concept: a critical analysis. *Health Policy Plan.* 2008;23:369–375.

13. Hoffman SJ. The evolution, etiology and eventualities of the global health security regime. *Health Policy Plan.* 2010;25:510–522.

14. Lakoff A. Two regimes of global health. *Humanity.* 2010;1:59–79.

15. Fitzmaurice AG, Mahar M, Moriarty LF, et al. Contributions of the US Centers for Disease Control and Prevention in implementing the Global Health Security Agenda in 17 partner countries. *Emerg Infect Dis.* 2017;23:S15–S24.

16. Yazbeck AS. *An Idiot's Guide to Prioritization in the Health Sector.* Washington DC: World Bank; 2002.

17. *Thirteenth General Programme of Work 2019–2023.* Geneva: World Health Organization; 2018.

18. *Ten Threats to Global Health in 2019.* Geneva: World Health Organization; 2019.

19. Glassman A, Chalkidou K, eds. *Priority-Setting in Health: Building Institutions for Smarter Public Spending.* Washington DC: Center for Global Development; 2012.

20. *The Case for Investing in Public Health: A Public Health Summary Report for EPHO 8.* Copenhagen: World Health Organization, Regional Office for Europe; 2014.

21. Horton S, Gelband H, Jamison D, Levin C, Nugent R, Watkins D. Ranking 93 health interventions for low- and middle-income countries by cost-effectiveness. *PLoS One.* 2017;12:e182951.

22. Mock C, Donkor P, Gawande A, Jamison D, Kruk M, Debas H. Essential surgery: key messages of this volume (chapter 1). In: Debas HT, Donkor P, Gawande A, Jamison DT, Kruk ME, Mock CN, eds. *Essential Surgery.* Vol 1. 3rd ed. Washington DC: IBRD/World Bank; 2015; 1–18.

23. Varmus H, Klausner R, Zerhouni E, Acharya T, Daar AS, Singer PA. Grand challenge in global health. *Science.* 2003;302:398–399.

24. *Convention on the Rights of the Child.* New York: United Nations; 1989.

25. Koplan JP, Fleming DW. Current and future public health challenges. *JAMA.* 2000;284:1696–1698.

26. Harris D, Moore M, Schmitz H. *Country Classifications for a Changing World.* Brighton, UK: Institute of Development Studies at the University of Sussex; 2009.

27. Hulme D. *The Making of the Millennium Development Goals: Human Development Meets Results-Based Management.* Manchester UK: Institute for Development Policy and Management, University of Manchester; 2007.

28. *The Millennium Development Goals Report 2015.* New York: United Nations; 2015.

29. *Health in 2015: From MDGs, Millennium Development Goals to SDGs, Sustainable Development Goals.* Geneva: World Health Organization; 2015.

30. Waage J, Banerji R, Campbell O, et al. The Millennium Development Goals: a cross-sectoral analysis and principles for goal setting after 2015. *Lancet.* 2010;376:991–1023.

31. *Transforming Our World: The 2030 Agenda for Sustainable Development.* New York: United Nations; 2015.

32. *Tier Classification for Global SDG Indicators.* New York: Inter-agency Expert Group on SDG Indicators; 2017.

33. Dietler D, Leuenberger A, Bempong NE, et al. Health in the 2030 Agenda for Sustainable Development: from framework to action, transforming challenges into opportunities. *J Global Health.* 2019;9:020201.

34. United Nations Economic and Social Council. *Report of the Inter-Agency and Expert Group on Sustainable Development Goal Indicators (E/CN.3/2021/2).* New York: United Nations; 2021.

35. Murray CJ, Frenk J. Health metrics and evaluation: strengthening the science. *Lancet.* 2008;371:1191–1199.

36. United Nations Department of Economic and Social Affairs. *World Population Prospects: The 2019 Revision.* New York: United Nations; 2019.

37. GBD 2019 Demographics Collaborators. Global age-sex-specific fertility, mortality, healthy life expectancy (HALE), and population estimates in 204 countries and territories, 1950–2019: a comprehensive demographic analysis for the Global Burden of Disease Study 2019. *Lancet.* 2020;396:1160–1203.

38. GBD 2019 Diseases and Injuries Collaborators. Global burden of 369 diseases and injuries in 204 countries and territories, 1990–2019: a systematic analysis for the Global Burden of Disease Study 2019. *Lancet.* 2020;396:1204–1222.

39. *International Statistical Classification of Diseases and Related Health Problems.* 11th ed. Geneva: World Health Organization; 2020.

40. Chen A, Jacobsen KH, Deshmukh AA, Cantor SB. The evolution of the disability-adjusted life year (DALY). *Socioecon Plann Sci.* 2015;49:10–15.

41. Prüss-Üstün A, Mathers C, Corvalán C, Woodward A. *Assessing the Environmental Burden of Disease at National and Local Levels: Introduction and Methods.* Geneva: World Health Organization; 2003.

42. Gold MR, Stevenson D, Fryback DG. HALYs and QALYs and DALYs, oh my: similarities and differences in summary measures of population health. *Annu Rev Public Health.* 2002;23:115–134.

43. Sassi F. Calculating QALYs, comparing QALY and DALY calculations. *Health Policy Plan.* 2006; 21:402–408.

44. AbouZahr C, Boerma T. Health information systems: the foundations of public health. *Bull World Health Organ.* 2005;83:578–583.

45. *SCORE for Health Data Technical Package: Global Report on Health Data Systems and Capacity, 2020.* Geneva: World Health Organization; 2021.

46. GBD 2019 Risk Factors Collaborators. Global burden of 87 risk factors in 204 countries and territories, 1990–2019: a systematic analysis for the Global Burden of Disease Study 2019. *Lancet.* 2020;396:1223–1249.

47. *Human Development Report 2020: The Next Frontier.* New York: United Nations Development Programme; 2020.

48. Ong LL. Burgernomics: the economics of the Big Mac standard. *J Int Money Finance.* 1997;16:865–878.

49. World Development Indicators. World Bank. Accessed 2020. https://data.worldbank.org/

50. GBD 2015 SDG Collaborators. Measuring the health-related Sustainable Development Goals in 188 countries: a baseline analysis from the Global Burden of Disease Study 2015. *Lancet.* 2016;388:1813–1850.

51. *2020 Social Progress Index.* Washington DC: Social Progress Imperative; 2020.

52. Helliwell JF, Layard R, Sachs JD, De Neve JE, eds. *World Happiness Report 2021.* New York: Sustainable Development Solutions Network; 2021.

53. Wilkinson RG, Pickett KE. Income inequality and population health: a review and explanation of the evidence. *Soc Sci Med.* 2006;62:1768–1784.

54. *National Human Development Report 2015: Human Security and Human Development in Nigeria.* Abuja: United Nations Development Programme; 2015.

CHAPTER 3

Socioeconomic Determinants of Health

Populations are healthiest when the ability of their members to be healthy is not inhibited by income level, educational level, gender, employment, race, ethnicity, immigration status, or other socioeconomic and political factors. The goal of health equity is to reduce the health disparities between low- and high-income populations while improving health status in all population groups.

3.1 Health Equity and the Sustainable Development Goals

Socioeconomic status (SES), also called socioeconomic position (SEP), describes an individual's standing in a society based on individual and household income, education, gender, occupation, ethnicity and race, and other characteristics that exist within broader cultural, social, political, and policy environments.[1] There is no one measure of SES, but proxies such as ownership of various assets (like a car, television, or livestock), amount of education, type of job, residential area, and other characteristics can be used to evaluate a person's relative position in a community or a larger population group. At the individual level, there is a lot of variability in health status. Many low-income individuals are quite healthy, and some high-income people suffer from serious illnesses even at a young age. At the population level, however, there is clear evidence that lower SES populations have significantly lower health status than wealthier socioeconomic groups.[2]

The less favorable health status of populations with lower SES is largely a function of economic, social, and political environments, and it is not caused by innate biological differences.[3] The personal factors and community conditions that enable or hinder access to health are collectively called the **social determinants of health**,[4] and they can be summarized using the acronym PROGRESS: **p**lace of residence, **r**ace and ethnicity, **o**ccupation and employment status, **g**ender and sex, **r**eligion, **e**ducation, **s**ocial capital, and other **s**ocioeconomic indicators (**Figure 3.1**).[5] Interventions that alleviate the socioeconomic circumstances that limit an individual's ability to access healthcare services and other tools for health can yield significant benefits for physical and mental health. Progress toward achieving the socioeconomic Sustainable Development

P	Place of residence (rural or urban; state/province; housing characteristics)
R	Race, ethnicity, culture, and language
O	Occupation and employment status
G	Gender and sex
R	Religion
E	Education
S	Socioeconomic position (income, wealth, and other measures)
S	Social capital (neighborhood, community, and family support and other aspects of social relationships and networks)
Plus	Age, disability, sexual orientation, involvement in the criminal justice system, and other characteristics

Figure 3.1 The PROGRESS-Plus framework for the social determinants of health.

Data from Kavanagh J, Oliver S, Lorenc T. Reflections on developing and using PROGRESS-Plus. *Equity Update.* 2008;2:1–3.

Goals (SDGs) of ending poverty (SDG 1), ensuring quality education for all (SDG 4), achieving gender equality (SDG 5), promoting employment and decent work for all (SDG 8), reducing inequalities within and among countries (SDG 10), and promoting peaceful societies and good governance (SDG 16) will improve the health of many millions of people.

Health equity is the principle that everyone should have an equal opportunity to be as healthy as possible.[6] Health equity is closely tied with **social justice**, the principle that moving toward greater equality in the distribution of income and wealth, opportunities for education and employment, access to health and security, and involvement in civic and political activities is valuable for human flourishing.[7] A health **inequality** (or health disparity) is a remediable difference in health status or access to health services between population groups. When an inequality is considered to be unfair and unjust, the difference is classified as an **inequity**.[8] Health equity advocates champion efforts to raise the health status of every subgroup within every population, and they call for disadvantaged populations to receive additional resources because health equity cannot be realized without the elimination of health disparities.[9]

Gaps in health status can be observed when comparing lower- and higher-SES populations within one country or comparing lower-income and higher-income countries. While high-income countries have undergone a series of health transitions that improved their health and longevity, low-income countries are still in the early stages of many health transitions. Globalization has exacerbated some health disparities within and between countries, but it has also created opportunities to close those gaps by improving the health status of disadvantaged populations even as the healthiest populations continue to make progress on extending the years of healthy life that their residents enjoy. When the health status of low-SES populations within one country improves, those health equity gains raise the health status of the whole country. Similarly, when the health status of lower-income countries improves, those health equity gains yield benefits for overall world health.

3.2 Economics

The economic status of a household is a function of both income and wealth. **Income** is the amount of take-home pay earned by household members in a week, year, or other time period. **Wealth** is the accumulated worth of a household's resources. Wealth can include a house, a car, a bicycle, livestock, a television, a radio, and other consumer goods. When someone in a high-income or wealthy household has a health concern, that person usually has the resources to immediately access high-quality medical care, including accurate diagnostic tests and effective therapies. Attending to health issues early can often prevent mild concerns from becoming severe problems. By contrast, low-income households generally have very little wealth, so they have few resources to draw on when someone in the household is injured or develops a severe illness.

People living in low-resource households may not be able to afford care for health problems that are not immediately life threatening or disabling. The direct costs of medical care add up quickly when they include transportation to a healthcare facility, fees for clinical consultations, and payment for medications and supplies like bandages, which often are not provided by healthcare facilities and must be purchased by the patient. There are also indirect costs associated with lost wages for patients and caregivers, especially when outpatients must sit in a waiting area for a full day before seeing a clinician and when families of hospitalized patients must provide all food and most personal care for inpatients. The facilities where poor people can access health services are often underfunded, understaffed, and understocked, and they rarely have the clinical specialists, support staff, and equipment necessary to be able to offer advanced care.[10] Disparities in access to health services contribute to significant gaps in health status between the average person from a high-income or wealthy household and the average person living in a low-income household.

Extreme poverty is defined as surviving on less income than an international poverty line, typically set at an income of less than $1 or $2 per person per day. Many of the world's poorest people live in remote rural areas, where they try to grow enough as subsistence farmers

with a small plot of land to feed all household members. Others are the urban poor, who often live in unplanned settlements that have no trash removal, running water, electricity, or other utilities. The percentage of the world's people living in extreme poverty decreased from approximately 35% in 1990 to 10% in 2015 (**Figure 3.2**).[11] This reduction in extreme poverty during the Millennium Development Goals (MDGs) era was so significant that the number of people living in extreme poverty dropped even as the world's population increased by nearly 2 billion people over those 25 years.[12] However, 750 million people were still living in extreme poverty at the end of 2015.

Relative poverty occurs when people are living on less than the nationally defined poverty line in their own countries. People living in relative poverty may have limited opportunities for education, employment, and engagement in social and political processes, and low-income communities are often especially vulnerable to environmental hazards such as extreme weather events.[13] These aspects of poverty are associated with an increased risk of disease, disability, and early death. In countries without universal health coverage, a single medical crisis can push a vulnerable household into poverty.[14] The cycle of illness and poverty can be difficult to overcome.

Poverty is about more than just income and consumption.[15] Economic factors are intertwined with a variety of sociocultural, political, and environmental conditions that enable some

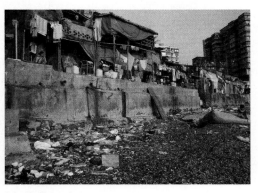

© Sam DCruz/Shutterstock

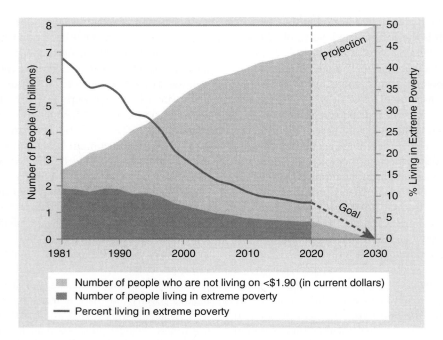

Figure 3.2 The percentage of the world's population living in poverty has decreased significantly.

Data from World Development Indicators. World Bank. Accessed 2020. https://data.worldbank.org/

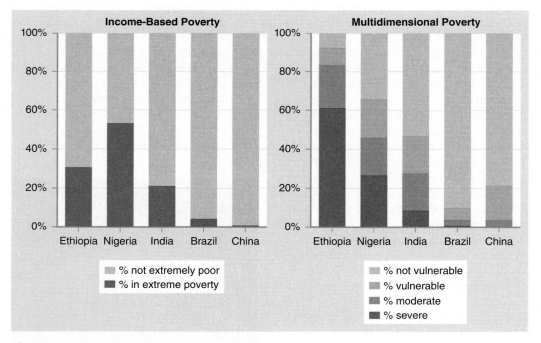

Figure 3.3 Income-based versus multidimensional poverty.

Data from *Global Multidimensional Poverty Index 2020: Charting Pathways Out of Multidimensional Poverty: Achieving the SDGs.* New York: United Nations Development Programme; 2020.

people to thrive and leave others to struggle. The United Nations Development Programme (UNDP) uses a Multidimensional Poverty Index (MPI) to capture the various dimensions of poverty, including hunger; limited formal education; lack of access to electricity, drinking water, and toilets; use of substandard materials to construct residences; and other indicators of reduced standards of living. When the MPI is used as a measure of poverty rather than income alone, a large proportion of people living in lower-income countries are classified as living in poverty (**Figure 3.3**).[16] Like other economic measures, the MPI varies significantly between countries and within national borders. For example, rates of poverty and severe poverty in Nigeria are higher in rural areas than in cities and much higher in the north than in the south.[17] Regions with more poverty have less favorable health metrics.

Just as the health status of individuals and households is related to their income, wealth, and overall SES, the health status of communities and nations is linked to their economic and development status. Investments in public health stimulate economic growth, and economic growth facilitates improvements in population health status.[18] SDG 1 sets an ambitious goal of "ending poverty in all its forms everywhere" by 2030.[19] The specific targets for ending poverty include eradicating extreme poverty, defined as living on less than $1.25 per day (SDG 1.1); reducing by half the proportion of people living in relative poverty according to national definitions (SDG 1.2); and implementing social protections for vulnerable populations, such as children, older adults, and people with disabilities (SDG 1.3).[20] Even though SDG 1 will not be achieved by 2030, global efforts to eradicate poverty will enable many millions more people to live healthier lives over the coming decade.

3.3 Education

Literacy is the ability to read and write and apply those communication skills. Literacy exists along a spectrum from minimal recognition of written words to the advanced fluency gained through higher education. **Functional literacy** is the ability to understand written words well enough to complete routine daily tasks.[21] Functional literacy allows readers to learn about food preparation and exercise programs in newspapers and magazines, comprehend health and safety warnings on consumer products, access air and water quality reports, read posters advertising immunization and screening campaigns, follow directions on medicine containers and hospital discharge orders, understand the health benefits packages offered by employers and the government, apply for aid and benefits, read brochures about their health conditions, use signs to navigate hospitals, and seek out additional information online or at libraries.

Health literacy is the ability to access, understand, and apply health information.[22] People who cannot read or have low literacy levels will have difficulty accessing health services and completing other health-related activities. They may delay seeking care for a health problem because they worry about being unable to complete paperwork at a doctor's office or being ridiculed for not knowing how to read or write. They may have difficulty taking their prescribed medications properly if their healthcare providers have not fully explained dosage and timing and they do not understand the instructions

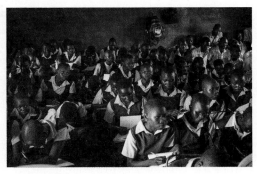

© Punghi/Shutterstock

on the label. They may not understand the safety information provided by a pharmacist or know when to return for a follow-up examination.

Both the ability to read and a higher number of years of formal education are correlated with higher health status for adults and their children.[23] For example, women with more formal schooling are more likely to give birth at a healthcare facility, which means that both mothers and newborns have an improved likelihood of survival if there are complications during or after delivery.[24] The children of women with more education are also more likely to receive preventive medical services, such as vaccines, and to receive skilled clinical care for illnesses. Because women who have several years of formal education are equipped to access the information they need to keep their children healthy and nourished,

their children are more likely to survive past their fifth birthdays.

Improved access to education in recent decades has enabled most boys and girls to learn how to read, including children who live in countries where the literacy rate is low among older adults (**Figure 3.4**).[25] However, there are still gaps in educational access. Most high- and upper-middle-income countries have strong school enrollment from early childhood education through secondary school and beyond, but in low-income countries many children and adolescents are not attending school (**Figure 3.5**).[26] Since many schools in lower-income countries have school health programs that provide hygiene and health education, nutritional support, treatment for intestinal worm infections, and other health services, children who are not in school miss critical

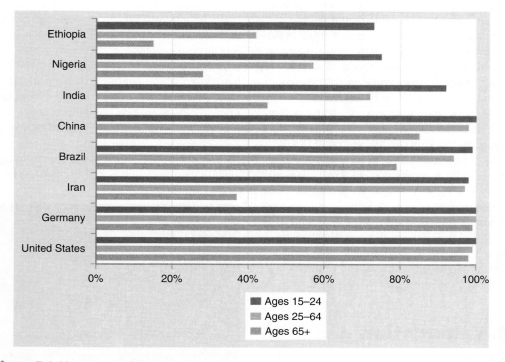

Figure 3.4 Literacy rates by age group.
Data from UNESCO Institute for Statistics database. UNESCO. Accessed 2020. http://data.uis.unesco.org/

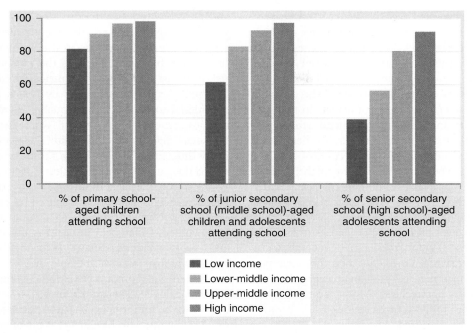

Figure 3.5 School enrollment by grade and country income level.

Data from *Global Education Monitoring Report Summary 2020: Inclusion and Education: All Means All.* Paris: UNESCO; 2020.

opportunities for both learning and healthy development.[27]

SDG 4 aims to "ensure inclusive and equitable quality education and promote lifelong learning opportunities for all," starting with access to early childhood education (SDG 4.2) and continuing with access for all girls and boys to primary and secondary education (SDG 4.1) and then to technical, vocational, or university education (SDG 4.3).[19] Increasing the proportion of children worldwide who complete at least a basic education (typically about seven years of primary school) and reaching the target that "all youth and a substantial proportion of adults, both men and women, achieve both literacy and numeracy" by 2030 (SDG 4.6)[19] will generate significant long-term benefits for the economic status and quality of life of those individuals and their communities. Those socioeconomic improvements will also yield major benefits for the health and well-being of current populations and future generations.

3.4 Gender

Sex refers to the biological classification of people as male or female based on genetics (such as the presence of XY or XX sex chromosomes) and reproductive anatomy. Males and females also have different body chemistry, hormones, physiology, and brain function. These differences mean that males and females sometimes have different symptoms for the same disease and different prognoses and pathways to recovery. For example, males are more likely to have dramatic heart attacks with crushing chest pain, while females often have subtle symptoms like feeling more tired than usual.[28] This difference is a key reason why heart disease in women has traditionally been underdiagnosed.

Gender refers to social, cultural, and psychological aspects of expressing maleness or femaleness. **Gender roles** describe how a cultural group expects men and women to behave based on their genders. For example, women may be expected to cook, clean, and take care of children, but not to work with heavy machinery or serve as religious leaders. Some cultures enforce strict rules about what women can wear in public and whether they can be in public spaces unaccompanied by a male. This can limit the ability of women to participate in the marketplace and government, attend school and religious meetings, and acquire medical attention and information. Some cultures consider women to be under the authority of their fathers or other male relatives until marriage and under the authority of their husbands after marriage. In these places, laws may restrict women's ability to own property and manage their own finances. Gender roles also define the social and behavioral norms for men. For example, young men may feel pressure to engage in risky behaviors like reckless driving, excessive alcohol consumption, or hazardous work in order to demonstrate their masculinity.[29]

Men and boys encounter different health challenges than women and girls because of both biological characteristics related to sex and social structures related to gender (**Figure 3.6**).[30] These differences in health status must be considered when planning for

and implementing health education and preventive, diagnostic, and therapeutic health services.[31] Some differences in the burden of disease are biological, such as the increased risk of breast cancer among females. The differential rate of breast cancer by sex is not considered to be a health inequality because it is a function of biology and is not due to the social determinants of health.[32] However, many differences in population health by sex and gender arise from sociocultural factors.[33] For example, the rates of adverse health outcomes related to alcohol use, tobacco use, and occupational hazards are higher among men than women. Differences in health status that are due to gender-associated behaviors and risks are remediable health disparities.[34]

When the Human Development Index (HDI) is calculated separately by sex, females often lag behind males because they earn smaller incomes and have fewer years of education (**Figure 3.7**).[35] SDG 5 aims to "achieve gender equality and empower all women and girls." The targets include eliminating "all forms of violence against all women and girls in the public and private spheres, including trafficking and sexual and other types of

MALES have a higher proportion of DALYs than females from...	FEMALES have a higher proportion of DALYs than males from...
■ Cancers of the lung, liver, stomach, and esophagus ■ Chronic respiratory diseases, such as chronic obstructive pulmonary disease and pneumoconiosis ■ Alcohol and drug use disorders ■ Cirrhosis and other chronic liver diseases ■ Autism spectrum disorders ■ Tuberculosis ■ Hernias ■ Unintentional injuries, such as road traffic injuries and drowning ■ Physical violence	■ Cancers of the breast and thyroid ■ Musculoskeletal disorders, including osteoarthritis, rheumatoid arthritis, and low back pain ■ Depression ■ Anxiety disorders ■ Headache disorders, such as migraines ■ Nutritional deficiencies, such as iron-deficiency anemia ■ Gallbladder and biliary (bile duct) disease ■ Dermatitis ■ Sexual violence

Figure 3.6 Examples of differences in the age-standardized disability-adjusted life years (DALYs) attributed to various health conditions by sex.

Data from GBD 2019 Diseases and Injuries Collaborators. Global burden of 369 diseases and injuries in 204 countries and territories, 1990–2019: a systematic analysis for the Global Burden of Disease Study 2019. *Lancet.* 2020;396:1204–1222.

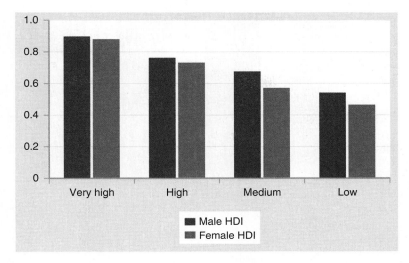

Figure 3.7 Human Development Index (HDI) values for males and females by country human development index level.

Data from *Human Development Report 2020: The Next Frontier: Human Development and the Anthropocene.* New York: United Nations Development Programme; 2020.

exploitation" (SDG 5.2) and ending harmful practices "such as child, early, and forced marriage and female genital mutilation" (SGD 5.3).[19] The language of SDG 5 focuses on women's empowerment, but the goal of health equity requires identifying and reducing the numerous preventable health issues that disproportionately affect women and girls and, at the same time, taking action to reduce the burden from avoidable health conditions that disproportionately burden men and boys. Ideally, integrating gender-equity perspectives into new health policies, strategies, and plans will reduce within-country health disparities and improve overall population health status.[36]

3.5 Employment

Three of the key components that contribute to the SES of an individual or household—economic security, educational level, and employment and occupational category—are inextricably linked to each other and to health status (**Figure 3.8**). An intervention aimed at one of these three categories may positively

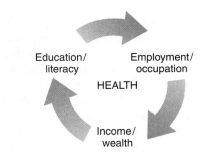

Figure 3.8 Employment, economics, and education are interrelated.

impact the others. For example, new reading skills may lead to a better job, increased job skills may lead to a higher hourly wage, and extra income may be used to pay for additional training. An improvement in any one of these dimensions of SES can lead to increased health.

Employment of at least one wage earner per household is generally critical for keeping a household out of poverty. In low-income countries, the agricultural sector—farming, fishing, and forestry—is the dominant area of employment (**Figure 3.9**).[37] Many subsistence farmers

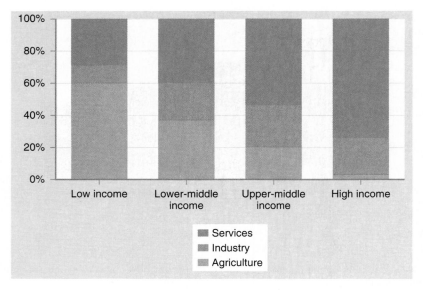

Figure 3.9 Employment by sector and country income level.

Data from *World Employment and Social Outlook: Trends 2020*. Geneva: International Labour Organization; 2020.

are part of the informal workforce rather than drawing a salary and benefits, but their work still enables them to house and feed their families. In middle-income countries, the industrial sector is growing, and jobs in manufacturing, construction, and related areas account for an increasing share of the workforce. In high-income countries, most jobs are in the service sector, with many people working in areas such as retail trade. In addition to the monetary income from working, formal employment may provide healthcare coverage, disability insurance, transportation subsidies, free food during working hours, housing allowances, assistance with school fees for employees and their children, and additional benefits. The financial and other benefits of formal employment can have a significant, positive impact on the health of workers and their families.

However, not all jobs are equally beneficial for health. People working as manual laborers have higher all-cause mortality rates, cardiovascular mortality rates, and cancer mortality rates than people the same age who are working in nonmanual professional jobs.[38] Men and women who work in manual jobs also report

lower self-rated health than same-age peers who work as managers or in other professional positions.[39] Among people doing manual labor, unskilled workers have higher mortality rates and lower self-rated health than skilled workers. People with limited job skills often have the most dangerous jobs, receive little compensation for their labor, and have little or no job security. Low-skilled workers who are injured or ill may not receive adequate treatment for their health problems when they cannot afford to take time off to consult with a medical professional and recuperate at home or they cannot afford to pay for healthcare services.

Unemployment is the inability of a person who is not working for pay to secure a paid position despite actively seeking a paid job. People who are retired, have opted not to work outside the home, or are not seeking employment for other reasons are not considered to be unemployed. **Underemployment** typically describes a situation in which a person is involuntarily working part-time rather than full-time or is a low-wage worker whose earnings are below the local poverty level even after working long hours.[40] (In international contexts, underemployment does not refer to people who are employed full-time and earning a living wage but are underutilizing their education and training in their current positions.) Being unemployed, being underemployed, or having unstable employment can be detrimental to mental and physical health status.[41,42] All-cause mortality rates are higher among unemployed men and women than employed people of the same age.[43] People who have lost their jobs are more likely than working peers to develop depression and other mental health disorders.[44] Unemployed people are more likely to adopt unhealthy behaviors like smoking and harmful use of alcohol,[45] and those risk behaviors can increase the risk of chronic diseases and injuries. This reduced health status can then cause prolonged unemployment.

SDG 8 aims to "promote sustained, inclusive, and sustainable economic growth, full and productive employment, and decent work for all."[19] Decent work means eradicating forced labor and ending child labor (SDG 8.7) as well as protecting labor rights and promoting safe working environments (SDG 8.8). Full employment means that everyone who wants to work can safely earn a living wage, including young adults, older adults, migrant workers, and people with disabilities. Employment and the income earned from working are associated with improved health status.

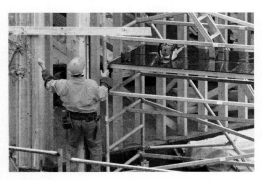

© Ari N/Shutterstock

3.6 Culture, Discrimination, and Health

Culture is a way of living, believing, behaving, communicating, and understanding the world that is shared by members of a social unit. Culture encompasses a group's norms, values, morals, rules, and customs as well as the foods people eat, the clothes they wear, the language they use, the ways they interact with those inside and outside the cultural group, and how they describe and experience adverse health situations.[46] The term **illness** describes a person's perception of his or her own experience of having an adverse health condition. **Sickness** describes the ways in which a person with a physical or mental health condition relates to and is regarded by his or her community. Culture frames the ways that health, illness, and sickness are experienced across the life span, from the way childbirth is approached to decisions about end-of-life care.

Culture shapes health beliefs, affects health behaviors, and steers decisions about when and where to seek healthcare services. In cultures that take a mechanistic approach to health, the human body is expected to function like a well-oiled machine, and disease is viewed as a malfunction or breakdown of the machinery. A moralistic perspective considers health to be the result of clean living and disease to be a type of punishment for wrongdoing. A supernatural viewpoint blames illness on demonic possession, evil eye, or the anger of God or the gods or ancestors. A disequilibrium approach considers disease to be caused by imbalances within the body, such as an imbalance between hot and cold, yin and yang, or the four humors. Disease may also be attributed to energy or qi imbalances; to emotions like fright or grief or jealously; or to stress, weather, food, germs, sex, genes, or age. These cultural beliefs about the causes of disease influence the interpretation of symptoms and diagnoses, the timeline for seeking treatment, the type of healer who is consulted (such as a physician or nurse, a counselor, a religious advisor, a massage therapist, or an herbalist), and even the types of therapy that will be effective.

Celebrations of the various cultural traditions that exist within a nation or a community can strengthen bonds among people with diverse backgrounds. However, cultural differences can also be used to divide people. At worst, these divisions can lead to abuse, violence, hate crimes, war, and genocide. People who belong to minority racial, ethnic, tribal, religious, or other groups may systematically be treated less favorably than members of majority groups in the workplace, the marketplace, and the healthcare system. Medical practitioners may be unfamiliar with the special health needs of patients from other backgrounds. Patients may be uncomfortable discussing health concerns and being examined by a medical professional who is not a member of their group or is not sensitive to their cultural beliefs and practices. For example, women from some cultural and religious groups may be unwilling to be examined by a male clinician. Some barriers to healthcare access are legally sanctioned, such as when proof of legal residency is required before health care can be offered. Because of these obstacles to accessing health care, the health status of minority populations tends to be worse than that of majority populations.

Significant differences in health status exist between countries and between different population groups within countries.[47] Some of these health disparities are a product of differences in SES, and some are a function of prejudice and discrimination against people from marginalized groups.[48] **Prejudice** is a perception about an individual based solely on preconceived notions about a sociocultural group to which that person belongs. Racism, sexism, classism, ageism, and ableism (prejudice against people with disabilities) are all forms of prejudice. **Discrimination** encompasses the actions taken against an individual because

of that person's membership in a sociocultural group. Unfair hiring and pay practices, restrictions on access to housing and services, and harassing "jokes" and insults are examples of discriminatory practices. Prejudice is a set of beliefs and attitudes. Discrimination is a set of practices and behaviors. While not all people who hold prejudicial beliefs act on them, prejudiced thoughts are the basis for discrimination.

Prejudice and discrimination are often related to race and ethnicity. **Ethnicity** is a social grouping based on many dimensions of cultural heritage, nationality, language, religion, tribal affiliation, and other factors. **Race** refers to superficial categories that group individuals based primarily on physical attributes like skin color. Significant cultural and genetic diversity is present within most racial groups. For example, the U.S. government typically collects and reports data for five racial categories and one ethnic category.[49] The five racial categories are American Indian or Alaska Native, Asian, Black or African American, Native Hawaiian or other Pacific Islander, and White. The "Asian" category groups people with ancestors from countries as diverse as China, India, the Philippines, and Thailand. The "White" category includes most people whose ancestors were from Europe, North Africa, the Middle East as well as many with ancestors from other countries in the Americas. The only ethnic category classifies people as "Hispanic or Latino" versus "Not Hispanic or Latino." People who identify as "Hispanic or Latino" might have ancestry in places as diverse as Bolivia, Cuba, Mexico, and Spain.

Significant differences in health status often exist between different racial and ethnic groups within the same country. An assortment of explanations each partly explains the reasons for these health disparities.[50] Racial and ethnic categories may capture some genetic differences between population groups, including some differential risks for heritable genetic disorders. Ethnicity may be a marker for some health-related behaviors.

If members of a population group tend to have similar dietary preferences and favorite foods, alcohol and tobacco use habits, and physical activity routines, these practices may account for some of the health differences observed between populations. Race and ethnicity may also be associated with socioeconomic factors. Members of marginalized population groups may have lower SES than other people in their town or city, and poverty is associated with reduced health status. Additionally, discrimination because of race, ethnicity, or other characteristics may cause chronic psychosocial stress that contributes to adverse health outcomes.[51] All of these factors except for genetics are modifiable ones. Health equity for all racial and ethnic groups is achievable.

For example, Indigenous communities tend to have less favorable health status than other population groups within their countries.[52] An **Indigenous population** is a group that has maintained unique cultural traditions (and often also languages) for many generations after the colonization or domination of their traditional homeland by another group. More than 400 million people worldwide identify as members of Indigenous communities.[53] These groups include, among many others, the Cherokee and Navajo of the United States, the Hmong of Southeast Asia, the Maasai of Kenya, the Quichua of Ecuador, the Sami of Scandinavia, the Tangata Whenua (Māori) of New Zealand, and the Torres Strait Islanders of Australia.[54] Indigenous populations usually have morbidity and premature mortality rates that exceed the national averages in their countries of residence.[55] The reduced health status of Indigenous populations is due partly to high rates of poverty,[56] but it also arises from social exclusion, lack of political and legal power, and health systems that are not aligned with Indigenous cultures.[57] Achieving health equity for Indigenous populations can be realized with economic growth, sociopolitical empowerment, laws against discrimination, and structural changes that increase access to culturally sensitive health care.[58]

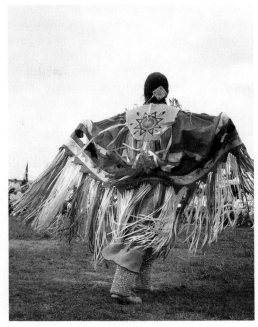

© Knumina Studios/Shutterstock

SDG 10 aims to "reduce inequality within and among countries" by taking steps to reduce poverty (SDG 10.1), ensure equal opportunities through the elimination of discriminatory laws (SDG 10.3), and "empower and promote the social, economic, and political inclusion of all, irrespective of age, sex, disability, race, ethnicity, origin, religion, or economic or other status" (SDG 10.2).[19] Actions to increase equity across these domains are expected to reduce health disparities by increasing the health status of currently disadvantaged groups.

3.7 Migrant and Refugee Health

An international **migrant** is a person who has moved across an international border and is residing in a new country. By 2020, there were nearly 270 million people worldwide who were living in a country that was not their original homeland.[59] Some international migrants intend to settle permanently in their new host country, while others are temporary residents or guest workers. An **immigrant** is a person who has settled in a new country and intends to stay there permanently. An **expatriate** is a person who is temporarily living in another country and intends to return to his or her home country. For example, people working in a foreign country for their home government, a business, the press corps, a nongovernmental organization, or another entity are usually considered to be guest workers or "expats" rather than immigrants.

Most international migrants voluntarily move from one country to another to be closer to family, start a new job, or pursue educational opportunities. The typical voluntary international migrant moves from a middle-income country to a high-income destination country where the prospects for economic prosperity are greater (**Figure 3.10**).[60] Moving to a new country and establishing legal residency there is often an expensive process, so voluntary migration is rarely an option for individuals

and families with very low incomes. Immigrants to high-income countries are often highly educated and entrepreneurial, and they represent a disproportionately high share of professionals working in information technology, health care, and other highly skilled fields in high-income countries, in addition to having high representation in hospitality and agricultural work.[61] Voluntary migrants tend to be healthier than the general population.[62]

However, not all migration is voluntary. Some migrants are forced to move because of violence, persecution, or natural disasters. Some are involved in **trafficking**, the crime of arranging for a person to relocate with the intention of forcing that migrant into sex work, debt bondage, slavery, or other types of forced labor. The experience of being an involuntary migrant is often accompanied by adverse health effects.[63] Smuggled migrants, victims of trafficking, and people fleeing conflict and persecution may experience violence and nutritional deprivation as well as other traumas during their travels. While some migrants gain greater access to healthcare services when they move from a country with poor health infrastructure to a country with a high-quality healthcare system, many migrants encounter new health challenges as they settle into their new places of residence.[64] **Acculturation** is the complex process of adopting the practices, traditions, values, and identity of a new community after migrating.[65] Acculturation generally brings improved ability to navigate the healthcare system of the host country and access the tools for health.

A **refugee** is a person who has been forced to move across an international border because of security concerns like war, civil conflict, political strife, or persecution based on race, tribe, religion, political affiliation, or membership in some other group. Refugees typically secure permission to move to a new country prior to arriving in that country. An **asylum seeker** is an involuntary migrant who asks for protection from a host country after arriving in that country rather

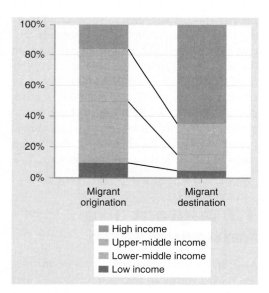

Figure 3.10 Most migrants originate in middle-income countries and move to high-income countries.

Data from *International Migration 2019*. New York: United Nations Department of Economic and Social Affairs; 2019.

than waiting for a refugee application to be processed prior to traveling. Asylum seekers are often included in the refugee category in reports about involuntary international migration because the lived experiences of refugees and asylum seekers are similar. The primary difference between the groups is the status of their legal documents.

There are currently more than 25 million refugees worldwide who are living outside their home countries, about 40% of whom are children and adolescents.[66] About 75% of refugees move from their country of origin to a neighboring country. For example, during recent crises, many Syrians relocated to Turkey and many Venezuelans relocated to Colombia. Nearly all refugees originate in low- or middle-income countries, and about 85% are hosted by low- or middle-income countries (**Figure 3.11**).[66] One of the reasons that low-income countries are overrepresented as countries of origin for refugees is that the circumstances that lead to mass emigration also

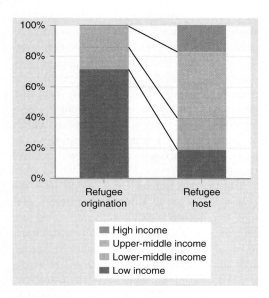

Figure 3.11 Most refugees and asylum seekers originate in low-income countries and relocate to middle-income countries.

Data from *Global Trends: Forced Displacement in 2019*. Geneva: United Nations High Commissioner for Refugees; 2020.

cause economic deterioration. Syria dropped from being a lower-middle-income country to a low-income country because of its civil war, and the crisis in Venezuela caused it to drop from a high-income country status to an upper-middle-income status.

The Office of the United Nations High Commissioner for Refugees (UNHCR) and other humanitarian organizations, both governmental and private, help meet the basic needs of refugees by providing water, food, sanitation, shelter, fuel, and health care for sick, pregnant, and vulnerable individuals. When possible, these organizations also offer treatment for malnutrition, resolve violence and security issues, and provide therapy for post-traumatic stress and other mental health disorders. Fewer than half of refugees access these services in "camps" that provide long-term shelter for children, women, and the elderly. Most refugees settle in cities or rural areas where they live alongside local residents and rely on local social services for health care and other types of assistance.[67]

To be classified as a refugee or asylum seeker, an involuntary migrant must cross an international border. An **internally displaced person (IDP)** is a person who fled his or her home community because of civil war, famine, natural disaster, or another crisis but did not cross into another country. IDPs usually do not live in camps or special shelters for displaced people. Most move to new cities or rural areas. There are an estimated 50 million IDPs worldwide, of whom about 90% were displaced by conflict and violence and about 10% by natural disasters.[68] In total, involuntary migrants and IDPs account for about 1% of the world's population. IDPs and refugees share the experience of having lost their homes, jobs, social support networks, and some of their independence and sense of security, but IDPs are not afforded the same protection and assistance as refugees. Because IDPs have remained in their home countries, they are often not eligible for assistance from UNHCR and other international groups.

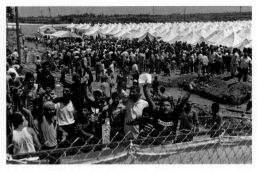

© Thomas Koch/Shutterstock

The services provided to involuntary migrants early in the cycle of displacement are not intended to be long-term solutions. Millions of today's refugees will be able to return to their home countries within the next several years. Returning home after a period of displacement is often the preferred option, even though returnees may face challenges related to the destruction of houses, healthcare facilities, schools, and other community buildings; the loss of farmland to environmental damage and to hazards like unexploded ordnance; and the displacement of their family members, neighbors, and other members of their community. However, many refugees will not be able to return home. Those who settle in new areas often face challenges associated with learning new cultural practices and adapting to them, overcoming language and communication barriers, having limited occupational options, and potentially having limited access to health care.[69] The ultimate goal is for involuntary migrants, including refugees and IDPs, to secure permanent living situations and become self-sufficient by integrating into their host countries and communities, resettling in a secondary host country or community (such as relocating from a refugee camp to a new permanent country of residence), or returning to their home communities.

Several of the SDGs specifically relate to the well-being of migrants. One of the SDG targets for reducing inequality is to "facilitate the orderly, safe, regular, and responsible migration and mobility of people, including through the implementation of planned and well-managed migration policies" (SDG 10.7).[19] Other SDG targets aim to protect migrants from being trafficked (SDG 5.2), forced into slavery (SDG 8.7), and working in unsafe environments (SDG 8.8). Policies and practices that pertain to these issues and the other aspects of inequality covered by SDG 10 will improve the health of refugees and other migrants as well as the health of their neighbors.

3.8 Governance and Politics

Access to health care and other services is associated with wealth, education, and employment, and it is also related to power. **Power** is the authority to control or influence the actions of others. Power can be conferred by political position and by socioeconomic advantages. Government officials may have the authority to demand certain services for themselves. Business leaders may have the money and connections to access care that is denied to others. Power can also be conferred by cultural systems. A tribal or religious leader may have the power to mobilize people and resources at will. A husband may have the power to control his wife's movements and activities. Powerful people can choose to limit or grant access to goods and resources like property, technology, social networks, and health care.

In many countries, some people have the power to secure health for themselves and their families while others without power have limited or no access to the resources they need to be safe and healthy. Ethnic, racial, religious, and tribal minorities; immigrants, refugees, and IDPs; people with mental health disorders, physical impairments, or other disabilities; older adults; people in prison; and members of other potentially vulnerable groups may not have the power to demand access to an equitable level of health care.

Governance consists of the processes and structures that enable governments to set policies, provide services, and protect human rights. Good governance equips public agencies and other organizations with the resources they need to be well managed, and sound management ensures that health and social services are reliably delivered to the people who need them. **Corruption** occurs when politically powerful people abuse their positions for personal gain. Corruption can occur in government, business and finance, news media, the legal system, sports, healthcare systems, and other sectors of civil society. Lower-income countries tend to have less functional governance structures and more fraud, theft, bribery, kickbacks, and other types of corruption than high-income countries (**Figure 3.12**), but every government and public-serving organization can continue to work toward improved effectiveness and transparency.[70]

SDG 16 focuses on peace, justice, and strong institutions and aims to "promote peaceful and inclusive societies for sustainable development, provide access to justice for all, and build effective, accountable, and inclusive

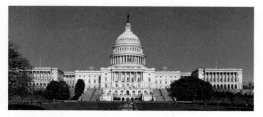
Courtesy of Pixabay

institutions at all levels."[19] Countries with good governance have low rates of violence (SDG 16.1), child abuse and human trafficking (SDG 16.2), organized crime (SDG 16.3), corruption and bribery (SDG 16.4), and discrimination (SDG 16.b). They have freedom of the press (SDG 16.10) and justice systems that quickly and fairly enforce laws (SDG 16.3), and they are transparent (SDG 16.6) and allow diverse representatives to participate in decision-making (SDG 16.7). None of the other SDGs can be achieved when functioning governance systems are not in place to ensure that everyone has access to clinical health services, education, clean drinking water, and other tools for health.

An inclusive society is one in which all people have equitable access to governmental

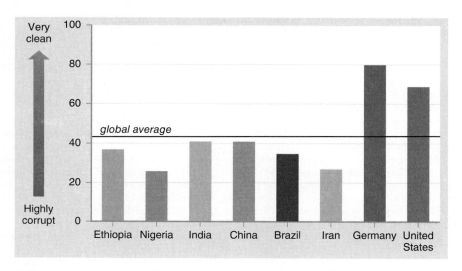

Figure 3.12 Perceptions of corruption in a country's public sector (0 = highest level of perceived corruption, 100 = lowest level of perceived corruption).

Data from *Corruption Perceptions Index 2019*. Berlin: Transparency International; 2020.

institutions and services, including health-related services. Improvements in the health status of low-resource groups do not harm the health status of groups with greater access to resources. Instead, improvements to the health status of any population group can raise the health status of the whole population. Everyone benefits when contagious infections are not circulating within a country's borders. Everyone benefits when workers have enough food to be strong and productive. Everyone benefits when health issues like cardiovascular disease, diabetes, and depression can be detected early and managed well so that those individuals can remain active in their communities. Population health is optimized when everyone has an equal opportunity to be maximally healthy regardless of socioeconomic status.[71]

References

1. *World Health Organization Commission on Social Determinants of Health. Closing the Gap in a Generation: Health Equity Through Action on the Social Determinants of Health.* Geneva: World Health Organization; 2008.
2. Wilkinson R, Marmot M. *Social Determinants of Health: The Solid Facts.* Copenhagen: World Health Organization; 2003.
3. Braveman P, Gottlieb L. The social determinants of health: it's time to consider the causes of the causes. *Public Health Rep.* 2014;129(Suppl 2):19–31.
4. Marmot M. Social determinants of health. *Lancet.* 2005;365:1099–1104.
5. Kavanagh J, Oliver S, Lorenc T. Reflections on developing and using PROGRESS-Plus. *Equity Update.* 2008;2:1–3.
6. Braveman P, Gruskin S. Defining equity in health. *J Epidemiol Community Health.* 2003;57:254–258.
7. United Nations Department of Economic and Social Affairs. *Social Justice in an Open World: The Role of the United Nations.* New York: United Nations; 2006.
8. Gwatkin DR. Health inequalities and the health of the poor: What do we know? What can we do? *Bull World Health Organ.* 2000;78:3–18.
9. Braveman P. What are health disparities and health equity? We need to be clear. *Public Health Rep.* 2014;129(S2):5–8.
10. Berendes S, Heywood P, Oliver S, Garner P. Quality of private and public ambulatory health care in low and middle income countries: systematic review of comparative studies. *PLoS Med.* 2011;8:e1000433.
11. *World Development Indicators 2020.* Washington DC: World Bank; 2020.
12. United Nations Department of Economic and Social Affairs. *World Population Prospects: The 2019 Revision.* New York: United Nations; 2019.
13. United Nations Department of Economic and Social Affairs. *World Social Report 2020.* New York: United Nations; 2020.
14. Wagstaff A, Flores G, Smitz MF, Hsu J, Cepynoga K, Eozenou P. Progress on impoverishing health spending in 122 countries: a retrospective observational study. *Lancet Glob Health.* 2018;6:e180–e192.
15. Benatar S. Politics, power, poverty and global health: systems and frames. *Int J Health Policy Manag.* 2016;5:599–604.
16. *Global Multidimensional Poverty Index 2020.* New York: United Nations Development Programme; 2020.
17. *2019 Poverty and Inequality in Nigeria.* Abuja: National Bureau of Statistics; 2020.
18. Jamison DT, Summers LH, Alleyne G, et al. Global health 2035: a world converging within a generation. *Lancet.* 2013;382:1898–1955.
19. *Transforming Our World: The 2030 Agenda for Sustainable Development.* New York: United Nations; 2015.
20. United Nations Economic and Social Council. *Report of the Inter-Agency and Expert Group on Sustainable Development Goal Indicators* (E/CN.3/2021/2). New York: United Nations; 2021.
21. Berkman ND, Davis TC, McCormack L. Health literacy: what is it? *J Health Commun.* 2010;15 (Suppl 2):9–19.
22. Nutbeam D. Health literacy as a public health goal: a challenge for contemporary health education and communication strategies into the 21st century. *Health Promot Int.* 2000;15:259–267.
23. Kickbusch IS. Health literacy: addressing the health and education divide. *Health Promot Int.* 2001;16:289–297.
24. Cleland JG, van Ginneken JK. Maternal education and child survival in developing countries: the search for pathways of influence. *Soc Sci Med.* 1988;27:1357–1368.
25. UNESCO Institute for Statistics database. UNESCO. Accessed 2020. http://data.uis.unesco.org/
26. *Global Education Monitoring Report Summary 2020.* Paris: UNESCO; 2020.
27. Bundy D, Schultz L, Sarr B, Banham L, Colenso P, Drake L. The school as a platform for addressing health in middle childhood and adolescence (chapter 20). In: Bundy DAP, De Silva N, Horton S, Jamison DT, Patton

GC, eds. *Child and Adolescent Health and Development.* Vol. 8. 3rd ed. Washington DC: IBRD/World Bank; 2017:269–286.

28. Arslanian-Engoren C, Engoren M. Physiological and anatomical bases for sex differences in pain and nausea as presenting symptoms of acute coronary syndromes. *Heart Lung.* 2010;39:386–393.

29. *Gender Equality, Work and Health: A Review of the Evidence.* Geneva: World Health Organization; 2006.

30. GBD 2019 Diseases and Injuries Collaborators. Global burden of 369 diseases and injuries in 204 countries and territories, 1990–2019: a systematic analysis for the Global Burden of Disease Study 2019. *Lancet.* 2020;396:1204–1222.

31. Johnson JL, Greaves L, Repta R. Better science with sex and gender: facilitating the use of a sex and gender-based analysis in health research. *Int J Equity Health.* 2009;8:14.

32. Bird CE, Rieker PP. Gender matters: an integrated model for understanding men's and women's health. *Soc Sci Med.* 1999;48:745–755.

33. Langer A, Meleis A, Knaul FM, et al. Women and health: the key for sustainable development. *Lancet.* 2015;386:1165–1210.

34. Hawkes S, Buse K. Gender and global health: evidence, policy, and inconvenient truths. *Lancet.* 2013;381:1783–1787.

35. *Human Development Report 2020.* New York: United Nations Development Programme; 2020.

36. *Integrating Equity, Gender, Human Rights and Social Determinants into the Work of WHO: Roadmap for Action (2014–2019).* Geneva: World Health Organization; 2015.

37. *World Employment and Social Outlook: Trends 2020.* Geneva: International Labour Organization; 2020.

38. Toch-Marquardt M, Menvielle G, Eikemo TA, et al. Occupational class inequalities in all-cause and cause-specific mortality among middle-aged men in 14 European populations during the early 2000s. *PLoS One.* 2014;9:e108072.

39. Aldabe B, Anderson R, Lyly-Yrjänäinen M, et al. Contribution of material, occupational, and psychosocial factors in the explanation of social inequalities in health in 28 countries in Europe. *J Epidemiol Community Health.* 2011;65:1123–1131.

40. Dooley D. Unemployment, underemployment, and mental health: conceptualizing employment status as a continuum. *Am J Community Psychol.* 2003;32:9–20.

41. Wilson SH, Walker GM. Unemployment and health: a review. *Public Health.* 1993;107:153–162.

42. Benach J, Vives A, Amable M, Vanroelen C, Tarafa G, Muntaner C. Precarious employment: understanding an emerging social determinant of health. *Annu Rev Public Health.* 2014;35:229–253.

43. Roelfs DJ, Shor E, Davidson KW, Schwartz JE. Losing life and livelihood: a systematic review and meta-analysis of unemployment and all-cause mortality. *Soc Sci Med.* 2011;72:840–854.

44. Paul KI, Moser K. Unemployment impairs mental health: meta-analyses. *J Vocational Behav.* 2019;74:264–282.

45. Dooley D, Fielding J, Levi L. Health and unemployment. *Annu Rev Public Health.* 1996;17:449–465.

46. Boyd KM. Disease, illness, sickness, health, healing and wholeness: exploring some elusive concepts. *Med Humanities.* 2000;26:9–17.

47. Braveman P, Tarimo E. Social inequalities in health within countries: not only an issue for affluent nations. *Soc Sci Med.* 2002;54:1621–1635.

48. Stuber J, Meyer I, Link B. Stigma, prejudice, discrimination and health. *Soc Sci Med.* 2008;67:315–317.

49. *Revisions to the Standards for the Classification of Federal Data on Race and Ethnicity.* Washington DC: Office of Management and Budget; 1997.

50. Dressler WW, Oths KS, Gravlee CC. Race and ethnicity in public health research: models to explain health disparities. *Ann Rev Anthropol.* 2005;34:231–252.

51. Pascoe EA, Smart Richman L. Perceived discrimination and health: a meta-analytic review. *Psychol Bull.* 2009;135:531–554.

52. Gracey M, King M. Indigenous health part 1: determinants and disease patterns. *Lancet.* 2009;374:65–75.

53. *The Indigenous World 2020.* Copenhagen: International Work Group for Indigenous Affairs; 2020.

54. Bartlett JG, Madariaga-Vignudo L, O'Neil JD, Kuhnlein HV. Identifying indigenous peoples for health research in a global context: a review of perspectives and challenges. *Int J Circumpolar Health.* 2007;66:287–307.

55. King M, Smith A, Gracey M. Indigenous health part 2: the underlying causes of the health gap. *Lancet.* 2009;374:76–85.

56. United Nations Department of Economic and Social Affairs. *State of the World's Indigenous Peoples: Indigenous Peoples' Access to Health Services.* New York: United Nations; 2015.

57. Hernández A, Ruano AL, Marchal B, San Sebastián M, Flores W. Engaging with complexity to improve the health of indigenous people: a call for the use of systems thinking to tackle health inequity. *Int J Equity Health.* 2017;16:26.

58. United Nations Department of Economic and Social Affairs. *State of the World's Indigenous Peoples: Implementing the United Nations Declaration on the Rights of Indigenous Peoples.* New York: United Nations; 2019.

59. *World Migration Report 2020.* Geneva: International Organization for Migration; 2019.

60. United Nations Department of Economic and Social Affairs. *International Migration 2019*. New York: United Nations; 2019.

61. *International Migration Outlook 2020*. Paris: Organisation for Economic Co-operation and Development; 2020.

62. Aldridge RW, Nellums LB, Bartlett S, et al. Global patterns of mortality in international migrants: a systematic review and meta-analysis. *Lancet.* 2018;392:2553–2566.

63. *International Migration, Health and Human Rights*. Geneva: International Organization for Migration; 2013.

64. Gushulak BD, MacPherson DW. The basic principles of migration health: population mobility and gaps in disease prevalence. *Emerg Themes Epidemiol.* 2006;3:3.

65. Fox M, Thayer Z, Wadhwa PD. Assessment of acculturation in minority health research. *Soc Sci Med.* 2017;176:123–132.

66. *Global Trends: Forced Displacement in 2019*. Geneva: United Nations High Commissioner for Refugees; 2020.

67. Spiegel PB, Checchi F, Colombo S, Paik E. Health-care needs of people affected by conflict: future trends and changing frameworks. *Lancet.* 2010;375:341–345.

68. *Global Report on Internal Displacement 2020*. Geneva: Internal Displacement Monitoring Centre, Norwegian Refugee Council; 2020.

69. Abubakar I, Aldridge RW, Devakumar D, et al. The UCL–Lancet Commission on Migration and Health: the health of a world on the move. *Lancet.* 2018;392:2606–2654.

70. *Corruption Perceptions Index 2019*. Berlin: Transparency International; 2020.

71. Ottersen OP, Dasgupta J, Blouin C, et al. The Lancet–University of Oslo Commission on Global Governance for Health: the political origins of health inequity: prospects for change. *Lancet.* 2014;383:630–667.

Environmental Determinants of Health

Human health is dependent on healthy environments. Environmental health concerns related to drinking water, sanitation, indoor air pollution, occupational safety, and unplanned urbanization can often be improved through practice and policy interventions at the local or national level, but transnational problems like outdoor air pollution and climate change will only be solved through global cooperation.

4.1 Environmental Health and the Sustainable Development Goals

The **environment** consists of the surroundings in which humans and other organisms live. The **natural environment** includes aspects of the biological and physical world that are not created by humans. Human health is affected by environmental biology (such the types of vegetation and animals that are native to a location), geography (such as whether a location is desert, tropical, arctic, or something more moderate), geology (such as the presence of earthquake fault lines or volcanoes), and climate (such as the usual weather and temperature patterns in an area). The **built environment** includes all structures built by humans for human use, including buildings, roads, bridges, sidewalks, recreational areas,

and even public artwork. Where people live and work; the materials used to construct residential, industrial, and commercial buildings; what people eat and where that food comes from; the source and quality of drinking water; the quality of the air that is breathed, both indoors and outdoors; whether hazardous substances like cleaning agents, fertilizers, and motor oil are stored in or near the home or workplace; and numerous other components of the built home and work environments all play a role in health status.

Environmental health is the public health discipline that studies the connections between human health and environmental exposures, such as poor water quality, air pollution, solid and hazardous waste, unsafe food, vermin and infection-transmitting insects, radiation, noise, and residential and industrial hazards. Humans have long recognized the environment's role in disease etiology. For many centuries before microscopes allowed people to observe bacteria, communities recognized that some illnesses were linked to environmental exposures, and they took care to dispose of human waste, protect water sources, and bury the carcasses of diseased animals. During much of the 19th century, for example, the prevailing theory of disease causation in Western countries was that epidemics were spontaneously generated in places with poor sanitation.[1] The term **miasma** was used to describe the foul-smelling gases of poorly managed waste that were thought to cause disease prior to the discovery of pathogenic microorganisms. When cholera outbreaks occurred in England in the mid-1800s, investigators found a higher infection rate in places of low altitude, especially places near marshes that had an abundance of pungent odors, and they blamed the spread of cholera on contact with those offensive gases.[2] Later studies determined that bacterially contaminated drinking water was the true cause of the outbreaks and malodorous places were more likely than other locations to have dirty water, but conclusions based on miasma theory were sufficient to enable behavior changes that reduced the risk of infection.

The most important environmental health advances in the 19th and early 20th centuries arose from the discovery that microscopic bacteria, viruses, and parasites cause infectious diseases. After the origination of germ theory, public health efforts in various countries focused primarily on sanitation and cleanliness, with special attention on actions to reduce epidemics that were thought to be associated with urban crowding and its associated grime.[3] As scientific discoveries provided more information about how infectious agents and parasites were spread, additional environmental health interventions were developed and deployed. For example, the determination that mosquitoes and other biting insects could transmit germs to humans made vector control strategies a higher priority. Today, outbreaks are no longer blamed on miasmas, but good hygiene (like frequent handwashing) and the avoidance of known environmental hazards remain very important for preventing infections and injuries.

Many of the biggest advancements in environmental health science in the 20th century grew out of new evidence linking environmental hazards to noncommunicable diseases.[4] Even after most medical scientists shifted their efforts from the identification of social and environmental risk factors for disease to the identification of specific disease-causing microorganisms and genes,[5] one of the biggest public health breakthroughs of the century was a series of studies published in the 1950s that confirmed that cigarette smoking was a major cause of lung cancer, emphysema, and cardiovascular disease.[6] Subsequent studies showed that exposure to secondhand smoke was also a risk factor for lung disease.[7] Additional 20th century research provided evidence that environmental and occupational hazards were associated with many other types of heart and lung disease, cancer, and other noncommunicable conditions. These discoveries led to regulations that reduced exposure to tobacco smoke, radon, leaded gasoline, noise, and other dangers.

Today, in the early 21st century, about one in five deaths is still attributable to water pollution, air pollution, occupational hazards, unsafe buildings and roads, and other modifiable environmental exposures (**Figure 4.1**).[8] Lack of access to safe drinking water, sanitation, and hygiene causes many cases of diarrheal diseases. Failure to control insects and other pests increases the risk of malaria and other vector-borne diseases. Air pollution contributes to respiratory infections as well as heart disease, strokes, lung cancer, chronic obstructive pulmonary disease (COPD), and asthma. Occupational hazards cause low back pain and hearing loss. Unsafe work, home, and community environments contribute to the burden from road traffic injuries, falls, drowning, and other injuries. Numerous other factors contribute to other types of infections, noncommunicable diseases, and injuries (**Figure 4.2**).[9] Climate change is likely

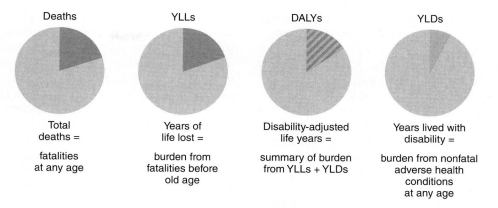

Figure 4.1 Percentage of global population health outcomes attributed to environmental and occupational risk factors.

Data from GBD 2019 Risk Factors Collaborators. Global burden of 87 risk factors in 204 countries and territories, 1990–2019: a systematic analysis for the Global Burden of Disease Study 2019. *Lancet.* 2020;396:1223–1249.

Disease	Population Attributable Fraction (%)	Major Environmental Contributor(s)
Intestinal worm infections	100	Sanitation
Drowning	73	Safety of home and community environments, occupational risks
Diarrheal diseases	57	Drinking water, sanitation, and hygiene
Asthma	44	Air pollution and occupational risks
Malaria	42	Environmental vector management
Road traffic injuries	39	Occupational risks, built environment, traffic regulation, and land use
Acute lower respiratory infections (pneumonia)	35	Indoor air pollution
Chronic obstructive pulmonary disease	35	Air pollution
Cardiovascular diseases (such as ischemic heart disease and stroke)	31	Air pollution
Falls	30	Built environment and occupational risks
Back and neck pain	27	Occupational risks
Hearing loss	22	Occupational noise
Self-harm	21	Chemicals, built environment, gun control, home and community safety
Cancers	20	Air pollution and many other factors

Figure 4.2 Percentage of disability-adjusted life years from selected conditions attributable to environmental risk factors.

Data from Prüss-Ustün A, Wolf J, Corvalán C, Bos R, Neira M. *Preventing Disease Through Healthy Environments: A Global Assessment of the Burden of Disease from Environmental Risks.* Geneva: World Health Organization; 2016.

to exacerbate many of these environmental health challenges in the coming decades.

Everyone is vulnerable to the adverse effects of environmental hazards, but environmental health problems place a particularly high burden on residents of low- and middle-income countries (**Figure 4.3**).[8] The lowest-income communities and households are the most vulnerable to environmental threats. Poverty affects the type of dwelling a household lives in (which can be unstable, unventilated, and built with harmful materials); how crowded the home is (which can facilitate the spread of contagious diseases like tuberculosis); and whether it is in proximity to schools, healthcare facilities, public transportation, and waste dumps. Low-income communities often do not have access to reliably safe drinking water, functioning toilets, or enough water to practice good hygiene, so residents of those areas have a high risk of contracting infections. In some places, the dwindling availability of wood for fuel limits the ability of households to boil water and cook food. Without electricity for refrigeration, it is

difficult to store food safely. A lack of infrastructure for communication and transportation can make it difficult to access health education and healthcare services. The tools for disease prevention, such as soap and mosquito netting, can be unaffordable luxuries for households that must dedicate all income to immediate survival needs like food, housing, clothing, and emergency medical care. Low-income communities are also often situated in places that are especially vulnerable to extreme weather events, such as flooding and heat waves.

Population health requires safe home, work, and community environments, and it is also dependent on healthy ecosystems at grander national, regional, and global scales.[10] One of the health-specific Sustainable Development Goals (SDGs) targets focuses specifically on environmental health, aiming to "substantially reduce the number of deaths and illnesses from hazardous chemicals; air, water, and soil pollution; and contamination" (SDG 3.9).[11] Many other SDG targets are also related to environmental health, including

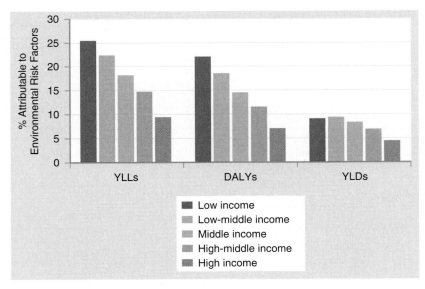

Figure 4.3 Percentage of the burden of disease attributed to environmental and occupational risk factors, by country sociodemographic group.

Data from GBD 2019 Risk Factors Collaborators. Global burden of 87 risk factors in 204 countries and territories, 1990–2019: a systematic analysis for the Global Burden of Disease Study 2019. *Lancet.* 2020;396:1223–1249.

ones focused on sustainable agriculture (2.4), drinking water (6.1), sanitation (6.2), clean energy (7.1), urban pollution (11.6), hazardous waste (12.4), and climate-related hazards (13.1). Making progress toward achieving the environmental SDGs of ensuring drinking water and sanitation for all (SDG 6), ensuring modern energy for all (SDG 7), building resilient infrastructure (SDG 9), making cities safe and sustainable (SDG 11), ensuring responsible consumption and production patterns (SDG 12), and taking action to combat climate change and its impacts (SDG 12), along with the related goals of ocean conservation (SDG 14) and ecosystem restoration (SDG 15), will be necessary for achieving and maintaining poverty reduction and improvements in global health status.[12]

4.2 Water, Sanitation, and Hygiene

The most fundamental necessities for life are water, food, shelter, and fuel for heat and cooking. Everyone needs access to an adequate daily supply of water for drinking; cooking; hygiene; and cleaning tasks, such as washing clothes, scrubbing cooking pots, and cleaning homes. A household has access to **safe drinking water** when there is an adequate supply of affordable clean drinking water in or near the home. Water access is a function of water quality, reliability, quantity, proximity, and cost (**Figure 4.4**).[13]

Quality: Drinking water needs to be free of bacteria, viruses, and parasites that can

Service Level	Quality and Reliability	Quantity per Person per Day	Proximity	Hygiene Needs Met?	Level of Health Concern
No access	Neither quantity nor quality ensured	May be less than 5 liters	More than 1 kilometer or 30 minutes round trip	No, because only available at source	Very high
Basic access	Quantity ensured but quality not ensured	About 20 liters	Between 100 and 1,000 meters or 5–30 minutes round trip	Yes, for handwashing and food hygiene; no, for laundry and bathing	High
Intermediate access	Quantity and quality usually assured	About 50 liters	Water delivered through one tap that is within 100 meters or 5 minutes round trip	Yes	Low
Optimal access	Quantity and quality ensured	About 100 liters	Continuous supply through multiple taps	Yes	Very low

Figure 4.4 Water service level (quality, reliability, quantity, and proximity) and health effects.

Data from Howard G, Bartram J. *Domestic Water Quantity, Service Level and Health.* Geneva: World Health Organization; 2003.

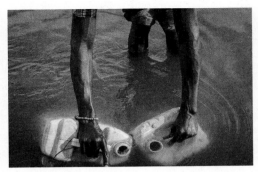

© Punghi/Shutterstock

cause diarrhea and other infectious diseases, and it must also be free of harmful chemicals and sediments.[14] The water should not appear cloudy, dirty, or strangely colored and it should not cause problems with cooking (such as giving food a strange flavor, color, or texture) or washing.[15] To be classified as an improved water source, the water must be protected, which means that people should not wash clothes or bathe in the vicinity where drinking water is collected and animals, sewage, and garbage should be kept away from the water source.

Reliability: The water source must be available and functioning all the time, or the household must have access to adequate water storage and water treatment methods, such as filtering, boiling, or using chemicals like chlorine.

Quantity: **Hygiene** is the practice of maintaining cleanliness in order to prevent disease. Personal hygiene behaviors include handwashing (hand hygiene), tooth brushing (oral hygiene), and bathing (body hygiene). Enough water must be available each day so people can stay hydrated and clean. The average minimum amount of water needed by one person each day just to survive is about 4–5 gallons (15–20 liters), including part of a gallon (about 1–3 liters) for drinking, part of a gallon (2–3 liters) for food preparation and cleanup, 1–2 gallons (4–6 liters) for laundry, and 1–2 gallons (6–7 liters) for personal cleanliness.[16] For healthy living, rather

than mere survival, a minimum of about 13 gallons (50 liters) of water per person per day is recommended.[13] (As a comparison, the typical American uses about 82 gallons daily at his or her residence for indoor and outdoor purposes.[17])

Proximity: To be considered accessible, the water source must be close enough to the home so that distance does not prevent people from using the water they need for health. At best, water is piped directly into an individual house. Public water taps, boreholes, and protected (and lined) dug wells that bring water near to homes, but not inside them, are also considered to be improved water sources (**Figure 4.5**).[18] In some places, it is possible for households to supplement their water access by collecting and storing rainwater for drinking and domestic use. To achieve universal basic access to water, every person should live within one kilometer (about 0.6 miles) of a safe drinking water source.[13] When water sources are farther from the home, women and children may have to spend several hours each day walking to a water source, waiting for their turn to fill a container, and walking home.

Cost: Water must be affordable enough that people have access to at least the minimum amount of water necessary for healthy living. This does not mean that water must be free. Households using a community water system may be asked to pay a reasonable fee so that the system can be maintained. These fees also promote water conservation if they are tied to the amount of water drawn from the pump by a household. However, it is problematic for public health when the prices charged by water providers are exorbitant.

Sanitation is the safe disposal of human excreta (feces). A household has access to sanitation when there is a toilet in the home or a latrine near the home that can be used without a per-use payment.[18] Open defecation occurs when people defecate in a field, a street, or another place that is not a toilet facility. Rural

Unimproved			Improved
WATER			
• Surface water from a river, dam, lake, pond, stream, canal, irrigation channel, or other water body	• Unprotected dug well • Unprotected spring • Water from mobile vendors, such as tanker trucks or carts with a small tank or drum • Bottled water (when used as a primary source of water)	• Public tap or standpipe • Tube well or borehole • Protected dug well • Protected spring • Rainwater collection	• Clean drinking water piped into the user's home or yard
SANITATION			
• Open defecation (using a field, forest, bush, open body of water, beach, or other open space as a toilet)	• Pit latrine without a slab or platform • Hanging latrine • Bucket (or bag) latrine • Flush or pour toilet that drains into a street, yard, open sewer, ditch, or drainage way	• Shared or public sanitation facilities	• Flush or pour toilet that diverts waste to a piped sewer system, a septic tank, or a pit latrine • Ventilated improved pit (VIP) latrine • Pit latrine with slab • Composting toilet

Figure 4.5 Examples of improved and unimproved drinking water sources and sanitation facilities.

Data from *Progress on Sanitation and Drinking Water: 2015 Update and MDG Assessment*. New York: UNICEF/World Health Organization Joint Monitoring Programme for Water Supply and Sanitation; 2015.

residents without access to sanitation systems may be able to go to an outdoor defecation site away from their living areas. Urban residents without access to a toilet or latrine often have no choice but to defecate at the side of a road or into a bag that is thrown outside, a waste disposal method that is sometimes called a "flying toilet." A desire for privacy means that many people without access to an improved sanitation facility, especially women, wait until dark to defecate, even though it is often dangerous for them to be out at night.

Compared to open defecation, an improved toilet facility provides greater comfort, privacy, cleanliness, safety, and protection from dangers at night and from snakes and pests.[19] One of the simplest sanitation facilities is a pit latrine, which is a hole in the ground covered by an outhouse or encircled by a privacy blind. A ventilation-improved pit (VIP) latrine has some sort of slab or platform over the hole to prevent people from falling into it and has vents that carry fumes away from the outhouse and keep flies out of it. Even something as simple as a VIP latrine is considered to be an "improved" sanitation facility. Septic tanks and sewer connections are more advanced sanitation technologies that use water to remove waste from indoor toilets.

People who live in communities where open defecation is practiced have a significantly increased risk of bacterial, viral, and protozoal diarrheal diseases and helminthic (worm) infections due to contact with fecal matter.[20] In lower-income countries where many residents do not have reliable access to safe drinking water and sanitation, there is a substantial mortality rate associated with

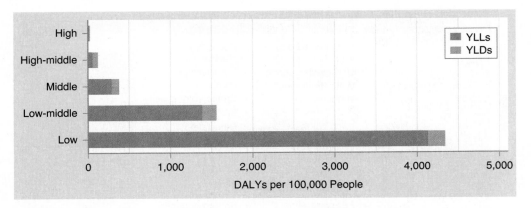

Figure 4.6 All-ages burden of disease attributed to unsafe water, sanitation, and handwashing per 100,000 people, by country sociodemographic group.

Data from GBD 2019 Risk Factors Collaborators. Global burden of 87 risk factors in 204 countries and territories, 1990–2019: a systematic analysis for the Global Burden of Disease Study 2019. *Lancet.* 2020;396:1223–1249.

lack of access to these tools for health (**Figure 4.6**).[8] A **community-led total sanitation** (CLTS) program is a set of public health interventions that encourage toilet use in places where residents are accustomed to open defecation and have not yet adopted new sanitation behaviors.[21] CLTS programs also promote frequent handwashing with soap and other healthy behaviors associated with toileting. A community is declared to have **open defecation free** (ODF) status when all members are consistently using designated toilet facilities and no one is defecating outside. Becoming an ODF community requires toilets to be present and used by all community members every time they need to relieve themselves.

A **WASH program** combines improved access to **wa**ter and **s**anitation systems with **h**ygiene promotion. The most effective interventions for reducing the public health burden from diarrheal diseases and intestinal parasites are WASH programs that build infrastructure while providing health education that encourages handwashing and consistent use of toilets.[22] WASH interventions are cost-effective mechanisms for reducing the burden of water- and sanitation-related diseases in low- and middle-income countries.[23] Increased access to these utilities is associated with both economic growth and improvements in population health status.[24]

Millennium Development Goal (MDG) 7 aimed to reduce the proportion of people without access to improved water sources and sanitation facilities by half between 1990 and 2015. The percentage of the world's people with access to an improved water source increased from about 76% in 1990 to 88% in 2015 and 91% in 2020, and the MDG target for water was met.[18] If current trends continue, about 98% of people will have access to at least a basic water service by 2030.[25] Access to an improved sanitation facility increased from about 54% of the world's people in 1990 to 73% in 2015 and 78% in 2020, and good progress was made toward achieving the MDG target for sanitation even though it was not met (**Figure 4.7**).[18]

SDG 6 has the even more ambitious goal of ensuring "available and sustainable management of water and sanitation for all."[11] Achieving this goal would require 100% of the world's people to have reliable access to safe drinking water and sanitation. While the MDGs counted all "improved" water sources and sanitation facilities as meeting its targets, the SDGs require access to "safely managed" utilities. Safely managed drinking water services are free from contamination; available

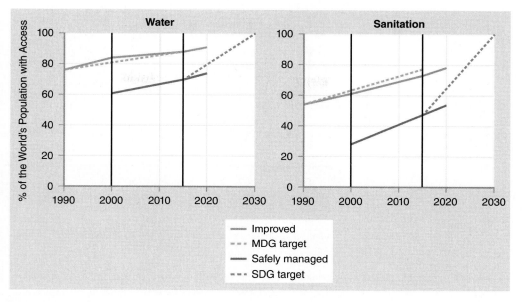

Figure 4.7 Progress toward achieving Millennium Development Goal (MDG) targets for "improved" water and sanitation and Sustainable Development Goal (SDG) targets for "safely managed" water and sanitation.

Data from *Progress on Sanitation and Drinking Water: 2015 Update and MDG Assessment.* New York: UNICEF/World Health Organization Joint Monitoring Programme for Water Supply and Sanitation; 2015; and *Progress on Household Drinking Water, Sanitation and Hygiene, 2000–2020: Five Years into the SDGs.* New York: World Health Organization/UNICEF Joint Monitoring Programme for Water Supply and Sanitation; 2021.

when needed; and accessible on the premises of the home, yard, or plot.[25] Basic improved drinking water sources may be up to 30 minutes round-trip walking distance away from the home, but safely managed services must be immediately accessible. Safely managed sanitation services have toilets that are not shared by more than one household, and excreta must be safely treated and disposed of on-site (in covered pit latrines or septic tanks) or elsewhere (either by having the contents of pit latrines or septic tanks emptied and transported to a designated fecal sludge treatment facility or by using wastewater to carry excreta through sewer lines to a treatment facility).

The percentage of the world's people with safely managed drinking water increased from about 61% in 2000 to 70% in 2015 and 74% in 2020, the percentage with safely managed sanitation increased from about 28% in 2000 to 47% in 2015

and 54% in 2020, and the percentage who engage in open defecation decreased from about 21% in 2000 to 10% in 2015 and 6% in 2020.[25]

Even with the steady progress on WASH since the launch of the MDGs, in 2020 more than 750 million people did not have access to at least basic improved water sources; about 1.7 billion did not have access to at least basic improved sanitation facilities, including nearly 500 million people who still practiced open defecation; and about 2.3 billion people did not have a handwashing facility with soap and water at home.[25] Access to improved water and sanitation remained especially limited in rural areas (**Figure 4.8**).[25]

Critical gaps in access to these utilities are likely to remain even after the end of the SDG era in 2030.[26] The WHO/UNICEF Joint Monitoring Programme for Water Supply and Sanitation estimates that in 2030 only 81% of

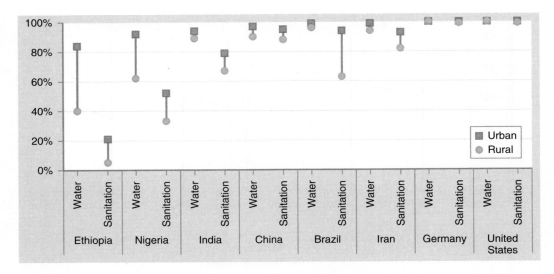

Figure 4.8 Access to at least basic drinking water and sanitation in rural and urban areas in 2020.

Data from *Progress on Household Drinking Water, Sanitation and Hygiene, 2000–2020: Five Years into the SDGs.* New York: World Health Organization/UNICEF Joint Monitoring Programme for Water Supply and Sanitation; 2021.

the world's people will have safely managed drinking water, 67% will have safely managed sanitation, and 78% will have access to basic hygiene, defined as having soap and water at home.[25] Reducing the global burden from diarrheal diseases will require greater investment in WASH in lower-income countries.[27]

4.3 Energy and Air Quality

Energy is necessary for at least three important purposes: cooking food and boiling water for safe consumption, providing a source of heat when outdoor temperatures are low, and providing a source of light at night. All fuels that are burned for energy release air pollutants, including carbon monoxide (CO), nitrogen oxides (NOx), sulfur dioxide (SO_2), ozone (O_3), volatile organic compounds, and particulate matter. **Particulate matter** describes substances that are small enough to remain suspended in the air for long periods of time and travel deep into the lungs. Air

pollutants can cause lung disease by triggering inflammation, damaging the cells that line the respiratory tract, and impairing immune system response.[28] They increase the risk of numerous respiratory diseases, including pneumonia, asthma, lung cancer, and other chronic respiratory diseases, and they exacerbate cardiovascular disorders.[29]

Both indoor and outdoor air pollution are hazardous to human health. **Household air pollution**, also called **indoor air pollution**, is the presence of harmful chemicals or other substances in the air inside or near buildings at concentrations above the thresholds established for human safety. Indoor air pollution is often generated by cooking inside with unclean fuels. **Biomass** is fuel from organic materials like wood, vegetation, or animal waste. Biomass is usually burned in open fires or in simple stoves that release most of the smoke from burning into the home or cooking shelter.[30] The health risks associated with indoor air pollution are especially high for women and young children who spend several hours a day near fires while cooking.[31] Use of solid fuels for cooking and other energy needs can have adverse effects on respiratory health as well as other body systems.[32] Children are at risk of burns from falling into open fires or knocking over pots of boiling water. Women and children often spend hours each week collecting sticks and brush to use as fuel, and they are susceptible to injuries related to carrying heavy loads over uneven terrain. As sources of biomass close to the home are used up, fuel gatherers must travel farther distances to find fuel. There are also environmental consequences since burning of solid fuels contributes to outdoor air pollution and the demand for wood and charcoal contributes to deforestation.

Ambient air pollution, also called **outdoor air pollution**, is the presence of harmful chemicals or other substances in the air outside buildings at concentrations above the thresholds established for human safety. Outdoor air pollution is created by power plants; the exhaust from motor vehicles; and the wastes produced by industrial processes, forest fires, and the disposal of solid waste. Electricity is not a pollution-free form of energy when the electricity is generated by burning coal or oil or other fuels. However, there are numerous health benefits associated with having electricity in the home and being able to cook with cleaner fuels, including cleaner indoor air, safer food storage because of refrigeration, and greater access to health and safety messages delivered through radios, televisions, or the Internet.

The percentage of the world's people with electricity in their homes increased from about 72% in 1990 to 90% today.[33] However, having electricity does not mean that electricity is the only source of household energy. About 35% of people worldwide use solid fuels like biomass as their primary source of energy for cooking (**Figure 4.9**).[33] Thus, while less than 1 billion people today do not

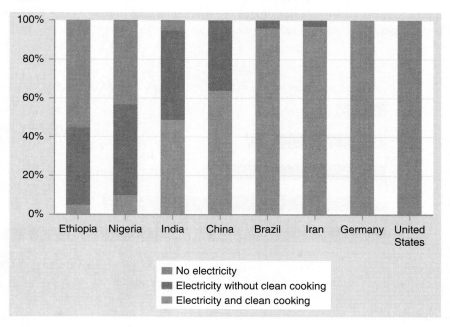

Figure 4.9 Access to electricity and clean cooking.

Data from *Tracking SDG 7: The Energy Progress Report 2020.* Washington DC: World Bank; 2020.

have electricity in their homes, nearly 3 billion people who live in low- and middle-income countries continue to cook with unclean fuels that generate indoor air pollution.[33]

Globally, more than 10% of deaths before old age are attributed to air pollution.[8] There is a substantial mortality rate associated with the combined effects of indoor and outdoor air pollution in many low- and middle-income countries,[34] and even in high-income countries this rate is not negligible (**Figure 4.10**).[8] Indoor air pollution is mostly a health problem in lower-income countries where solid fuels are used for cooking and heating, but outdoor air pollution is a health concern in countries of all income levels (**Figure 4.11**).[8]

SDG 7 is focused on ensuring "universal access to affordable, reliable, sustainable, and modern energy services" (SDG 7.1).[11] In lower-income countries, where cooking with solid fuels generates a lot of indoor air pollution, progress toward this goal will be met by increasing the proportion of households with electricity. There are also interventions that can reduce exposure to indoor air pollution among people without electricity, such as using cook

stoves with a flue that diverts pollutants out of the home.[35] When it is not possible to increase ventilation inside the home, moving the kitchen to the outside of the home reduces smoke inhalation (if the outside cooking area has good ventilation). Improved cooking devices such as those that use solar panels or other alternative energy sources generally create less smoke than biomass. Keeping children away from smoke and using pot lids also reduce the health risks associated with cooking.

In middle-income countries, which tend to have high levels of urban pollution and increasing production of outdoor air pollution, progress toward SDG 7 can be made by supporting smart infrastructure development.[36] As countries get richer, they usually shift from using biomass as the primary source of energy to using gas and other sources of energy that generate more outdoor air pollution.[33] While industrialization is critical for growing economies, reducing poverty, and raising standards of living, rising demands for energy can harm environmental and human health.[37] The hope is that gains in energy efficiency will reduce

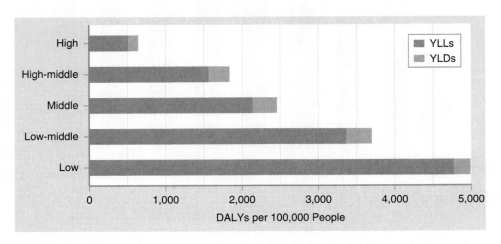

Figure 4.10 All-ages burden of disease attributed to air pollution per 100,000 people, by country sociodemographic group.

Data from GBD 2019 Risk Factors Collaborators. Global burden of 87 risk factors in 204 countries and territories, 1990–2019: a systematic analysis for the Global Burden of Disease Study 2019. *Lancet.* 2020;396:1223–1249.

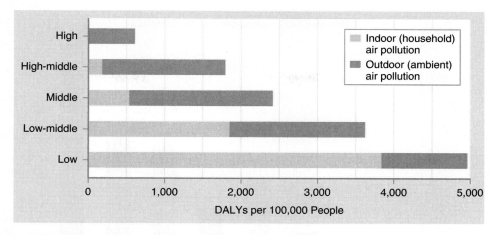

Figure 4.11 All-ages rate of the disability-adjusted life years (DALYs) attributed to indoor and outdoor air pollution per 100,000 people, by country sociodemographic group.

Data from GBD 2019 Risk Factors Collaborators. Global burden of 87 risk factors in 204 countries and territories, 1990–2019: a systematic analysis for the Global Burden of Disease Study 2019. *Lancet.* 2020;396:1223–1249.

the environmental damage that is likely to accompany further industrialization and intensified consumption (SDG 7.3).[38]

In high-income countries, contributions toward achieving SDG 7 will be made if a greater proportion of electricity is generated from renewable sources that release fewer emissions into the air (SDG 7.2). People in higher-income countries use more energy per person than people in lower-income countries,[39] so they also generate more air polluting emissions per person than less-industrialized countries. **Renewable energy** is energy derived from a source like wind or solar power that is not depleted when it is used. Wind, solar, ocean, geothermal, and other renewable sources of energy produce less environmental damage than combustible fossil fuel sources like oil and coal (**Figure 4.12**).[40] Most countries with high rates of electrification and high energy consumption generate only a small share of their current energy from renewable energy sources (**Figure 4.13**).[33] As renewable energy sources become more economical to install and manage, the proportion of energy generated from these sources is expected to increase significantly.

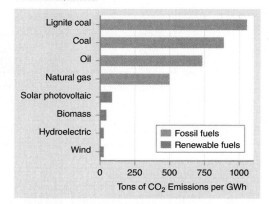

© Svetlana Eremina/Shutterstock

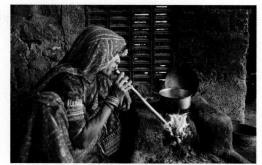

Figure 4.12 Renewable sources emit fewer greenhouse gases (CO_2 emissions per gigawatt hour [GWh]) than nonrenewable energy sources.

Data from *Comparison of Lifecycle Greenhouse Gas Emissions of Various Electricity Generation Sources.* London: World Nuclear Association; 2011.

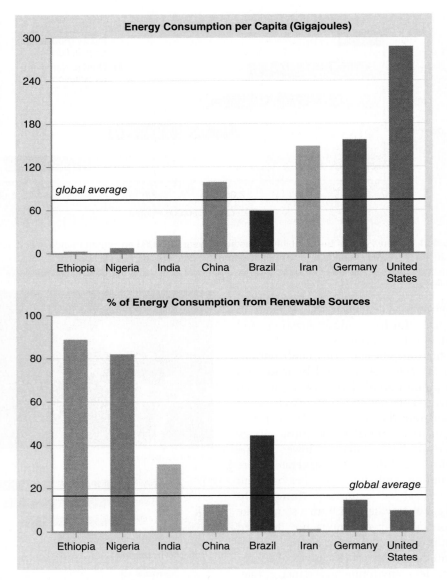

Figure 4.13 Use of renewable energy as a percentage of total consumption.

Data from *Tracking SDG 7: The Energy Progress Report 2020*. Washington DC: World Bank; 2020; and *Statistical Review of World Energy*. 69th ed. London: BP; 2020.

4.4 Occupational and Industrial Health

The field of **occupational health**, also called occupational safety, workplace health,

and a variety of other related names, is an applied public health field focused on primary prevention of injuries and other work-related health problems. Occupational health was one of the first public health specialty fields.[41] In 1713, Bernardino

Ramazzini published *Diseases of Workers*, a book that detailed the environmental hazards encountered in 52 occupations, listing poisoning, respiratory diseases, problems related to prolonged postures and repetitive tasks, and psychological stress as some of the many on-the-job threats to health. In 1753, James Lind published the results of an experiment that supported the hypothesis that sailors could prevent scurvy if they consumed citrus fruit during long journeys.[42] (After this discovery, sailors were sometimes called "limeys" for the citrus fruit carried on ships.) In 1775, Percivall Pott identified chimney soot as the cause of elevated rates of scrotal cancer in chimney sweeps who had constant exposure to coal tar due to rarely bathing or changing their trousers.[43] New occupational risks continue to be identified today.

Many workers are exposed to a mix of biological, chemical, physical, mechanical, and psychosocial challenges at work.[44] Some occupations carry risks specific to the type of work being done.[45] Workers exposed to loud noises are at risk of permanently impaired hearing. Office and factory workers have an increased risk of repetitive strain injuries, such as carpal tunnel syndrome, that can develop after repeatedly performing the same tasks. Some workers who have long-term exposure to industrial chemicals are at increased risk of developing certain types of cancers. Those who work in manufacturing may be at risk of crush wounds from moving parts. Medical workers are at risk of contracting infectious diseases from needle sticks and contact with body fluids. All workers may be subjected to stress that may impair mental health.[46]

Every year there are more than 350 million on-the-job injuries that are severe enough to keep the injured person away from work for at least four days.[47] An even larger number of workers experience disability from long-term exposures to workplace hazards. Occupational risks are estimated to be responsible for 24% of years lived with disability from low back pain, 17% of hearing loss, 12% of chronic respiratory diseases, and 11% of injuries worldwide.[8] Some workplace events and exposures cause injuries or chronic diseases that lead to early death. An estimated 1.9 million people die each year from adverse health conditions related to occupational exposures, including more than 450,000 who die from work-related chronic respiratory diseases, such as emphysema, asthma, and pneumoconiosis, which is caused by inhalation of silica, asbestos, coal dust, and other substances; more than 300,000 who die from occupational injuries; and more than 250,000 who die from lung cancer and other cancers attributed to workplace exposure to asbestos, other harmful substances, or radiation.[48]

Most occupational injuries, diseases, and deaths could be prevented if worksite managers and government officials enforced compliance with safety regulations.[49] **Industrial hygiene** is the process of assessing and mitigating workplace hazards. Specialists in industrial and occupational hygiene issue ear protection to workers in factories with high noise levels, make sure that people who spend their days in front of a computer have ergonomically designed chairs and are taking steps to minimize repetitive motion injuries, provide education about proper use of heavy machinery and hazardous materials, equip healthcare workers with personal protective equipment, provide wellness coaching, and work to reduce other risks specific to particular worksites.[50]

Toxicology is the study of the harmful effects that chemicals and other environmental materials can have on living things. Hazardous exposures in the workplace may include radiation, chemical pollutants, and toxic substances like polychlorinated biphenyls (PCBs), dioxins, asbestos, lead, mercury, cadmium, organic solvents, and pesticides. Many of these are released into the environment through industrial activities (**Figure 4.14**).[51] Chemicals and other substances produced, handled, stored, transported, or disposed of at work and chemicals released from work activities can pose both acute (immediate) and long-term health risks to people exposed to them. Toxicologists study the effect of exposure frequency (how often a person is exposed), duration (the length of exposure at a given time), and dose (the amount of hazardous substance contacted) on health. They also assess the various exposure routes (like inhalation, ingestion, and absorption through the skin) and pathways (through air, water, food, soil, or other mechanisms) related to hazardous exposures. A **carcinogen** is a substance that can cause genetic mutations that lead to cancer. A **teratogen** is a substance that can cause birth defects. Carcinogens, teratogens, and other hazards can be regulated or banned.

Hazardous substances cause an estimated 350,000 deaths worldwide each year, including about 240,000 deaths attributable to asbestos, 65,000 attributable to silica exposure, 20,000 attributable to diesel engine exhaust, and 10,000 attributable to arsenic.[8] Most of these deaths are due to cancer caused by exposure to a carcinogenic agent, but some are deaths from acute poisoning. Although hazardous substances are

Substance	Uses
Arsenic	Used to make "pressure-treated" lumber, as a pesticide for cotton plants, and in copper and lead smelting
Lead	Used in the production of batteries, ammunition, metal products (solder and pipes), and devices to shield X-rays; released from the burning of fossil fuels and during mining and manufacturing; used in some gasoline, paints, caulks, and ceramic products
Mercury	Used in thermometers, dental fillings, batteries, and some antiseptic creams and ointments
Vinyl chloride	Used to make polyvinyl chloride (PVC), plastic products like pipes, wire and cable coatings, and packaging materials
Polychlorinated biphenyls (PCBs)	Used as coolants and lubricants in transformers, capacitors, and other electrical equipment
Benzene	Used to make other chemicals that form plastics, resins, nylon and synthetic fibers, rubbers, lubricants, dyes, detergents, drugs, and pesticides
Cadmium	Extracted during the production of metals like zinc, lead, and copper for use in batteries, pigments, metal coatings, and plastics
Polycyclic aromatic hydrocarbons (PAHs), such as benzo(a)pyrene and benzo(b)fluoranthene	A group of more than 100 different chemicals that are formed during incomplete burning of coal, oil, gas, garbage, tobacco, charbroiled meat, and other organic substances; also found in coal tar, crude oil, creosote, roofing tar, some medicines and dyes, plastics, and pesticides

Figure 4.14 Examples of harmful substances at worksites.

Data from *ATSDR's substance priority list 2019*. Atlanta GA: U.S. Agency for Toxic Substances and Disease Registry; 2019.

used and produced in industrial settings in countries across the income spectrum, workers in lower-income countries have greater risks from occupational exposure. Many highly toxic substances that are heavily regulated or banned in high-income countries are still used in lower-income countries, and most workers in low-income countries where occupational regulations are rarely enforced do not have access to protective gear and safety training.[52] Furthermore, in some places where paid jobs are scarce, work that requires repeated exposure to dangerous chemicals may be seen as the only alternative to unemployment. The industries producing the most pollution-related health problems worldwide include used lead acid battery recycling, mining and ore processing, lead smelting, tannery operating, artisanal small-scale gold mining, industrial and municipal dumping, chemical and product manufacturing, and the dye industry.[53]

Ecotoxicology examines the impact of toxic exposures on populations, communities, and ecosystems. When an industrial disaster occurs, it often affects people who do not work at the site of the incident. The pollutants, toxins, and other substances released into air or water as a result of an industrial incident can affect the local community and may spread to a larger area. A gas leak at a chemical plant in Bhopal, India, in December 1984 released liquid and vapor methyl isocyanate. Several thousand people died when they were exposed to the fumes, some in their beds and others in the street after they staggered out of their homes to try to escape from the chemical. Hundreds of thousands of people sustained lung injuries.[54] The radioactivity released during the meltdown of the nuclear reactor at Chernobyl in Ukraine (then part of the USSR) in April 1986 spread a radioactive cloud across most of Europe. One health-related outcome of the meltdown was an increase in the incidence of thyroid cancer among children in the most contaminated regions.[55] Routine industrial practices may also put entire communities

at risk, especially in lower-income countries with few regulations to prevent environmental contamination.[52]

Chemical hazards in the home and community and at worksites can be especially dangerous for children who are still developing and growing. The risk of exposure to hazardous materials and other dangerous conditions is especially high for children who are sent to work at an early age. **Child labor** is violation of child rights that occurs when a child has an excessive workload, unsafe work conditions, or extreme work intensity. The International Labour Organization (ILO) makes a distinction between acceptable participation of children in economic activity and unacceptable employment of children as laborers.[56] Economic activity consists of working (for pay or not) on activities other than household chores or schooling. Rural children are allowed to work alongside their parents on the family farm. It is permissible for children aged 12 years and older to spend a few hours per week doing light paid work that is not hazardous, and older children are permitted to work longer hours. However, it is not acceptable for children to spend long hours doing agricultural work, domestic labor, or factory work that harms their physical health, mental health, or moral development. At worst, a child may be sold by his or her family into bonded labor, forced into sex work, or forced into armed conflict. In 2000, about 16% of all children between 5 and

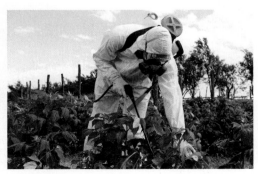

© Hedgehog94/Shutterstock

17 years old were engaged in child labor, about 245 million children total.[57] Today, less than 10% of children are engaged in child labor, but there are still about 150 million children doing child labor, including more than 70 million children who are doing hazardous work.[58]

Both SDG 8 and SDG 9 include targets that focus on occupational health. SDG 8 aims to end child labor (SDG 8.7) and "promote safe and secure working environments for all workers" (SDG 8.8), and SDG 9 aims to "build resilient infrastructure, promote inclusive and sustainable industrialization, and foster innovation" with "increased resource-use efficiency and greater adoption of clean and environmentally sound technologies and industrial processes" (SDG 9.4).[11] Many countries from all income levels have enacted occupational and environmental health and safety laws,[59] but meeting the SDG targets will require more attention on occupational health and safety, including protecting children from harmful labor, preventing workplace injuries and work-related diseases and disabilities, and safeguarding the health and safety of communities located near industrial sites.

4.5 Urbanization

Urbanicity is the degree to which a particular location is urban, and it is a function of total population size, density, diversity, and access to city services like retail facilities and public transportation.[60] Urbanicity is the opposite of **rurality**, the degree to which a particular location is rural. The percentage of the world's people who live in urban areas grew from about 30% in 1950 to 39% in 1980, 47% in 2000, and 56% in 2020, and it is expected to rise to about 68% by 2050 (**Figure 4.15**).[61]

The governments of large population centers are responsible for supporting public health in their cities by maintaining a safe built environment, managing water and sanitation services, disposing of waste, minimizing pollutants,

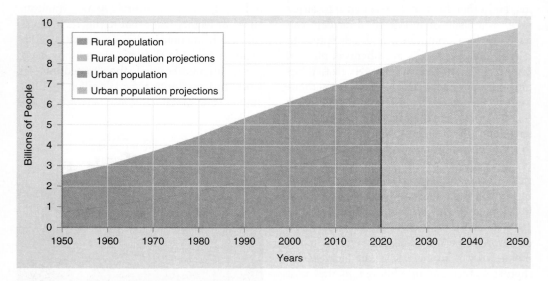

Figure 4.15 World urban and rural population estimates, 1950–2050.

Data from United Nations Department of Economic and Social Affairs. *World Urbanization Prospects: The 2018 Revision.* New York: United Nations; 2018.

providing access to parks and other recreational areas, and ensuring access to health and social services.[62] On average, urban residents have greater access than rural residents to safe drinking water and sanitation facilities, a relatively reliable public transportation system, and healthcare providers and health technologies. Electricity in cities reduces cooking time and makes it easier to store food safely. Communications systems broadcast news and entertainment shows as well as emergency warnings and health messages. There are more opportunities to pursue additional education and find employment outside the home in cities than in rural areas. Pregnancy in cities is safer because of greater access to antenatal care and assistance by medical professionals during delivery, and similar benefits extend to other acute infections and injuries that require urgent care as well as chronic diseases that benefit from frequent monitoring by clinicians.

However, the benefits of urbanicity are not available to all urban residents (**Figure 4.16**). Many people who move to cities end up living in unplanned settlements (sometimes called shantytowns, slums, or squatter camps) where the quality of life is generally worse than rural life.[63] In low- and middle-income countries, clusters of temporary structures are often quickly erected at the outskirts of large cities to accommodate rural-to-urban migrants. The structures are often built with cardboard or scraps of metal, wood, or other found objects, and they may provide little comfort or privacy and only minimal protection from the sun, rain, wind, and other elements. These dwellings may eventually be replaced with shacks built from blocks or bricks with a tin or asbestos roof or with sturdier houses constructed from cement, but many more years may pass before these growing communities have access to critical utilities. Informal dwellings are often built in floodplains or on other vulnerable lands, and they usually lack drainage and sewer systems. During storms, floodwaters may carry feces and other waste into homes. Trash and human waste might collect near homes and attract rodents and insects, increasing the risk of infectious diseases. Cooking with solid fuels generates high levels

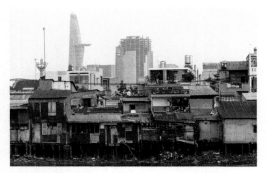

© Stephane Bidouze/Shutterstock

of air indoor pollution, and unplanned communities in urbanizing cities are often located in undesirable locations near noisy and polluted highways or industrial centers that generate outdoor air pollution at levels that exacerbate asthma and cardiovascular conditions. Urban workers may face new occupational hazards and might not have access to affordable emergency healthcare services. Violence related to crowding and road traffic accidents (often of the motor vehicle versus pedestrian variety) might occur often.[64] It might be difficult to grow or purchase nutritious foods, and there may be little time or space for exercising.

Despite the challenges of daily life in unplanned urban areas, thousands of people each day move from rural areas to cities in search of higher incomes, better jobs, more social opportunities, and greater conveniences. **Urbanization** is a shift toward more people living in cities and fewer people living in rural areas.[65] In nearly every country, the proportion of the population that lives in cities is increasing and is expected to continue to rise (**Figure 4.17**).[61] In lower-income countries, both rural and urban populations are growing due to high birth rates and increasing life expectancies, but there is so much rural-to-urban migration that the urban population is growing much faster than the rural population (**Figure 4.18**).[61] This process of urbanization affects both urban and rural residents. Rural women may bear a heavy burden when their husbands move to

Sector	Rural	Unplanned Urban	Planned Urban
Water	■ May have minimal access to improved water sources ■ Risk of microbial contamination	■ May have minimal access to affordable clean water ■ Risk of microbial exposure and industrial and agricultural chemical contamination	■ Reliable access to safe, clean drinking water
Sanitation	■ May have inadequate sanitation facilities ■ Open defecation in a field away from the house may be common	■ May have inadequate sanitation facilities ■ Open defecation in the street may be common	■ Sewage system
Trash disposal	■ Solid waste is burned or buried	■ No collection of solid waste ■ Trash heaps create a habitat for insect and rodent vectors	■ Solid waste is collected and removed
Chemical hazards	■ Potential exposure to agrochemicals like fertilizer and pesticides	■ Potential exposure to industrial waste	■ Little exposure to industrial or agricultural hazards
Fuel	■ Solid fuels, which may be able to be collected locally	■ Solid fuels, which may be expensive	■ Electricity
Air quality	■ Indoor air pollution from burning biomass	■ Both indoor and outdoor air pollution ■ Noise pollution	■ Some outdoor air pollution ■ Some indoor air pollution from building materials
Nutrition	■ May have limited ability to purchase food ■ Can usually grow, gather, or hunt for food	■ May have limited access to afford-able, healthy foods ■ May not have space for a garden	■ Adequate access to healthy and safe dietary choices
Health facilities	■ Facilities may be far from home and may provide only basic care	■ Facilities may be crowded and understaffed	■ Basic, emergency, and specialty healthcare (including mental health and rehabilitation) facilities are available

Figure 4.16 Comparison of health risks associated with living in rural, unplanned urban, and planned urban areas.

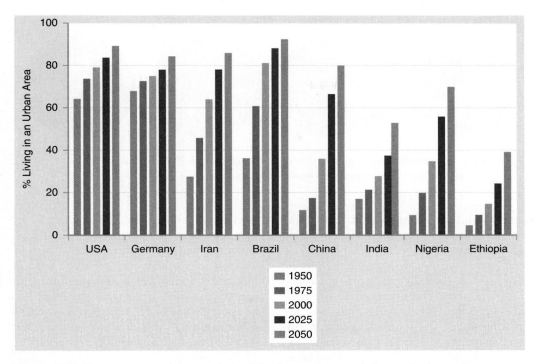

Figure 4.17 The percentage of the population living in an urban area is increasing in nearly every country and is projected to continue to increase.

Data from United Nations Department of Economic and Social Affairs. *World Urbanization Prospects: The 2018 Revision.* New York: United Nations; 2018.

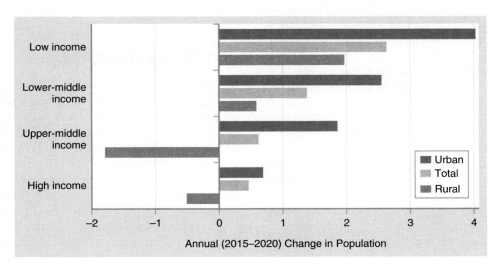

Figure 4.18 Average annual rate of change in the size of urban and rural populations between 2015 and 2020, by country income level.

Data from United Nations Department of Economic and Social Affairs. *World Urbanization Prospects: The 2018 Revision.* New York: United Nations; 2018.

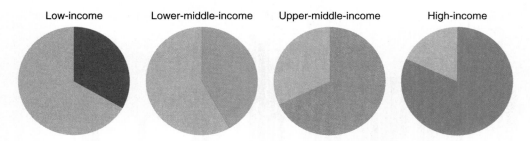

Figure 4.19 Percentage of the population living in an urban area in 2020, by country income level.

Data from United Nations Department of Economic and Social Affairs. *World Urbanization Prospects: The 2018 Revision.* New York: United Nations; 2018.

cities to find wage employment, leaving the women with the responsibility of completing all household chores. Parents who move to a city may have to leave their children in the care of rural-dwelling grandparents, which puts a strain on three generations. In higher-income countries, urban populations are growing while rural populations shrink. This is exacerbating inequalities in income and access to health services between urban areas, where most work is in the service sector, and rural areas, where agriculture remains the dominant sector.

A **megacity** is a metropolitan area with 10 million or more inhabitants. The number of megacities increased from 10 in 1990 to 29 in 2015 and is expected to rise to 41 by 2030.[66] Although high-income countries have the most urbanized populations (**Figure 4.19**), nearly all megacities are located in middle-income countries.[61] A metacity (or hypercity) is a megacity with 20 million or more residents. Several cities are at or near that size already, including Tokyo, Japan; Delhi, India; Shanghai, China; São Paulo, Brazil; Mexico City; Cairo, Egypt; Mumbai, India; Beijing, China; and Dhaka, Bangladesh. By 2030, Kinshasa, in the Democratic Republic of Congo; Lagos, Nigeria; and Karachi, Pakistan, are likely to be added to this list. Only one metacity is in a high-income country. Megacities and metacities in low- and middle-income countries often experience major challenges associated with rapid

population growth that is not matched by increased resources for social, educational, environmental, and health services.[67]

SDG 11 has an aim of "making cities and human settlements inclusive, safe, resilient, and sustainable" through targets related to housing (SDG 11.1), transportation (SDG 11.2), air quality and waste management (SDG 11.6), and open public spaces (SDG 11.7).[11] Because the majority of the world's people live in cities, urban health is a core component of global public health.[68] As the world urbanizes, the ability to achieve global health goals will depend on cities being healthy.[69]

4.6 Sustainability

Sustainability is a concept that emphasizes the need to provide for current human needs without compromising the ability of future generations to meet their needs.[70] Sustainability is central to the SDGs, which aim to reduce poverty and disease for today's people while ensuring that future generations inherit a healthy planet that allows them to enjoy long, healthy lives.[71] Sustainable development promotes economic growth while simultaneously protecting the environment from the adverse effects that typically accompany industrialization.[72] Sustainability has previously been described as a combination of "3 Es": ethics (or equity), environment, and economics.[73] In the SDGs, these concepts have been expanded to include "5 Ps": people, planet, prosperity (or profit), peace, and partnership.[11] People/ethics, planet/environment, and prosperity/economics are dependent on stable nations (peace) and are best able to be achieved through global collaboration (partnerships).

Sustainability principles are integrated into all 17 SDG goals, but SDG 12 has a specific focus on "ensuring sustainable consumption and production patterns" through targets related to management of natural resources (SDG 12.2), reduction of food waste (SDG 12.3), management of hazardous waste (SDG 12.4), and improvements in recycling and reuse (SDG 12.5).[11] Concerns about environmental protection and the prudent use of natural resources have increased in recent decades as human population growth accelerated. The potential dangers of population growth can be illustrated by comparing Earth to an island. Picture a small island in the middle of an ocean. At first, 10 people settle on the island. They build homes, develop a system for collecting fresh water (because ocean water is too salty to drink or use for irrigation), and begin to farm the land. They also begin to have children, and eventually those

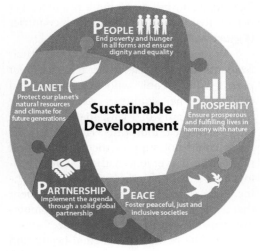

children have children. Soon the population has reached 100, and then it grows to 1,000. The amount of land available for farming decreases as more homes are built, but the need for food is greater because there are more people who need to eat. Access to drinking water on the island may become a source of conflict as more people compete for a finite resource. Water quality may decrease as waste pollutes water sources. Solid energy sources may become depleted as demand for energy increases. Some plant and animal species may be threatened and at risk of disappearing from the island due to overharvesting and habitat destruction. These types of environmental health challenges could be expected to become even worse as the population continues to grow.

Overpopulation occurs when a population becomes so large that the amount of food and other environmental resources available are insufficient to support all members of the population. In 1798, Thomas Malthus hypothesized that overpopulation leads to catastrophes like famines, epidemics, and wars.[74] In the 21st century, this idea is expressed in terms of concerns about the unequal distribution of food and natural resources, the risks associated with the increased pollution and congestion that will occur with continued population growth, and the likelihood of increased crime and conflict as resources in some regions of the world become scarce. For example, many countries are already facing water scarcity crises, especially small island nations and desert countries where internal freshwater resources are extremely limited, and water wars are seen as a possibility in the coming decades as more people compete for control over the world's finite supply of the fresh water that is essential for survival.[75]

The size of the human population remained relatively steady for millennia, but recent growth has been exponential. A plot of the world's population shows a "J-shaped" growth pattern (**Figure 4.20**).[76] It took only

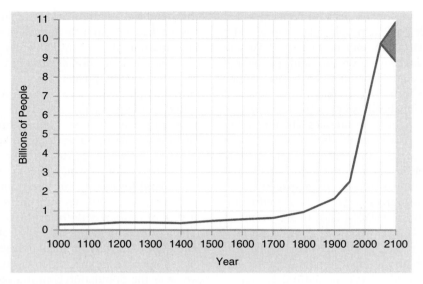

Figure 4.20 The "J-shaped curve" for world population growth.

Data from United Nations Department of Economic and Social Affairs. *World Population to 2300*. New York: United Nations; 2004; United Nations Department of Economic and Social Affairs. *World Population Prospects: The 2019 Revision*. New York: United Nations; 2019; GBD 2019 Demographics Collaborators. Global age-sex-specific fertility, mortality, health life expectancy (HALE), and population estimates in 204 countries and territories, 1950–2019: a comprehensive demographic analysis for the Global Burden of Disease Study 2019. *Lancet*. 2020;396:1160–1203; Vollset SE, Goren E, Yuan CW, et al. Fertility, mortality, migration, and population scenarios for 195 countries and territories from 2017 to 2100: a forecasting analysis for the Global Burden of Disease Study. *Lancet*. 2020;396:1285–1306.

40 years—from 1950 until 1990—for the number of humans to double from 2.5 billion to 5 billion. The current world population is approaching 8 billion, and demographers project that the global population may rise to nearly 10 billion by 2050 and up to 11 billion by 2100.[77] The population is expected to stabilize after that time, but it might also grow or shrink depending on numerous socioeconomic and environmental factors that will unfold over the coming decades.[78]

Carrying capacity is the maximum human population the Earth can sustain. There is no easy way to calculate the carrying capacity because it depends on the standard of living and cultural factors in addition to population density (measured as land area per person or as arable land area per person, which includes only farmable land in the estimation), climate, and the land and natural resources that are available. However, carrying capacity can be approximated based on estimations of the per capita area of land

needed to meet a population's consumption patterns. One example of this type of metric is the **ecological footprint**, which measures how much burden human consumption places on the biosphere. People in high-income countries have large ecological footprints and use many more resources per person than people in low-income countries (**Figure 4.21**).[79]

As countries' economies grow, their residents tend to use more resources per person. Most people who live in low- and middle-income countries aspire to the higher standards of living that come with larger ecological footprints. However, Earth likely could not support the current world population if everyone had the typical ecological footprint of today's residents of high-income countries. Economic development that depletes natural resources and promotes overconsumption is not sustainable,[80] and it can generate new environmental health and population health problems.

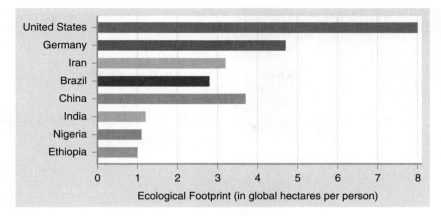

Figure 4.21 Ecological footprints per capita (in units of global hectares).

Data from *National Footprint and Biocapacity Accounts 2021*. Oakland CA: Global Footprint Network; 2021.

4.7 Ecosystem Health

Ecology describes the relationships of living things to one another and the environments in which they live. An **ecosystem**, or ecological system, consists of all the living things that share a particular environment, including animals, plants, and microorganisms. Some ecosystems are terrestrial (land based), like forests, grasslands, and deserts. Some are aquatic, like oceans, lakes, and rivers. All of the living (biotic) organisms in an ecosystem are dependent on one another and on the nonliving (abiotic) components of the ecosystem, such as its geological formations and weather systems. A sustainable ecosystem maintains its structure and function over time. This often involves deriving energy from the sun; using energy and nutrients to produce biomass; and cycling carbon, oxygen, nitrogen, phosphorus, and other elements so they can be reused. **Biodiversity** is the presence of a wide variety of plant and animal species within a particular ecosystem. A sustainable ecosystem can maintain its biodiversity and level of productivity indefinitely.

Ecosystem services are the benefits that humans receive from various ecosystems. They include provisioning services like fresh water, food, and fuel; regulation services such as pollination, decomposition, and flood control; cultural services such as artistic inspiration and recreational opportunities; and supporting services like photosynthesis, soil formation, nutrient cycling, and water cycling.[81] Many of these functions are essential for human survival. Global health partnerships have tended to focus on human health without adequately considering the dependency of human health on ecosystem health. Humans are dependent on plants and animals for food, so human lives are threatened when agricultural crops, livestock, wildlife, and ecosystems are harmed by environmental degradation and disease.

The **One Health** concept emphasizes the interconnectedness of human health, animal health, and ecosystem health.[82] The One Health model is most often applied when working to prevent and control the infectious diseases that cycle between humans, domestic animals, and wildlife.[83] For example, influenza viruses are routinely exchanged between humans, domestic and wild birds, pigs, and other animals, and the recent epidemics of Ebola and COVID-19 likely originated when viruses circulating in animal populations crossed species and began causing human

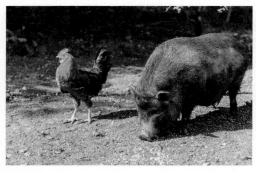

© Lightix/Shutterstock

disease. Many infectious diseases of animals have the potential to spill over into human populations,[84] so changes in animal behaviors and animal health associated with habitat degradation, biodiversity loss, pollution, and climate change can also become threats to human health.[85]

The emerging field of **planetary health** emphasizes the dependence of human health on the Earth and seeks to understand the damage that human actions impose on ecosystem health.[86] Threats to the health of the planet include habitat loss and degradation, species overexploitation, invasive plant and animal species that crowd out native species in a location, the dissemination of pathogens in new areas due to human transportation systems, pollution, and climate change.[87] Humans can support planetary health by preserving and restoring natural resources, producing energy and goods more efficiently and less wastefully, and utilizing resources more wisely.[88]

In a globalized world, everyone has a stake in contributing to planetary health.[89] Individuals can reduce their consumption of energy and consumer goods, reuse items when possible, recycle products that are no longer usable, and rethink the actions that increase their ecological footprints. Communities and corporations can conduct risk–benefit assessments for planned activities that include health and environmental evaluations, as well as economic ones, so that informed decisions

can be made.[90] Governments can formulate strategic plans that protect both population and ecosystem health.[91] Millions of local decisions to support ecosystem health will add up to actions that enable planetary health.

4.8 Climate Change and Health

At the local level, it is easy to observe the impact of human actions that alter the environment. Erecting buildings, installing electrical lines and sewers, and paving streets usually improves the quality of life for local residents, but these environmental changes typically result in the loss of undeveloped and recreational areas. Cutting down forests to create farmland, operating surface mines, and extracting fossil fuels may generate resources that are valuable to humans, but these activities can permanently damage local ecosystems. Any intentional change to the local environment may have some expected and unexpected side effects that adversely affect human health.[92] For example, building a dam may prevent flooding and improve agricultural productivity, but having a larger body of water nearby may increase the risk of some parasitic and insect-transmitted infections.[93]

The immediate effects of most human activities are local, but the distinction between local and global environmental change is getting blurrier.[94] In a globalized world, the choices any person makes about where to live, work, and travel and what to purchase can have an impact on people who live in distant lands. The air pollution created by millions of commuters driving to work each day in one city does not just damage their airspace but also that of their neighbors. When electronic waste (e-waste) and other types of garbage are discarded by people in high-income countries, the potentially toxic materials may be shipped to dumps in lower-income countries.[95] Deforestation and habitat destruction, soil erosion and salinization, water management problems, overhunting and overfishing, invasive species (which may crowd out local flora and fauna), human population growth, and increasing use of resources per capita can all have global as well as local impacts.[96]

Climate change is a long-term shift in weather patterns and average temperatures. The **Intergovernmental Panel on Climate Change (IPCC)** is a scientific board that reviews and synthesizes scientific data about climate and weather under the auspices of the United Nations. The IPCC has expressed certainty that global climate changes are occurring and will continue to occur for centuries to come.[97] The IPCC has also concluded that the observed changes in recent decades are very likely due to human activity,[98] such as the intensified use of natural resources across the planet.

While cycles of climate change have occurred throughout history, the rapid rate at which observable changes are occurring now is concerning.[99] The impacts of global climate change include land degradation, water and air quality issues, biodiversity loss, and temperature and precipitation extremes. The IPCC predicts that climate change will mean more frequent hot days and nights, fewer cold days and nights, an increasing frequency of heat waves, an increase in the frequency of heavy precipitation events in some areas and an increase in droughts in others, an increase in tropical cyclone (hurricane) activity, and an increase in the incidence of extremely high sea levels (**Figure 4.22**).[100]

Many of these expected climate changes could have significant adverse impacts on human health (**Figure 4.23**).[101] Extreme heat increases the rate of cardiovascular disease mortality.[102] Extreme precipitation events increase the risk of drowning and other types of injuries. Ecosystem changes can increase the risks of insect-borne infections, diarrheal diseases, and respiratory diseases associated with having more particulates and pollen in the air.[103] Floods, droughts, heat waves, and other weather extremes might also reduce agricultural productivity, and ocean acidification might reduce aquacultural productivity, leading to greater levels of food insecurity.[104] The negative impacts of climate change are likely to be especially detrimental to the world's lowest-income people, who often live in places with greater environmental vulnerability and fewer resources to prepare for and respond to extreme weather events.[105] This may lead to mass involuntary migration as some places become unsuitable for human habitation. More than 200 million people may be displaced by climate change between 2020 and 2050.[106]

One component of climate change is **global warming**, a gradual increase in the temperature of the Earth's atmosphere. A **greenhouse gas** (GHG) is a gas in the atmosphere that traps heat and causes

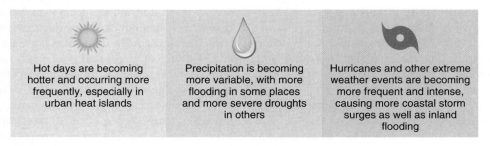

Hot days are becoming hotter and occurring more frequently, especially in urban heat islands

Precipitation is becoming more variable, with more flooding in some places and more severe droughts in others

Hurricanes and other extreme weather events are becoming more frequent and intense, causing more coastal storm surges as well as inland flooding

Figure 4.22 Examples of hazards associated with climate change.

Data from Field CB, Barros VR, Mastrandrea MD, et al., eds. *Climate Change 2014: Impacts, Adaptation, and Vulnerability. Contribution of Working Group II to the 5th Assessment Report of the Intergovernmental Panel on Climate Change.* Cambridge UK: Cambridge University Press; 2014.

Direct impacts of climate and weather on health	■ Increased rate of heat-related mortality from cardiovascular, respiratory, and kidney diseases exacerbated by heat waves ■ Increased risk of drowning from floods ■ Increased risk of injury from wildfires
Health impacts of ecosystem changes	■ Increased risk of vector-borne (insect- and arachnid-transmitted) infectious diseases, such as malaria, dengue fever, and tick-borne diseases ■ Increased risk of food- and waterborne infections, such as cholera ■ Increased risk of allergies and respiratory diseases associated with decreased air quality
Health impacts of economic and social disruption	■ Increased risk of undernutrition from diminished food production ■ Decreased mental health associated with higher levels of stress ■ Increased violence and conflict from population displacement ■ Decreased labor productivity associated with heat exhaustion

Figure 4.23 Examples of the likely impacts of climate change on human health.

Data from Smith KR, Woodward A, Campbell-Lendrum D, et al., Human health: impacts, adaptation, and co-benefits (chapter 11). In: Field CB, Barros VR, Mastrandrea MD, et al., eds. *Climate Change 2014: Impacts, Adaptation, and Vulnerability. Contribution of Working Group II to the 5th Assessment Report of the Intergovernmental Panel on Climate Change.* Cambridge UK: Cambridge University Press; 2014:709–754.

surface temperatures to increase. The GHGs of greatest concern include carbon dioxide (CO_2), methane (CH_4), nitrous oxide (N_2O), and fluorinated gases such as sulfur hexafluoride (SF_6), hydrofluorocarbons, and perfluorocarbons. The United Nations **Framework Convention on Climate Change (FCCC)** is an international environmental treaty that seeks to reduce greenhouse gas emissions.[107] The FCCC was negotiated in 1992 at the United Nations Conference on Environment and Development, colloquially called the Earth Summit, which was held in Rio de Janeiro, Brazil, and went into force in 1994. The 1997 Kyoto Protocol sought to toughen the FCCC commitments to reduce GHG emissions by the high-income signatory countries that generate the most emissions.[108] The 2015 Paris Agreement is a legally binding set of additional commitments from signatories across the income spectrum to reduce global warming and promote development that does not further exacerbate environmental damage.[109]

Other international agreements have also sought to combat climate change. For example, three of the SDGs tackle macro-level concerns about global environmental health: SDG 13 aims to "take urgent action to combat climate change and its impacts," with a focus on strengthening resilience to respond to "climate-related hazards and natural disasters" (SDG 13.1); SDG 14 aims to "conserve and sustainably use the oceans, seas, and marine resources"; and SDG 15 aims to "protect, restore, and promote sustainable use of terrestrial ecosystems, sustainably manage forests, combat desertification, and halt and reverse land degradation and halt biodiversity loss."[11]

Regardless of arguments about the precise causes of global warming and other aspects of climate change, the alarming trends documented by the IPCC support the value of humans treading more lightly on the Earth.[110] For example, alternative energy sources that harness solar, wind, or wave power may be able to produce energy that creates less pollution and less ecosystem damage than carbon-based fuels, hydroelectric power (which requires the building of massive dams and flooding of large swaths of land), and nuclear power (which remains dangerous because of the risk of a meltdown). Even if global climate change was not happening—though scientists agree that it is—cleaner air and ecosystem conservation are good for human and environmental health.

The predictions about the likely impacts of climate change are horrific:

Arctic habitats lost, coral reefs destroyed, islands and coastal areas submerged due to sea level rise, mass extinction, and other traumas. This can make it seem like the situation is a hopeless one, but it is still possible for these trajectories to be slowed and perhaps even reversed. When a hole in the ozone layer was discovered over the Antarctic region in the 1980s, there was widespread concern that this stratospheric barrier that absorbs much of the sun's ultraviolet radiation had been irreversibly damaged. Countries around the world quickly pledged to reduce production of the industrial chlorofluorocarbons (CFCs) that were driving this change. Since then, the ozone hole has begun to heal.[111] While global climate change is a more complex issue—one that includes the ozone layer as just one of many interconnected, urgent concerns—it is possible to achieve shared global environmental health goals if people from across the globe choose to work together to solve these pressing issues.

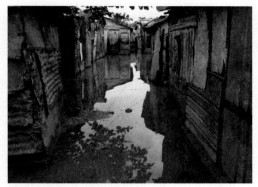

CDC/ Venecia Ramírez, Dominican Republic

References

1. Susser M, Susser E. Choosing a future for epidemiology: I. eras and paradigms. *Am J Public Health*. 1996;86:668–673.

2. Bingham P, Verlander NQ, Cheal MJ. John Snow, William Farr and the 1849 outbreak of cholera that affected London: a reworking of the data highlights the importance of the water supply. *Public Health*. 2004;118:387–394.

3. Shryock RH. The early American public health movement. *Am J Public Health*.1937;27:965–971.

4. Gochfeld M, Goldstein BD. Lessons in environmental health in the twentieth century. *Annu Rev Public Health*. 1999;20:35–53.

5. Pearce N. Traditional epidemiology, modern epidemiology, and public health. *Am J Public Health*. 1996;86:678-683.

6. Doll R, Hill AB. Lung cancer and other causes of death in relation to smoking. *Br Med J*.1956;2:1071–1081.

7. Hackshaw AK, Law MR, Wald NJ. The accumulated evidence on lung cancer and environmental tobacco smoke. *BMJ*. 1997;315:980–988.

8. GBD 2019 Risk Factors Collaborators. Global burden of 87 risk factors in 204 countries and territories, 1990–2019: a systematic analysis for the Global Burden of Disease Study 2019. *Lancet*. 2020;396:1223–1249.

9. Prüss-Ustün A, Wolf J, Corvalán C, Bos R, Neira M. *Preventing Disease Through Healthy Environments: A Global Assessment of the Burden of Disease from Environmental Risks*. Geneva: World Health Organization; 2016.

10. *Compendium of WHO and Other United Nations Guidance on Health and Environment*. Geneva: World Health Organization; 2021.

11. *Transforming Our World: The 2030 Agenda for Sustainable Development*. New York: United Nations; 2015.

12. United Nations Economic and Social Council. *Report of the Inter-Agency and Expert Group on Sustainable Development Goal Indicators (E/CN.3/2021/2)*. New York: United Nations; 2021.

13. Howard G, Bartram J. *Domestic Water Quantity, Service Level and Health*. Geneva: World Health Organization; 2003.

14. *Safer Water, Better Health*. Geneva: World Health Organization; 2019.

15. *Guidelines for Drinking-Water Quality: Fourth Edition Incorporating the First Addendum*. Geneva: World Health Organization; 2017.

16. *Water for Life: Community Water Security*. New York: Hesperian Foundation and United Nations Development Programme; 2005.

17. Dieter CA, Maupin MA, Caldwell RR, et al. *Estimated Use of Water in the United States in 2015*. Reston VA: U.S. Geological Survey; 2018.

18. *Progress on Sanitation and Drinking Water: 2015 Update and MDG Assessment.* New York: UNICEF/World Health Organization Joint Monitoring Programme for Water Supply and Sanitation; 2015.

19. *Guidelines on Sanitation and Health.* Geneva: World Health Organization; 2018.

20. *Preventing Diarrhoea Through Better Water, Sanitation and Hygiene: Exposures and Impacts in Low- and Middle-Income Countries.* Geneva: World Health Organization; 2014.

21. Kar K, Chambers R. *Handbook on Community-Led Total Sanitation.* London: Plan UK; 2008.

22. Mara D, Lane J, Scott B, Trouba D. Sanitation and health. *PLoS Med.* 2010;7:e1000363.

23. Watkins D, Dabestani N, Nugent R, Levin C. Interventions to prevent injuries and reduce environmental and occupational hazards: a review of economic evaluations from low- and middle-income countries (chapter 10). In: Mock CN, Nugent R, Kobusingye O, Smith KR, eds. *Disease Control Priorities: Injury Prevention and Environmental Health.* Vol. 7. 3rd ed. Washington DC: IBRD/World Bank; 2017:199–211.

24. Hutton G, Chase C. Water supply, sanitation, and hygiene (chapter 9). In: Mock CN, Nugent R, Kobusingye O, Smith KR, eds. *Disease Control Priorities: Injury Prevention and Environmental Health.* Vol. 7. 3rd ed. Washington DC: IBRD/World Bank; 2017:171–198.

25. *Progress on Household Drinking Water, Sanitation and Hygiene, 2000–2020: Five Years into the SDGs.* New York: World Health Organization/UNICEF Joint Monitoring Programme for Water Supply and Sanitation; 2021.

26. *State of the World's Sanitation: An Urgent Call to Transform Sanitation for Better Health, Environments, Economies and Societies.* New York: UNICEF/World Health Organization; 2020.

27. *WHO Water, Sanitation and Hygiene Strategy 2018–2025.* Geneva: World Health Organization; 2018.

28. Kampa M, Castanas E. Human health effects of air pollution. *Environ Pollut.* 2008;151:362–367.

29. Brunekreef B, Holgate ST. Air pollution and health. *Lancet.* 2002;360:1233–1242.

30. *WHO Global Air Quality Guidelines: Particulate Matter (PM2.5 and PM10), Ozone, Nitrogen Dioxide, Sulfur Dioxide and Carbon Monoxide.* Geneva: World Health Organization; 2021.

31. Gordon SB, Bruce NG, Grigg J, et al. Respiratory risks from household air pollution in low and middle income countries. *Lancet Respir Med.* 2014;2:823–860.

32. *Burning Opportunity: Clean Household Energy for Health, Sustainable Development, and Wellbeing of Women and Children.* Geneva: World Health Organization; 2016.

33. *Tracking SDG 7: The Energy Progress Report 2020.* Washington DC: World Bank; 2020.

34. Landrigan PJ, Fuller R, Acosta NJR, et al. The Lancet Commission on pollution and health. *Lancet.* 2018;391:462–512.

35. Smith KR, Pillarisetti A. Household air pollution from solid cookfuels and health (chapter 7). In: Mock CN, Nugent R, Kobusingye O, Smith KR, eds. *Disease Control Priorities: Injury Prevention and Environmental Health.* Vol. 7. 3rd ed. Washington DC: IBRD/World Bank; 2017:133–152.

36. Wilkinson P, Smith KR, Joffe M, Haines A. A global perspective on energy: health effects and injustices. *Lancet.* 2007;370:965–978.

37. Ezzati M, Bailis R, Kammen DM, et al. Energy management and global health. *Annu Rev Environ Resour.* 2004;29:383–419.

38. Haines A, Smith KR, Anderson D, et al. Policies for accelerating access to clean energy, improving health, advancing development, and mitigating climate change. *Lancet.* 2007;370:1264–1281.

39. *Statistical Review of World Energy.* 69th ed. London: BP; 2020.

40. *Comparison of Lifecycle Greenhouse Gas Emissions of Various Electricity Generation Sources.* London: World Nuclear Association; 2011.

41. Abrams HK. A short history of occupational health. *J Public Health Policy.* 2001;22:34–80.

42. Hughes RE. James Lind and the cure of scurvy: an experimental approach. *Med Hist.* 1975;19:342–351.

43. Waldron HA. A brief history of scrotal cancer. *Br J Ind Med.* 1983;40:390–401.

44. Abdalla S, Apramian S, Cantley L, Cullen M. Occupation and risk for injuries (chapter 6). In: Mock CN, Nugent R, Kobusingye O, Smith KR, eds. *Disease Control Priorities: Injury Prevention and Environmental Health.* Vol. 7. 3rd ed. Washington DC: IBRD/World Bank; 2017:97–132.

45. *Encyclopaedia of Occupational Health & Safety.* 4th ed. Geneva: International Labour Organization; 1998.

46. Leka S, Jain A. *Health Impact of the Psychosocial Hazards of Work: An Overview.* Geneva: World Health Organization; 2010.

47. *Time to Act for SDG 8: Integrating Decent Work, Sustained Growth and Environmental Integrity.* Geneva: International Labour Organization; 2019.

48. *WHO/ILO Joint Estimates of the Work-Related Burden of Disease and Injury, 2000–2016.* Geneva: World Health Organization/International Labour Organization; 2021.

49. Wolf J, Prüss-Ustün A, Ivanov I, et al. *Preventing Disease Through a Healthier and Safer Workplace.* Geneva: World Health Organization; 2018.

50. *A 5 Step Guide for Employers, Workers and Their Representatives on Conducting Workplace Risk Assessments.* Geneva: International Labour Organization; 2014.

51. *2019 ATSDR Substance Priority List*. Atlanta GA: U.S. Agency for Toxic Substances and Disease Registry; 2019.

52. *Pollution Knows No Borders: How the Pollution Crisis in Low- and Middle-Income Countries Affects Everyone's Health, and What We Can Do to Address It*. New York: Pure Earth; 2019.

53. *The World's Worst Pollution Problems 2016: The Toxics Beneath Our Feet*. New York: Pure Earth; 2016.

54. Mehta PS, Mehta AS, Mehta SJ, Makhijani AB. Bhopal tragedy's health effects: a review of methyl isocyanate toxicity. *JAMA*. 1990;265:2781–2787.

55. Shibata Y, Yamashita S, Masyakin VB, Panasyuk GD, Nagataki S. 15 years after Chernobyl: new evidence of thyroid cancer. *Lancet*. 2001;358:1965–1966.

56. *Ending Child Labour by 2025: A Review of Policies and Programmes*. Geneva: International Labour Organization; 2018.

57. *Marking Progress Against Child Labour: Global Estimates and Trends 2000–2012*. Geneva: International Labour Organization; 2013.

58. *Global Estimates of Child Labour: Results and Trends, 2012–2016*. Geneva: International Labour Organization; 2017.

59. *WHO Global Plan of Action on Workers' Health (2008–2017): Baseline for Implementation*. Geneva: World Health Organization; 2013.

60. Dahly DL, Adair LS. Quantifying the urban environment: a scale measure of urbanicity outperforms the urban-rural dichotomy. *Soc Sci Med*. 2007;64:1407–1419.

61. United Nations Department of Economic and Social Affairs. *World Urbanization Prospects: The 2018 Revision*. New York: United Nations; 2018.

62. Galea S, Vlahov D. Urban health: evidence, challenges, and directions. *Annu Rev Public Health*. 2005;26:341–365.

63. Moore M, Gould P, Keary BS. Global urbanization and impact on health. *Int J Hyg Environ Health*. 2003;206:269–278.

64. McMichael AJ. The urban environment and health in a world of increasing globalization: issues for developing countries. *Bull World Health Organ*. 2000;78:1117–1126.

65. Vlahov D, Galea S. Urbanization, urbanicity, and health. *J Urban Health*. 2002;79(Suppl 4):S1–S12.

66. United Nations Department of Economic and Social Affairs. *World Urbanization Prospects: The 2014 Revision*. New York: United Nations; 2014.

67. World Health Organization/United Nations-Habitat. *Global Report on Urban Health: Equitable Healthier Cities for Sustainable Development*. Geneva: World Health Organization; 2016.

68. *Health as the Pulse of the New Urban Agenda: United Nations Conference on Housing and Sustainable Urban Development, Quito, October 2016*. Geneva: World Health Organization; 2016.

69. Rydin Y, Bleahu A, Davies M, et al. Shaping cities for health: complexity and the planning of urban environments in the 21st century. *Lancet*. 2012;379:2079–2108.

70. *Our Common Future*. Geneva: World Commission on Environment and Development; 1987.

71. *Inheriting a Sustainable World? Atlas on Children's Health and the Environment*. Geneva: World Health Organization; 2017.

72. Lélé SM. Sustainable development: a critical review. *World Dev*. 1991;19:607–621.

73. Goodland R. The concept of environmental sustainability. *Annu Rev Ecol Systematics*. 1995;26: 1–24.

74. Nekola JC, Allen CD, Brown JH, et al. The Malthusian–Darwinian dynamic and the trajectory of civilization. *Trends Ecol Evol*. 2013;28:127–130.

75. Shiva A. *Water Wars: Privatization, Pollution, and Profit*. Cambridge MA: South End Press; 2002.

76. United Nations Department of Economic and Social Affairs. *World Population to 2300*. New York: United Nations; 2004.

77. United Nations Department of Economic and Social Affairs. *World Population Prospects: The 2019 Revision*. Vol. 1. New York: United Nations; 2019.

78. Vollset SE, Goren E, Yuan CW, et al. Fertility, mortality, migration, and population scenarios for 195 countries and territories from 2017 to 2100: a forecasting analysis for the Global Burden of Disease Study. *Lancet*. 2020;396:1285–1306.

79. *National Footprint and Biocapacity Accounts 2021*. Oakland CA: Global Footprint Network; 2021.

80. Barbier EB. The concept of sustainable economic development. *Environ Conserv*. 1987;14:101–110.

81. Millennium Ecosystem Assessment. *Ecosystems and Human Well-Being: A Framework for Assessment*. Washington DC: Island Press; 2003.

82. Zinsstag J, Schelling E, Waltner-Toews D, Tanner M. From "one medicine" to "one health" and systematic approaches to health and well-being. *Prev Vet Med*. 2011;101:148–156.

83. Gibbs EPJ. The evolution of One Health: a decade of progress and challenges for the future. *Vet Rec*. 2014;174:85–91.

84. Coker R, Rushton J, Mounier-Jack S, et al. Towards a conceptual framework to support one-health research for policy on emerging zoonoses. *Lancet Infect Dis*. 2011;11:326–331.

85. Millennium Ecosystem Assessment. *Ecosystems and Human Well-Being: Synthesis*. Washington DC: Island Press; 2005.

86. Whitmee S, Haines A, Beyrer C, et al. Safeguarding human health in the Anthropocene epoch: report of

the Rockefeller Foundation–Lancet Commission on planetary health. *Lancet*. 2015;386:1973–2028.

87. *Living Planet Report 2020: Bending the Curve of Biodiversity Loss*. Geneva: World Wildlife Federation; 2020.

88. *São Paulo Declaration on Planetary Health*. São Paulo: Planetary Health Alliance; 2021.

89. McMichael AJ, Beaglehole R. The changing global context of public health. *Lancet*. 2000;356:495–499.

90. *WHO Guidance to Protect Health from Climate Change Through Health Adaptation Planning*. Geneva: World Health Organization; 2014.

91. Frumkin H, Hess J, Luber G, Malilay J, McGeehin M. Climate change: the public health response. *Am J Public Health*. 2008;98:435–445.

92. McMichael AJ, Campbell-Lendrum DH, Corvalán CF, et al., eds. *Climate Change and Human Health: Risks and Responses*. Geneva: World Health Organization; 2003.

93. Morse SS. Factors in the emergence of infectious diseases. *Emerg Infect Dis*. 1995;1:7–15.

94. Friel S, Marmot M, McMichael AJ, Kjellstrom T, Vågerö D. Global health equity and climate stabilisation: a common agenda: *Lancet*. 2008;372:1677–1683.

95. Heacock M, Kelly CB, Asante KA, Birnbaum LS, Bergman Å, Bruné MN. E-waste and harm to vulnerable populations. *Environ Health Perspect*. 2016;124:550–555.

96. Diamond J. *Collapse: How Societies Choose to Fail or Succeed*. New York: Viking; 2005.

97. Pachauri RK, Meyer LA, eds. *Climate Change 2014: Synthesis Report. Contribution of Working Groups I, II and III to the 5th Assessment Report of the Intergovernmental Panel on Climate Change*. Cambridge UK: Cambridge University Press; 2014.

98. Stocker TF, Qin D, Plattner GK, et al., eds. *Climate Change 2013: The Physical Science Basis. Contribution of Working Group I to the 5th Assessment Report of the Intergovernmental Panel on Climate Change*. Cambridge UK: Cambridge University Press; 2013.

99. Ebi KL, Hess JJ, Watkiss P. Health risks and costs of climate variability and change (chapter 8). In: Mock CN, Nugent R, Kobusingye O, Smith KR, eds. *Disease Control Priorities: Injury Prevention and Environmental Health*. Vol. 7. 3rd ed. Washington DC: IBRD/World Bank; 2017:153–169.

100. Field CB, Barros VR, Mastrandrea MD, et al., eds. *Climate Change 2014: Impacts, Adaptation, and Vulnerability. Contribution of Working Group II to the 5th Assessment Report of the Intergovernmental Panel on Climate Change*. Cambridge UK: Cambridge University Press; 2014.

101. Costello A, Abbas M, Allen A, et al. Managing the health effects of climate change. *Lancet*. 2009;373:1693–1733.

102. Luber G, McGeehin M. Climate change and extreme heat events. *Am J Prev Med*. 2008;35:429–435.

103. *Quantitative Risk Assessment of the Effects of Climate Change on Selected Causes of Death, 2030s and 2050s*. Geneva: World Health Organization; 2014.

104. Watts N, Adger WN, Ayeb-Karlsson S, et al. The Lancet Countdown: tracking progress on health and climate change. *Lancet*. 2017;389:1151–1164.

105. Watts N, Adger WN, Agnolucci P, et al. Health and climate change: policy responses to protect public health. *Lancet*. 2015;386:1861–1914.

106. Clement V, Rigaud KK, de Sherbinin A, et al. *Groundswell Part 2: Acting on Internal Climate Migration*. Washington DC: World Bank; 2021.

107. *United Nations Framework Convention on Climate Change*. New York: United Nations; 1992.

108. *Kyoto Protocol to the United Nations Framework Convention on Climate Change*. New York: United Nations; 1998.

109. *Adoption of the Paris Agreement* (FCCC/CP/2015/L.9/Rev.1). New York: United Nations; 2015.

110. Tortell PD. Earth 2020: science, society, and sustainability in the Anthropocene. *Proc Natl Acad Sci U. S. A.* 2020;117:8683–8691.

111. Solomon S, Ivy DJ, Kinnison D, Mills MJ, Neely RR III, Schmidt A. Emergence of healing in the Antarctic ozone layer. *Science*. 2016;353:269–274.

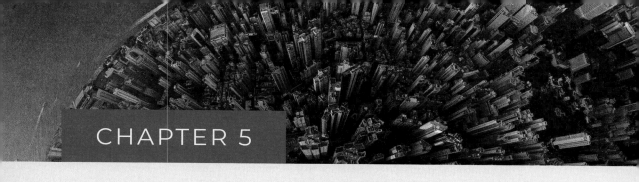

Health and Human Rights

The Universal Declaration of Human Rights and other international agreements establish that all of the world's people have the right to health services, essential medicines, and basic human needs like water, including survivors of natural disasters, people in prison, and people with disabilities. Progress toward health equity advances the realization of other human rights.

5.1 Health and Human Rights

The preamble to the Constitution of the World Health Organization (WHO), which has been affirmed by all of the nearly 200 countries that have membership in the United Nations (UN), lists nine foundational principles for the field of global health (**Figure 5.1**). The boldest claim is that "the enjoyment of the highest attainable standard of health is one of the fundamental rights of every human being" (principle 2).[1] This statement calls for quality health services to be accessible and affordable so that everyone has access to at least basic medical and psychological care (principle 7), especially children and people who are members of vulnerable population groups (principles 2 and 6). The preamble also notes that health is linked with peace (principle 3) and security (principles 4 and 5),

that everyone is at risk of outbreaks of infectious disease (principle 5), and that both the public (principle 8) and governments (principle 9) must take active responsibility for public health.

Two key terms in the preamble require careful definition: human rights and standard of health. **Human rights** are entitlements that are due to every person simply because that person is human. Human rights are considered to be universal, which means that they apply to every person of any age in all circumstances. The term **standard of health** refers to targets that governments set for improving the health of the populations they govern. The standard of health is not currently considered to be universal.[2]

The **Universal Declaration of Human Rights** (UDHR) is an international agreement unanimously adopted by the member states of the UN in 1948 that spells out more than

1	Health is a state of complete physical, mental, and social well-being and not merely the absence of disease or infirmity.
2	The enjoyment of the highest attainable standard of health is one of the fundamental rights of every human being without distinction of race, religion, political belief, economic, or social condition.
3	The health of all peoples is fundamental to the attainment of peace and security and is dependent upon the fullest cooperation of individuals and States.
4	The achievement of any State in the promotion and protection of health is of value to all.
5	Unequal development in different countries in the promotion of health and control of disease, especially communicable disease, is a common danger.
6	Healthy development of the child is of basic importance; the ability to live harmoniously in a changing total environment is essential to such development.
7	The extension to all peoples of the benefits of medical, psychological, and related knowledge is essential to the fullest attainment of health.
8	Informed opinion and active cooperation on the part of the public are of the utmost importance in the improvement of the health of the people.
9	Governments have a responsibility for the health of their peoples which can be fulfilled only by the provision of adequate health and social measures.

Figure 5.1 Health principles articulated in the Preamble to the Constitution of the World Health Organization.

Reproduced from *Constitution of the World Health Organization.* New York: United Nations; 1946.

two dozen civil, political, economic, social, and cultural human rights (**Figure 5.2**).[3] **Civil rights** are liberties that are granted by governments, such as the freedom to assemble peacefully and the right to equitable participation in governance. Articles 3–21 of the UDHR define the civil and political rights that protect the foundational freedoms of humans, such as the right to privacy and the right to freedom from torture. These rights are about protections rather than provisions, and they can be granted and upheld with limited financial costs to governments. Articles 22–28 of the UDHR outline the economic, social, and cultural rights that, if realized, would contribute to human flourishing. These rights, such as the right to social security, the right to education, and the right to a standard of living adequate for health and well-being, obligate governments to provide certain services to their people.[4] Because these rights carry real monetary costs, they are

somewhat aspirational. However, countries are called to make progress toward increasing the economic, social, and cultural rights of their populations.

Values are general principles that define what is good or evil and what is meaningful. **Morals** are the beliefs and customs that shape how a society defines what is right and wrong. Morals express the behaviors that are acceptable or unacceptable in a community based on collective values. **Ethics** are the principles that guide appropriate conduct in specific situations. Ethics put values and morals into action in real-life circumstances. For example, professional ethics codes guide the practice of medicine, law, education, engineering, and other fields. **Laws** are rules that define enforceable standards of behavior. Ethics often describe standards for optimal behavior, while laws establish minimum standards of acceptable behavior. The UDHR establishes a set of

Human Right	UDHR Articles
Right to equal dignity and human rights for all humans	1, 2
Right to life, liberty, and security of person	3
Freedom from slavery and servitude	4
Freedom from torture and cruel, inhuman, or degrading treatment or punishment	5
Right to recognition as a person	6
Freedom from discrimination	7
Right to legal protection of human rights	8
Freedom from arbitrary arrest, detention, or exile	9
Right to a fair trial	10
Right to be presumed innocent until proven guilty	11
Right to privacy	12
Freedom of movement	13
Right to asylum	14
Right to a nationality	15
Right to marry and found a family	16
Right to own property	17
Freedom of thought, conscience, and religion	18
Freedom of opinion and expression	19
Freedom of peaceful assembly and association	20
Right to participate in government	21
Right to social security	22
Right to work	23
Right to rest and leisure	24
Right to a standard of living adequate for the health and well-being, including food, clothing, housing, medical care, and necessary social services, and the right to security in the event of unemployment, sickness, disability, widowhood, or old age	25
Right to education	26
Right to participate in the cultural life of a community	27

Figure 5.2 Key articles in the Universal Declaration of Human Rights.

Data from *The Universal Declaration of Human Rights.* New York: United Nations; 1948.

shared global morals and serves as a foundational document for international human rights law.[5] Human rights are upheld when they are codified in the laws enacted, implemented, and enforced by governments.[6]

The UDHR does not state that people have a right to be healthy. No government can guarantee health for anyone. For many diseases and disorders, there are currently no effective preventive methods or curative treatments, so there is no way for any entity to alleviate the burden from those health issues. The UDHR does state that all people have the right to medical care and the underlying tools for health, such as safe drinking water and adequate nutrition, no matter where they live.[7] All governments can strive to increase access to preventive, diagnostic, and therapeutic services, starting with a basic package of healthcare services (such as antenatal care, childhood vaccinations, treatment of infectious diseases, and access to clean water) and then expanding the range of services that are available to the entire population.[8] Achieving the "highest attainable standard of health" requires governments to make steady progress toward health equity by increasing access to healthcare services and the tools for health.[9]

Health and human rights are intertwined. People who are denied their human rights are unable to advocate for their health, and populations that are unhealthy are unable to advocate for their rights.[10] By adopting the UDHR, all UN member countries have affirmed their agreement that human rights are universal.[11] This globalized approach to human rights means that when people in one country are being denied their human rights, people in other countries have the obligation to call attention to those violations. The goals of the field of health and human rights include providing education about rights, exposing human rights violations, increasing accountability for governments and other organizations involved in health and human services, and improving access to health and related services.[12]

5.2 Access to Health Services

The right to medical care is one of many human rights recognized in the Universal Declaration of Human Rights. Article 25 states that "everyone has the right to a standard of living adequate for the health and well-being of himself and of his family, including food, clothing, housing, and medical care and necessary social services."[1] Several key criteria are used to evaluate access to medical care, including availability, accessibility, affordability, acceptability, and quality.[13] Health services are available when there are an adequate number of medical facilities that are functioning, staffed, and stocked with the necessary supplies. They are accessible when they are geographically and physically reachable by everyone, regardless of residential location and physical ability. Health services are affordable when they are economically accessible and payment for services is commensurate with ability to pay. They are acceptable when clinical care providers are respectful of patients from all population groups and cultures. The quality of healthcare services is based on having well-maintained facilities that are stocked with appropriate supplies and staffed by appropriately skilled workers. These criteria set a minimum standard for access to medical care. They do not specify what constitutes an acceptable level of access to health personnel, clinical specialists, tests and procedures, medications, and health technology. Those details are expected to be defined by each country for its own people.

The right to health does not mean the right for everyone to have access to every health resource on demand. The economic reality is that most health systems cannot provide organ transplants to everyone who needs one to stay alive, expensive high-tech cancer treatments for everyone whose life could be extended by them, or years of intensive rehabilitation for everyone whose quality of life would improve with long-term care. Countries must make difficult decisions about which routine preventive health services and screenings will be covered by the national health plan, what types of emergency care will be provided to everyone with life-threatening injuries, which medications will be part of the health system's formulary, who will be eligible for particular surgical procedures, and countless other considerations. These selections are typically made after evaluating the effectiveness and cost-effectiveness of various medications, devices, and procedures aimed at improving survival and quality of life.[14] The right to health requires equitable access to covered services, so the services included in a national health plan must be in alignment with the resources available, such as the number of medical specialists and support staff available to implement covered procedures.[15]

The level of access to quality health services is a major social, economic, and political concern in countries across the income spectrum. The United States has sought for decades to figure out how to increase the proportion of the population with health insurance plans, regulate private health insurance plans, and contain rising healthcare costs.[16] Brazil, India, and China are all committed to providing universal access to healthcare services, but they are struggling to fund their health systems, improve the quality of care, and ensure access in rural areas.[17] Every country must make decisions about what healthcare services should be provided and who should pay for those services, and these decisions have human rights implications.

The shared commitment to ensuring that everyone has the basic tools for survival and health has already been recognized in numerous international agreements. However, before the concept of the right to health that is expressed in the UDHR can be fully integrated into national health strategies and operationalized at the global level, four key questions will need to be answered: (1) What are the services and goods that every person is guaranteed access to under the UDHR? (2) What responsibilities do governments have for the health of their own populations? (3) What obligations do governments have for the health of people in other countries? and (4) What kind of global governance for health would help ensure that all governments fulfill their responsibilities for the health of their own people and the world?[18]

5.3 Access to Essential Medicines

A **clinical trial** is a research study that experimentally tests the safety and efficacy of a health intervention. After a candidate medication or vaccine has been rigorously tested in a laboratory, it may progress through a series of phase 1, 2, and 3 trials that evaluate its safety and efficacy in several thousand human volunteers.[19] Candidate drugs and vaccines that perform well in clinical trials are then submitted for governmental review.

Research studies are expected to demonstrate the core biomedical research ethics principles of respect for persons, beneficence, and justice.[20] **Respect for persons** emphasizes autonomy, informed consent, voluntariness, and protection of potentially vulnerable individuals. **Autonomy** means that only the individual (or his or her legal guardian) is authorized to decide whether to volunteer to participate in a research study and that participation cannot be coerced. **Informed consent** describes an individual's voluntary decision to participate in a research study after reviewing essential information about the project. **Beneficence** is the ethical imperative for a research study to maximize possible benefits to individuals and society. Beneficence is often paired with **nonmaleficence**, the ethical imperative for a research study to do no harm. The benefits and risks of research must be carefully considered before a study begins recruiting participants. **Distributive justice** is the ethical principle that needed resources in a population should be fairly allocated. In research, this means that the benefits and burdens of research are fairly distributed.

A rigorous testing and approval process for medications, vaccines, and medical devices ensures the quality and safety of licensed products, but it makes the creation and testing of potential new products a long and expensive process.[21] In the United States, it takes an average of about 15 years and $1.4 billion in expenditures to move a new product through the process of development, testing, and review by the U.S. Food and Drug Administration (FDA).[22] It is similarly costly to move a new product from discovery through the regulatory review process in Europe.[23]

A **patent** is the exclusive legal right for one company to sell a new product for several years before other companies are allowed to produce and sell the product. In exchange for its research and development (R&D) investments, a pharmaceutical company with a newly approved product is typically granted a patent for at least 20 years (or another period of time negotiated with governmental and intergovernmental agencies).[24] This provides the company with a window of opportunity in which to recoup R&D costs and possibly make a profit. A **generic drug** is a medication with the same active ingredient as a brand-name drug. Generic medications usually cost less than brand-name ones, but generics cannot be sold legally until after the expiration of the exclusivity period granted to the patent recipient.

The **World Trade Organization (WTO)** is a UN-related organization that negotiates and enforces trade agreements among UN member nations. Several WTO-sponsored international agreements spell out the rules for trade in goods, services, and intellectual property.[25] Additional patent protections are provided to pharmaceutical and medical device companies through the World Intellectual Property Organization (WIPO) and some trade agreements between two or more countries. For example, trade agreements might extend the duration of

a patent on a medication or device and enforce rules that prohibit generic versions of the products from being manufactured or imported.

Having a highly regulated international pharmaceutical industry with strict manufacturing and packaging regulations protects public safety by ensuring the quality and safety of all licensed brand-name and generic medications. A **counterfeit** is an illegal product that is marketed deceptively. Some counterfeit products are ineffective because they do not contain any active pharmaceutical ingredient, and some counterfeit drugs are dangerous because they contain harmful contaminants. Some counterfeit drugs are sugar pills packaged in boxes with the name of brand-name medications on them, and some are legally produced medicines that are past their expiration dates and have been repackaged in new containers marked with dates that make it look like the product was just manufactured. Government regulations help ensure that medicines and vaccines are safe and legal products, not counterfeits. However, trade agreements that regulate pharmaceutical products may restrict the ability of low- and middle-income countries to legally produce or procure low-cost versions of patented medications.

An **essential medicine** is a drug that has been identified as a high priority for a country's health system to have in stock at all times because it is a cost-effective treatment for a frequently occurring health issue.[26] The WHO core list of essential medicines that healthcare systems should stock includes more than 400 anti-infective, anti-allergic, analgesic, antipsychotic, and hormonal drugs along with medications for noncommunicable diseases such as migraines, cancer, cardiovascular diseases, gastrointestinal diseases, diabetes, and asthma.[26] Most low-income countries omit many of the essential medicines from the WHO list from their national formularies, while high-income countries tend to include hundreds of additional medications in their national formularies.[27] People in high-income countries spend much more each year on medicines per person

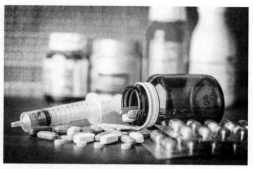

© Adul10/Shutterstock

(public and private spending combined) than people in low- and middle-income countries.[21] This gap is partly due to high-income country residents having access to more types of medications. People who live in high-income countries also have more access to diagnostic tools such as laboratory tests (including microscopy, immunoassays, antimicrobial susceptibility testing, nucleic acid testing, and other tests) and imaging tools like ultrasounds, X-rays, computed tomography (CT) scans, and magnetic resonance imaging (MRI) scans.[28]

In global health, the ethical principle of distributive justice calls for critical resources to be fairly allocated to the global population, not just the country where new scientific discoveries were made. The right to health in the UDHR implies that signatories have an ethical responsibility to expand the availability of free or affordable vaccines, diagnostic tests, and medicines in low-income countries.[29] This ethical imperative is considered to be especially relevant when products are tested in lower-income countries, which happens often even when high-income countries are expected to be the primary market for the new products.[30]

Concerns about access to essential medicines in low- and middle-income countries became a prominent global health issue as the HIV/AIDS epidemic expanded in the 1990s. New antiretroviral medications (ARVs) that were saving lives in high-income countries were too expensive to be widely dispensed in low- and middle-income countries. The **TRIPS Agreement** on trade-related aspects of intellectual property rights is

an international agreement negotiated through the WTO that protects patents, copyrights, registered trademarks, and industrial designs across international boundaries. As TRIPS signatories, countries like Brazil, India, and South Africa that tried to produce generic versions of patented ARVs or that imported generic medications produced elsewhere faced penalties for violating international intellectual property regulations.[31]

The 2001 Doha Declaration clarified that the TRIPS Agreement "does not and should not prevent members from taking measures to protect public health" and that "the Agreement can and should be interpreted and implemented in a manner supportive of WTO members' right to protect public health and, in particular, to promote access to medicines for all." It further noted that countries facing a "national emergency or other circumstances of extreme urgency" could issue "compulsory licenses" for medications to be manufactured locally.[32] This has helped increase legal access to critical medications.[33] The global AIDS crisis of the early 2000s also prompted pharmaceutical companies, governmental health agencies, and advocacy groups to begin working more closely together to make patented medications available at lower prices in low- and middle-income countries.

The Sustainable Development Goals (SDGs) recognize the continued importance of access to essential medicines.[34] This is expressed in the SDG target that aims to "support the research and development of vaccines and medicines for the communicable and non-communicable diseases that primarily affect developing countries, provide access to affordable essential medicines and vaccines, in accordance with the Doha Declaration on the TRIPS Agreement and Public Health, which affirms the right of developing countries to use the full provisions in the Agreement on Trade-Related Aspects of Intellectual Property Rights regarding flexibilities to protect public health, and, in particular, provide access to medicines for all" (SDG 3.b).[35] However, this does not mean that waivers of intellectual property protections are granted readily or that access to medical products is equitable. In the year after the first coronavirus vaccines were approved for widespread use, most vaccine doses were delivered in high-income countries even though ethicists recommended a global strategy that prioritized healthcare workers, other essential workers at high risk of infection, and individuals with a high risk of severe disease and death no matter where they happened to live.[36]

5.4 People with Disabilities

An **impairment** is a difference or limitation in an anatomical structure, mental or sensory function, or physiological function that constrains the capacity of an individual to do a task or action. Examples of impairments include motor impairments such as those related to missing limbs, arthritis and other types of joint inflammation, paralysis, and other musculoskeletal and neurological disorders; cognitive impairments such as memory loss; visual impairments such as color blindness, low vision, and blindness; and hearing impairments.

A **disability** is an activity limitation or participation restriction that is related to an impairment.[37] Disability usually refers to limitations associated with long-term impairments,[38] but burden of disease metrics like YLDs (years lived with disability) and DALYs (disability-adjusted life years) use the term to encompass both short- and long-term reductions in productivity at home, school, and work that can occur as a result of illnesses and injuries.[39] Burden of disease metrics do not just count the incidence or prevalence of various types of impairments. They seek to estimate the level and duration of reduced activity and participation associated with various adverse health conditions.

Disability is a function of the social context and environment in which a person with an impairment lives, learns, and works (**Figure 5.3**). The local environment and resources available to a person with a physical, cognitive, sensory, or other impairment, or a

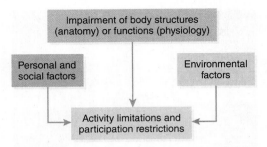

Figure 5.3 Disabilities are a function of biological, social, and environmental factors.

combination of impairments, shape how that individual interacts with other people and the world. A person who uses a wheelchair may easily access public transportation, sidewalks, and public buildings in Germany but might find it impossible to navigate the unpaved pathways of rural Ethiopia. An American with a severe visual impairment will usually have access to corrective lenses, electronic magnifiers, Braille editions of books, and audio recordings, but a low-income resident of Nigeria might not have access to any of these tools. Some people who grow up hard of hearing or deaf never have the opportunity to learn a language, attend school, or be fully involved in the lives of their families and communities. For those individuals, being deaf is a disability because it causes activity limitations and participation restrictions. Some children who grow up Deaf (with the capitalized term used to indicate Deaf culture and identity) are part of a vibrant community with a shared culture and language, typically a local form of sign language, especially if they are born into a Deaf family. For these individuals, deafness is not considered to be a disability.[40]

People with disabilities are entitled to all human rights, including the right to be treated with dignity, to have the autonomy to make decisions for themselves (if they are cognitively capable of doing so), and to be active members of society.[41] **Activities of daily living (ADLs)** are the routine daily self-care functions that are required for health and survival, such as dressing, eating, ambulating, using the toilet, and taking care of personal hygiene (**Figure 5.4**).

Instrumental activities of daily living (IADLs) are functions required for independent living, such as shopping, housekeeping, managing personal finances, preparing foods, and navigating transportation. People with disabilities may experience challenges related to ADLs, IADLs, and domains such as learning and communication (**Figure 5.5**).[42] When individuals with disabilities need assistance with these activities, providing that assistance is an important part of protecting the dignity and safety of those persons and enabling them to be included to the

Activities of Daily Living (ADLs): Self-care	Instrumental Activities of Daily Living (IADLs): Independence
Dressing	Shopping
Eating	Housekeeping
Ambulating (mobility)	Accounting (personal finances)
Toileting	Food preparation
Hygiene	Transportation

Figure 5.4 Activities of daily living (ADLs) and instrumental activities of daily living (IADLs).

Domain	Activities
Learning and applying knowledge	Watching, listening, learning to read, learning to write, learning to calculate, solving problems
General tasks and demands	Undertaking a single task, undertaking multiple tasks
Communication	Receiving spoken messages, receiving nonverbal messages, speaking, producing nonverbal messages, conversation
Mobility	Lifting and carrying objects, fine hand use (such as picking up objects or grasping them), walking, moving around using equipment (such as a wheelchair), using transportation
Self-care	Washing oneself (such as washing hands, bathing, and using a towel), caring for body parts (by brushing teeth, shaving, and grooming), toileting, dressing, eating, drinking, looking after one's own health
Domestic life	Acquisition of goods and services (such as by shopping), preparation of meals (such as by cooking), doing housework (such as cleaning house, washing dishes, doing laundry, and ironing), assisting others
Interpersonal interactions and relationships	Basic interpersonal interactions, complex interpersonal interactions, relating to strangers, formal relationships, informal social relationships, family relationships, intimate relationships
Major life areas	Informal education, school education, higher education, remunerative employment, basic economic transactions, economic self-sufficiency
Community, social, and civic life	Community life, recreation and leisure, religion and spirituality, human rights, political life, and citizenship

Figure 5.5 Domains of activity and participation from the *International Classification of Functioning, Disability, and Health.*

Data from *International Classification of Functioning, Disability and Health (ICF).* Geneva: World Health Organization; 2001.

fullest extent possible in the activities of their families and communities. Maximizing inclusion enables human rights to be realized.

About 15% of the world's people—more than 1 billion people total—have a moderate or severe disability.[37] About 3% have a severe disability. Many people with disabilities are able to live and work independently, especially when they have access to technologies that facilitate independence. An **assistive device**, also called assistive technology, is a tool that helps with the performance of a task. Assistive devices such as wheelchairs and canes, prostheses for people with missing arms or legs, orthotics and braces for people with various types of musculoskeletal disorders, eyeglasses, and hearing aids can enable independence and fuller participation in social activities. However, only about 10% of people worldwide who would benefit from medical assistive devices have them.[43] This causes significant levels of preventable disability. For example, millions of people are unable to attend school or work simply because they do not have eyeglasses to correct for refractive vision disorders.[44]

A safe and accessible physical environment and a strong social network are critical for maximizing the activities and social participation of all people who have impairments and disabilities (**Figure 5.6**).[42] Access to health technologies and health services, including (re)habilitation, is also important. **Habilitation** is the process of learning, maintaining, or improving functional abilities in order to maximize independence and quality of life. **Rehabilitation** is the process of restoring lost function to the greatest extent possible in order to maximize independence and quality of life. Adults and children of all ages who have impairments can benefit from timely access to appropriate physical therapy, occupational therapy, speech–language therapy, and other types of (re)habilitation services.[45] In a typical year about one in three people—about 2.4 billion individuals—experience low back pain, a bone fracture, a stroke, or another condition that could benefit from rehabilitative services.[46] Few of these individuals are able to access rehabilitation therapy. A condition that

Environment	Environmental Characteristics
Products and technology	Products for personal consumption (food, medicines), for personal use in daily living, for personal indoor and outdoor mobility and transportation, for communication; design, construction, and building materials of buildings for public use and buildings for private use
Natural environment and human-made changes to the environment	Climate, light, sound
Support and relationships	Support of and relationships with immediate family, friends, acquaintances, peers, colleagues, neighbors, community members, people in positions of authority, personal care providers and personal assistants, healthcare professionals
Attitudes	Individual attitudes of immediate family members, friends, personal care providers and personal assistants, healthcare professionals; societal attitudes; social norms, practices, and ideologies
Services, systems, and policies	Services, systems, and policies related to housing, communication, transportation, legal, social, health, education and training, labor and employment

Figure 5.6 Environmental characteristics that relate to activities and participation.

Data from *International Classification of Functioning, Disability and Health (ICF)*. Geneva: World Health Organization; 2001.

might be preventable or treatable in a high-income country where rehabilitation facilities are routinely accessible might cause permanent disability in a low-income country where rehabilitation services are not available.

People with disabilities have an increased risk of living in poverty. The direct costs associated with paying for medical care and assistance with ADLs and IADLs can be overwhelming. Health issues restrict the ability of some people with disabilities to work, and family caregivers may need to limit their paid employment and home productivity. These economic factors are exacerbated when people with disabilities have limited access to the public services, education, and employment opportunities that would enable a higher standard of living. The

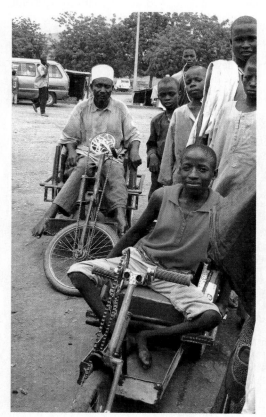

CDC/Paul Chenoweth. https://phil.cdc.gov/Details.aspx?pid=19443. Reference to specific commercial products, manufacturers, companies, or trademarks does not constitute its endorsement or recommendation by the U.S. Government, Department of Health and Human Services, or Centers for Disease Control and Prevention.

Convention on the Rights of Persons with Disabilities, which has been signed by most of the world's countries, calls for full equality for people with disabilities, including access to social protections, inclusive education, reasonable accommodations that enable participation in the workplace, and (re)habilitation and needed health services provided as close as possible to home communities.[47] The SDGs feature numerous targets geared toward increasing the ability of people with disabilities to access social protections (SDGs 1.3 and 10.2), education (SDGs 4.5 and 4.a), work (SDG 8.5), transportation (SDG 11.2), public spaces (SDG 11.7), and civic events (SDG 16.7).[48] These international agreements are intended to help ensure that the human rights of individuals with disabilities are honored.

Global health is founded on the principle that all people have the right to the highest attainable standard of health. The WHO's definition of health as "a state of complete physical, mental, and social well-being"[1] implies that any action that improves the social well-being of members of a community will improve the overall health status of the community. Reducing stigma and increasing the inclusion of people with disabilities in communal events yield health benefits for those individuals and their families and communities. Advocating for the human rights of all people, including people with disabilities, is a core part of making progress toward shared global health goals.

5.5 Health in Prisons

Prisons, jails, and detention centers house convicted criminals as well as suspects waiting for trial, juvenile offenders, and undocumented immigrants. People who are incarcerated are entitled to all fundamental human rights, including the right to be treated with dignity and the right to be protected from medical neglect, starvation, abuse, forced medical experimentation, and other civil rights violations.[49] When some rights are legally restricted, such as the right to freedom of movement during incarceration, there are ways to preserve other freedoms.[50] For example, prisoners should not be held in isolation for long periods of time and visitation should be allowed, when feasible, so that prisoners can maintain relationships with their children and other family members.

Incarcerated people are entitled to medical and dental care, adequate nutrition, protection from infectious diseases, and safe conditions.[51] Despite the protections that are supposed to be in place, incarceration may exacerbate existing health conditions and create new health problems as a result of exposure to severe overcrowding, poor ventilation, poor nutrition, unhygienic conditions, lack of access to medical care, abuse by guards, and prisoner-on-prisoner violence, including beatings and sexual assault.[52] Many people entering prison already have health problems related to addiction and other mental health disorders,[53] and depression, drug dependence, and other psychiatric issues may not be adequately diagnosed and treated during incarceration. A lack of mental health

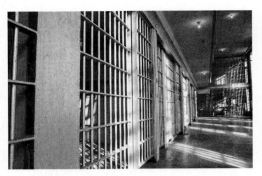

© Txking/Shutterstock

services in prisons contributes to the rates of self-harm and suicide being much higher among incarcerated people than the general population.[54] Prison populations also have higher rates of HIV, tuberculosis, viral hepatitis, and other chronic infectious diseases than the general population.[55] People receiving antibiotic therapy for tuberculosis prior to incarceration may have interruptions in treatment that facilitate the development of dangerous drug-resistant strains that have the potential to spread to other

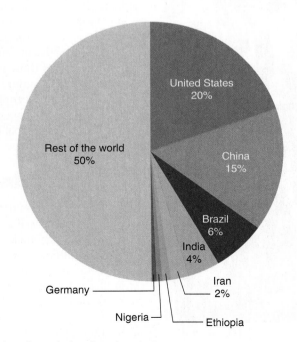

Figure 5.7 Distribution of people in prison by country.

Data from Walmsley R. *World Prison Population List.* 12th ed. London: Institute for Crime & Justice Policy Research; 2018.

prisoners and eventually into the community.[56] Contracting a potentially life-threatening infection is not part of any prisoner's sentence.

On any given day, more than 11 million people across the globe are incarcerated, including more than 2.1 million people in the United States (**Figure 5.7**).[57] The incarceration rate varies considerably between countries, but the country with the highest rate, by far, is the United States (**Figure 5.8**).[57] In the United States, local jails typically house pretrial detainees and individuals sentenced to less than a year of confinement while state and federal prisons typically house convicted felons sentenced to more than a year of confinement. At any given time, about 1.3 million Americans are in state prisons; about 630,000 are in local jails; and several hundred thousand are in federal prisons, youth correctional facilities, immigrant detention centers, and other places of confinement. Over the course of one year, several million Americans spend time in jail. Almost 75% of the individuals in local jails at any given time have not been convicted of a crime.[58] Many of those pretrial detainees remain in jail because they cannot afford bail. Worldwide, about 30% of incarcerated people are pretrial

or remanded detainees who have not been convicted of crimes and sentenced to spend time in prison.[59] Under international law, all incarcerated people—whether they are pretrial detainees or have been sentenced to spend the rest of their lives in prison—have the right to the same standard of health as the general population.[60]

5.6 Health Workforce

The SDGs aim to "substantially increase health financing and the recruitment, development, training, and retention of the health workforce in developing countries and small island developing states" (SDG 3.c).[35] The WHO estimates that about 4.45 doctors, nurses, and nurse-midwives per 1,000 people is the minimum ratio required for sustainable development.[61] Higher ratios allow for higher-quality services to be provided. At present, there is a very uneven distribution of health workers across the globe. After adding in all types of health professionals—physicians, nurses and midwives, dentists, pharmacists, clinical laboratory scientists, environmental and public health workers, community health

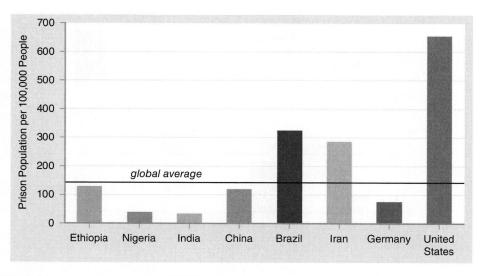

Figure 5.8 Incarceration rates per 100,000 residents.

Data from Walmsley R. *World Prison Population List*. 12th ed. London: Institute for Crime & Justice Policy Research; 2018.

workers, health managers, nutritionists, occupational and physical therapists, medical imaging technicians, optometrists, and others who work in the health sector—there are about 14 skilled health professionals per 1,000 people in high-income countries, 6 per 1,000 in upper-middle-income countries, 4 per 1,000 in lower-middle-income countries, and only 1.5 per 1,000 in low-income countries (**Figure 5.9**).[62]

One of the factors contributing to these inequalities in access to human resources for health is **brain drain**, the migration of healthcare professionals trained in low- and middle-income countries to higher-paying jobs in high-income countries.[63] About 16% of physicians and 7% of nurses working in the 22 high-income countries that are members of the Organisation for Economic Co-operation and Development (OECD) were trained in other countries.[64] (This is an average, and there is a lot of variability in the rate by country. For example, the percentage of physicians trained in another country is 11% in Germany and 25% in the United States.) Hundreds of thousands of physicians and nurses trained in India, China,

Iran, Nigeria, and other low- and middle-income countries work in OECD countries.[65] Low- and middle-income countries bear the cost of training these clinicians and then high-income countries reap the benefits of that investment in education. While it would be unethical to deny health professionals the opportunity to emigrate, it is problematic when skilled clinicians in countries with insufficient numbers of medical professionals are actively recruited by high-income countries.[66] The health SDGs will not be able to be met by 2030 if there is not a rapid expansion in the number of students enrolled in educational programs in medicine, nursing, and other health professions both in the lower-income countries that have the lowest clinician-per-population ratios as well as in the high-income countries that rely on foreign-born clinicians because they are not training enough clinicians within their own educational systems.[61]

The health workforce also has ongoing challenges related to diversity, equity, and inclusion. Many roles within the health sector are not equitably distributed across genders and other demographic groups.[67] For example, nearly 90%

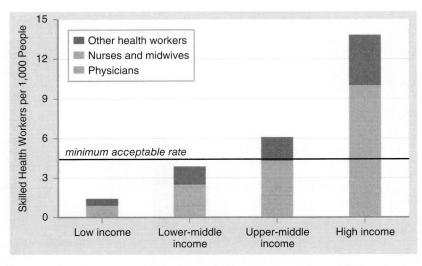

Figure 5.9 Physicians/surgeons, nurses/midwives, and other skilled health workers per 1,000 residents, by country income level.

Data from *Health Workforce Requirements for Universal Health Coverage and the Sustainable Development Goals.* Geneva: World Health Organization; 2016.

of nurses are women,[68] while most physicians, dentists, and pharmacists are men. Jobs typically staffed by women pay less on average than jobs typically staffed by men, and women tend to be paid less than men even when they work in the same occupation and work the same number of hours per week.[69] Women are more likely than men to experience sexual harassment and gender-based discrimination, and they have fewer pathways into leadership roles.[70] Women make up about 70% of the health workforce but fill only about 25% of leadership positions.[70]

Lack of representation in leadership roles is not just observed in clinical practice. It is also visible among the intergovernmental agencies, nonprofit organizations, corporations, and public–private partnerships that are the most prominent players in global health. Most of the executive officers, board members, and other leaders of high-profile global health organizations are men from high-income countries who attended elite institutions of higher education.[71] **Intersectionality** describes the overlapping identities and experiences related to socioeconomic status, gender, sexuality, race, (dis)ability, and other characteristics that align with social privilege or systemic discrimination.[72] More proportional inclusion of women, professionals who were born and trained in low- and middle-income countries, and individuals who represent other types of diversity and intersectionality in leadership roles is likely to improve innovation and productivity in global health.[73]

5.7 Access to Basic Human Needs

The most fundamental human right is the right to life. Human survival is dependent on having enough food, water, and air to support physiological processes and having sufficient shelter and clothing to protect the body from external exposures. These basic human needs are incorporated into the SDGs in targets that seek to "ensure that all men and women, in particular the poor and vulnerable, have equal rights to economic resources, as well as to basic services" (SDG 1.4) and to "ensure access for all to adequate, safe, and affordable housing and basic services" (SDG 11.1).[35] Additional aspects of meeting these basic human needs are included in targets specific to health and nutrition, education, water and sanitation, energy, housing, and other goals.

Because drinking water is something that everyone requires on a daily basis just to survive, access to water is considered to be a human right.[74] This does not mean that everyone has a right to an unlimited amount of free water, but it does mean that everyone has a right to an adequate quantity of clean water for consumption and hygiene at a reasonable cost.[75] Increasing access to water requires investments in water system infrastructure,[76] which usually means digging new groundwater wells and protecting surface water sources, installing miles of pipelines and pumps to transport water from sources to consumers, and constructing facilities to store and treat water. These improvements can be expensive, and the costs of building and maintaining the water system must usually be recouped through taxes or user fees. Additionally, user fees help promote conservation, which is important in places where freshwater resources are limited. Fresh water is therefore considered to be both an essential human need and a consumer good.[77]

Low-income households may struggle to access the water they need. For example, massive protests occurred in 2000 in Cochabamba, Bolivia's third largest city, after the government leased the city's water rights to a U.S.-based corporation in order to improve services and satisfy a condition of a World Bank loan.[78] To raise capital for modernizing the water system, the company significantly increased user fees. For many low-income households, the higher cost of water was an unbearable burden. There was no legal way to reduce the cost of the household's water. Residents were banned from using personal wells and storage tanks, and they were even

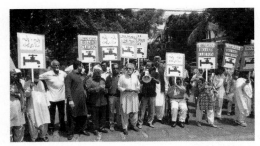

Residents of Karachi, Pakistan, protest drinking water shortages.

© Asianet-Pakistan/Shutterstock

forbidden to collect rainwater without a paid permit.[79] After several months of escalating protests, the water system was re-nationalized. Water privatization plans in many countries continue to generate concerns about how to guarantee that the poorest residents can access safe drinking water.[80]

To sustain healthy life, households must have access to an adequate quantity of affordable water that is safe to consume and use. Water that is contaminated with pathogens and toxins does not satisfy the human need for water. For example, parts of Bangladesh have long had a problem with arsenic-contaminated water.[81] This is a natural phenomenon that occurs when the groundwater that supplies drinking water wells flows through fluvial deposits that contain arsenopyrites.[82] Millions of residents remain at risk of **arsenicosis**, chronic arsenic poisoning from being exposed to contaminated water over a long period of time. The most visible symptoms are a change in skin color (hyperpigmentation) and the formation of hard skin patches (keratosis), but arsenicosis can also cause skin cancer and cancers of the lung, kidney, and bladder as well as liver damage and peripheral vascular disease. Low-cost filter systems can remove arsenic from drinking water, but even a very low-cost filter is more expensive than many Bangladeshi families can afford, and the filters are only a temporary solution because they produce toxic waste. Deeper wells that bypass the geological formations that contain arsenic might solve the problem, but

digging a deeper well is an expensive solution in low-income communities.[83]

Problems with equitable access to affordable and safe drinking water are not limited to low- and middle-income countries. In 2015 alone, tens of thousands of households in both Detroit and Philadelphia, two large cities in the United States, had their water supplies shut off,[84] and the discovery of high levels of lead in the municipal water system in Flint, Michigan, triggered a state of emergency that forced tens of thousands of households to rely on bottled water for drinking, cooking, and hygiene.[85] In many western U.S. states, where a growing human population and agricultural intensification have placed extreme demands on the watershed, the ownership of various supplies of water is determined based on so-called water rights that were sold many decades ago to cities, farmers, ranchers, and miners. It is illegal for people who do not own rights to the local watershed to use river water or collect rainwater.[86] When large cities like Los Angeles and Las Vegas require additional water for their growing populations, they can buy water rights from distant sources. Large volumes of water from those source rivers are then rerouted to the purchasing city. In some places, diversion of water and excessive use of water by upstream consumers has left downstream communities that have historically had adequate water supplies with an insufficient amount of water.[87] It can be difficult for those downstream populations to make a legal case for their right to the missing water, especially if the water crosses a state or national border (such as the U.S.–Mexico border). These ethical and legal challenges will become more pressing as more people move to dry climates.

Growing concerns about water scarcity in many countries and regions require conservation of precious freshwater resources (including the reduction of water loss during transport), clarification of the laws that govern water markets and water use, and a commitment to ensuring adequate water access to vulnerable populations. Similar considerations apply to other basic human needs, such as food and shelter.

5.8 Emergency Management

Both natural and human-generated disasters can create urgent needs for humanitarian assistance (**Figure 5.10**). **Emergency management**, also called disaster management, is the process of overseeing all the resources and responsibilities related to emergencies and disasters, including prevention, preparedness, response, and recovery. Emergency management is about more than just responding to events after they happen.[88] The steps of the emergency management cycle include 4 Rs: (1) Reduction of risks, (2) Readiness, (3) Response, and (4) Recovery (**Figure 5.11**):

- Reduction of risks, or **mitigation**, is the process of implementing preemptive measures to protect people and property from hazards, such as by enforcing building codes.
- Readiness (or preparedness) for responding to an emergency includes the creation and refinement of emergency operations plans, the establishment of emergency

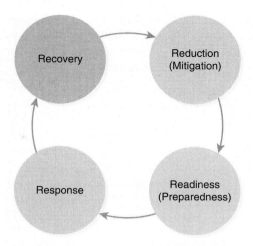

Figure 5.11 Four stages of the emergency management cycle.

communication infrastructure, and the training of public employees and emergency response volunteers.

- Response to an imminent, ongoing, or recent threat includes provision of emergency medical assistance, shelter, and other critical services.

Natural Disasters	Human-Generated Disasters
Weather-related disasters	Intentional
▪ Floods	▪ War
▪ Landslides/mudslides	▪ Genocide/ethnic cleansing
▪ Hurricanes/cyclones/typhoons	▪ Terrorism
▪ Tornadoes	▪ Refugee crises
▪ Winter storms	▪ Internally displaced person crises
Geophysical disasters	Unintentional
▪ Earthquakes	▪ Transportation accidents
▪ Tsunamis	▪ Industrial accidents
▪ Volcanic eruptions	▪ Hazardous materials spills
Climate-related disasters	▪ Explosions/fires
▪ Droughts	▪ Radiation
▪ Extreme heat	▪ Structural collapses (buildings, bridges, dams, and tunnels)
▪ Extreme cold	
▪ Wildfires and forest fires	
Biological disasters	
▪ Pandemic disease	
▪ Insect infestations	

Figure 5.10 Examples of types of disasters.

- Recovery is a phase in which continued efforts focus on rebuilding affected communities and attending to other aspects of reconstruction and rehabilitation.

Resilience is the ability of a community or nation to resist, survive, adapt to, and recover from natural disasters and other adverse events. Mitigating risks and preparing for potential critical incidents before they happen are the best ways to enable a smooth response and recovery when a natural or human-generated disaster does occur. However, preparedness requires investment in supplies, logistics, and trained emergency management personnel. Low-income communities, states, and countries may not have the finances to support risk assessment, equipment, infrastructure, training, and other tools that support operational readiness.[89]

The urgent needs during and immediately after any critical incident include water, sanitation, and hygiene; food; shelter and essential nonfood items, such as personal care items, clothing, bedding, cooking and eating utensils,

fuel, and lighting; and essential health services for injuries, infections, sexual and reproductive health, mental health, and noncommunicable diseases.[90] The amount of humanitarian support required after a critical incident is a function of the scale of the incident (**Figure 5.12**).[91] A **crisis** is a small-scale incident that can easily be managed with local resources, like when a tornado damages several homes in a small town and neighbors provide aid to the affected households. An **emergency** is a critical incident that stresses local resources but can still be managed locally. A **disaster** occurs when the need for assistance after a critical incident exceeds local capacity. A **catastrophe** is a large-scale critical incident that overwhelms local response networks and requires extensive outside assistance.[92] An international event requires a much different level of support than an incident affecting just one small community (**Figure 5.13**).[93]

Most responses to emergencies and disasters are managed by local and national authorities.

Category	Scale	Need	Response
1	Crisis	Capacity > demand	Local response is sufficient.
2	Emergency	Capacity = demand	Local response is sufficient.
3	Disaster	Demand > capacity	Outside assistance is necessary.
4	Catastrophe	Demand >> capacity	Extensive outside assistance is necessary.

Figure 5.12 The scale of critical incidents depends on capacity and demand.

Data from Quarantelli EL. Just as a disaster is not simply a big accident, so a catastrophe is not just a big disaster. *J Am Soc Prof Emerg Planners*. 1996;3:68–71.

PICE Stage	Potential for Additional Casualties	Effect on Local Resources	Extent of Geographic Involvement	Projected Need for Outside Assistance	Status of Outside Help
0	Static	Controlled	Local	Little to none	Inactive
1	Dynamic	Disruptive	Regional	Small	Alert
2	Dynamic	Paralytic	National	Moderate	Standby
3	Dynamic	Paralytic	International	Great	Dispatch

Figure 5.13 PICE (potential injury-creating event) nomenclature.

Data from Koenig KL, Dinerman N, Kuehl AE. Disaster nomenclature—a functional impact approach: the PICE system. *Acad Emerg Med*. 1996;3:723–727.

In the United States, for example, the **National Incident Management System (NIMS)** is an emergency response framework that specifies how various governmental agencies and nongovernmental organizations work together to respond to a disaster.[94] Under NIMS, the **Incident Command System (ICS)** is the organizational structure used in the field to provide a clear chain of command for responders. The national response plan also identifies 15 **Emergency Support Functions (ESFs)**, critical service areas that require immediate attention after a critical incident: (1) transportation; (2) communications; (3) public works and engineering; (4) firefighting; (5) emergency management; (6) mass care, emergency assistance, housing, and human services; (7) logistics management and resource support; (8) public health and medical services; (9) search and rescue; (10) oil and hazardous materials response; (11) agriculture and natural resources; (12) energy; (13) public safety and security; (14) long-term community recovery; and (15) external affairs. A specific lead agency is responsible for each ESF during a disaster response.

A well-managed international response to a disaster or catastrophe begins when an affected country invites the UN and other organizations to assist. A lead agency, usually the UN Office for the Coordination of Humanitarian Affairs (OCHA), is designated to coordinate the response by other UN agencies, government agencies (including militaries), the national Red Cross or Red Crescent society, and nongovernmental organizations. These groups work together to meet essential needs that have been designated as humanitarian response "clusters" (**Figure 5.14**).[95]

Cluster		Lead UN Agency
Overall Coordination		OCHA
Technical Clusters	Camp coordination and management	IOM (International Organization for Migration) and UNHCR
	Early recovery	UNDP (United Nations Development Programme)
	Education	UNICEF (and Save the Children)
	Food security	WFP (UN World Food Programme) and FAO (Food and Agriculture Organization of the United Nations)
	Health	WHO
	Nutrition	UNICEF
	Protection	UNHCR (United Nations High Commissioner for Refugees)
	Shelter	IFRC (International Federation of Red Cross and Red Crescent Societies) and UNHCR
	Water, sanitation, and hygiene	UNICEF
Support Clusters	Emergency telecommunications	WFP
	Logistics	WFP

Figure 5.14 Humanitarian response clusters.

Data from Stumpenhorst M, Stumpenhorst R, Razum O. The UN OCHA cluster approach: gaps between theory and practice. *J Public Health*. 2011;19:587–592.

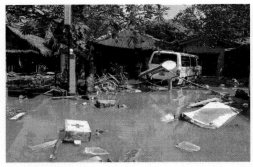

© Stefano Ember/Shutterstock

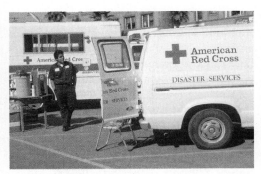

© Joseph Sohm/Shutterstock

Interagency coordination helps facilitate a timely and comprehensive response and ensures that volunteers and their host organizations complete appropriate training before traveling to the disaster site and are prepared to fully provide for themselves in the field.[96] If the various responders do not coordinate their efforts, the result can be chaos. In the weeks after the massive earthquake in Haiti in 2010, thousands of well-intentioned volunteers flew to Port-au-Prince to assist. Many of these spontaneous volunteers were unaffiliated with a Haiti-based host organization and arrived without adequate personal supplies, so they ended up being a burden rather than a help.[97] Supplies remained stockpiled at the airport because the Haitian government, local institutions, and various international governmental and nongovernmental organizations had difficulty communicating about on-the-ground needs, securing local transportation, and coordinating distribution efforts. Similar logistical issues have occurred after other large-scale natural disasters, including the devastating tsunami that hit Southeast Asia in 2004.[98]

The **Sendai Framework** for Disaster Risk Reduction is a global agreement that aims to significantly diminish the number of deaths and the magnitude of destruction caused by natural disasters.[99] The priority areas with the Sendai Framework include increasing awareness of disaster risks, strengthening emergency management capacities in all countries, promoting investment in risk reduction, and

enhancing the effectiveness of response and recovery efforts, including ensuring that the rebuilt structures are more resilient to future hazardous events.[100] The SDGs incorporate disaster preparedness and response into several targets (including SDGs 1.5, 2.4, 9.1, 11.5, 13.1, and 16.1), including ones that emphasize the need to implement the Sendai Framework (SDG 11.b) and "strengthen the capacity of all countries, in particular developing countries, for early warning, risk reduction, and management of national and global health risks" (SDG 3.d).[35] Global health preparedness enables communities and countries to save lives that might otherwise be lost to a variety of hazards.[101]

5.9 International Health Regulations

Globalization means that humans are tied together more tightly than ever before and a problem in one part of the world can quickly become a global issue.[102] One of the roles of global health agencies is to prevent dangerous outbreaks from spreading across national borders and causing widespread morbidity and mortality. The **International Health Regulations (IHR)** are a global health security agreement among all UN members that mandates reporting of outbreaks of infectious diseases of potential international concern. Under the IHR, all countries agree to notify the WHO immediately about situations that might become public health emergencies and to share critical information with all member nations when outbreaks are occurring.[103] The member nations also agree to develop and maintain public health systems that are able to monitor population health status, identify emerging problems, and respond to health crises, and they pledge to engage in travel and transportation practices that protect global public health.

The IHR are derived from agreements negotiated in the mid-1800s by several European countries that worked together to prevent cholera outbreaks without stifling international shipping and trade.[104] The WHO was established in 1948. In 1951, the member nations adopted a set of International Sanitary Regulations that were based on the existing cholera control frameworks. These international laws governing global health security were renamed the International Health Regulations in 1969 and were updated to focus on controlling six infectious diseases: cholera, plague, relapsing fever, smallpox, typhus, and yellow fever. Modifications made in 1973 and 1981 reduced the number of reportable diseases to just three: cholera, plague, and yellow fever. A major overhaul of the IHR adopted in 2005 increased requirements for shared communication about and coordinated responses to influenza, viral hemorrhagic fevers, and other emerging infectious diseases and events of potential international public health concern.[105] The 2005 updates to the IHR mandate more communication about all types of

health risks and events from member nations and obligate countries to strengthen their surveillance and response activities.[106]

Health **surveillance** is the process of continually monitoring health events in a population so that emerging problems can be detected and appropriate control measures can be implemented quickly. Surveillance is the first step in a public health approach to responding to threats (**Figure 5.15**).[107] Surveillance systems, which are usually run by governments, track infectious disease reports from hospitals and other information sources to look for possible outbreaks or clusters of disease, which occur when there is an unusually high incidence of disease in a particular place (spatial clustering) or time (temporal clustering).[108] The health statistics collected as part of surveillance allow communities, states and provinces, and nations to know which adverse health issues cause the most disability in their populations and to recognize when an unusual health situation is emerging. Baseline data about incidence and prevalence from routine surveillance allow epidemiologists to identify when an atypically large number of cases of a disease are being diagnosed.

It is not necessary for surveillance systems to track an entire population. **Sentinel surveillance** is the continuous collection and analysis of high-quality data from a limited number of clinics or hospitals so that public health officials will be able to detect changes in health status in the larger population from which the sentinel sites were sampled. If an outbreak is suspected based on data from

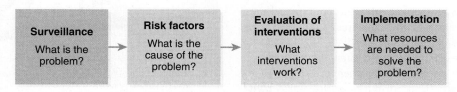

Figure 5.15 Surveillance is the first step in a public health approach to responding to threats to health.

Data from Holder Y, Peden M, Krug E, Lund J, Gururaj G, Kobusingye O, eds. *Injury Surveillance Guidelines.* Geneva: World Health Organization; 2001.

sentinel sites, a more rigorous investigation involving additional clinics, hospitals, and laboratories can be conducted. **Passive surveillance** is the compilation of mandatory reports of notifiable disease diagnoses from medical laboratories. **Active surveillance** is the process of public health officials contacting healthcare providers to ask about how often they are diagnosing prioritized diseases. **Syndromic surveillance** is the process of tracking potential outbreaks or other disease events based on reports of symptoms, school absentee reports, spikes in Internet searches for particular diseases, and other types of data rather than relying solely on counts of laboratory-confirmed diagnoses. International ethical guidelines call for public health surveillance of any type to be conducted only for legitimate public health purposes and only when the government is transparent about its health surveillance activities and shares relevant results with the public.[109] Minimizing the harms and injustices that could occur as a result of data collection and use is critical. Names and other personal identifiers should only be recorded when there is a true need for that information, and identifiable data must be secured.[109]

Surveillance enables epidemiologists to describe how often diseases are occurring in a population. An **endemic** disease is an adverse health condition that is always present in a human population. For example, malaria and dengue are constant threats to health in many parts of the world and are considered to be endemic in those places. An **outbreak** is characterized by at least several people becoming ill from a disease that is not usually present in a population, as happens when dozens of people contract a foodborne illness after eating at the same restaurant. An **epidemic** occurs when an adverse health condition is occurring more often than usual in a human population and there are more than a few sporadic occurrences of disease. A **pandemic** is a worldwide epidemic. Pandemics

of highly pathogenic infectious diseases are global health priorities because they have the potential to wreak havoc on global travel and trade in addition to causing widespread illness and death. Historic pandemics of influenza, cholera, and other infections that cause severe disease have shaped international health agreements and global preparedness and response plans.[110]

A **PHEIC** is a **p**ublic **h**ealth **e**mergency of **i**nternational **c**oncern that can be declared under the 2005 IHR when an infectious disease outbreak is causing serious illnesses, is likely to (or has already) spread to other countries, and would benefit from a coordinated global response. Several events have been declared to meet the PHEIC criteria,[111] including the 2009 H1N1 influenza pandemic, a resurgence of polio that occurred in 2014, the 2014 West African outbreak of Ebola virus, the spread of Zika virus in the Americas in 2016, the spread of Ebola in the Democratic Republic of the Congo in 2019, and the coronavirus that was first identified in China in 2019 and caused a pandemic in 2020. PHEIC status enables international resources to be released to support the response to the disease event and obligates the affected countries to act on the disease control recommendations issued by the WHO. If the right to life is paramount, then coordinated responses to PHEICs are critical for protecting human rights.

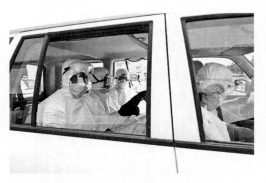

Umid Sharapov, M.D./CDC Connects. https://phil.cdc.gov/Details.aspx?pid=20980. Reference to specific commercial products, manufacturers, companies, or trademarks does not constitute its endorsement or recommendation by the U.S. Government, Department of Health and Human Services, or Centers for Disease Control and Prevention.

References

1. *Constitution of the World Health Organization*. New York: United Nations; 1946.
2. Gostin LO, Friedman EA, Buse K, et al. Towards a framework convention on global health. *Bull World Health Organ*. 2013;91:790–793.
3. *Universal Declaration of Human Rights*. New York: United Nations; 1948.
4. Leckie S. Another step towards indivisibility: identifying the key features of violations of economic, social and cultural rights. *Human Rights Q*. 1998;20:81–124.
5. Gostin LO, Meier BM, Thomas R, Magar V, Ghebreyesus TA. 70 years of human rights in global health: drawing on a contentious past to secure a hopeful future. *Lancet*. 2018;392:2731–2735.
6. Gostin LO, Sridhar D. Global health and the law. *New Engl J Med*. 2014;370:1732–1740.
7. Hunt P. The human right to the highest attainable standard of health: new opportunities and challenges. *Trans R Soc Trop Med Hyg*. 2006;100:603–607.
8. *International Covenant on Economic, Social and Cultural Rights* (A/RES/21/2200). New York: United Nations; 1966.
9. Gostin LO, Monahan JT, Kaldor J, et al. The legal determinants of health: harnessing the power of law for global health and sustainable development. *Lancet*. 2019;393:1857–1910.
10. Mann JM, Gostin LO, Gruskin S, Brennan T, Lazzarini Z, Fineberg HV. Health and human rights. *Health Hum Rights*. 1994;1:6–23.
11. *Global Health Ethics: Key Issues*. Geneva: World Health Organization; 2015.
12. Farmer P. Pathologies of power: rethinking health and human rights. *Am J Public Health*. 1999;89:1486–1496.
13. United Nations Committee on Economic, Social and Cultural Rights. *General Comment 14: The Right to the Highest Attainable Standard of Health* (E/C 12/2000/4). Geneva: United Nations Office of the High Commissioner for Human Rights; 2000.
14. Spiegelhalter DJ, Gore SM, Fitzpatrick R, Fletcher AE, Jones DR, Cox DR. Quality of life measurements in health care. III: resource allocation. *BMJ*. 1992;305:1205–1209.
15. *A Universal Truth: No Health without a Workforce*. Geneva: World Health Organization/Global Health Workforce Alliance; 2014.
16. Berwick DM, Nolan TW, Whittington J. The triple aim: care, health, and cost. *Health Aff*. 2008;27:759–769.
17. Marten R, McIntyre D, Travassos C, et al. An assessment of progress towards universal health coverage in Brazil, Russia, India, China, and South Africa (BRICS). *Lancet*. 2014;384:2164–2171.
18. Gostin LO, Friedman EA, Ooms G, et al. The joint action and learning initiative: towards a global agreement on national and global responsibilities for health. *PLoS Med*. 2011;8:e1001031.
19. *Good Review Practice: Clinical Review of Investigational New Drug Applications*. Silver Spring MD: U.S. Food and Drug Administration; 2013.
20. National Commission for the Protection of Human Subjects of Biomedical and Behavioral Research. *The Belmont Report: Ethical Principles and Guidelines for the Protection of Human Subjects of Research*. Washington DC: U.S. Department of Health, Education, and Welfare; 1979.
21. *The Pharmaceutical Industry and Global Health: Facts and Figures 2017*. Geneva: International Federation of Pharmaceutical Manufacturers & Associations; 2017.
22. DiMasi JA, Grabowski HG, Hansen RW. Innovation in the pharmaceutical industry: new estimates of R&D costs. *J Health Econ*. 2016;47:20–33.
23. Van Norman GA. Drugs and devices: comparison of European and U.S. approval processes. *JACC Basic Transl Sci*. 2016;1:399–412.
24. *Managing Access to Medicines and Health Technologies* (MDS-3). Arlington VA: Management Sciences for Health; 2012.
25. Fidler DP, Drager N, Lee K. Managing the pursuit of health and wealth: the key challenges. *Lancet*. 2009;373:325–331.
26. *World Health Organization Model List of Essential Medicines: 22nd List*. Geneva: World Health Organization; 2021.
27. Persaud N, Jiang M, Shaikh R, et al. Comparison of essential medicines lists in 137 countries. *Bull World Health Organ*. 2019;97:394–404.
28. Fleming KA, Horton S, Wilson ML, et al. The Lancet Commission on diagnostics: transforming access to diagnostics. *Lancet*. 2021;398:1997–2050.
29. Lee JY, Hunt P. Human rights responsibilities of pharmaceutical companies in relation to access to medicines. *J Law Med Ethics*. 2012;40:220–233.
30. Glickman SW, McHutchison JG, Peterson ED, et al. Ethical and scientific implications of the globalization of clinical research. *N Engl J Med*. 2009;360:816–823.
31. 't Hoen E, Berger J, Calmy A, Moon S. Driving a decade of change: HIV/AIDS, patents and access to medicines for all. *J Int AIDS Soc*. 2011;14:15.
32. World Trade Organization (Doha WTO Ministerial 2001). *Declaration on the TRIPS Agreement and Public Health*. Geneva: World Trade Organization; 2001.
33. Smith RD, Correa C, Oh C. Trade, TRIPS, and pharmaceuticals. *Lancet*. 2009;373:684–691.
34. Wirtz VJ, Hogerzeil HV, Gray AL, et al. Essential medicines for universal health coverage. *Lancet*. 2017;389:403–476.

35. *Transforming Our World: The 2030 Agenda for Sustainable Development*. New York: United Nations; 2015.

36. Jecker NS, Wightman AG, Diekema DS. Vaccine ethics: an ethical framework for global distribution of COVID-19 vaccines. *J Med Ethics*. 2021;47:308–317.

37. *World Report on Disability 2011*. Geneva: World Health Organization; 2011.

38. Leonardi M, Bickenbach J, Ustun TB, Kostanjsek N, Chatterji S, MHADIE Consortium. The definition of disability: what is in a name? *Lancet*. 2006;368: 1219–1221.

39. Mont D. Measuring health and disability. *Lancet*. 2007;369:1658–1663.

40. Jones M. Deafness as culture: a psychosocial perspective. *Disability Stud Q*. 2002;22:51–60.

41. *Convention on the Rights of Persons with Disabilities and Optional Protocol*. New York: United Nations; 2006.

42. *International Classification of Functioning, Disability and Health (ICF)*. Geneva: World Health Organization; 2001.

43. *Priority Assistive Products List*. Geneva: World Health Organization; 2016.

44. *World Report on Vision*. Geneva: World Health Organization; 2019.

45. *WHO Global Disability Action Plan 2014–2021: Better Health for All People with Disability*. Geneva: World Health Organization; 2014.

46. Cieza A, Causey K, Kamenov K, Hanson SW, Chatterji S, Vos T. Global estimates of the need for rehabilitation based on the Global Burden of Disease Study 2019: a systematic analysis for the Global Burden of Disease Study 2019. *Lancet*. 2020;396:2006–2017.

47. *Convention on the Rights of Persons with Disabilities: Training Guide*. New York: United Nations Office of the High Commissioner on Human Rights; 2014.

48. United Nations Economic and Social Council. *Report of the Inter-Agency and Expert Group on Sustainable Development Goal Indicators* (E/CN.3/2021/2). New York: United Nations; 2021.

49. Møller L, Stöver H, Jürgens R, Gatherer A, Nikogosian H, eds. *Health in Prisons: A WHO Guide to the Essentials in Prison Health*. Copenhagen: World Health Organization Europe; 2007.

50. Coyle A, Fair H. *A Human Rights Approach to Prison Management: Handbook for Prison Staff*. 3rd ed. London: Institute for Criminal Policy Research; 2018.

51. *The United Nations Standard Minimum Rules for the Treatment of Prisoners*. Geneva: Office of the United Nations High Commissioner for Human Rights; 1977.

52. *Global Prison Trends 2019*. London: Penal Reform International; 2019.

53. Baranyi G, Scholl C, Fazel S, Patel V, Priebe S, Mundt AP. Severe mental illness and substance use disorders in prisoners in low-income and middle-income countries: a systematic review and meta-analysis of prevalence studies. *Lancet Glob Health*. 2019;7:e461–e471.

54. Fazel S, Hayes AJ, Bartellas K, Clerici M, Trestman R. Mental health of prisoners: prevalence, adverse outcomes, and interventions. *Lancet Psychiatr*. 2016;3:871–881.

55. Dolan K, Wirtz AL, Moazen B, et al. Global burden of HIV, viral hepatitis, and tuberculosis in prisoners and detainees. *Lancet*. 2016;388:1089–1102.

56. Kamarulzaman A, Reid SE, Schwitters A, et al. Prevention of transmission of HIV, hepatitis B virus, hepatitis C virus, and tuberculosis in prisoners. *Lancet*. 2016;388:1115–1126.

57. Walmsley R. *World Prison Population List*. 12th ed. London: Institute for Crime & Justice Policy Research; 2018.

58. Wagner P, Sawyer W. *Mass Incarceration: The Whole Pie 2020*. Northampton MA: Prison Policy Initiative; 2020.

59. Walmsley R. *World Pre-trial/Remand Imprisonment List*. 4th ed. London: Institute for Crime & Justice Policy Research; 2020.

60. Lines R. The right to health of prisoners in international human rights law. *Int J Prison Health*. 2008;4:3–53.

61. *Global Strategy on Human Resources for Health: Workforce 2030*. Geneva: World Health Organization; 2016.

62. *Health Workforce Requirements for Universal Health Coverage and the Sustainable Development Goals*. Geneva: World Health Organization; 2016.

63. Taylor AL, Hwenda L, Larsen BI, Daulaire N. Stemming the brain drain: a WHO Global Code of Practice on International Recruitment of Health Personnel. *N Engl J Med*. 2011;365:2348–2351.

64. *Recent Trends in International Migration of Doctors, Nurses and Medical Students*. Paris: Organisation for Economic Co-operation and Development; 2019.

65. Dumont J, Lafortune G. *International Migration of Doctors and Nurses to OECD Countries: Recent Trends and Policy Implications*. Geneva: World Health Organization, High-Level Commission on Health Employment and Economic Growth; 2016.

66. *User's Guide to the WHO Global Code of Practice on the International Recruitment of Health Personnel*. Geneva: World Health Organization; 2010.

67. Dhatt R, Thompson K, Lichtenstein D, Ronsin K, Wilkins K. The time is now: a call to action for gender equality in global health leadership. *Glob Health Epidemiol Genom*. 2017;2:e7.

68. *State of the World's Nursing 2020*. Geneva: World Health Organization; 2020.

69. Boniol M, McIsaac M, Xu L, Wuliji T, Diallo K, Campbell J. *Gender Equity in the Health Workforce: Analysis of 104 Countries*. Geneva: World Health Organization; 2019.

70. *Delivered by Women, Led by Men: A Gender and Equity Analysis of the Global Health and Social Workforce.* Geneva: World Health Organization; 2019.

71. *The Global Health 50/50 Report 2020: Power, Privilege and Priorities.* London: Global Health 50/50; 2020.

72. Zeinali Z, Muraya K, Govender V, Molyneux S, Morgan R. Intersectionality and global health leadership: parity is not enough. *Hum Resour Health.* 2019;17:29.

73. Shannon G, Jansen M, Williams K, et al. Gender equality in science, medicine, and global health: where are we at and why does it matter? *Lancet.* 2019;393:560–569.

74. Gliek PH. The human right to water. *Water Policy.* 1998;1:487–503.

75. Howard G, Bartram J. *Domestic Water Quantity, Service Level and Health.* Geneva: World Health Organization; 2003.

76. *The United Nations World Water Development Report 2020: Water and Climate Change.* Paris: UNESCO World Water Assessment Programme; 2020.

77. Bleumel EB. The implications of formulating a human right to water. *Ecol Law Q.* 2004;31:957–1006.

78. Nickson A, Vargas C. The limitations of water regulation: the failure of the Cochabamba concession in Bolivia. *Bull Latin Am Res.* 2002;21:99–120.

79. Morgan B. Water: Frontier markets and cosmopolitan activism. *Soundings J Polit Nat.* 2004;28:10–24.

80. Mirosa O, Harris LM. Human right to water: contemporary challenges and contours of a global debate. *Antipode.* 2012;44:932–949.

81. Smith AH, Lingas EO, Rahman M. Contamination of drinking-water by arsenic in Bangladesh: a public health emergency. *Bull World Health Organ.* 2000;78:1093–1103.

82. Nordstrom DK. Worldwide occurrences of arsenic in ground water. *Science.* 2002;296:2143–2144.

83. Ahmed M, Jakariya M, Quaiyum M, Mahmud SN. *An Implementation Guide for the Arsenic Mitigation Program.* Dhaka: BRAC; 2002.

84. Jones PA, Moulton A. *The Invisible Crisis: Water Unaffordability in the United States.* Cambridge MA: Unitarian Universalist Service Committee; 2016.

85. Markel H. Remember Flint. *Milbank Q.* 2016; 94:229–236.

86. Hundley N Jr. *Water and the West: The Colorado River Compact and the Politics of Water in the American West.* Los Angeles CA: University of California Press; 2009.

87. Glennon R. Water scarcity, marketing, and privatization. *Texas Law Rev.* 2005;83:1873–1902.

88. McLoughlin D. A framework for integrated emergency management. *Public Admin Rev.* 1985;45(Special Issue):165–172.

89. *A Strategic Framework for Emergency Preparedness.* Geneva: World Health Organization; 2017.

90. *The Sphere Handbook: Humanitarian Charter and Minimum Standards in Humanitarian Response.* 2018 ed. Rugby UK: Sphere; 2018.

91. Quarantelli EL. Just as a disaster is not simply a big accident, so a catastrophe is not just a big disaster. *J Am Soc Prof Emerg Planners.* 1996;3:68–71.

92. Holguín-Veras J, Jaller M, Van Wassenhove LN, et al. On the unique features of post-disaster humanitarian logistics. *J Oper Manag.* 2012;30:494–506.

93. Koenig KL, Dinerman N, Kuehl AE. Disaster nomenclature—functional impact approach: the PICE system. *Acad Emerg Med.* 1996;3:723–727.

94. *National Incident Management System.* Washington DC: U.S. Department of Homeland Security; 2008.

95. Stumpenhorst M, Stumpenhorst R, Razum O. The UN OCHA cluster approach: gaps between theory and practice. *J Public Health.* 2011;19:587–592.

96. Krin CS, Giannou C, Seppelt IM, et al. Appropriate response to humanitarian crises. *BMJ.* 2010;340:c562.

97. Jobe K. Disaster relief in post-earthquake Haiti: unintended consequences of humanitarian volunteerism. *Travel Med Infect Dis.* 2011;9:1–5.

98. VanRooyen M, Leaning J. After the tsunami: facing the public health challenges. *N Engl J Med.* 2005;352:435–438.

99. Aitsi-Selmi A, Egawa S, Sasaki H, Wannous C, Murray V. The Sendai Framework for Disaster Risk Reduction: renewing the global commitment to people's resilience, health, and well-being. *Int J Disaster Risk Sci.* 2015;6:164–176.

100. *Sendai Framework for Disaster Risk Reduction 2015–2030.* Geneva: United Nations Office for Disaster Risk Reduction; 2015.

101. Subbarao I, Lyznicki JM, Hsu EB, et al. A consensus-based educational framework and competency set for the discipline of disaster medicine and public health preparedness. *Disaster Med Public Health Prep.* 2008;2:57–68.

102. Bettcher D, Lee K. Globalisation and public health. *J Epidemiol Commun Health.* 2002;56:8–17.

103. *International Health Regulations (2005): Areas of Work for Implementation.* Geneva: World Health Organization; 2007.

104. Lee K, Dodgson R. Globalization and cholera: implications for global governance. *Glob Gov.* 2000;6:213–236.

105. *International Health Regulations 2005.* 3rd ed. Geneva: World Health Organization.

106. Fidler DP, Gostin LO. The new International Health Regulations: an historic development for international law and public health. *J Law Med Ethics.* 2006;34:85–94.

107. Holder Y, Peden M, Krug E, Lund J, Gururaj G, Kobusingye O, eds. *Injury Surveillance Guidelines.* Geneva: World Health Organization; 2001.

108. Mercy JA, Rosenberg ML, Powell KE, Broome CV, Roper WL. Public health policy for preventing violence. *Health Aff.* 1993;12:7–29.

109. *WHO Guidelines on Ethical Issues in Public Health Surveillance*. Geneva: World Health Organization; 2017.

110. Madhav N, Oppenheim B, Gallivan M, Mulembakani P, Rubin E, Wolfe N. Pandemics: risks, impacts, and mitigation (chapter 17). In: Jamison DT, Gelband H, Horton S, Jha P, Laxminarayan R, Mock CN, Nugent R, eds. *Disease Control Priorities: Improving Health and Reducing Poverty*. Vol. 9. 3rd ed. Washington DC: IBRD/World Bank; 2017:315–346.

111. Bennett B, Carney T. Public health emergencies of international concern: global, regional, and local responses to risk. *Med Law Rev*. 2017;25:223–239.

Global Health Financing

Trillions of dollars are spent each year on medical care and public health interventions, including billions invested in global health activities that are financed by governments, private foundations, and other donors. Some countries' health systems provide universal health coverage, while others deliver most medical services only to those who can pay out of pocket for them.

6.1 Medicine and Public Health

Medicine is the practice of preventing, diagnosing, and treating health problems in individuals and families. For thousands of years, various types of medical practitioners in cultures across the globe have cared for people with health concerns, including herbalists adept at treating fevers, midwives skilled in delivering babies, and numerous other people equipped to provide physical and spiritual comfort to people with various ailments. As modern medical science has developed, clinical professionals like physicians, surgeons, nurses, dentists, psychologists, and physical therapists have developed specialized methods for caring for patients. Examples of interventions in the medical field include antibiotics to treat infections, medications to manage chronic diseases (such as insulin for people with diabetes and inhaled bronchodilators for people with asthma), surgery to correct

traumatic injuries, counseling to ameliorate mental health concerns, and rehabilitation therapy to restore function after an injury.

Public health encompasses the actions taken at the population level to promote health and prevent illnesses, injuries, and early deaths (**Figure 6.1**).[1] Public health professionals work in epidemiology, health education, environmental health, health policy and management, public health administration, maternal and child health, public health nutrition, health economics, health communication, and many other fields of specialization. Examples of public health interventions include policies and practices that ensure that food and drinking water are safe, vaccination campaigns that prevent widespread outbreaks of infectious diseases, school nutrition programs that ensure that children have access to the nutritious food they need to grow and learn, community services that support individuals with addiction and other mental health disorders, traffic safety policies such as mandatory use of seat belts and child car seats,

1	Assess and monitor population health status, factors that influence health, and community needs and assets.
2	Investigate, diagnose, and address health problems and hazards affecting the population.
3	Communicate effectively to inform and educate people about health, factors that influence it, and how to improve it.
4	Strengthen, support, and mobilize communities and partnerships to improve health.
5	Create, champion, and implement policies, plans, and laws that impact health.
6	Utilize legal and regulatory actions designed to improve and protect the public's health.
7	Assure an effective system that enables equitable access to the individual services and care needed to be healthy.
8	Build and support a diverse and skilled public health workforce.
9	Improve and innovate public health functions through ongoing evaluation, research, and continuous quality improvement.
10	Build and maintain a strong organizational infrastructure for public health.

Figure 6.1 Essential public health services.

The Futures Initiative: The 10 Essential Public Health Services. Alexandria VA: Public Health National Center for Innovations; 2020.

and health education campaigns that promote active lifestyles for people of all ages.

The **Global Charter for the Public's Health**, which was launched by the World Health Organization (WHO) and partner associations in 2016, identifies protection, prevention, and promotion as the three core public health services and governance, advocacy, capacity, and information as the four core public health functions.[2]

- Protection includes environmental sustainability, emergency preparedness, infectious disease prevention and control, and other global health actions that require international coordination.
- Prevention describes the interventions that support access to primary, secondary, and tertiary prevention of adverse health conditions, such as vaccination, screening, medical services, and rehabilitation therapy.
- Promotion seeks to improve health equity through actions that focus on the socioeconomic, environmental, and other determinants of health across the life span. **Health promotion** is an applied social science that encourages individuals

and communities to take steps to improve their own health. The **Ottawa Charter** for Health Promotion is an international agreement sponsored by the WHO and approved at a conference in Canada in 1986 that identifies healthy public policies, supportive environments, strong communities, skilled personnel, and expanded access to preventive health services as core health promotion actions.[3]

Governance encompasses the processes that prioritize, fund, manage, and monitor public health laws and policies. Advocacy is used in this context to describe values like equity, ethics, community engagement, and communication that undergird public health. Capacity highlights the need for a skilled public health workforce. Information provides a foundation for evidence-based decision-making.

The lines between medicine and public health are blurry (**Figure 6.2**). Medicine tends to focus on the clinical care of individuals, while public health has a focus on larger populations. Public health usually emphasizes the prevention of health problems, while medicine has more of a focus on treating existing

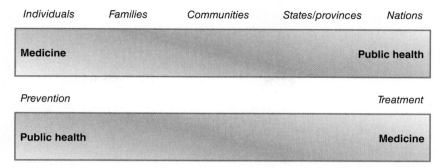

Figure 6.2 Comparing medicine and public health.

problems. However, many people who work in population health and provide preventive services trained in clinical fields (such as public health nurses and physicians specializing in preventive medicine), and many people who are dedicated to increasing access to treatment for individuals with critical health issues trained in public health. Medical research informs the design of public health interventions, and the information generated from public health research helps clinicians make differential diagnoses, prescribe appropriate therapies, and encourage healthy lifestyles for their patients.

Both medicine and public health play important roles in 21st century global health practice. Funding for global health supports a variety of individual-level interventions, such as providing daily medications to millions of individuals living with HIV and supplying mosquito nets to protect millions of households from malaria. Funding for global health also supports global population-level initiatives, such as those that seek to prevent dangerous emergent strains of influenza virus from causing pandemics and work to mitigate the anticipated future impacts of global warming.

6.2 Global Health Financing

Spending on health services can be divided into two categories: (1) money spent on personal health and (2) money spent on public health. Personal health expenses arise from medical services that are used by one individual or family, such as the cost of purchasing antibiotics to treat a bacterial infection, paying for a midwife to help deliver a baby, or buying test strips for self-monitoring of blood glucose levels by people with diabetes. Public health expenses relate to shared activities that protect a community, a nation, or the global population at large, such as the costs associated with investigating and containing outbreaks of infectious diseases, marketing the mass vaccination days that are part of the global polio eradication campaign, using insecticides in outdoor areas to kill the mosquitoes that can transmit dangerous pathogens to humans, and developing evidence-based clinical guidelines for managing chronic diseases.

Worldwide spending on health now exceeds $8 trillion per year and accounts for 10% of the world's total gross domestic product (GDP) (**Figure 6.3**).[4] This is nearly double the amount of money spent on health in 2000, even after adjusting for inflation, and spending on health is expected to continue to rise in absolute dollars and as a percentage of GDP.[5] High-income countries spend much more per resident on health than low-income countries do (**Figure 6.4**), and this difference remains significant even after adjusting for differences in the cost of living.[6]

There are a diversity of mechanisms for paying for medical expenses: some countries have a publicly funded healthcare system that is paid

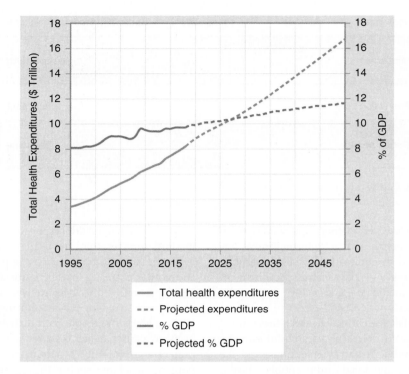

Figure 6.3 Worldwide spending on health. (Past and future health expenditures are inflation adjusted to today's constant dollars.)

Data from Global Burden of Disease Health Financing Collaborator Network. Health sector spending and spending on HIV/AIDS, tuberculosis, and malaria, and development assistance for health: progress towards Sustainable Development Goal 3. *Lancet.* 2020;396:693–724.

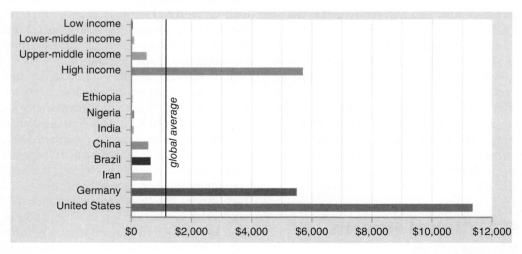

Figure 6.4 Distribution of total health spending per capita by country income level and for featured countries.

Data from Global Burden of Disease 2020 Health Financing Collaborator Network. Tracking development assistance for health and for COVID-19: a review of development assistance, government, out-of-pocket, and other private spending on health for 204 countries and territories, 1990–2050. *Lancet.* 2021;398:1317–1343.

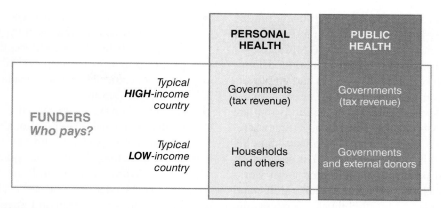

Figure 6.5 Governments in high-income countries use tax revenue to pay for most health services; in low-income countries, a more diverse set of funders pay for health activities.

for with tax revenue, some have a healthcare system in which the medical care of individuals is usually funded by private health insurance or the personal funds of the individual and his or her family, and some countries pay for medical services with a combination of public and private sources.[7] There is less diversity in which entities pay for public health functions. Most public health activities in higher-income countries are funded by taxes, and public health initiatives in lower-income countries are often financed with a combination of governmental and external support (**Figure 6.5**).

Financing is the provision of money for an activity and the management of that investment. Financing for global health is allocated to both personal and public health functions. Some global health funding helps lower-income countries expand the personal healthcare services that they offer to residents. For example, some donors have provided financing that enables more women in low-income countries to give birth at hospitals at no cost to the family, more children to be treated for intestinal worm infections through school-based programs, and more people living with HIV to access free and low-cost antiretroviral medications. Some global health funding supports global health governance,[8] pandemic preparedness and response, the development and dissemination of new health

technologies, and other public health functions.[9] There are also expenses that blend the personal and public health categories, like the costs associated with educating healthcare workers, ensuring that clinicians are licensed and staying up to date on best practices, and building and maintaining hospitals to ensure that everyone has access to essential health services. These activities are public health functions that enable individuals to access quality personal health care.

6.3 Health Systems

A **health system** includes all the people, facilities, products, resources, and organizational structures that deliver health services to a population. The health system model that a country uses shapes how all its residents pay for and access medical care.

- An entrepreneurial or market-driven model typically requires households to pay for services at the time of care or to sign a legally binding agreement to pay for care in installments.[10] Those who cannot pay are denied care. Under this model, most personal healthcare services are privately paid for and delivered at privately managed facilities, but some targeted populations (such as pregnant women and young children) receive publicly funded care. This model is used in most low- and middle-income countries (LMICs).

- A cost-sharing insurance fund model typically requires all workers and employers to contribute to nonprofit "sickness funds" or social health insurance funds that are heavily regulated by the government and cover all residents. The "private" funding in this multipayer system is mandatory, and payments into the fund cover workers as well as children, older adults, and people with disabilities. Services are typically delivered by private providers at private clinics and hospitals. This decentralized model is used today in countries such as Germany, Japan, and Switzerland. It is sometimes called the Bismarck model because it was first deployed in 1883 when Otto von Bismarck was the chancellor of Prussia.[11]

- A national health insurance system is a single-payer system that is fully funded through taxes but delivers services through private providers at private facilities, as occurs in countries such as Canada, South Korea, and Taiwan.[12]

- A comprehensive or socialized medicine model is a single-payer national health system that is paid for with taxes and is publicly managed, like the systems in Cuba, Spain, Sweden, and the United Kingdom. Under this model, most healthcare facilities are owned and operated by the government, and healthcare workers are often government employees. Patients never receive medical bills because all services are funded by taxes. This health system approach is sometimes called the Beveridge model in honor of William Beveridge, who helped establish the UK's National Health Service (NHS).[12]

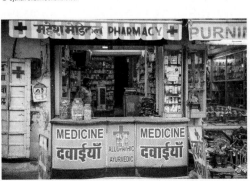

© Djohan Shahrin/Shutterstock

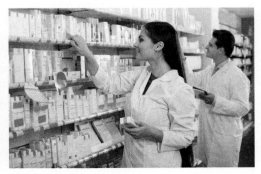

© Fivepointsix/Shutterstock.

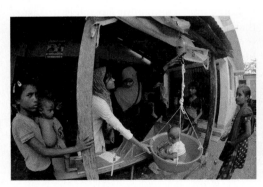

© Pablo Rogat/Shutterstock

© BearFotos/Shutterstock.

Every health system model allows high-income residents to access care, but only some ensure access for low-income residents (**Figure 6.6**).[13] In places where patients and their families pay directly for most medical services, the poorest households are often excluded from accessing skilled care. By contrast, countries that spread the cost of medical services across the entire population through tax revenue or mandatory participation in highly regulated insurance plans enable everyone to access the services that are included in the national health plan. These services typically include family planning (contraception), obstetric and newborn care, child vaccines, medications for infectious diseases and chronic conditions (such as high blood pressure and diabetes), care for acute injuries, and other services that have been identified as population priorities.[14]

The WHO has identified six core building blocks of health systems[15]:

- The provision of effective personal and population-based healthcare services
- A well-trained and productive health workforce that is able to provide quality care to all population groups

- A strong health information system that enables evidence-informed decision-making
- Access to essential medicines, medical devices, vaccines, and other health technologies
- A health financing system that enables everyone to access affordable services when they are needed while providing incentives to limit overuse of services
- Effective oversight of the system to ensure safety, efficiency, and accountability

A high-quality health system is equitable, resilient, and efficient.[16] Some of the WHO's building blocks are ones that can be financed and implemented effectively through either public or private sector funding and implementation models, but some oversight and regulatory functions are most efficiently managed by governments.

Universal health coverage (UHC) is a population-level status achieved when everyone in a country has access to high-quality health services (including preventive care, diagnosis, treatment, and rehabilitation) and everyone is protected from major health-associated financial shocks via a tax-based financing system or a health insurance plan.[17]

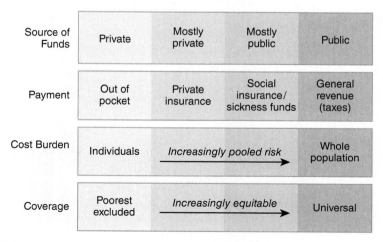

Source of Funds	Private	Mostly private	Mostly public	Public
Payment	Out of pocket	Private insurance	Social insurance/ sickness funds	General revenue (taxes)
Cost Burden	Individuals	*Increasingly pooled risk* →		Whole population
Coverage	Poorest excluded	*Increasingly equitable* →		Universal

Figure 6.6 Universal health coverage spreads the cost burden for health services across the entire population.

Data from *The World Health Report 1999: Making a Difference*. Geneva: World Health Organization; 1999.

The Sustainable Development Goals (SDGs) aim by 2030 to "achieve universal health coverage, including financial risk protection, access to quality essential healthcare services, and access to safe, effective, quality, and affordable medicines and vaccines for all" (SDG 3.8).[18]

Every health system has finite financial reserves, so it is not possible for national health systems to provide every procedure for every condition to every person even if they have adopted a UHC system. Priority setting is a necessary step toward achieving UHC.[19] Government officials and others with health leadership responsibilities in countries aiming to achieve UHC must make difficult decisions about which goods and services will be provided to everyone.[20] For example, health system leaders must decide which procedures will and will not be available in public hospitals and which medications will and will not be included in the national formulary. Resource limitations may mean that only part of a comprehensive strategy for improving population health status can be publicly funded. Budgeting authorities might determine that it is possible to improve access to in-hospital trauma care for injured people but there is not sufficient funding to simultaneously support injury prevention activities, train and equip more emergency responders, and provide more physical therapy and rehabilitation services for survivors. The decision to increase coverage for one type of service sometimes requires decreases in support for other types of health services. UHC does not require full provision of all possible services, but it does require equitable coverage of high-priority services.[21]

Government officials must also make critical determinations about how much funding can be allocated to the health system and how much must be dedicated to maintaining other necessary services. Funding decisions have a very tangible impact on the quality of services that are provided. Increases in government spending on health often require decreases in funding for education and other social services and vice versa. The governments of high-income countries with aging populations usually allocate more of their budget to health than to education, while the governments of LMICs with a large proportion of children in their populations usually allocate similar amounts of funding to health and education (**Figure 6.7**).[22] Health system strengthening requires a process of identifying priorities and resources, strategizing about the policies that will achieve key goals, transforming those ideas into operational action plans, and then implementing changes and tracking progress toward meeting the targets.[23]

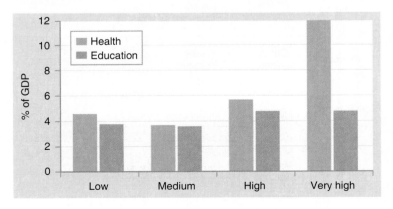

Figure 6.7 Government spending on health and education as a percentage of gross domestic product (GDP), by country Human Development Index level.

Data from *Human Development Report 2020: The Next Frontier: Human Development and the Anthropocene.* New York: United Nations Development Programme; 2020.

6.4 Paying for Personal Health

Out-of-pocket payments are cash disbursements made by patients and their families in order to receive health services. The amount of money that individuals must spend on medical services if they or a household member becomes ill is a function of their countries' health systems. There are some general patterns by country income level (**Figure 6.8**),[5] but each country has a unique mix of strategies for paying for medical expenses.

In most low-income countries, some basic clinical services that have been deemed necessary for achieving high-priority global health goals are financed by domestic governments and international donors to ensure that these services are available to everyone who needs them. For other health conditions, both public and private healthcare facilities may charge user fees and require additional payments for medications and supplies.[24] When subsidized healthcare services are unavailable or the quality of local medical services is poor, families are often unable to access any type of skilled care.

The health services that are affordable and accessible to residents of low-income countries are a function of the health conditions that have been prioritized by their health systems. Some low-income countries have prioritized maternal and newborn survival. In some of those countries, all pregnant women can give birth for free at public hospitals (if they can afford transportation to a hospital, which is not always possible for women who live in rural areas). In low-income countries that have not prioritized maternal health, women must pay out of pocket to give birth at a hospital or must pay midwives out of pocket to help deliver their babies at home. When families cannot afford to pay for help, women must deliver at home without a trained birth assistant. Some low-income countries have prioritized distribution of HIV medications. In those countries, everyone with HIV can access free

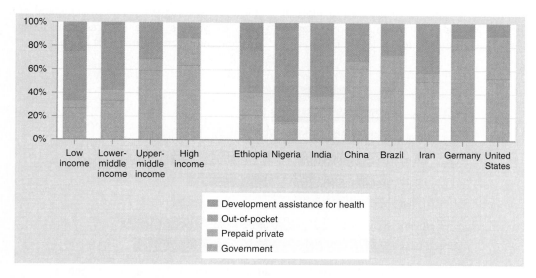

Figure 6.8 Distribution of source of funding for health by country income level and for featured countries. (Prepaid private spending includes private insurance and spending by nongovernmental organizations.)

Data from Global Burden of Disease Health Financing Collaborator Network. Health sector spending and spending on HIV/AIDS, tuberculosis, and malaria, and development assistance for health: progress towards Sustainable Development Goal 3. *Lancet*. 2020;396:693–724.

or low-cost antiretroviral medications, with the price tied to income to ensure free access to low-income individuals. In low-income countries that have not prioritized HIV, antiretroviral medications might be available only to people who can afford to pay out of pocket for them. Increasing access to affordable health services for the most vulnerable populations is one of the major goals for health system strengthening in most low-income countries. Priority-setting processes determine which services will be subsidized and which will not.

In most middle-income countries, governments pay for a portion of medical care costs, but the remaining money spent on health is expended in the form of out-of-pocket payments.[5] Out-of-pocket spending can be especially burdensome to households in lower-middle-income countries, where government expenditures tend to cover only a small portion of healthcare costs. In upper-middle-income countries, the services covered by government health plans vary considerably by country. Some health systems pay for all the expenses of hospitalization for a range of causes, while others require patients to pay part or most of the cost of their hospital stays. Some health systems require users to pay fees at the time of

service and pay out of pocket for prescription medications and therapy, while others do not. Only a few government health plans include dental care and vision care in their health packages. In places where private healthcare coverage is available to supplement government services, there are substantial variations in the prices of private plans and differences in the quality of services covered by the plans.

Most high-income countries have a government-sponsored healthcare system that is paid for through general tax revenue, mandatory payments into a government-run social security system, or other types of compulsory contributions. Medical services are typically provided at government health facilities or at private facilities that receive most of their funds from the government. These types of health systems usually seek to ensure that all residents have access to quality medical care and are not at risk of bankruptcy from medical bills. (The health financing and delivery system in the United States is a notable exception to the general global trend for high-income countries.) High-income countries invest more money in their health systems and are able to provide more services than lower-income countries (**Figure 6.9**).[25]

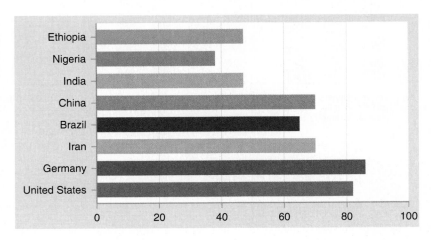

Figure 6.9 UHC effective coverage index, calculated from coverage rates for 23 types of health services and presented on a scale from 0 (worst) to 100 (best).

Data from GBD 2019 Universal Health Coverage Collaborators. Measuring universal health coverage based on an index of effective health coverage of health services in 204 countries and territories, 1990–2019: a systematic analysis for the Global Burden of Disease Study 2019. *Lancet.* 2020;396:1250–1284.

6.5 Health Insurance

Insurance is a risk management strategy that protects purchasers against major financial losses. Health insurance is intended to protect insured people from incurring overwhelming expenses if they happen to develop an expensive health condition. Health insurance systems, whether private or public, are funded based on the principle of pooled risk. **Pooled risk** assumes that if many low-risk people and a few high-risk people pay premiums to an insurance system over many years, there will be a pot of money that can be used to pay for major illnesses and injuries when they occur. Only a few people will develop a very serious chronic condition or suffer a catastrophic injury. However, because everyone is at risk of unexpected health crises, most people are willing to pay additional taxes or purchase insurance that protects them against the small possibility of needing to forgo essential medical care because they cannot afford it or acquiring a lifetime of unmanageable, impoverishing debt as a result of one medical incident.[26]

The country that spends the most on health each year, by far, is the United States, which has a health system that is unique among high-income countries because it is not a universal health coverage system. Nearly all medical services are provided at private facilities, and a mix of private insurance and government funding is used to pay for healthcare services. Pooled risk was at the core of the U.S. Patient Protection and Affordable Care Act (ACA) of 2010, which made participation in an insurance plan mandatory for those who could afford it and provided financial support for lower-income households to purchase private coverage or gain access to government-sponsored health coverage plans. The proportion of Americans who were uninsured decreased after the ACA insurance mandate went into effect in 2014, but the percentage of uninsured people did not reach 0%; in 2015, about 9% of Americans had no health insurance.[27]

Among insured Americans, about two-thirds have private health insurance and about one-third are on a government plan.[28] Most working-age Americans and their children have employment-based private health insurance. The majority of adults who are employed full-time (and some who are employed part-time) receive healthcare coverage for themselves, their spouses, and their minor children through an employer's plan. Insurance plans that cover the full spectrum of care, including medications, preventive care, clinic visits for minor conditions, hospitalizations for serious illnesses, and surgeries, are often expensive for businesses and employees. Most plans require the employee to pay for a portion of the coverage through a **premium**, a monthly fee paid for health insurance. Most plans also have deductibles. A **deductible** is the amount that an insured person must spend out of pocket on medical care each year, in addition to premiums, before the insurance company begins paying for health services. Insurance plans with lower premiums have higher deductibles, which means that patients are reimbursed for expenses only after they have paid thousands of dollars out of pocket. After meeting the deductible for a plan year, patients sometimes must continue to pay out of pocket copays or co-insurance payments until they reach the maximum out-of-pocket amount for the plan year. A **copay** is usually a fixed fee that is paid when receiving routine medical services, such as a fee of $50 for each clinic visit or $25 for each prescription for a generic medication. **Co-insurance** is a percentage of the costs of healthcare services that an insured patient must pay for out of pocket, such as 20% of the total cost. Copays and co-insurance are intended to discourage overuse of the health system.

The major governmental insurance plans in the United States provide healthcare coverage for older adults, low-income households, and military personnel. **Medicare** is the federal health funding system in the United States that provides coverage for people who are

65 years old and older as well as some younger people with serious permanent disabilities. Medicare coverage is based on age and disability status, and it is not tied to income. **Medicaid** is a federal program that provides funding to states to support state-sponsored health coverage for very low-income citizens. Tricare is the health plan for military personnel, their families, and military retirees. Medicare, Medicaid, and Tricare plans enable members to access medical services at participating private providers. The government also provides direct government-managed healthcare services to injured military veterans through the Veterans Administration hospital system and to some Native Americans through the Indian Health Service.

Health insurance in the United States was originally designed to cover only the catastrophic expenses that arise from serious illnesses or injuries. Today, many insurance plans also pay for preventive care and treatment of minor health problems. This is because health economists have determined that health systems save money when minor conditions are treated before they become major problems. For example, an insurance company may calculate that it is cheaper to pay for thousands of people to be screened for early-stage cancer, which can usually be treated at a relatively low cost, than it is to pay for expensive treatment for one person with advanced-stage cancer. If screening many people and treating several patients with early-stage cancer will prevent a few insured people from requiring expensive treatments for cancers that were not detected until they were at an advanced stage, the insurance company may conclude that encouraging all of its clients to participate in the cancer screening program will yield financial benefits for the company. Similarly, a health insurance company may calculate that it is cheaper to pay for frequent routine checkups for people with chronic diseases like diabetes and asthma than it is to pay for emergencies that require hospitalization. The company may provide incentives for people with these chronic conditions to participate in disease management programs that detect emergent problems early and avert the need for expensive emergency care.

Some other high-income countries use a form of health insurance as part of their strategies for achieving universal health coverage. For example, every resident of Germany must belong to a highly regulated "sickness fund."[29] All sickness funds provide the same services to members at the same cost to users, and out-of-pocket payments for health services are minimal. Employers pay half of the sickness fund costs for employees, and the government covers the full cost for children and unemployed adults. Inpatient care is provided at both public and private hospitals, and most outpatient care is provided at private clinics. The payments that providers receive for their services are identical no matter where they work.

Health insurance is also being used by a growing number of residents of middle-income countries so they can access advanced care from high-quality private healthcare providers.[30] For example, lower-income households in Brazil usually receive healthcare services at public facilities that are funded by tax revenue, but a large proportion of higher-income households (or their employers) purchase private insurance plans and seek medical and surgical care at private facilities.[31] Everyone in Brazil can access free primary and emergency medical care at public facilities—this is an important right guaranteed under Brazil's constitution—but the public health system offers a limited range of services and technologies.[32] Health insurance allows wealthier households to access a greater range of health services, procedures, medications, and equipment from their preferred providers, and having those individuals use the private health system allows the public medical system to allocate more of its resources to care for the lowest-income residents.

6.6 Paying for Global Health Interventions

The money spent on public health initiatives comes from a different set of sources than the money that pays for individual medical care. Most public health interventions are funded through local or national taxes collected in the country where the public health services are being implemented. International and global public health activities are funded by a combination of grants from one country to another; grants and loans from intergovernmental agencies; and gifts from private sector foundations, businesses, and individuals. Small donations may be given directly to implementing groups, but large donations are typically channeled through first-level recipient organizations that manage the process of distributing funds to the second-level recipient groups that actually implement projects (**Figure 6.10**).

In a typical year, about $40 billion of the more than $8 trillion spent on health is global health financing that originates from high-income country governments and other donors

and funds global health initiatives, including supporting medical services in lower-income countries.[33] (In 2020, that number increased to about $55 billion as additional funds were allocated to COVID-19 response.[6]) For the governments of high-income countries, health funding for lower-income countries is often part of foreign policy strategies for building trade alliances and protecting homeland security.[34]

Other donors to global health programs have varied motivations for giving.[35] Philanthropic organizations focused on reducing poverty and promoting human flourishing may view global health as a tool for achieving their missions. Disease-specific charities may be able to multiply their impact by working worldwide rather than limiting their work to a single country or region. Expanding their project portfolios may also attract new donors and volunteers. Multilateral lending groups, such as the World Bank and other development banks, may consider global health projects to be good financial investments, especially when aid is provided in the form of loans that will be repaid with interest.

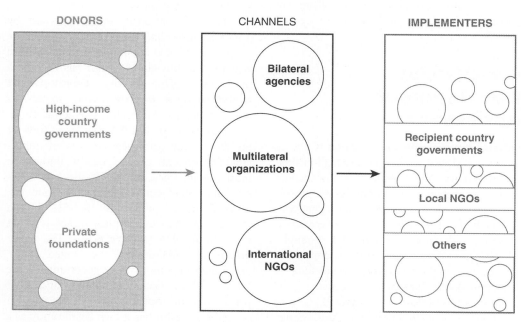

Figure 6.10 Typical pathway from global health funders to implementers.

Large corporations may use global health work to cultivate customer loyalty in new markets, take advantage of tax breaks, and foster a shared sense of purpose among employees. Most of these rationales for funding global health involve benefits for both the recipients and the donors. The best global health projects achieve goals that are beneficial to all involved parties.

Sustainable global health programs aim to generate long-term health benefits that endure even after specific projects end. A program that is fully dependent on outside donors and does not involve recipients in planning, decision-making, and evaluation is not sustainable. The preferred financing mechanisms for new global health initiatives are sources that are stable and sustainable over time, that are new funding lines rather than money redirected from other health programs, and that are managed efficiently without demanding heavy administrative costs or burdening recipient populations.[36] Ideally, global health programs should encourage the self-sufficiency of participating communities by building local technical capacity and facilitating the integration of effective externally funded programs into the routine services offered by internally funded national systems.[37]

6.7 Official Development Assistance

Official development assistance (ODA) is money given by the government of a high-income country to the government of a low-income country to support socioeconomic development. Although some ODA is given simply to fight poverty, aid is often tied to the political and economic interests of the donor country. For example, bilateral food aid agreements may require food to be purchased in the donor country and shipped by donor-country carriers to the recipient (as is the case for most U.S. food assistance[38]).

Foreign aid spending by the United States provides an illustration of how ODA is allocated (**Figure 6.11**).[38] In a typical recent year, the United States spent more than $45 billion on foreign aid, which is about 1% of the total national government spending.[38] The U.S. government considers foreign aid to be a critical contributor to national security because aid supports economic growth, promotes stability, and combats illegal activities.[38] The top recipients of foreign assistance from the United States in recent years include Afghanistan, Jordan, Ethiopia, Syria, Kenya, and Nigeria,[38] all of which were engaged in civil conflicts or were located adjacent to conflict areas and were housing large refugee populations. The major channels for distribution of ODA include the U.S. Agency for International Development (USAID), the Department of Defense, the Department of State, and other national agencies. Billions of foreign aid dollars are invested each year in military and security assistance, which primarily consists of providing military training and equipment to allies. Aid is also given in the form of cash transfers, equipment and commodities (such as food), training and expert advice, and infrastructure development (such as building schools and medical clinics in post-conflict areas).

The amount spent on foreign aid by donor countries and the project areas that are supported by ODA can vary considerably from year to year, but global health has become a prominent ODA priority. **Development assistance for health** (DAH), sometimes called donor aid for health, is external funding designated for health activities in low- or middle-income countries. DAH is an important component of the health budget in most low-income countries,[39] and it is a sizable portion of current foreign aid budgets. More than $25 billion of the $40 billion invested in DAH in a typical recent year has come from ODA (**Figure 6.12**).[5] The major donors of DAH include the United States, other high-income country governments, the Bill & Melinda Gates Foundation, and other private philanthropies.[33]

Global health has grown significantly as a share of U.S. ODA since 2000.[38] In recent years,

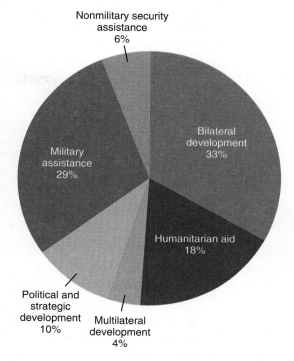

Figure 6.11 Foreign aid expenditures by the United States in recent years, including military and security assistance.

Data from Lawson ML, Morgenstern EM. *Foreign Aid: An Introduction to U.S. Programs and Policy.* Washington DC: Congressional Research Service; 2020.

nearly $10 billion of the U.S. foreign aid budget has been allocated to global health activities (**Figure 6.13**).[5] That makes the United States the largest contributor of DAH worldwide both in terms of the percentage of its foreign aid budget assigned to DAH and the total budget for DAH. In a typical recent year, about 60% of U.S. funding for DAH was distributed by U.S. agencies (such as USAID and the Department of Defense) to second-level implementers, about 25% was channeled through nonprofit organizations that managed second-level implementers, about 6% went to United Nations agencies (such as the WHO and UNICEF), about 5% went to the Global Fund, about 3% to Gavi to support child vaccination programs, and less than 1% went to the World Bank and other development banks.[33] HIV/AIDS programs received the largest share of funding (more than 60% of total

U.S. DAH).[33] Other supported activities targeted newborn and child health, reproductive and maternal health, malaria, tuberculosis, other infectious diseases (such as neglected tropical diseases), and health systems strengthening as well as areas such as digital health (health informatics), nutrition, humanitarian responses, and water, sanitation, and hygiene.[40]

In recent years, the five donor nations that have consistently provided the greatest amount of ODA in total dollars were the United States, Germany, the United Kingdom, Japan, and France.[41] Most ODA is donated to LMICs by high-income countries that are members of the Development Assistance Committee (DAC) of the Organisation for Economic Co-operation and Development (OECD). Some upper-middle-income countries also include small amounts of ODA in their annual budgets.

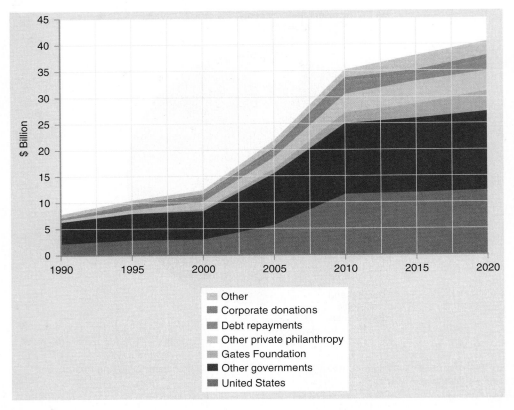

Figure 6.12 Donors of funding for development assistance for health (DAH).

Data from Global Burden of Disease Health Financing Collaborator Network. Health sector spending and spending on HIV/AIDS, tuberculosis, and malaria, and development assistance for health: progress towards Sustainable Development Goal 3. *Lancet.* 2020;396:693–724.

The SDGs call for "developed countries to implement fully their official development assistance commitments, including the commitment by many developed countries to achieve the target of 0.7% of gross national income (GNI) for ODA to developing countries and 0.15%–0.20% of GNI to least developed countries" (SDG 17.2).[18] The countries that spent at least 0.7% of their GNI on ODA in a typical recent year were Luxembourg, Norway, Sweden, Denmark, the United Kingdom, and Turkey (which directed nearly all of its ODA funds toward humanitarian and food aid in Syria).[41] By contrast, the United States spent less than 0.2% of its GNI on ODA, a rate far below the 0.7% target in the SDGs, even though the United States had the world's largest ODA budget.[41]

The SDGs emphasize that ODA is only part of the plan for funding development activities, and they call for action to "strengthen domestic resource mobilization, including through international support to developing countries, to improve domestic capacity for tax and other revenue collection" (SDG 17.1) and to "mobilize additional financial resources for developing countries from multiple sources," including foreign direct investments and remittances (SDG 17.3).[18] **Foreign direct investment** (FDI) is a business investment made by a corporation or an individual in another country. **Remittances** are funds transferred by international

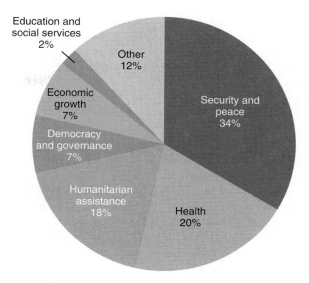

Figure 6.13 Program areas for foreign aid expenditures from the United States in recent years.

Data from Lawson ML, Morgenstern EM. *Foreign Aid: An Introduction to U.S. Programs and Policy.* Washington DC: Congressional Research Service; 2020.

workers to family members in their home communities. The total amount of ODA globally by 2020 neared $170 billion annually, which was about 0.3% of GNI in DAC countries.[41] That was a much lower amount than the money distributed to lower-income countries through FDI and remittances. Before 2020, the annual volume of FDI invested in LMICs neared $1.5 trillion,[42] and the annual value of remittances sent to LMICs was nearly $550 billion.[43] The amount of new FDI and remittances decreased in 2020 due to the coronavirus pandemic, but the values were expected to rebound as the global economy recovered.

6.8 Foundations and Corporate Donations

A **foundation** is a charitable trust that gives grants to other nonprofit organizations. A private foundation is one that is established and funded by an individual, family, or corporation as a mechanism for making tax-deductible donations to entities that align with values of the funders. Public charities that solicit financial

support from individuals, foundations, and government agencies in order to engage in nonprofit activities may also be described as foundations. The particular regulations that apply to various types of foundations are specific to each country, but tax laws typically require public charities to have a diverse board of directors and disburse a set percentage of their assets each year in order to maintain their tax-exempt status.

An **endowment** is a large donation made to a nonprofit organization so that the funds can be invested and the interest from the investments can be used to support the operation of the charity. The **Bill & Melinda Gates Foundation** is the largest private foundation in the world. The Gates Foundation has more than $40 billion in assets; other foundations with endowments of at least several billion dollars that fund global health projects include, among others, the Wellcome Trust (based in the United Kingdom), Ford Foundation, Robert Wood Johnson Foundation, Bloomberg Family Foundation, and W. K. Kellogg Foundation.[44] These foundations' endowments are so large that they enable the foundations to give away large sums of money each year. The Gates Foundation, for example, has distributed more than $5 billion annually in recent years, with a large portion of that total allocated to health projects.[45] The recipients of Gates Foundation funding included, among others, the WHO, UNICEF, and other United Nations organizations; public–private partnerships such as the Global Fund, the International AIDS Vaccine Initiative, the Global Alliance for TB Drug Development, and the Coalition for Epidemic Preparedness Innovations; nongovernmental organizations such as the Clinton Health Access Initiative, END Fund, PATH, and Population Services International; and research institutes working on agricultural health technologies, such as the International Centre for Diarrhoeal Disease Research, Bangladesh (ICDDR,B), as well as technology companies and universities.[45]

Many large companies have established corporate foundations to do charitable work related to their areas of expertise, and many also support other forms of benevolent engagement. A **corporate social responsibility** (CSR) plan spells out the positive social and environmental actions a company voluntarily supports. For example, a company may choose to build its facilities with sustainable materials and implement a recycling program even when these actions are not legally required, or it may sponsor local charities that are important to employees. The major multinational companies that manufacture food and beverage products and produce personal care items are among the many corporations with CSR strategies that support global health. For example, Nestlé, Unilever, Danone, Mars, PepsiCo, the Kellogg Company, and Mondelēz (formerly Kraft Foods) have made commitments to improve access to nutritious food products, and all of them are taking action to improve their social and environmental practices.[46]

In-kind donations of goods or services related to the corporation's core business are often part of CSR programs. Pharmaceutical companies are some of the largest donors to global health initiatives. Each year, GlaxoSmithKline (GSK), Novartis, Johnson & Johnson, Pfizer, Sanofi, Takeda, AstraZeneca, Merck KGaA, Roche, NovoNordisk, and other drug companies donate millions of doses of medications to disease control programs.[47] For example, many millions of people have been treated through Merck and Co.'s Mectizan® (ivermectin) donation program that targets onchocerciasis (river blindness), Pfizer's Zithromax® (azithromycin) program for trachoma, and GSK's Zentel® (albendazole) program for lymphatic filariasis.

In addition to being an expression of humanitarian values, and often a tax deduction, corporate donations help develop international markets and increase brand recognition among potential customers. Populations with increased incomes and decreased health expenditures as a result of charitable health initiatives have more money to spend on other goods and services. By investing in helping potential and current consumers become healthy and maintain their health, companies are doing good work while expanding their markets and gaining brand loyalty.

6.9 Personal Donations

Charitable donations are crucial sources of funding for a diversity of health-related projects, and many people all over the world have been and continue to be generous in their support of nonprofit entities. For example, in a typical recent year people in the United States donated more than $400 billion to charity, with about 70% of this total given by individuals, 15% by foundations, 10% from bequests (donations released to a charity from the estate of a deceased person who named the charity in his or her will), and 5% by corporations.[48] In total, those donations represent about 2.1% of the country's total GDP, and individual donations account for nearly 2% of all disposable income in the United States. The major recipients of funding were religious groups (about 30% of donations), educational institutions (14%), human services organizations (12%), and health charities (9%).[48] Because many of the nonprofit organizations within all of these categories provide services that support health and the tools for health, a large proportion of all donations went toward activities related to health promotion.

The generosity of individual donors is especially visible after major natural disasters, when charities may receive millions of dollars of donations in the days immediately after the event.[49] The American Red Cross received $488 million in designated donations after the massive earthquake in Haiti in 2010,[50] $581 million in designated donations after the devastating Indian Ocean tsunami in 2004,[51] and $2.1 billion after Hurricane Katrina hit the Gulf Coast of the United States in 2005.[52] These amounts represent only a fraction of all donated funds since the Red Cross was just one of numerous organizations receiving humanitarian donations after these catastrophes. Americans gave billions of dollars to charities providing humanitarian services in the affected areas, and individuals from other countries were also generous with their donations.

Another popular giving option for individual donors is **child sponsorship**, a charitable donation model in which a donor selects a child to sponsor and then receives regular updates about that child (often including an annual photograph and a thank-you letter written by the child) in exchange for continued monthly contributions to the host organization. Some child sponsorship programs make direct cash transfers to the families of sponsored children, but many use the funds to support community development projects (like clean water and sanitation projects and school improvement projects) that benefit both sponsored and nonsponsored children in a community. Well-run child sponsorship programs are effective at increasing the educational attainment of participating children and improving their employment opportunities in adulthood.[53]

While many of the recipients of individual donations are charities that work on a small scale, some have budgets of hundreds of millions of dollars and are prominent channels of funding for global health initiatives as well as being on-the-ground implementers. Some nonprofit organizations have large budgets because they receive generous donations from many foundations and individuals. While some of these charities have relatively modest fundraising budgets, some spend much more than 10¢ on advertising for each $1 raised. For example, the American Cancer Society spends more than 20¢ of each $1 donation on fundraising, and the national American Red Cross spends about 18¢ to raise $1.[54]

Some nonprofit organizations have large budgets because they compete with for-profit corporations for governmental contracts to implement international health and development projects. These groups typically report that a large portion of their annual revenue is from government grants. For example, Catholic Relief Services, the International Rescue Committee, and Mercy Corps report that more than half of their budget in recent years came from government grants. World Vision and Save the Children also have large budgets and receive several hundred million dollars in U.S. government contracts in a typical year. By contrast, some groups refuse most government funds, such as Compassion International (which declines government funds for religious reasons) and Doctors Without Borders USA (which declines most government funds and corporate donations for philosophical reasons).

Some nonprofit organizations have large budgets because they manage donations of goods rather than cash. For example, Americares and Direct Relief (both of which work to quickly deliver medical supplies to places affected by natural disasters) and Feeding America (a nationwide network of food banks in the United States) report donations valued at more than $1 billion per year with very low administrative and fundraising expenses (less than 1% of the budget total). Most of their donations are in the form of medical supplies and food, so the accounting is not directly comparable to that of cash-based charities.

The annual reports of registered charities enable potential donors to evaluate the financial performance of organizations before contributing. Organizations' websites and other online tools—such as Charity Navigator, GiveWell, GreatNonprofits, and GuideStar (run by Candid)—also allow potential donors to assess and compare the importance and effectiveness of the organizations' work.[55] The best-rated charities spend a relatively small proportion of their budgets on administration and fundraising, and they apply most of their income to direct program expenses.

References

1. *The Futures Initiative: The 10 Essential Public Health Services*. Alexandria VA: Public Health National Center for Innovations; 2020.
2. Lomazzi M. A Global Charter for the Public's Health—the public health system: role, functions, competencies and education requirements. *Eur J Public Health*. 2016;26:210–212.
3. *The Ottawa Charter for Health Promotion*. Ottawa: First International Conference on Health Promotion; 1986.
4. *Global Spending on Health: Weathering the Storm*. Geneva: World Health Organization; 2020.
5. Global Burden of Disease Health Financing Collaborator Network. Health sector spending and spending on HIV/AIDS, tuberculosis, and malaria, and development assistance for health: progress towards Sustainable Development Goal 3. *Lancet*. 2020;396:693–724.
6. Global Burden of Disease 2020 Health Financing Collaborator Network. Tracking development assistance for health and for COVID-19: a review of development assistance, government, out-of-pocket, and other private spending on health for 204 countries and territories, 1990–2050. *Lancet*. 2021;398:1317–1343.
7. Kutzin J, Witter S, Jowett M, Bayarsaikhan D. *Developing a National Health Financing Strategy: A Reference Guide*. Geneva: World Health Organization; 2017.
8. Frenk J, Moon S. Governance challenges in global health. *N Engl J Med*.2013;368:936–942.
9. Schäferhoff M, Fewer S, Kraus J, et al. How much donor financing for health is channeled to global versus country-specific aid functions? *Lancet*. 2015; 386:2436–2441.
10. Roemer MI. National health systems throughout the world. *Ann Rev Public Health*. 1993;14:335–353.
11. Busse R, Blümel M, Knieps F, Bärnighausen T. Statutory health insurance in Germany: a health system shaped by 135 years of solidarity, self-governance, and competition. *Lancet*. 2017;390:882–897.
12. Reid TR. *The Healing of America: A Global Quest for Better, Cheaper, and Fairer Health Care*. New York: Penguin Books; 2010.
13. *The World Health Report 1999: Making a Difference*. Geneva: World Health Organization; 1999.
14. *Tracking Universal Health Coverage: First Global Monitoring Report*. Geneva: World Health Organization/World Bank; 2015.
15. *Everybody's Business: Strengthening Health Systems to Improve Health Outcomes: WHO's Framework for Action*. Geneva: World Health Organization; 2007.
16. Kruk ME, Gage AD, Arsenault C, et al. High-quality health systems in the Sustainable Development Goals era: time for a revolution. *Lancet Glob Health*. 2018;6:e1196–e1252.
17. *The World Health Report 2013: Research for Universal Health Coverage*. Geneva: World Health Organization; 2013.
18. *Transforming Our World: The 2030 Agenda for Sustainable Development*. New York: United Nations; 2015.
19. Norheim OF. Ethical perspective: five unacceptable trade-offs on the path to universal health coverage. *Int J Health Policy Manag*. 2015;4:711–714.
20. Frenk J. The global health system: strengthening national health systems as the next step for global progress. *PLoS Med*. 2010;7:e1000089.
21. *Making Fair Choices on the Path to Universal Health Coverage: Final Report of the WHO Consultative Group on Equity and Universal Health Coverage*. Geneva: World Health Organization; 2014.
22. *Human Development Report 2020: The Next Frontier: Human Development and the Anthropocene*. New York: United Nations Development Programme; 2020.
23. Schmets G, Rajan D, Kadandale S, eds. *Strategizing National Health in the 21st Century: A Handbook*. Geneva: World Health Organization; 2016.
24. Basu S, Andrews J, Kishore S, Panjabi R, Stuckler D. Comparative performance of private and public healthcare systems in low- and middle-income countries. *PLoS Med*. 2012;9:e1001244.
25. GBD 2019 Universal Health Coverage Collaborators. Measuring universal health coverage based on an index of effective health coverage of health services in 204 countries and territories, 1990–2019: a

systematic analysis for the Global Burden of Disease Study 2019. *Lancet*. 2020;396:1250–1284.

26. Gottret P, Schieber G. *Health Financing Revisited: A Practitioner's Guide*. Washington DC: World Bank; 2006.

27. Barnett JC, Vornovitsky MS. *Health Insurance Coverage in the United States: 2015*. Washington DC: U.S. Census Bureau; 2016.

28. Keisler-Starkey K, Bunch LN. *Health Insurance Coverage in the United States: 2019*. Washington DC: U.S. Census Bureau; 2020.

29. Busse R, Blümel M. Germany: health system review. *Health Syst Transit*. 2014;16:2.

30. Mills A. Health care systems in low- and middle-income countries. *N Engl J Med*. 2014;370:552–557.

31. Paim J, Travassos C, Almeida C, Bahia L, Macinko J. The Brazilian health system: history, advances, and challenges. *Lancet*. 2011;377:1778–1797.

32. Macinko J, Harris MJ. Brazil's family health strategy: delivering community-based primary care in a universal health system. *N Engl J Med*. 2015;372:2177–2181.

33. *Financing Global Health 2019: Tracking Health Spending in a Time of Crisis*. Seattle: Institute for Health Metrics and Evaluation; 2020.

34. Yach D, Bettcher D. The globalization of public health, II: the convergence of self-interest and altruism. *Am J Public Health*. 1998;88:738–741.

35. Stuckler D, McKee M. Five metaphors about global-health policy. *Lancet*. 2008;372:95–97.

36. *Fast-Track: Ending the AIDS Epidemic by 2030*. Geneva: UNAIDS; 2014.

37. Shediac-Rizkallah MC, Bone LR. Planning for the sustainability of community-based health programs: conceptual frameworks and future directions for research, practice and policy. *Health Educ Res*. 1998;13:87–108.

38. Lawson ML, Morgenstern EM. *Foreign Aid: An Introduction to U.S. Programs and Policy*. Washington DC: Congressional Research Service; 2020.

39. Bendavid E, Ottersen T, Peilong L, et al. Development assistance for health (chapter 16). In: Jamison DT, Gelband H, Horton S, Jha P, Laxminarayan R, Mock CN, Nugent, R, eds. *Disease Control Priorities: Improving Health and Reducing Poverty*. Vol. 9. 3rd ed. Washington DC: IBRD/World Bank; 2017:299–314.

40. *Response, Recovery and Resilience: The Power of U.S. Investments in Global Health*. Washington DC: Global Health Council; 2021.

41. *Development Co-operation Report 2020*. Paris: Organisation for Economic Co-operation and Development; 2020.

42. *World Investment Report 2020*. Geneva: United Nations Conference on Trade and Development; 2016.

43. Ratha D, De S, Kim EJ, et al. *Phase II: COVID-19 Crisis through a Migration Lens: Migration and Development Brief 33*. Washington DC: KNOMAD-World Bank; 2020.

44. *The Investment Guide to Private Foundations: Portfolios, People and Investment Performance*. New York: Foundation IQ; 2021.

45. *2019 Annual Tax Return (Form 990-PF)*. Seattle: Gates Foundation; 2020.

46. *Access to Nutrition Index: Global Index 2021*. Utrecht: Access to Nutrition Initiative; 2021.

47. *Access to Medicine Index 2021*. Amsterdam: Access to Medicine Foundation; 2021.

48. *Giving USA 2020: The Annual Report on Philanthropy for the Year 2019*. Chicago: The Giving Institute; 2020.

49. *Global Humanitarian Assistance Report 2020*. Bristol UK: Development Initiatives Ltd.; 2020.

50. *Haiti Earthquake Response: Five-Year Update (January 2015)*. Washington DC: American Red Cross; 2015.

51. *Tsunami Recovery Program: Five-Year Report*. Washington DC: American Red Cross; 2009.

52. *The Face of Recovery: The American Red Cross Response to Hurricanes Katrina, Rita, and Wilma*. Washington DC: American Red Cross; 2007.

53. Wydick B, Glewwe P, Rutledge L. Does international child sponsorship work? A six-country study of impacts on adult life outcomes. *J Political Econ*. 2013;121:393–436.

54. Charity Navigator. 2021. https://www.charitynavigator.org

55. MacAskill W. *Doing Good Better: How Effective Altruism Can Help You Help Others, Do Work That Matters, and Make Smarter Choices about Giving Back*. New York: Gotham Books; 2015.

CHAPTER 7

Global Health Implementation

Global health financing is channeled through international cooperation agencies like USAID, United Nations organizations such as the World Health Organization, public–private partnerships such as the Global Fund, development banks, and other groups that distribute funds to national and local governments, nonprofit organizations, corporate contractors, and other groups that implement global health projects.

7.1 Global Health Channels and Implementers

The groups that set global health priorities and fund global health activities usually are distinct from the entities that implement health projects at the national and community levels.[1] The typical funding pathway for a global health initiative is for a donor (usually a high-income country government or a large foundation) to give money to a first-level recipient (such as an international cooperation agency, a United Nations organization, or a global partnership) that serves as a channel, which then passes funding along to numerous second-level recipients (such as government agencies, nongovernmental organizations, and private sector contractors) that implement the projects (**Figure 7.1**).

For example, funding from the U.S. government might be channeled through USAID (a U.S. government agency) to nonprofit organizations and for-profit USAID contractors that will deliver funded goods and services in partner countries. The Bill & Melinda Gates Foundation might award a contract to a channel such as the World Health Organization (WHO) or the Coalition for Epidemic Preparedness Innovations (a global partnership), and the selected channel might then offer subcontracts to the governments of lower-income countries, which will implement the selected interventions. Alternately, high-income country governments might channel funds through the World Bank, which then provides loans to the governments of lower-income countries to implement prioritized interventions, such as building new clinics or upgrading the infrastructure of existing healthcare facilities. The channels provide technical and logistical

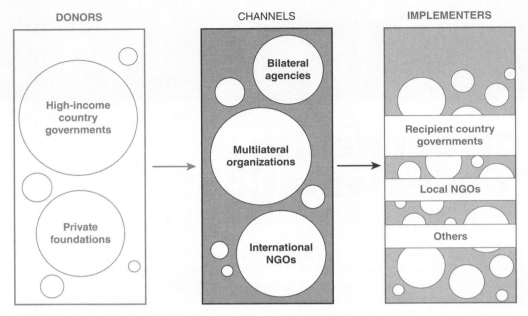

Figure 7.1 Typical pathway from global health funders to implementers.

support to second-level recipients as well as having responsibility for budget and management oversight.

The largest channels of development assistance for health (DAH) include bilateral aid agencies in high-income countries; United Nations (UN) organizations, including the WHO; public–private partnerships; and nongovernmental organizations (**Figure 7.2**).[2] Global health implementers include governmental agencies in low- and middle-income countries (LMICs), large nonprofit organizations, and businesses specializing in international development. Large implementing groups may work in several functional areas in multiple world regions. Smaller implementing groups may focus on one thematic area of expertise and work within a limited geographic zone.

The major funders often use terms like strategy and action plan to describe the outputs they generate. A **strategy** is a big-picture plan for how to achieve a major goal. An **action plan** describes all of the steps that will be taken to achieve strategic goals and implement approved policies. A **scheme** is an

operationalized plan that spells out the desired outcomes and completion timelines for an action plan. These documents guide the allocation of funding to channels and implementers. Funding may be offered to existing partners to implement part or all of an action plan, or a call for proposals might request bids from groups that are prepared to implement one or more of the components of an action plan.

By contrast, implementers more often use terms like project and program to describe their work. A **project** is a series of coordinated tasks that are completed within a limited time period in order to achieve a specific target. A **program** is a portfolio of related projects that together achieve part of an action plan. A **deliverable** is a product, service, or other result of a project that fulfills the terms of a contract or other agreement. Most funded projects have outcomes that must be achieved by the project implementation team to fulfill the terms of the contract between the funder and the recipient. **Project management** is the process of initiating, planning, executing, monitoring, and closing out projects.[3]

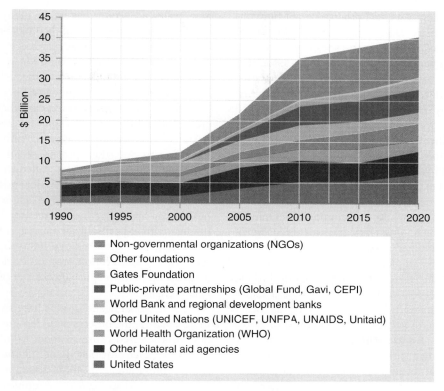

Figure 7.2 Channels of funding for development assistance for health (DAH).

Data from Global Burden of Disease Health Financing Collaborator Network. Health sector spending and spending on HIV/AIDS, tuberculosis, and malaria, and development assistance for health: progress towards Sustainable Development Goal 3. *Lancet.* 2020;396:693–724.

A project manager is responsible for ensuring that deliverables are completed on time and within budget. The same series of project management steps are implemented for nearly all global health projects, even when they have very different objectives.

7.2 Global Health Interventions

Global health implementers provide services in a diversity of specialty areas. For example, they may have expertise in fast responses to crises or long-term engagements that grow and sustain health-related programs, they may specialize in interventions for one disease or have strengths at growing the general capacity of primary healthcare facilities to manage a

variety of illnesses, they may have skills related to developing and advocating for health policies, or they may have excellent supply chain management capabilities. Global health implementers build on organizational strengths related to timing, clinical approaches, and logistics as they deliver interventions. Some large implementers work in multiple areas, but many implementing groups choose to focus only on the activities that align with their core strengths.

Some agencies and organizations have expertise in responding quickly to emergencies, and others have experience in working alongside communities to promote lasting economic growth. **Relief** is aid that meets the immediate needs of people who might otherwise not have access to water, food, shelter, emergency medical care, and other urgent necessities after major natural disasters and during wars and other types of humanitarian crises. **Development** is a long-term process of improving the socioeconomic and environmental conditions that are associated with suboptimal population health status. Some development programs are designed centrally by professionals and disseminated to participating localities. Some use a slower **community development** process in which community members identify their own priorities and take action to achieve them with the support of partner organizations. Relief groups quickly deliver the material goods needed for survival, while community development groups make long-term investments in capacity building and sustainable change.

Many implementation groups provide clinical care at hospitals and clinics or through community-based healthcare providers. Clinical initiatives are often described as being horizontal or vertical.[4] In the context of global health, a **horizontal program** strengthens an existing health system so that it can deliver additional health services. Horizontal programs are often described as integrating newly funded packages of health services into existing primary care delivery systems. A **vertical program** delivers disease-specific services that are not fully integrated into the health system. Vertical programs are often implemented when global health priorities like disease eradication efforts demand an intensive but time-limited series of coordinated efforts. For example, routine childhood vaccinations given to young children when their parents take them to regularly scheduled health and nutrition checkups are received through horizontal programs, while childhood vaccinations delivered during special national immunization days are distributed through vertical programs.[5]

A **policy** is a set of principles and procedures established by governments or other groups to guide decision-making and resource allocation. **Public policy** is the process by which laws, regulations, policies, and government-sponsored programs are developed, implemented, enforced, funded, administered,

and evaluated. Policymakers in many fields are becoming more aware of the links between health and all other policy areas, and they are incorporating health promotion strategies into their recommendations using a "health in all policies" (HiAP) framework.[6] A policy or partnership is **multisectoral** when it is created and advanced by representatives and resources from governments (the "public sector"), businesses (the "private sector"), and nonprofit groups (sometimes called the "civic sector" or the civil society, independent, or voluntary sector).[7] A HiAP approach to global health may bring together multisectoral stakeholders with expertise in finance, agriculture, education, sanitation, energy, transportation, security, communication, and other domains to work on solutions to complex population health challenges.[8]

Some global health groups have strengths in **advocacy**, the process of increasing awareness of a selected cause in order to influence policies related to that issue. Rather than merely providing education about a health issue to individuals and communities, advocates lobby for political support and social acceptance for desired policies.[9] For example, some global health implementers have expertise in advocating for human rights and building support for social change. A variety of communication tactics are used for advocacy. **Social media** are electronic communication tools that allow users to generate and share content, and they are often used to rally public support for legislative resolutions prior to votes on them. The goal is to change public opinions and persuade constituents to contact their elected officials to express support for or against a proposed law, policy, or regulation.

Some global health implementers have expertise in **logistics**, the process of coordinating complex operations, especially the movement of supplies and equipment. Logistics specialists are able to efficiently procure or produce, package, transport, store, and deliver food, medications, medical devices, and other goods to people and communities in need.

Advocacy calls for an action to be taken, and logistics enable that action to happen after funding for the activity has been secured.

7.3 International Cooperation

Foreign policy describes the strategies and approaches a country uses to engage with other nations and protect its own interests as they pertain to security, trade, and other critical functions.[10] The "3 Ds" of foreign policy have been described as diplomacy, defense, and development.[11] Health can be a component of all three areas:

- **Diplomacy** is the process of negotiating agreements between countries, resolving disputes peacefully, and navigating other aspects of international relations.[12] **Health diplomacy** uses health projects as part of meeting foreign policy goals.[13]

- Defense is carried out by militaries. Some military and security aid supports humanitarian assistance and disaster relief (HADR) activities.

- Development in the foreign policy context is often called development cooperation or **international cooperation**, and it includes financial assistance, technical support, capacity building, and other actions implemented by a donor country in a recipient partner country as part of a foreign policy strategy. Development aid directly supports medical and public health interventions, and it also improves population health status by financing health-related socioeconomic and environmental interventions.

International cooperation is about more than high-income donor countries (and a growing number of upper-middle-income countries) sending money to a low- or middle-income recipient country to alleviate poverty and improve health. Development projects are integral parts of donor countries' overall foreign policy strategies. Funded projects seek to improve the economic situation in lower-income countries while promoting stability and fostering future opportunities for expanded trade. The targeted recipient countries, goals, and methods are selected based on the political situations and historic connections of the donor nation. For example, the United Kingdom's Foreign, Commonwealth & Development Office (previously called the Department for International Development, or DFID) works especially closely with members of the Commonwealth of Nations (formerly the British Commonwealth), which are almost exclusively former British colonies or protectorates,[14] and the Japan International Cooperation Agency (JICA) works worldwide but is especially active in the Asian countries with which it has strong economic ties.[15]

Most high-income countries have a specialized agency that leads their international cooperation efforts (**Figure 7.3**), although some implement these initiatives through a ministry of foreign affairs (or an equivalent agency). For example, **USAID**, the United States Agency for International Development, is the lead international cooperation agency in the United States. USAID is a major channel for U.S. government funds allocated to global health activities, and it also operates

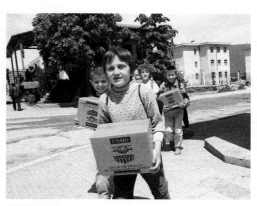

© Northfoto/Shutterstock

Country	Abbreviation	Agency
Austria	ADA	Austrian Development Agency
Belgium	Enabel	Enabel (Belgian Development Agency)
Czech Republic	CzDA	Czech Development Agency
France	AFD	Agence Française de Développement
Germany	GIZ	Deutsche Gesellschaft für Internationale Zusammenarbeit
Iceland	ICEIDA	Icelandic International Development Agency
Ireland	Irish Aid	Irish Aid
Japan	JICA	Japan International Cooperation Agency
Republic of Korea	KOICA	Korea International Cooperation Agency
Luxembourg	LuxDev	Lux-Development
Norway	Norad	Norwegian Agency for Development Cooperation
Spain	AECID	Agencia Española de Cooperación Internacional para el Desarrollo (Spanish Agency for International Development Cooperation)
Sweden	Sida	Swedish International Development Cooperation Agency
Switzerland	SDC	Swiss Agency for Development and Cooperation
United Kingdom	FCDO	Foreign, Commonwealth & Development Office
United States	USAID	U.S. Agency for International Development

Figure 7.3 Examples of international development and cooperation agencies.

global health programs, partners with other groups to implement global health activities, engages in global health diplomacy, supports research and development, and provides technical assistance related to global health.[16] USAID has been active for several decades in supporting maternal and child health programs, infection control efforts, and health systems strengthening as well as other aspects of global health.[17] The U.S. Department of State and the Millennium Challenge Corporation also engage in health diplomacy on behalf of the United States. USAID and other countries' development cooperation agencies typically send representatives to partner countries to oversee projects, provide technical and logistical support, and build "friendships" between the two nations.

7.4 The United Nations

The **United Nations** is the world's largest intergovernmental organization. The UN was founded by 51 member states in 1945, at the end of World War II, and the membership list has expanded to include more than 190 member nations. The goals of the UN are "to maintain international peace and security," "to develop friendly relations among nations," and "to achieve international co-operation in solving international problems of an economic, social, cultural, or humanitarian character."[18] The UN is governed by its main bodies: the UN General Assembly, which is the chief policy-setting group for the UN and is composed of one voting representative from each member state; the 15-member UN Security Council, which is responsible for peace building, mediation, and security operations; the Economic and Social Council; the International Court of Justice, which provides legal judgments and advisory opinions; and the UN Secretariat, which is run by the Secretary-General of the UN and manages numerous departments and offices, such as the Department of Economic and Social Affairs, the Department of Political and Peace-building Affairs, the Office for the Coordination of Humanitarian Affairs, the Office for Disaster Risk Reduction (UNDRR), and the UN Office on Drugs and Crime (UNODC). The UN also hosts programs and funds, specialized agencies, and several UN-related organizations, including the International Atomic Energy Agency (IAEA), the International Organization for Migration (IOM), and the World Trade Organization (WTO).

The programs and funds of the UN are overseen by the General Assembly and financed through voluntary contributions from member nations (**Figure 7.4**). These entities include:

- **UNDP**, the UN Development Programme, which focuses on poverty reduction.
- **UNEP**, the UN Environment Programme, which promotes healthy ecosystems and sustainable use of natural resources.[19]
- **UNFPA**, the UN Population Fund (formerly the UN Fund for Population Activities), which supports reproductive health programs.

UN Entity		Designation	Primary Work Area
UNDP	UN Development Programme	Program	Poverty reduction and resilience
UNEP	UN Environment Programme	Program	Environmental health
UNFPA	UN Population Fund	Fund	Reproductive health
UN-Habitat	UN Human Settlements Programme	Program	Urban development
UNICEF	UN Children's Fund	Fund	Children and mothers
WFP	World Food Programme	Program	Nutrition
ITC	International Trade Centre	Other	Business development
OHCHR	Office of the High Commissioner for Human Rights	Other	Human rights
UNAIDS	Joint UN Programme on HIV/AIDS	Other	HIV/AIDS
UNCTAD	UN Conference on Trade and Development	Other	International trade
UNHCR	UN High Commissioner for Refugees	Other	Refugees
UNOPS	UN Office for Project Services	Other	Project management
UNRWA	UN Relief and Works Agency for Palestinian Refugees	Other	Palestinian refugees
UN-Women	UN Entity for Gender Equality and the Empowerment of Women	Other	Women

Figure 7.4 United Nations funds, programs, and other entities.

- UN-Habitat, the United Nations Human Settlements Programme, which advises on sustainable urban development.
- **UNICEF**, the UN Children's Fund (formerly the UN International Children's Emergency Fund), which advocates for children's rights and provides humanitarian assistance for children as part of its commitment to end preventable deaths of children, newborns, and their mothers and promote the healthy development of all children from birth through adulthood.[20]
- The **World Food Programme** (WFP), which aims to eliminate hunger and malnutrition associated with natural disasters and armed conflict.

The specialized agencies of the UN are autonomous international organizations that work with the UN and are funded through both assessed contributions and voluntary donations (**Figure 7.5**). **FAO**, the Food and Agriculture Organization of the UN, is the UN's lead agency for improving nutrition and agricultural productivity. FAO, the World Bank, and many of the other specialized agencies also work on sociopolitical, economic, and environmental issues that are related to health.

The **World Health Organization** (WHO) is a specialized agency of the UN that was launched in 1948 and serves as the UN's primary health agency. The WHO is governed by the World Health Assembly (WHA), composed of one representative from each UN member state. The WHA convenes every May to approve a budget, make policy decisions, and approve conventions, agreements, and regulations. The core functions of the

Agency		Primary Work Area
FAO	Food and Agriculture Organization	Nutrition
ICAO	International Civilian Aviation Organization	Aviation
IFAD	International Fund for Agricultural Development	Rural development
ILO	International Labour Organization	Labor rights
IMF	International Monetary Fund	Economic growth
IMO	International Maritime Organization	Shipping
ITU	International Telecommunication Union	Information and communication technologies
UNESCO	UN Educational, Scientific and Cultural Organization	Culture
UNIDO	UN Industrial Development Organization	Industrial development
UNWTO	World Tourism Organization	Tourism
UPU	Universal Postal Union	Postal services
WHO	World Health Organization	Health
WIPO	World Intellectual Property Organization	Intellectual property
WMO	World Meteorological Organization	Meteorology
World Bank Group	World Bank	Poverty reduction

Figure 7.5 United Nations specialized agencies.

WHO are to provide leadership for the health work being done across the UN; identify global health research priorities; develop standards of practice, such as child growth charts and recommendations for laboratory and diagnostic procedures; formulate evidence-based policy recommendations; provide technical support to UN member nations; and monitor disease epidemics and compile health statistics.[21] Current priority areas include universal health coverage and other aspects of health systems strengthening, health promotion across the life span, and emergency preparedness and response.[22]

The COVID-19 pandemic drew attention to the challenges that arise from the WHO's limited legal authority and financial resources. Under the International Health Regulations (IHR) adopted in 2005, countries are obligated to notify the WHO of outbreaks of concerning infectious diseases within 24 hours of national public health officials becoming aware of the threat, but the WHO cannot penalize countries that do not comply with that rule. The IHR do not allow the WHO to receive and act on reports of outbreaks from nongovernmental entities, and they allow member nations to choose whether to allow the WHO to send independent reviewers to their countries to examine surveillance data and investigate pandemic origins.[23] In November 2021, the WHO convened the first official meeting to begin negotiating a possible new pandemic preparedness and response accord that could improve compliance with and enforcement of the IHR and increase the resources available for preventing, detecting, and containing emerging infectious diseases in countries of all income levels.[24]

The WHO also supports global health through partnerships with other UN organizations and with external groups. **UNAIDS**, the Joint UN Programme on HIV/AIDS, is an entity co-sponsored by 10 UN system agencies—UNHCR, UNICEF, WFP, UNDP, UNFPA, UNODC, the International Labour Organization (ILO), UNESCO, the WHO, and the World Bank—to advance HIV/AIDS prevention and control. The **World Organisation for Animal Health** (known as **OIE**, the acronym for the Office International des Epizooties, the organization's original name in French) is an intergovernmental group that helps to control the spread of zoonotic infectious diseases and to promote food safety. OIE is not part of the UN system, but it works closely with FAO and the WHO on One Health efforts that integrate human, animal, and ecosystem health.

7.5 Development Banks

There are two main categories of official development assistance (ODA): bilateral aid and multilateral aid. **Bilateral aid** is money given directly from the government of one country (usually a high-income country) to the government of another country (usually a lower-income country) to support development activities. **Multilateral aid** is funding for development activities that is pooled from many donor countries. The largest multilateral organizations include the UN, the World Bank and other development banks, and the European Union. These multilateral groups typically serve as channels of global health funding, with high-income country governments serving as the funders and LMIC governments serving as the implementers.

Multilateral organizations, sometimes called intergovernmental organizations, receive two types of funds from member nations. Assessed contributions are mandatory dues calculated from each country's economic and population statistics. Voluntary contributions are extra funds that countries opt to donate. Mandatory funds go to the general budget of multilateral organizations. Voluntary contributions can be designated as core (unrestricted) or noncore (restricted) funding. Core funding can be used by the recipient multilateral organization on any projects the organization deems to be priorities. Some of these projects respond to the specific needs of selected low-income countries, but many are global initiatives that are of value to all countries (such as support for outbreak prevention and control). Noncore funding is given for a specific purpose by the donor and must be spent on the designated activity. In recent years, about 60% of total ODA has been bilateral ODA channeled through bilateral agencies, about 25% has been core multilateral aid from assessed and voluntary contributions, and about 15% has been earmarked (noncore) aid that was channeled through multilateral organizations to designated recipient countries.[25]

Two multilateral institutions have played a unique role in financing economic development projects, the World Bank and the International Monetary Fund (IMF). Both institutions were founded in 1944 during a summit held at Bretton Woods, New Hampshire, in the United States. Both are headquartered in Washington, DC. Both are owned by their nearly 180 member nations. Both offer loans and grants. A **loan** is borrowed money that must be repaid with interest. A **grant** is a gift of money that does not have to be repaid. Both the World Bank and the IMF may require recipient countries to implement economic policy reforms as a condition of receiving loans, such as raising taxes, reducing government spending, devaluing the country's currency, eliminating price controls and subsidies, and increasing the production of exports. However, the two institutions have distinct functions and modes of operating.[26] (They also have some distinct traditions. For example, the World Bank president has always been a U.S. citizen, while the IMF's managing director has always been a European.)

The **World Bank** is a multilateral investment bank that offers loans to developing countries. Its board of governors is composed of representatives from each member country, typically member countries' ministers of finance (or the equivalent, such as the Secretary of the Treasury of the United States). Most World Bank loans are expected to be

repaid with interest. Debt repayments are usually used to offer new loans for development projects in other countries, including projects focused on health.

The World Bank Group includes five institutions. The World Bank's primary lending institute is the International Bank for Reconstruction and Development (IBRD), which issues bonds so that it can fund loans to middle-income member countries. These loans carry an interest rate that is slightly above the market rate, and they are usually supposed to be repaid within 15 years. Most IBRD loans are for specific infrastructure projects, although funds can also be used for other economic development purposes. The International Development Association (IDA) makes interest-free loans to low-income member nations using money that has been donated from high-income countries. IDA loans are usually supposed to be paid back over a 25- to 40-year period. The World Bank Group is also home to the International Finance Corporation, which supports private sector development; the Multilateral Investment Guarantee Agency, which supports foreign direct investment in LMICs; and the International Centre for Settlement of Investment Disputes.

The **International Monetary Fund (IMF)** is a multilateral organization that provides a structure for international monetary policy and currency exchanges and makes loans to countries of any income level that have a balance of payment need and would otherwise not be able to make payments on their other international loans. The IMF is funded by membership fees (called quotas) paid by its member countries, and it operates like a credit union. The goal of IMF loans is to allow countries to rebuild their monetary reserves, stabilize their currencies, continue paying for imports, and create conditions for economic growth and high employment rates. The interest rates for IMF funds are usually slightly below market rates, and loans from the IMF are usually supposed to be paid back within a few years.

A major criticism of the international loan system is that interest payments divert money away from education, health, clean water, and other essential human services in lower-income countries. When interest rates are high, countries that are allocating large portions of their annual budgets to interest payments may still not be making good progress toward lowering the amount of principal that must be repaid in the future. The Sustainable Development Goals (SDGs) acknowledge the significant problems associated with overwhelming debt in low-income countries, and they aim to "assist developing countries in attaining long-term debt sustainability through coordinated policies aimed at fostering debt financing, debt relief, and debt restructuring, as appropriate, and address the external debt of highly indebted poor countries to reduce debt distress" (SDG 17.4).[27] The World Bank and the IMF have established plans for debt forgiveness in the poorest, most indebted countries so that those countries can devote more of their resources to their own health and educational systems rather than requiring those countries to prioritize debt repayment. However, concerns about debt burden are one of the reasons that development banks are now playing less of a role as channels of global health funding than they did in the past.

7.6 Global Partnerships

A **public–private partnership (PPP)** is a long-term collaboration in which the costs, risks, and benefits are shared by governmental and nongovernmental entities. For global health PPPs, the public partners typically are the national governments of countries from across the income spectrum that use PPPs as channels for dispersing DAH.[28] In 2000, more than 15% of DAH was channeled through development banks; by 2020, that percentage had decreased to about 5% as the share of funds distributed through public–private

partnerships grew from 0% to about 10%.[2] The private partners in global health PPPs include nonprofit foundations and for-profit corporations such as pharmaceutical companies.[29] Global health PPPs are developing new products (such as new medications, vaccines, and diagnostic tools), improving the quality and regulation of products, distributing donated and subsidized health products, educating the public about health issues, strengthening health services and health informatics systems, and coordinating complex global health efforts.[30]

Public–private partnerships often target development of medications and vaccines for diseases that for-profit companies are unlikely to invest in because of the limited revenue expected from a product created primarily for use in LMICs.[31] When these partnerships are funded by governments or philanthropic organizations rather than for-profit companies, the medications and vaccines the partnerships produce can be made available at an affordable price as soon as they are proven to be safe and effective. Other global health partnerships work to accelerate the timeline for making existing medicines, vaccines, and diagnostic tools legally available at affordable prices in LMICs.[32]

A health product is only valuable for global health when the intended users can afford the product and they choose to use the product for its intended purposes. Increasing the number of individuals who choose to use a new product requires the product to gain local acceptance and be adopted by end users. A **stakeholder** is a person who has an interest in the success or failure of a group and can influence or be affected by that group's decisions or actions. Increasing use of health technologies is a process that requires product advocacy and buy-in from a variety of stakeholders, including donors, policymakers, and end users.[33] **Social marketing** is the use of advertising strategies to change behaviors in targeted populations. After a new product is developed by the research partners in a PPP, partners with expertise in social marketing can increase demand for the new product, and partners with expertise in manufacturing can ensure that there are enough supplies to meet demand.

Dozens of PPPs are currently working to set and accomplish goals for selected global health issues. The largest global health partnerships are the Global Fund; Gavi, the Vaccine Alliance; and the Coalition for Epidemic Preparedness Innovations.[28]

- The **Global Fund**—more formally the Global Fund to Fight AIDS, Tuberculosis and Malaria—was founded in 2002 to support infectious disease control initiatives in LMICs. Applicant countries propose their own sets of projects, and they manage the implementation of funded programs. The Global Fund provides technical support and negotiates with pharmaceutical companies and other manufacturers to procure medications and other health products at low costs. The Global Fund is able to make these goods affordable by signing contracts to purchase massive quantities of commonly desired products—enough to meet the demand in many countries—and guaranteeing that the manufacturer will receive payment for its products.[34]
- **Gavi**, the Vaccine Alliance (formerly known as the Global Alliance for Vaccines and Immunization) was launched in 2000 and works with lower-income countries to identify vaccine priorities and then procure and distribute the vaccines. Gavi negotiates with manufacturing companies to increase the production of desired vaccines, and then Gavi and the recipient countries share the costs of the vaccines. Countries pay larger shares of the costs as their economies grow until they are fully sustaining their own vaccination programs.[35]
- **CEPI**, the Coalition for Epidemic Preparedness Innovations, was established

in 2016 to coordinate development of new vaccines that protect against emerging infectious diseases and to ensure that those products are available to everyone. In 2020, COVAX was launched by CEPI, Gavi, and the WHO as a mechanism for pooling resources for development of vaccines that protect against COVID-19 and sharing the risks of investments not yielding viable vaccine candidates. CEPI leads research and development of COVID vaccines for the partnership, Gavi is responsible for procurement and deployment of vaccines, and the WHO oversees equitable allocation.[36]

Successful global health partnerships yield benefits for all of the partners who contribute to research, production, and distribution activities. The governments of high-income countries attain an effective mechanism for achieving their foreign policy, scientific, and humanitarian goals. Corporate partners make a profit on reduced-price products by selling a larger volume of products than they would sell if they were not part of the partnership, and they also benefit when subsidized health products open up new markets to the company and enhance their reputations. Most importantly, the health of the world's people is advanced when partnerships increase the visibility of specific health issues, raise funds to support research and development, implement new treatment protocols and technical standards, and improve access to health care and the tools for health.[37]

7.7 Local and National Governments

In most countries, clinical health services are provided at government-owned and -operated medical facilities or at private nonprofit or for-profit medical facilities that are regulated by governments. Governments certify healthcare facilities, license healthcare practitioners, and approve medicines and other medical products. Governments also decide, at least in part, the list of services that are covered by public funds, social security, or health insurance schemes and the choices (if any) that people have about which healthcare facilities and clinicians provide their care. Governments are also responsible for the public health system (**Figure 7.6**).[38] Government public health agencies protect residents from unsafe medications, medical products, foods, and environmental hazards; provide recommendations and regulations about nutrition, vaccination, screening tests, worker safety, and other actions that promote health and prevent disease; and respond to outbreaks and other threats to public health.[39]

The lead governmental health agency in a country is often called the **ministry of health**. In most countries, clinical health services and public health programs are implemented by national ministries of health and their state or provincial and district health offices or with the approval of these agencies.[40] The national health agency also typically takes the lead on communicating about health-related issues with intergovernmental agencies (such as the WHO), global partnerships, and other external groups. For example,

the IHR require a country's lead health agency to submit timely reports about outbreaks of dangerous infectious diseases. Under the IHR, international teams cannot be deployed to support epidemic containment efforts until after a country's health minister submits a formal request for assistance.[41] Ministries of health also oversee the training and licensure of all clinicians working within their borders, including ensuring that visiting clinicians providing patient care are qualified practitioners.

In the United States, the Department of Health and Human Services (HHS) performs the functions of a health ministry plus additional tasks. The lead health protection agency in the United States is the U.S. **Centers for Disease Control and Prevention (CDC)**. One of the many roles of CDC is responding to outbreaks and other public health emergencies, including participating in international responses when foreign governments invite CDC to collaborate.[42] CDC also works with partners in other countries to conduct research, set up monitoring and surveillance systems, and train public health workers. Although CDC often participates in and leads responses to international health threats, it is not a multinational organization; CDC is an American governmental agency that is overseen by HHS.

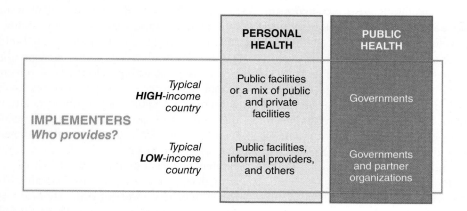

Figure 7.6 Governments are responsible for implementing most public health activities.

The **National Institutes of Health (NIH)** is the lead health research agency within the U.S. Department of Health and Human Services. Although most NIH research is conducted at study sites within the United States, NIH research may be conducted internationally when the research protocol meets the rigorous standards for ethical research established by NIH and by host country governments. Other operating divisions of HHS include the Agency for Healthcare Research and Quality (AHRQ), the Agency for Toxic Substances and Disease Registry (ATSDR), the Centers for Medicare & Medicaid Services, the Food and Drug Administration (FDA), the Health Resources and Services Administration (HRSA), the Indian Health Service, and the Substance Abuse and Mental Health Services Administration (SAMHSA), among others. Other countries have similarly complex organizational structures within their health ministries.

7.8 The Nonprofit Sector

A **nonprofit organization** (NPO) is a mission-driven group that reinvests surplus revenue in the organization rather than distributing extra income to owners or shareholders. Some NPOs are led by unpaid volunteers, but many have paid staff. A **nongovernmental organization** (NGO), sometimes called a private voluntary organization (PVO), is a nonprofit organization that is privately managed and receives at least some of its funding from private sources. NGOs from countries across the income spectrum are involved in providing clinical care and public health services, disseminating relief aid, supporting community development work, engaging in advocacy, and managing logistics for health programs and projects.

NGOs with global health portfolios may serve as channels of global health funding and often serve as implementers of health-related projects. NGOs may focus on one key health issue (such as specializing in providing surgical services or raising awareness about HIV prevention), or they may work on multiple issues in a particular location (such as delivering various socioeconomic development, environmental sustainability, and health interventions in one country or a smaller geographic area). An **international NGO** (INGO) is a large NGO with a diverse portfolio of projects that are implemented in numerous countries. A **faith-based organization** (FBO) is an NGO sponsored by a religious or religiously affiliated entity. FBOs rarely require that aid recipients adhere to a particular faith or listen to an evangelistic message, but they openly represent a particular religious tradition. Examples of FBOs include the American Jewish World Service, Catholic Relief Services, Church World Service, Islamic Relief, and World Vision.

Most large global health NGOs raise funds from individuals, private foundations, and governmental sources. One challenge for many NGOs is balancing the goals of donors and the desires and needs of recipients.[43] Directed donations are ones in which the donor stipulates that the contributed funds or supplies must be used in a particular way. Sometimes this works well, but when donors are not aware of conditions in the recipient community, the donation may not generate the intended outcome. A community that wants to upgrade its local health clinic by adding a solar panel to provide electricity to the building may instead receive a microscope that cannot be used without electricity. A nursing school may receive a donation of textbooks written in a language not spoken by any of the students or containing obsolete content. Or a donor may send used medical equipment that cannot be maintained by the community, expired medications that must be discarded immediately, or a water pump that cannot be locally repaired. (**Appropriate technology** is affordable and environmentally sustainable technology that can be locally operated and maintained.) Donors may also demand input into operational decisions. For example, they may insist that expatriates, rather than host-country staff, manage projects and oversee budgets, even if that inhibits capacity building in host communities.

Both large and small NGOs function best when their leaders communicate regularly with local government officials and other community leaders in the places where the NGO is implementing projects. For example, suppose that a nonprofit organization based in the United States wants to distribute free insecticide-treated bednets in rural communities in Nigeria. A typical first step toward implementation would be for representatives from the nonprofit organization and their Nigerian partner organization(s) to meet with leaders from the local government and other community organizations, including religious groups, to ask for their support. If the project is deemed to be one that will benefit the targeted communities, these local leaders and other community representatives will be able to help the nonprofit group design an appropriate distribution system and spread the word about the free bednets to members of the participating communities. The local leaders will also be able to tell American visitors if their community members do not need or do not want bednets, if the visitors are scheduled to come at a bad time (such as arriving during harvest time or on the day of a special event), or if hosting the visitors, who might need meals and places to sleep, will place an undue burden on some communities. Without doing these sorts of pre-implementation checks, visiting groups might inconvenience recipient communities, violate laws about taxation of imported products, duplicate existing malaria control programs, undermine the community health outreach programs of local hospitals and clinics, financially harm local vendors who sell bednets, or encounter other preventable problems.

The well-intentioned efforts of NGOs and other implementing groups working in global health (including for-profit international development companies) can sometimes have harmful side effects, including inadvertent social and political consequences.[44] The presence of a relief NGO in a conflict area may exacerbate instability by providing supplies that allow violence to continue or by encouraging displaced people to congregate in one area that could be targeted for attack. The long-term presence of a community development NGO may promote a "culture of dependency" and slow the development of governmental and commercial service providers. Those unplanned outcomes are not a reason for groups to stop delivering lifesaving relief supplies and supporting development activities, but they highlight the need for implementers to think ahead of time about how to maximize good and minimize harm.

Skills in effective cross-cultural communication are a requirement for everyone working in global health, especially for INGO leaders who must navigate complex political terrains. For example, some of the largest U.S.-based INGOs receive a substantial portion of their budgets from the U.S. government. Their workers may be seen by host communities as agents of a foreign government. Other challenges arise from the political situations in host countries. INGOs must decide how closely they will work with officials from host countries and how they will handle potential problems with corruption and mismanagement. Some humanitarian groups feel that it is important to remain publicly neutral about political matters, while others feel compelled to speak openly about any injustices they witness.

NGOs that successfully maneuver these complex landscapes play a very important role in global health implementation. Since NGOs often work for decades in the same communities, their employees and volunteers build relationships and trust with community members. NGOs can then serve as points of connection between communities and donors (and channel organizations), with NGOs using their networks to help new projects and programs quickly reach their target audiences. For example, Rotary International members worldwide have worked together on the global polio eradication campaign, with local Rotary

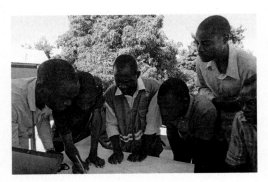

A polio vaccination team in Mozambique.

CDC/Theresa Roebuck. https://phil.cdc.gov/Details.aspx?pid=22756. Reference to specific commercial products, manufacturers, companies, or trademarks does not constitute its endorsement or recommendation by the U.S. Government, Department of Health and Human Services, or Centers for Disease Control and Prevention.

clubs in endemic areas facilitating vaccination campaigns in their own communities.[45] NGOs are often the organizations that actually deliver global health interventions to the people who will most benefit from them.

7.9 The Corporate Sector

A variety of businesses serve as global health channels and implementers. Some companies receive contracts to manage the delivery of global health services. Some companies are the private partners in PPPs, and they are paid to manufacture the medications, vaccines, and other products that are distributed as part of global health initiatives. (These companies might also donate some of their products as part of their corporate social responsibility plans, but that is a separate function from participation in contracted manufacturing of health products.) Some companies excel at **supply chain management**, the process of coordinating all the steps from selecting and procuring products through the logistics of transporting, storing, and delivering them.[46]

USAID is one of the major channels for disbursing global health funding from the U.S. federal government to companies that serve as implementing partners. USAID does not have the staff to implement all of its own projects, so many of its projects are managed by outside groups. Several of the leading USAID contractors are for-profit companies, such as Chemonics, DAI (formerly Development Alternatives Incorporated), Abt Associates, and Tetra Tech (and its wholly owned subsidiary ARD, formerly Associates in Rural Development). Most of the other leading USAID contractors are nonprofit organizations that receive nearly all of their funds from government contracts and are therefore not dependent on fundraising from private donors, such as FHI 360 (formerly Family Health International), Jhpiego, and RTI International. These groups are incorporated as nonprofits, but they are not charities. Only a few of the major recipients of USAID funding are charities that manage large government contracts but still rely on private donations for a large portion of their operating expenses. All of these groups compete with one another for USAID contracts.

Among the global health implementing groups that have annual budgets of millions of dollars, the functional differences between for-profits and nonprofits are often minimal. For example, both for-profit and nonprofit contractors typically offer their professional staff from high-income countries professional-level salaries and compensation packages, no matter what setting they are working in. Professional staff from LMICs who are working in their home countries—"host-country nationals," in international development lingo—typically earn salaries that are locally competitive but lower than the salaries of their peers from high-income countries,[47] even though these pay differentials can become a source of workplace tension.[48] Charities that are dependent on private donors tend to offer smaller compensation packages to employees.

Many companies that are not primarily focused on global health play a role in influencing health behaviors and health status, whether they are multinational corporations or smaller businesses. Food and beverage companies, manufacturers of hygiene supplies and personal care products, pharmaceutical companies, manufacturers of medical devices, and other corporations that produce health-related goods and provide health-related services play an important role in facilitating health for populations around the world. These businesses are typically not part of the funder–channel–implementer pathway for large-scale global health initiatives, but they are key contributors to achieving global health goals via market-based strategies. Any company may play a role in influencing health via marketing (especially if its products are ones that promote or inhibit health), lobbying, and corporate social responsibility activities.[49] Corporations can also play a role in health promotion by protecting the health and safety of their employees and the communities where they work, producing and selling healthy products, and participating in public health alliances.[50]

7.10 Research and the Academic Sector

Universities are generally considered to have three core missions: teaching, research, and service. Colleges and universities in countries across the income spectrum contribute to global health by educating future practitioners in medicine, nursing, dentistry, physiotherapy, pharmacology, counseling, other clinical disciplines, public health, engineering, statistics, informatics, business, marketing, public policy, public administration, law, international relations, education, the biomedical sciences, and all the other fields that contribute to improving human and environmental health directly or by improving the socioeconomic and environmental contributors to population health.

Many universities contribute to global health through **research**, the process of systematically investigating a topic in order to discover new insights about the world. **Quantitative research** is a research approach that uses structured, hypothesis-driven approaches to gather data that can be statistically analyzed. **Qualitative research** is a research approach that uses in-depth interviews, focus group discussions, participant–observation, and other unstructured or semistructured methods to explore attitudes and perceptions, identify themes and patterns, and formulate new theories. Academic researchers use quantitative and qualitative research methods to measure the epidemiological and economic burden from various health conditions; provide insight about the ways that people experience and understand health and disease; identify the socioeconomic, behavioral, environmental, and other risk factors for diseases and the protective factors that can keep people healthy; and carry out experimental trials to determine which interventions are the safest and most effective. Research at universities contributes to the development of new medications, vaccines, diagnostic tools, and medical devices.[51] The journal articles and other publications written by researchers in the academic sector and by people who work at research institutes, think tanks, and other organizations provide a critical foundation of scientific evidence that is used to develop global health strategies and design intervention plans. Researchers also contribute to needs assessments, prioritization exercises, and evaluations of the outcomes of global health initiatives.

While most of the global health funding that flows through universities is for educational and research activities, some universities also accept contracts to implement global health programs and subcontracts from other implementers to participate in some aspects of program implementation. Many students, trainees, professors, staff, and other members of university communities are also active in voluntary service that contributes to global health. All three of the traditional functions of universities—teaching, research, and service—are being used to advance global health.

7.11 Measuring Impact

Many packages of global health interventions would increase the quality of life of millions of people at a relatively low cost per person.

However, all of these interventions together add up to a lot of money, especially for low-income countries where the total amount spent on health per person per year is significantly less than $100. Trillions of dollars each year would be required to implement global health strategies for all of the various causes of disease, disability, and death. Difficult decisions must be made about how to allocate limited resources. Because resources for global health are scarce, funding recipients are expected to demonstrate to global health financers that their resources are being put to good use.

A typical project passes through planning, implementation, and evaluation stages, with assessment strategies applied throughout the project cycle. **Monitoring** is a process of ongoing assessment of a project or program to track progress toward achieving predefined targets. If the monitoring process reveals that a project or program is not fulfilling its mandate, adjustments can be made to increase the impact of the intervention. **Evaluation** is an assessment of how well a project, program, or policy has met its goals. Together, **M&E** (monitoring and evaluation) is the systematic collection of information about an ongoing intervention (process evaluation) and the determination of whether the intervention achieved its objectives (impact evaluation). Most contracts for global health implementation work mandate that the recipient group have a robust M&E plan that examines the inputs into a program, the processes used during the intervention period, the outputs generated during the implementation process, and the short-term outcomes and longer-term impacts that can be attributed to the program.

M&E uses quantitative indicators (numeric metrics) and qualitative indicators (descriptive observations) as measures of the success of a program. In addition to measuring population health outcomes like mortality and disability, M&E can be used to track the performance of health systems by quantifying the coverage rates for various interventions; tallying the financial, human, and material resources invested in health systems; evaluating the satisfaction of clients with health service providers and public health programs; determining which interventions are cost effective; and tracking the inequalities that may remain within a health system.[52] M&E can also examine whether progress is being made toward a program becoming locally sustainable.

Health policy analysis typically progresses through a series of steps such as defining the key health concern and the context in which it occurs; searching for evidence about the interventions that might improve the situation; evaluating the policy options and their likely outcomes; and making a decision about which option to prioritize for advocacy, funding, and implementation.[53] The planning phases that occur before implementation and evaluation include analysis of the policy options, considerations about how decision-makers and other stakeholders understand the problem and their readiness to support a policy change, and development of an action plan for communication, implementation, and evaluation.[54]

When "value for money" considerations in global health are being made, the best interventions are ones that are economical, effective, and efficient as well as being ethical and equitable.[55] Economical interventions use the fewest monetary and other resources. **Effectiveness** is a measure of the success of an intervention under real-world conditions. (By contrast, **efficacy** measures success in ideal, laboratory-controlled conditions.) An effective health intervention is one that generates significant improvements in the health of the target population. **Efficiency** is an evaluation of the cost effectiveness of an intervention that is based on both its effectiveness and resource considerations. Efficient interventions generate significant outputs, outcomes, and impacts (effectiveness) for the inputs (economics) invested in the project.

Cost-effectiveness analysis (CEA) is an economic analysis that compares the health gains from an intervention to the financial costs of that intervention. The goal of CEA is to confirm that the funds spent on a health initiative are achieving the planned outcomes and are making efficient use of financial and other resources. CEA works best when the goals of a project are specific and measurable. The most cost-effective global health interventions tend to be relatively inexpensive, can be easily distributed to many people, focus on prevention rather than treatment, and are targeted toward children and young adults so that they can avert many potential years of long-term disability or years lost to premature death. Some of the most cost-effective interventions include treating infectious diseases with antimicrobial medications, managing cardiovascular diseases with generic medications, and supporting child nutrition.[56] Expensive, high-tech solutions, such as coronary artery bypass surgery for treatment of ischemic heart disease, tend to be among the least cost-effective interventions.

CEA is not by itself sufficient for making decisions about health finance priorities and evaluating the value of global health programs. One limitation is that cost-benefit analyses tend to promote interventions that have already proven to be successful, and they tend to undervalue pioneering interventions that have not yet been proven to reliably achieve results. Innovation is necessary for improving global health practice, but creative ideas are sometimes considered to be risky uses of resources. For example, successful vaccine programs are very cost effective, but the upfront cost of research and development for a new vaccine is high and there is no guarantee that a safe, effective, licensed vaccine will be produced. It is important for some funding agencies and research organizations to be willing to risk failure so that new technologies and innovative approaches to solving global health problems can be developed and tested.

Some cost-effectiveness analyses compare the cost of action to the cost of inaction. The costs of inaction include lost lives, lost productivity due to disease and disability, and the direct and indirect costs of medical care that

are incurred when an intervention is not implemented to reduce the incidence and prevalence of preventable and treatable health conditions. When it is expensive to allow public health problems to continue, cost-effectiveness analyses can quantify the estimated long-term savings that will accrue when funds are invested in prevention and control activities. However, this reveals another shortcoming of cost-benefit analysis: CEA often requires analysts to make judgments about what a healthy life is worth. The calculations may require an estimate of how much it costs a disabled person to be unable to work, or they may demand an approximation of how much an additional year of life is worth for a 70-year-old compared to a 7-year-old. While these sorts of estimates may be helpful at the population level, they break down at the individual level. Estimates of lost wages do not capture the burden of lost self-sufficiency that may accompany a disability, and few families would put a price tag on grandpa and deem his year of life to be worth less than that of his grandchild.

Global health statistics, budget spreadsheets, and numbers-heavy progress reports sometimes seem to reduce real people to nameless, faceless masses: a few million children dying from preventable diseases like diarrhea and malaria, a few million people with treatable mental health disorders lacking access to therapy, a few million young adults with HIV infection gaining access to lifesaving antiretroviral medications, and a few million households gaining access to a reliable source of clean drinking water. But statistics cannot capture the profound grief experienced by families who lose a child, just as they cannot fully express how life changing a new water well can be. Many groups include photographs of people in their annual reports and other publications as a reminder that their work is about real people whose lives are being affected in very real ways by health problems and health interventions. Even when monitoring and evaluation activities appear to be coldly quantitative, empathy and shared humanity are central to the process.

References

1. McCoy D, Chand S, Sridhar D. Global health funding: how much, where it comes from and where it goes. *Health Policy Plan.* 2009;24:407–417.
2. Global Burden of Disease Health Financing Collaborator Network. Health sector spending and spending on HIV/AIDS, tuberculosis, and malaria, and development assistance for health: progress towards Sustainable Development Goal 3. *Lancet.* 2020;396:693–724.
3. *A Guide to the Project Management Body of Knowledge (PMBOK® Guide).* 5th ed. Newtown Square PA: Project Management Institute; 2013.
4. Oliveira-Cruz V, Kurowski C, Mills A. Delivery of priority health services: serving for synergies within the vertical versus horizontal debate. *J Int Dev.* 2003;15:67–86.
5. Msuya J. *Horizontal and Vertical Delivery of Health Services: What Are the Trade Offs?* Washington DC: World Bank; 2004.
6. *Health in All Policies (HiAP): Framework for Country Action.* Geneva: World Health Organization; 2014.
7. Woulfe J, Oliver TR, Siemering KQ, Zahner SJ. Multisector partnerships in population health improvement. *Prev Chronic Dis.* 2010;7:A119.
8. *Health in All Policies as Part of the Primary Health Care Agenda on Multisectoral Action.* Geneva: World Health Organization Technical Series on Primary Health Care; 2018.
9. Nutbeam D. Health promotion glossary. *Health Promot Int.* 1998;13:349–364.
10. Feldbaum H, Lee K, Michaud J. Global health and foreign policy. *Epidemiol Rev.* 2010;32:82–92.
11. *3D Planning Guide: Diplomacy, Development, Defense.* Washington DC: USAID; 2012.
12. Katz R, Kornblet S, Arnold G, Lief E, Fischer JE. Defining health diplomacy: changing demands in the era of globalization. *Milbank Q.* 2011;89:503–523.
13. Feldbaum H, Michaud J. Health diplomacy and the enduring relevance of foreign policy interests. *PLoS Med.* 2010;7:e1000226.
14. *Department for International Development Annual Report and Accounts 2019-20.* London: Department for International Development; 2020.
15. *Japan Bank for International Cooperation Annual Report 2020.* Tokyo: Japan International Cooperation Agency; 2020.
16. *Agency Financial Report Fiscal Year 2020: A Foundation Built on Decades of Global Health Investment.* Washington DC: USAID; 2020.
17. Himelfarb T. *50 Years of Global Health: Saving Lives and Building Futures.* Washington DC: USAID; 2013.
18. *Charter of the United Nations.* San Francisco CA: United Nations; 1945.
19. *Global Environmental Outlook 5 (GEO-5): Environment for the Future We Want.* Nairobi: United Nations Environment Programme; 2012.
20. *Strategy for Health (2016–2030).* New York: UNICEF; 2015.
21. *Twelfth General Programme of Work 2014–2019: Not Merely the Absence of Disease.* Geneva: World Health Organization; 2014.
22. *Thirteenth General Programme of Work 2019–2023: Promote Health, Keep the World Safe, Serve the Vulnerable.* Geneva: World Health Organization; 2018.
23. Taylor AL, Habibi R, Burci GL, et al. Solidarity in the wake of COVID-19: reimagining the International Health Regulations. *Lancet.* 2021;396:82–83.
24. Labonté R, Wiktorowicz M, Packer C, Ruckert A, Wilson K, Halabi S. A pandemic treaty, revised International Health Regulations, or both? *Global Health.* 2021;17:128.
25. *Development Co-operation Profiles 2020.* Paris: OECD Publishing; 2020.
26. Driscoll DD. *The IMF and the World Bank: How Do They Differ?* Washington DC: International Monetary Fund; 1996.
27. *Transforming Our World: The 2030 Agenda for Sustainable Development.* New York: United Nations; 2015.
28. *Financing Global Health 2020: The Impact of COVID-19.* Seattle: Institute for Health Metrics and Evaluation; 2021.
29. Storeng KT, de Bengy Puyvallée A, Stein F. COVAX and the rise of the 'super public private partnership' for global health. *Glob Public Health.* 2021. doi:10.1080/17441692.2021.1987502
30. Widdus R. Public–private partnerships for health: their main targets, their diversity and their future directions. *Bull World Health Organ.* 2001;79:713–720.
31. Howitt P, Darzi A, Yang GZ, et al. Technologies for global health. *Lancet.* 2012;380:507–535.
32. *Access to Medicine Index 2021.* Haarlem Netherlands: Access to Medicine Foundation; 2021.
33. Frost LJ, Reich MR. *Access: How Do Good Health Technologies Get to Poor People in Poor Countries?* Cambridge MA: Harvard Center for Population and Development Studies; 2008.
34. *Results Report 2020.* Geneva: The Global Fund; 2020.
35. *Gavi Progress Report 2019.* Washington DC: Gavi; 2020.
36. *Enabling Equitable Access to COVID-19 Vaccines: Summary of Equitable Access Provisions in CEPI's COVID-19 Vaccine Development Agreements.* Oslo: Coalition for Epidemic Preparedness Innovations; 2021.

37. Buse K, Harmer AM. Seven habits of highly effective global public–private health partnerships: practice and potential. *Soc Sci Med.* 2007;64:259–271.

38. Szlezák NA, Bloom BR, Jamison JT, et al. The global health system: actors, norms, and expectations in transition. *PLoS Med.* 2010;7:e1000183.

39. Frieden TR. Government's role in protecting health and safety. *N Engl J Med.* 2013;368:1857–1859.

40. Macfarlane S, Racelis M, Muli-Musiime F. Public health in developing countries. *Lancet.* 2000;356: 841–846.

41. Fidler DP, Gostin LO. The new International Health Regulations: an historic development for international law and public health. *J Law Med Ethics.* 2006;34:85–94.

42. *Strengthening Health Security Across the Globe: Progress and Impact of U.S. Government Investments in the Global Health Security Agenda: 2019 Annual Report.* Atlanta GA: Centers for Disease Control and Prevention; 2019.

43. Antrobus P. Funding for NGOs: issues and options. *World Dev.* 1987;15(Suppl 1):95–102.

44. Stein JG. In the eye of the storm: humanitarian NGOs, complex emergencies, and conflict resolution. *Peace Conflict Stud.* 2001;8:2.

45. Majiyagbe J. The volunteers' contribution to polio eradication. *Bull World Health Organ.* 2004;82:2.

46. *The Logistics Handbook: A Practical Guide for the Supply Chain Management of Health Commodities.* 2nd ed. Arlington VA: USAID; 2011.

47. Carr SC, McWha I, MacLachlan M, Furnham A. International–local remuneration differences across six countries: do they undermine poverty reduction work? *Int J Psychol.* 2010;45:321–340.

48. Bonache J, Sanchez JI, Zárraga-Oberty C. The interaction of expatriate pay differential and expatriate inputs on host country nationals' pay unfairness. *Int J Hum Resour Manage.* 2009;20:2135–2149.

49. Kickbusch I, Allen L, Franz C. The commercial determinants of health. *Lancet Glob Health.* 2016;4:e895–e896.

50. *The Bangkok Charter for Health Promotion in a Globalized World.* Geneva: World Health Organization; 2005.

51. Moran M. The grand convergence: closing the divide between public health funding and global health needs. *PLoS Biol.* 2016;14:e1002363.

52. Murray CJ, Frenk J. Health metrics and evaluation: strengthening the science. *Lancet.* 2008;371: 1191–1199.

53. Collins T. Health policy analysis: a simple tool for policy makers. *Public Health.* 2005;119:192–196.

54. *Supporting the Policy-Making Process.* Ottawa: Public Health Ontario; 2018.

55. *Better Value, Better Health: Towards a Strategy and Plan for Value for Money in WHO (A70/INF./6).* Geneva: World Health Organization; 2017 (May 16).

56. Horton S, Gelband H, Jamison D, Levin C, Nugent R, Watkins D. Ranking 93 health interventions for low- and middle-income countries by cost-effectiveness. *PLoS One.* 2017;12:e182951.

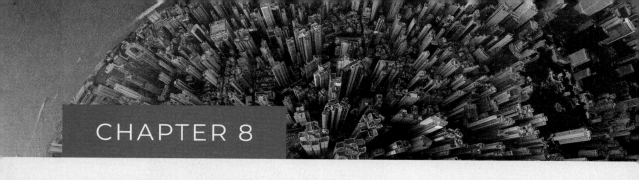

CHAPTER 8

HIV/AIDS and Tuberculosis

The new global partnerships and funding mechanisms that were established in the early 2000s in response to the HIV crisis transformed global health. Collaborative approaches to prioritizing, financing, and implementing global health programs are also being used to reduce the burden from tuberculosis, drug-resistant infections, and other dangerous infectious diseases.

8.1 HIV/AIDS, Tuberculosis, and Global Health

HIV/AIDS, tuberculosis (TB), and malaria are among the infections that cause the most deaths worldwide each year. These "big three" infectious diseases have been the target of numerous initiatives that aim to prevent, diagnose, and treat as many cases as possible. The rapid expansion of the global HIV epidemic during the 1980s and 1990s, in particular, was the primary driver of the shift from traditional international health practices to modern global health approaches.[1] Funding for infectious diseases accounted for less than 10% of the world's total development assistance for health (DAH) in 1990 and only about 20% in 2000, but the proportion grew to nearly 50% by 2010. In recent years, about 40% of DAH has been allocated to infectious diseases,

including about 33% just for the "big three" (**Figure 8.1**).[2]

The Global Fund to Fight AIDS, Tuberculosis and Malaria is a large public–private partnership founded in 2002 to support infectious disease prevention and control initiatives in low- and middle-income countries (LMICs). The Global Fund has spent more than $45 billion donated by the governments of high-income countries and other partner organizations to provide antiretroviral medications to millions of people with HIV, dispense antibiotics to millions of people with TB, distribute millions of bednets to people living in malaria-endemic areas, test and treat millions of cases of malaria, and strengthen health systems in LMICs, among other achievements.[3]

These three infectious diseases are also the focus of specialized multilateral organizations and agencies, like the Joint United Nations Programme on HIV/AIDS (UNAIDS); global partnerships and alliances, like the Stop TB

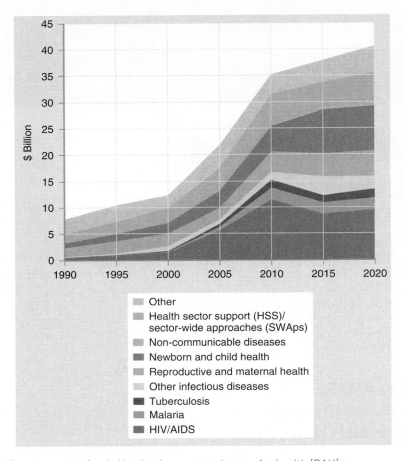

Figure 8.1 Program areas funded by development assistance for health (DAH).

Data from Global Burden of Disease Health Financing Collaborator Network. Health sector spending and spending on HIV/AIDS, tuberculosis, and malaria, and development assistance for health: progress towards Sustainable Development Goal 3. *Lancet.* 2020;396:693–724.

Partnership; diplomatic efforts, such as the President's Emergency Plan for AIDS Relief (PEPFAR) and the President's Malaria Initiative (PMI) in the United States; scientific collaborations like the International AIDS Vaccine Initiative (IAVI) and the TB Drug Accelerator Program; and countless charitable organizations. Investments in HIV/AIDS, TB, and malaria control are made for a variety of overlapping reasons, including the recognition that contagious diseases can easily spread across international borders, the humanitarian impulse to save lives, and the observation that healthier countries and communities tend to have stronger economies and more stable political systems.[4]

Most large-scale HIV, TB, and malaria programs have targeted just one of the diseases, and a comparison of the three conditions shows why integrated programs have not been the norm (**Figure 8.2**). Each of the three infections is caused by a different type of pathogen, so they require different types and durations of clinical care. Each has a distinct primary mode of transmission, which means that different prevention strategies are required. Each causes hundreds of thousands of deaths each year, so each demands a large-scale response. Each affects people of all ages, but children bear a greater share of the burden from malaria than from HIV and TB. However, there

Disease	HIV/AIDS	TB	Malaria
Type of pathogen	Virus	Bacterium	Protozoan
Name of the pathogenic agent	Human immunodeficiency virus (HIV)	*Mycobacterium tuberculosis*	Several *Plasmodium* species
Primary mode(s) of transmission	Sexual contact and injecting drug use	Airborne by droplet spread	Mosquito bites
Can it be cured with medication?	No	Yes	Yes
Approximate current number of deaths per year	700,000	1,400,000 (including 200,000 people with HIV)	600,000
Approximate percentage of deaths from the disease that occur among children	14%	16%	65%

Figure 8.2 Comparison of HIV/AIDS, TB, and malaria in typical recent years.

Data from *UNAIDS Data 2021*. Geneva: UNAIDS; 2021; *Global Tuberculosis Report 2021*. Geneva: World Health Organization; 2021; and *World Malaria Report 2021*. Geneva: World Health Organization; 2021.

are similarities across the disease control strategies, too, with all benefiting from the financial, technical, and operational support of dozens of players, including governmental agencies, nongovernmental organizations, businesses, charitable foundations, scientists and other researchers, health professionals, and local volunteers.

8.2 Viruses, Bacteria, and Fungi

The infectious disease epidemiology triad describes the agent, host, and environment characteristics that contribute to the spread of infectious diseases in human populations. An **agent** is a pathogen or a chemical or physical cause of disease or injury; a **host** is a human who is susceptible to an infection or another type of disease or injury; and the environment includes the external factors that facilitate or inhibit health, including social and political environments as well as natural and built environments. There are many pathogens that can be agents of infection, including viruses, bacteria, fungi, and parasites (**Figure 8.3**). Different infectious agents require

different methods of prevention and treatment. Interventions for HIV, TB, malaria, and other infections must be tailored to the type of infectious agent, its usual mode of transmission, and the technologies and other resources that are available to prevent and treat the infection.

A **virus** consists of a nucleic acid (DNA or RNA) encased in a protein shell called a capsid. A capsid is formed from protein subunits called capsomeres, and it may consist of a single or double shell. Viruses are grouped into dozens of families (including more than 20 families that are known to cause infections in humans) based on their shapes, modes of transmission, and other observations.

- Helical (or filamentous) viruses are shaped like long cylinders.
- Icosahedral (or isometric) viruses have roughly spherical shapes. A picornavirus, for example, is a nonenveloped icosahedral RNA virus named for its tiny round shape (with "pico-" being a prefix meaning 10^{-12}).
- Enveloped viruses have their capsids covered by an additional lipid (fatty acid) bilayer called an envelope. The envelopes

Type of Agent	Viruses	Bacteria	Fungi
Relative size	Small	Medium	Large
Number of cells	Acellular (noncellular)	Single celled	Single celled or multicellular
Nucleic acids	DNA or RNA (1 nucleocapsid)	DNA and RNA (1 chromosome)	DNA and RNA (2+ chromosomes)
Cell nucleus	None	Nucleoid region (prokaryote)	True nucleus (eukaryote)
Nuclear membrane	No	No	Yes
Cell organelles	No	No	Yes
Cellular membrane	No	Yes	Yes
Cell wall	No	Yes (peptidoglycan)	Yes (chitin)

Figure 8.3 Comparison of viruses, bacteria, and fungi.

typically have protein spikes on their outer surfaces. For example, a coronavirus is an enveloped helical RNA virus that has spikes of surface proteins that give it a halo- or crown-like appearance when it is viewed under a microscope.

- Complex viruses may have unusual or asymmetrical shapes or extra structures, such as protein tails.

Viruses are extremely tiny, and because they are acellular (not cells), they are generally not considered to be alive. They can only replicate by invading the cells of a living host and taking control of the cells' nuclei. After a virus particle attaches itself to the cell membrane of a human cell, its genetic material enters the cell and travels to the nucleus, where it directs the cell to make many new copies of the virus's genetic material and to form new viral proteins. A **virion**, or virus particle, is an assembled virus with nucleic acid and an outer protein coating. New virions are formed from the copied nucleic acids and proteins. These virions are then released from the cell either by gradual extrusion or by rupturing the host cell. After being liberated, the new virions travel to other parts of the body to infect additional

cells, or they are shed from the body to infect other people.

The human body will clear most acute viral infections on its own, but some viruses become chronic infections, such as HIV and hepatitis C virus. Viral infections cannot be cured by antibiotics designed to kill bacteria and parasites, but antiviral medications can reduce the number of virus particles present in the body and mitigate the symptoms of some types of infectious diseases. For example, antiviral medications can slow the progression of HIV infection, suppress the lesions caused by herpes virus, and make influenza symptoms less severe. However, the healthier option is for humans to avoid contracting viral infections. Vaccines protect against some viral diseases, including chickenpox, hepatitis B, human papillomavirus (HPV), measles, polio, and rotavirus. Personal hygiene and health practices such as handwashing often, using a high-quality face mask to protect against respiratory pathogens, and using barrier methods during sexual activities can reduce the risk of contracting many other viruses.

A **bacterium** is a single-celled organism that lacks a true nucleus. Bacteria can be differentiated based on their shapes, such as rods (bacilli), spheres (cocci), and spirals (spirochetes, vibrios, and spirilla); by relative size (although all are very small); and by the amount of a substance called peptidoglycan in their cell walls. The peptidoglycan on the surface of Gram-positive bacteria will bond to a special dye. Gram-negative bacteria have an outer membrane over the peptidoglycan layer, so the dye will not stain them. Bacteria are found nearly everywhere on the planet, from the arctic tundra to hot springs deep in the ocean. They play an important role in decomposition and chemical cycling, in the fixation of nitrogen into plants, and in the production of foods like cheese and yogurt. Millions of helpful bacteria line the human digestive tract and other body surfaces, crowding out harmful bacteria. However, some types of bacteria can cause disease. For example, some strains of *Escherichia coli* can cause severe diarrhea, and some strains of *Staphylococcus* can cause skin disease.

The stages of bacterial pathogenesis include contact with host tissue through a suitable portal of entry, adhesion to the cells of the host, invasion into new tissues and locations within the body after evading or overcoming the host's immune response, and multiplication. As bacteria are colonizing the body, they may release chemicals that cause their hosts to become ill. Some bacteria (usually Gram-positive ones, such as those that cause botulism and tetanus) produce and release exotoxins as they grow and metabolize, and these toxins can destroy cell walls and other structures. Many symptoms of gastrointestinal bacterial infections are the result of endotoxins that are released from the outer membrane of Gram-negative bacteria when the bacteria die and disintegrate.

Most bacterial infections can be cured with antibiotics, although a growing number of pathogenic (disease-causing) bacteria are becoming resistant to common antibiotics. Some types of bacterial diseases are vaccine preventable, including bacterial meningitis, pneumococcal pneumonia, tetanus, and whooping cough. The same types of health behaviors that prevent viral infections, such as hygiene and food safety practices, also help prevent bacterial infections.

A **fungus** is a spore-producing organism such as a mold, yeast, or mushroom. Fungi are heterotrophs, which means that they cannot make their own food, and they usually reproduce using both sexual and asexual reproduction cycles. Molds are composed of multicellular filaments called hyphae, and a network of hyphae is called a mycelium. Yeasts are single-celled fungi that reproduce by budding. Fungi are important decomposers used to make bread, beer, and some types of cheese, but some are pathogenic.

Fungal diseases frequently occur after the "healthy" bacteria that live in or on the body are disturbed by antibiotic use or immunosuppression. For example, *Candida albicans* is a yeast that is routinely found on human skin, especially around moist areas like the mouth, groin, and underarms. Sometimes an overgrowth of *Candida*, called **candidiasis**, presents as thrush (a white coating on the tongue), a vaginal yeast infection, or a diaper rash. Other examples of fungal infections include histoplasmosis (a fungal infection that affects the lungs) and dermatomycoses (fungal diseases of the skin) like ringworm and athlete's foot. Fungi thrive in moist, dark places, and are especially prevalent in the tropics. Antifungal medications can treat some fungal diseases.

8.3 HIV and AIDS

Human immunodeficiency virus (HIV) is a retrovirus that destroys specialized blood cells that are needed by the immune system to fight infection. A **leukocyte** is a white blood cell. There are several types of leukocytes, including neutrophils, lymphocytes, monocytes, eosinophils, and basophils. A **lymphocyte** is a type of white blood cell that attacks viruses, bacteria, and other pathogens. Lymphocytes include B cells, T cells, and natural killer (NK) cells. B cells form and mature in the bone marrow, while **T cells** are lymphocytes that form in the bone marrow, then mature in the thymus, a lymphatic system organ located behind the sternum (breastbone). Some T cells are "helper" cells that trigger the body's immune response, and some are "killer" cells that stimulate B cells to produce antibodies that combat viruses. **CD4** is a glycoprotein found on the surface of some types of immune system cells, including helper T cells. HIV targets CD4-positive (CD4[+]) T cells.

HIV can be transmitted from an infected individual to another person when body fluids like blood, semen, vaginal fluid, or breastmilk are exchanged during sexual contact; the sharing of needles used to inject drugs; or by mother-to-child transmission during childbirth or breastfeeding. HIV is not transmitted through casual contact like shaking hands, sharing eating utensils, or using the same toilet. Transmission of HIV through blood transfusions is rare now that donated blood and blood products can be tested for HIV. Most HIV infections are caused by HIV virus type 1, or HIV-1. There is also an HIV-2 virus that accounts for a small fraction of the HIV cases, primarily in West Africa.[5] HIV-2 progresses more slowly and causes milder symptoms than HIV-1.

AIDS is the **a**cquired **i**mmuno**d**eficiency **s**yndrome that occurs as a result of the destruction of immune system cells by the HIV virus.[6] A **sign** is an objective indicator of disease that can be clinically observed, such as a rash, cough, fever, or elevated blood pressure. A **symptom** is a subjective indication of illness that is experienced by an individual but cannot be observed by others, such as a headache, stomachache, pain, or fatigue. A **syndrome** is a collection of signs and symptoms that occur together. HIV is contagious because it is a transmissible virus; AIDS is not contagious because it is a syndrome related to HIV infection and is not an infectious agent. The secondary

infections associated with AIDS are called opportunistic infections. An **opportunistic infection** (OI) is one that occurs when the body's immune system is weakened enough to give a pathogen an opportunity to invade. The most frequently occurring OIs include tuberculosis, bacterial pneumonia, chronic diarrhea, and fungal infections such as *Cryptococcus*.[7]

A person newly infected with HIV may experience flu-like symptoms for a few days or weeks but is often asymptomatic (**Figure 8.4**). During this stage, the infected individual still has a normal number of CD4 cells, but there is a high viral load in the blood (with many virus particles per cubic millimeter) and it is possible to transmit the virus to others. The World Health Organization (WHO) has identified four clinical stages of HIV infection and AIDS disease that follow primary infection (**Figure 8.5**).[8] In stages 1 and 2, which can last from a few weeks to more than 20 years, the infected person is asymptomatic or has only minor symptoms like skin infections and recurrent respiratory infections. Stage 3 is marked by more severe symptoms like recurrent respiratory infections, persistent fevers, tuberculosis, mouth ulcers, and the loss of more than 10% of body weight due to chronic diarrhea. The CD4 count begins to fall, and the viral load in the blood begins to increase. In stage 4, serious OIs mark the onset of AIDS, and the CD4 count becomes very low (below 200 particles per mm[3]) and may fall to undetectable levels. Individuals with AIDS are vulnerable to OIs, many types of AIDS-associated cancers, and other comorbidities.

There is currently no HIV vaccine and no medication that can cure HIV infection. However, people who have contracted the virus can take medications that help manage the progression and symptoms of the infection. An **antiretroviral** (ARV) is a medication for a retroviral infection that suppresses the viral count and slows the progression of symptoms. **Antiretroviral therapy**

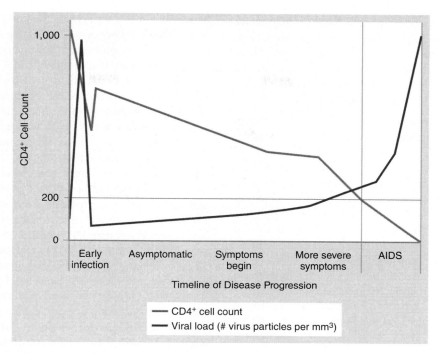

Figure 8.4 CD4+ cell count and viral load following HIV infection.

Stage	Primary HIV Infection	Clinical Stage 1	Clinical Stage 2	Clinical Stage 3	Clinical Stage 4 (AIDS)
HIV-associated symptoms	Mild	Asymptomatic	Mild	Advanced	Severe
Weight	Normal	Normal	Loss of less than 10% of body weight	Loss of more than 10% of body weight	HIV wasting syndrome
Activity level	Asymptomatic	Asymptomatic, normal activity	Symptomatic, normal activity	Bedridden less than 50% of the day in the last month	Bedridden more than 50% of the day during the last month
Examples of associated clinical conditions	Acute retroviral syndrome: flu-like symptoms about 2–4 weeks after initial infection that resolve within a few weeks	Persistent enlargement of lymph nodes in several parts of body	Minor skin problems (like fungal infections and mouth ulcers) and upper respiratory infections	Chronic diarrhea, chronic fevers, thrush, pulmonary TB, and severe bacterial infections like pneumonia and meningitis	Chronic diarrhea, chronic fevers, complex infections, and HIV-associated cancers

Figure 8.5 Clinical staging system for HIV/AIDS.

Data from *WHO Case Definitions of HIV for Surveillance and Revised Clinical Staging and Immunological Classification of HIV-Related Disease in Adults and Children.* Geneva: World Health Organization; 2007.

(ART), also called **HAART** (highly active antiretroviral therapy), uses combinations (sometimes called "cocktails") of three or more different types of medication that are taken together to combat HIV. The drugs used for ART include the following:

- Nucleoside/nucleotide reverse transcriptase inhibitors (NRTIs), such as abacavir (ABC), emtricitabine (FTC), lamivudine (3TC), tenofovir, and zidovudine (AZT)
- Non-nucleoside reverse transcriptase inhibitors (NNRTIs), such as efavirenz (EFV) and nevirapine (NVP)
- Protease inhibitors, such as atazanavir (ATV), darunavir (DRV), lopinavir (LPV), and ritonavir (RTV)
- Integrase inhibitors, such as dolutegravir (DTG) and raltegravir (RAL)
- Other types of medications, such as fusion inhibitors, attachment inhibitors, CCR5 antagonists, post-attachment inhibitors, and pharmacological enhancers

The WHO recommends that first-line therapy include an NRTI plus an integrase inhibitor (usually DTG).[9]

The **natural history of disease** describes the typical timeline for progression of an adverse health condition from onset to resolution (either recovery or death) if treatment is not received. The median survival time after infection with HIV if a person does not take ART is about 10 years, including an average of 2 years from onset of clinical AIDS to death.[10] Individuals may experience much shorter or longer than average durations of infection. Some people who contract HIV quickly progress to AIDS, while some survive for decades without disease progression. ART prolongs both the duration of time between infection and the onset of clinical AIDS and the time between onset of AIDS and death, extending the lives of people with HIV infection by years or even decades.[11]

The WHO recommends that treatment with ARVs begin immediately after diagnosis since earlier use of ARVs is associated with better outcomes than delayed treatment.[12] Use of prophylactic doses of co-trimoxazole (a combination of two antibiotics, sulfamethoxazole and trimethoprim) is recommended for people with advanced HIV to reduce the risk of bacterial, fungal, and protozoal OIs, and isoniazid can be used as preventive treatment in people with HIV who are at risk of TB disease.[12]

ART does not work for all people with HIV: some cannot tolerate the side effects, some do not adhere to the treatment regimen and skip too many doses for the medicines to be effective, and some have a drug-resistant strain of HIV.[13] Even when the medications reduce the viral load, they do not cure HIV infection or alleviate all of the symptoms. When someone with HIV stops taking ART, viral loads will rebound within just a few weeks.[14] However, for most people with HIV, ART is effective at managing HIV as a chronic condition and enabling many years of healthy life that would be impossible without the medicines. Even if one of the many HIV candidate vaccines under development proves to be highly effective and is added to the tools available for HIV prevention,[15] there will still be a continued need for HIV treatment services for individuals who already have HIV infections.[16]

8.4 HIV/AIDS Epidemiology

Phylogenetic analysis of stored serological specimens suggests that the first cases of HIV infection in humans probably occurred in the 1920s in central Africa in what is now the Democratic Republic of the Congo.[17] The first cases of AIDS were not diagnosed until 1981, when clusters of homosexual men in the United States were diagnosed with fungal *Pneumocystis carinii* pneumonia (PCP, now called *P. jirovecii* pneumonia)[18] and Kaposi's sarcoma, which until then had been a very infrequently observed type of cancer.[19] The HIV-1 virus was not identified by virologists until several years later.[20]

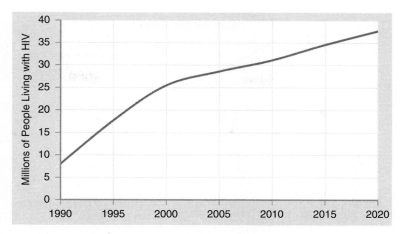

Figure 8.6 Number of people living with HIV worldwide.

Data from *UNAIDS Data 2021*. Geneva: UNAIDS; 2021.

Over the subsequent years, the epidemic spread across the globe, and the prevalence of HIV infection increased dramatically. By 1990, there were nearly 10 million people living with HIV. That number increased to 20 million by the late 1990s, more than 30 million by 2010, about 35 million by 2015, and about 38 million by 2020 (**Figure 8.6**).[21] One of the contributors to the increasing number of people living with HIV is expanded access to antiviral medications that enable people with HIV to live longer lives. However, the rising prevalence rate is also due to many people contracting HIV each year. In the absence of a cure for HIV, the long-term goal is to stabilize the prevalence of HIV by reducing the incidence of new HIV infections to zero and lowering the mortality rate from AIDS to zero. Once those goals are achieved, the prevalence of HIV will slowly decrease to zero as people with HIV die in older adulthood of diseases not related to HIV infection (or as HIV infections are able to be cured with new therapeutic regimens). Progress on HIV control is being monitored, in part, by tracking decreases in the incidence–prevalence ratio (IPR), which has a target of no more than 3 new cases per 100 prevalent cases per year, and the incidence–mortality ratio (IMR), which has a target of a <1:1 ratio (less than one new case per death).[22]

UNAIDS and its many partner organizations have established ambitious plans for dramatically reducing both the number of new HIV infections per year and the number of AIDS-related deaths each year between 2010 and 2030.[23] In 2016, the World Health Assembly called for action to reduce both the annual number of incident cases and the annual number of deaths to below 500,000 by 2020 and then to below 200,000 by 2030 as intermediate targets toward eventually reducing both incidence and mortality to zero.[24] Progress on reducing the number of new infections has been slow. New cases of HIV peaked at about 3 million per year around the turn of the century; by 2020, the incidence rate was still about 1.5 million per year, which was three times higher than the target for that year (**Figure 8.7**).[21] Progress toward reducing the mortality rate has been faster. The annual number of HIV deaths peaked at just below 2 million in 2005; by 2020, there were fewer than 700,000 HIV deaths.[21] However, this was still not a sufficient reduction to meet the global targets. About 1.5% of all deaths in a typical year were still attributable to HIV infection.[25]

One of the challenges of tracking progress toward achieving epidemiological goals is that

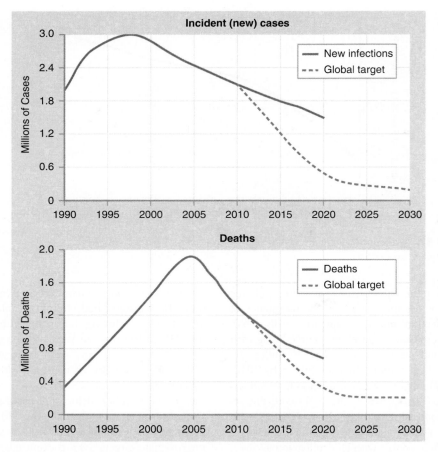

Figure 8.7 Number of new (incident) cases of HIV and HIV-related deaths per year.
Data from *UNAIDS Data 2021*. Geneva: UNAIDS; 2021.

many countries do not compile and disseminate reliable statistics about HIV prevalence, incidence, and mortality.[26] A related limitation is that it often takes several years to compile and analyze even routinely collected data. Preliminary reports generated from incomplete data sets provide funders and implementers with some information about trends, but accurate outputs are often not available for several years. For example, the preliminary HIV statistics for 2010 that were released by UNAIDS in 2011 estimated that 2.7 million people contracted new HIV infections that year, 1.8 million people died, and the prevalence was 34 million[27]; five years later, after they had

time to compile and analyze a more complete set of data, they concluded that the true numbers for 2010 were closer to 2.5 million new cases, 1.5 million deaths, and a prevalence of 33.3 million.[28] Most reports from UN organizations and research groups like the Global Burden of Disease Collaboration advise that outputs from different rounds of analysis should not be compared and newer estimates should be considered more reliable than older ones. Estimates of the peak HIV incidence and mortality rates have been revised downward over time, but the general trends for when those numbers peaked and how quickly or slowly they have decreased align with the original estimates.

About 0.6% of adults (ages 15+ years) worldwide are currently living with HIV infection.[21] Some countries have prevalence rates of less than 0.1%, but some countries in southern and eastern Africa have rates above 10%. In the 1990s and early 2000s, AIDS caused life expectancies to plummet in many sub-Saharan African countries, and it dramatically altered the social structure in communities with high incidence rates.[29] Because nearly all infections and deaths were occurring in young- and middle-aged adults, many older adults had to become caregivers for both their sick adult children and their young grandchildren. Orphans and vulnerable children (OVCs) without family caregivers often ended up homeless and living in extreme poverty.[30] Today, the majority of Africans living with HIV are taking medications that will enable them to raise their children and live into older adulthood if their access to the drugs is not interrupted. However, sub-Saharan Africa continues to be disproportionately burdened by HIV and AIDS. The high prevalence rate causes higher-than-average incidence rates. While the region accounts for only about 14% of the world population, it is home to 60% of incident HIV cases and two-thirds of prevalent HIV cases and AIDS deaths (**Figure 8.8**).[21]

More than half of the people living with HIV worldwide are females.[31] The all-ages rate of new infections is slightly higher in males than females, but among young adults the incidence and prevalence rates are higher among females then males (**Figure 8.9**).[21] The incidence rate among females rises sharply in adolescence and peaks in the 20s, while males experience peak incidence in their 30s (**Figure 8.10**).[25] Hormones and vaginal anatomy, physiology, and microbiology make

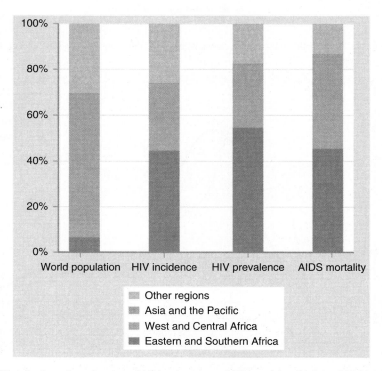

Figure 8.8 Distribution of total cases of HIV, new cases of HIV, and deaths from AIDS by world region.

Data from *UNAIDS Data 2021*. Geneva: UNAIDS; 2021; and United Nations Department of Economic and Social Affairs. *World Population Prospects: The 2019 Revision*. New York: United Nations; 2019.

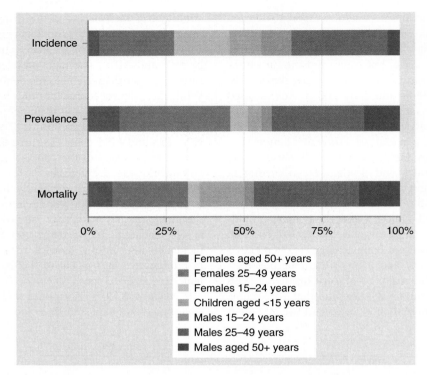

Figure 8.9 Distribution of total cases of HIV, new cases of HIV, and deaths from AIDS by sex and age group.

Data from *UNAIDS Data 2021*. Geneva: UNAIDS; 2021.

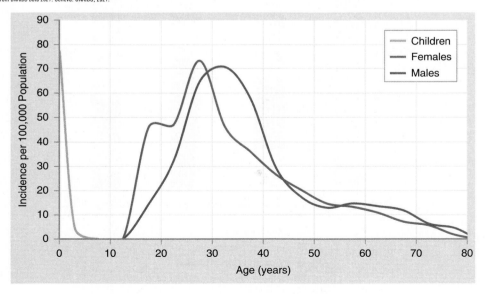

Figure 8.10 Rate of new (incident) cases of HIV per 100,000 people per year, by sex.

Data from GBD 2019 Diseases and Injuries Collaborators. Global burden of 369 diseases and injuries in 204 countries and territories, 1990–2019: a systematic analysis for the Global Burden of Disease Study 2019. *Lancet*. 2020;396:1204–1222.

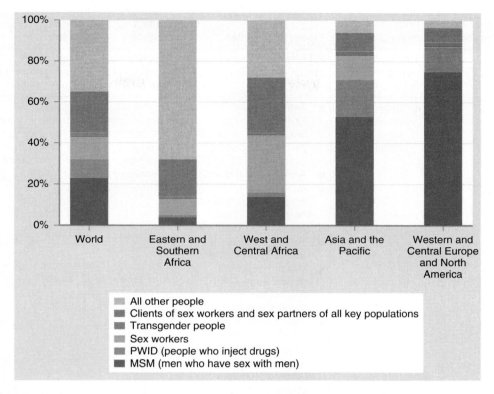

Figure 8.11 Proportion of new cases of HIV among people ages 15–49 years among key populations.
Data from *UNAIDS Data 2021*. Geneva: UNAIDS; 2021.

females more susceptible than males to sexually transmitted infections.[32] Women are at least twice as likely as men to acquire HIV from an act of heterosexual intercourse.[33] Women also face sociocultural risks for contracting HIV. Women generally marry at younger ages than men, they may not have the power to demand condom use, and they are more likely than men to be the victims of sexual violence.[34]

Some populations experience a significantly elevated rate of HIV infection because they have a higher than average likelihood of contact with HIV-infected blood and other body fluids, they are at high risk of being assaulted, and discrimination may limit their access to health care. Key populations with high vulnerability to HIV infection include men who have sex with men (MSM), people who inject drugs (PWID), sex workers, people in prison or other criminal justice detention centers, and transgender people.[35] About 60% of new infections worldwide occur among members of key populations and their sex partners (**Figure 8.11**).[21] In the sub-Saharan African countries with the highest HIV incidence rates, the majority of incident cases occur in women, and members of key populations account for only a minority of cases. In most high-income countries, MSM and PWID and their partners account for the majority of new infections, and most incident cases occur in men.

8.5 HIV Interventions

The ultimate goal for control of the global HIV epidemic is to reduce the incidence of new viral infections to zero cases while simultaneously

Level of Prevention	Primordial Prevention	Primary Prevention	Secondary Prevention	Tertiary Prevention
Goal	Prevent risk factors for HIV	Mitigate risk factors in people without HIV	Detect HIV before it becomes symptomatic	Manage HIV after it becomes symptomatic
Examples of interventions	■ Support inclusive and equitable communities	■ Reduce sexual risks by abstaining from sex, having few sexual partners, and using condoms ■ Avoid needle sharing ■ Use universal precautions to reduce contact with blood and body fluids ■ Treat other sexually transmitted infections ■ Use pre-exposure or post-exposure prophylaxis medications ■ Treat people with HIV with ART to lower viral loads and reduce the risk of transmission to others	■ Screen for asymptomatic HIV infection through voluntary counseling and testing services	■ Take antiretroviral therapy ■ Treat coinfections

Figure 8.12 Examples of interventions for HIV.

allowing all people who already have HIV infection to live long, healthy lives. A variety of interventions will be useful for reducing HIV incidence and supporting those who already have the infection (**Figure 8.12**).

The reduction in the HIV mortality rate in recent years is a direct function of increased access to ART. Individuals who are taking ARVs often reduce their viral counts to such low levels that there is almost no risk that they will pass the virus on to a sexual partner (even though the use of condoms and other precautions is still recommended) or other people. This makes treatment of existing HIV cases a critical component of HIV prevention strategies. The "15 by 15" goal of 15 million people taking ART daily by 2015 was achieved (**Figure 8.13**).[36] Because of that success,

ambitious "90–90–90" treatment targets were established:

● At least 90% of people with HIV infection know their status by 2020
● At least 90% of people with diagnosed HIV are taking ART by 2020 (so that at least 81% of all people with HIV are taking ART)
● At least 90% of people on ART are achieving viral suppression by 2020 (so that at least 73% of all people with HIV have achieved viral suppression)

For 2030, the aim is for all three measures to exceed 95%.[37]

By 2020, about 84% of people with HIV knew their status, 87% of people who knew they had HIV were taking medication (which

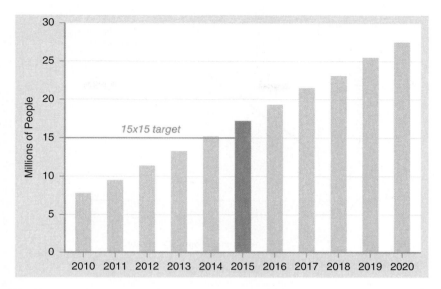

Figure 8.13 Number of people with HIV worldwide who are receiving antiretroviral therapy (ART).
Data from *UNAIDS Data 2021*. Geneva: UNAIDS; 2021.

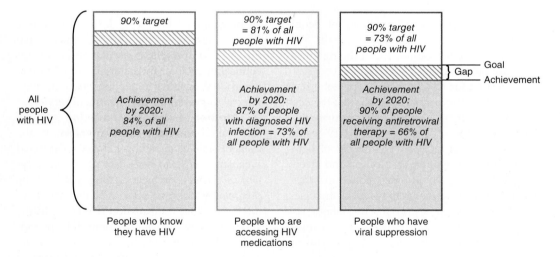

Figure 8.14 90–90–90 treatment targets for HIV worldwide by 2020 and actual achievements (shaded area) by 2020.
Data from *UNAIDS Data 2021*. Geneva: UNAIDS; 2021.

equals 73% of all people with HIV), and 90% of people taking medications had achieved viral suppression (which equals about 66% of all people with HIV) (**Figure 8.14**).[21] While this represented good progress in the percentage of people with HIV who were taking ART, it fell short of the 90–90–90 goal for 2020 (**Figure 8.15**).[21] An acceleration in the scale-up of ART programs will be necessary to get on track toward meeting the global targets

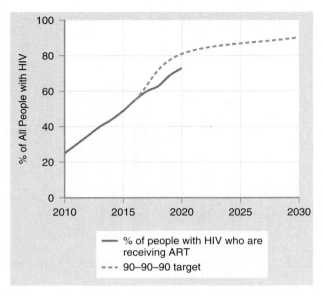

Figure 8.15 Percentage of people with HIV who are receiving antiretroviral therapy (ART).
Data from *UNAIDS Data 2021*. Geneva: UNAIDS; 2021.

for 2030. There are still millions of people with HIV infection who would benefit from access to ART but cannot afford the treatment or have other barriers to accessing it.

Testing for HIV enables people who have HIV infection to be diagnosed so that they can access treatment. **Voluntary counseling and testing** (VCT), also called HIV testing and counseling (HTC), is a process of being tested for HIV or another infection and receiving counseling about risk reduction, treatment referrals, and communication strategies. VCT includes pre-test counseling about risk assessment, the testing process, and planned prevention and coping strategies; performance of an HIV test, typically using a rapid diagnostic test of blood or oral fluids; receipt of test results; and post-test counseling about risk reduction and disclosure of HIV status.[38] Testing is recommended for everyone with known exposure to HIV, everyone who is a member of a high-risk population, everyone with symptoms consistent with HIV infection, everyone diagnosed with a sexually transmitted infection, everyone diagnosed with tuberculosis,

all pregnant women, and all blood donors.[39] All HIV testing services should ensure that the "5Cs" are present: consent, confidentiality, counseling before and after the test, correct (valid) test results, and connection through referral to prevention and treatment services.[39]

Mother-to-child transmission (MTCT), also called **vertical transmission**, is the transmission of a pathogen from an infected pregnant woman to her offspring during pregnancy, delivery, or breastfeeding. ARV use by pregnant women is a form of prevention of mother-to-child transmission (PMTCT). In the absence of any ARV interventions, a baby born to an HIV-infected mother has about a 15%–30% risk of contracting HIV during delivery; if the infant is breastfed for several months, the cumulative risk can be as high as 25%–45%.[40] If the mother takes ARVs during pregnancy and delivery—and in the weeks after delivery, if she is breastfeeding—the likelihood of transmission is much lower, only about 1% or 2%.[41] The WHO encourages new mothers with HIV who have undetectable HIV viral counts to breastfeed while continuing to take ART;

mothers with HIV infection who are not taking ART are encouraged to use formula instead of breastmilk when replacement feeding is acceptable, feasible, affordable, sustainable, and safe (AFASS).[42] When families cannot reliably afford formula or do not have consistent access to clean water, the risk of infant death due to diarrhea from unsafe water used to mix the formula may be greater than the risk of contracting HIV through breastmilk; in those situations, breastfeeding may be the safest option even for mothers with HIV who are not taking ART.

As the percentage of pregnant women accessing ARVs increased to 85%, the rate of MTCT decreased, but about 150,000 babies still contract HIV infection each year through MTCT (**Figure 8.16**).[21] Some pregnant women with HIV do not know their status, so they are not aware that they are at risk of transmitting the virus to their newborns. Some women who know they have HIV cannot afford ART or live too far from a formal health center to access it, some choose not to take ART because they are at risk of violence if their partners discover that they are taking HIV medications, and some choose not to take medications for other reasons.

ARVs are also used for prevention purposes by people who do not have HIV infection. **Pre-exposure prophylaxis (PrEP)** is the process of taking medications prior to a likely exposure to a pathogen in order to reduce the risk of contracting an infection. When both partners in a relationship undergo HIV testing and they are found to be discordant, with one member HIV positive and the other HIV negative, the HIV-negative partner can opt to take PrEP to reduce the risk of infection.[43] **Post-exposure prophylaxis (PEP)** is the process of taking medications after exposure to a pathogen in order to reduce the likelihood of contracting an infection. People with occupational exposures to HIV, such as healthcare workers who have sustained a needle stick injury while treating a patient with HIV, and those with other unexpected

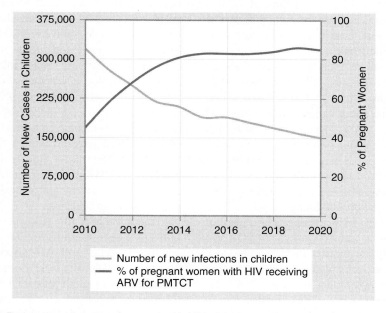

Figure 8.16 Percentage of pregnant women with HIV taking antiretroviral (ARV) medications for prevention of mother-to-child transmission (PMTCT) of HIV and number of infants contracting HIV each year.

Data from *UNAIDS Data 2021*. Geneva: UNAIDS; 2021.

potential exposures to HIV, such as the victims of sexual assaults, can complete a short course of ARVs as PEP to reduce the likelihood of infection.[44]

Several behavioral prevention methods are recommended for all people to reduce the risk of contracting HIV. One is **universal precautions**, the use of barriers like nitrile gloves to prevent contact with blood or body fluids when caring for a sick person or cleaning soiled laundry. Another is following the ABCs of HIV prevention: abstinence, being faithful to a partner if sexually active, and consistently and correctly using a condom during all sexual acts.[45] Although the risk of HIV per sexual act is usually low—less than 1 in 250 heterosexual contacts with a person who has HIV infection—the cumulative risk can be high, so consistent condom use is necessary.[46] Routine use of health services is also beneficial since detection and treatment of other sexually transmitted infections reduces biological vulnerability to HIV.[47] Health workers in all regions of the world must continue HIV/AIDS education efforts because the incidence of new cases tends to increase when people stop worrying about their risk.

Several other risk reduction strategies are also being used for HIV prevention. Male **circumcision** is the surgical removal of the foreskin of the penis. Voluntary male medical circumcision (VMMC) in countries with high levels of HIV transmission where circumcision of male infants has not been the traditional practice has been shown to reduce incidence of HIV infection in men who undergo the procedure.[48] (VMMC reduces the risk of HIV infection, but it does not negate the need to use condoms as protection against HIV and other sexually transmitted infections.) In some places, needle exchanges for injecting drug users have helped reduce incidence.[49] A combination of approaches is often the best option to ensure protection of individuals and communities. However, limited budgets for disease prevention and control mean that in most places only a few types of HIV services can be implemented.[50]

About 94% of new cases of HIV and 98% of AIDS deaths occur in LMICs.[25] In a typical recent year, about $20 billion total was spent on HIV prevention, treatment, and other activities in LMICs.[2] Nearly half of the funds were provided by the governments of LMICs, and most of the remaining funds came from DAH from high-income countries. About half of the DAH for HIV/AIDS in recent years has come in the form of bilateral aid from the United States.[51] **PEPFAR**, the U.S. President's Emergency Plan for AIDS Relief, provides financing for ART and other HIV prevention and treatment services in LMICs. PEPFAR was launched in 2003 when few people living with HIV in sub-Saharan Africa had access to ART. In the years since its founding, PEPFAR funding has enabled millions of people in LMICs to gain access to life-extending medications and has allowed millions of babies to be born HIV free to mothers with HIV infection. Each year, PEPFAR provides full courses of ART to millions of people, supports VCT programs that test tens of millions of people, sponsors VMMC programs in targeted regions, and funds programs that care for orphans and vulnerable children.[52] After PEPFAR, non-governmental organizations (funded by governments and philanthropies) and the Global Fund (a partnership funded mostly by high-income countries) are the second and third largest channels for DAH for HIV/AIDS.[51] The mix of funders and channels involved in HIV programming illustrates the complexity of current global health financing and delivery mechanisms.

Total funding for HIV interventions in LMICs exceeds funding for TB and malaria combined, and households pay out of pocket for a much smaller share of HIV prevention and treatment costs than they do for TB and malaria (**Figure 8.17**).[51] Even so, $20 billion per year is several billion dollars less than the amount required to be on track to meet global goals for reducing HIV incidence and mortality.[51]

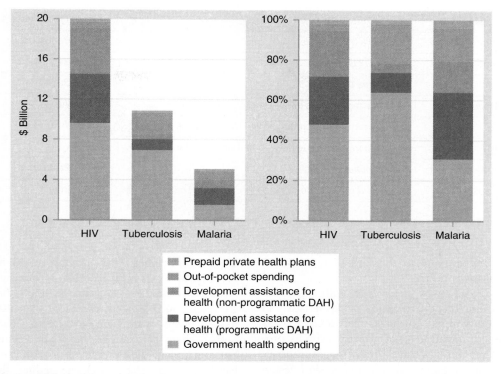

Figure 8.17 Health spending on HIV, tuberculosis, and malaria in low- and middle-income countries in a typical recent year.

Data from *Financing Global Health 2019: Tracking Health Spending in a Time of Crisis.* Seattle: Institute for Health Metrics and Evaluation; 2020.

8.6 Sexually Transmitted Infections

Besides HIV, several other pathogens can be transmitted through sexual contact (**Figure 8.18**).[53] A **sexually transmitted infection** (STI) is an infection spread through sexual intercourse or other types of sexual contact. STIs are often asymptomatic. When symptoms of an STI are present, the affected individual is considered to have a sexually transmitted disease (STD), also called a venereal disease.

Some of the most frequently occurring bacterial STIs worldwide are chlamydia,[54] gonorrhea,[55] and syphilis.[56] **Chlamydia** is an infection with *Chlamydia trachomatis*, obligate intracellular bacteria that can cause chronic urogenital or eye infections. **Gonorrhea** is an infection with diplococcus *Neisseria gonorrhoeae* bacteria. Chlamydia and gonorrhea are often asymptomatic, especially in women, but they may cause reproductive tract discharge and a burning sensation when urinating. If left undiagnosed and untreated, both infections can cause chronic health problems, such as **pelvic inflammatory disease**, an infection in the upper female reproductive system (the uterus, ovaries, and other structures) that can cause pain and lead to scarring and infertility. About 130 million new cases of chlamydia and 90 million new cases of gonorrhea occur worldwide each year.[57] Bacterial STIs can usually be cured with antibiotics, but cases of drug-resistant gonorrhea that

Disease	Agent Name	Type of Agent
Chlamydia	*Chlamydia trachomatis*	Bacterium
Gonorrhea	*Neisseria gonorrhoeae*	Bacterium
Syphilis	*Treponema pallidum*	Bacterium
Herpes	Herpes simplex virus (HSV-2, herpesvirus family)	Virus
HIV	Human immunodeficiency virus (HIV, retrovirus family)	Virus
HPV	Human papillomavirus (HPV, papillomavirus family)	Virus
Trichomoniasis	*Trichomonas vaginalis*	Protozoan
Crabs	*Pthirus pubis* (crab louse)	Insect

Figure 8.18 Examples of sexually transmitted infections (STIs).

do not respond to standard therapies are a growing concern.[58]

Syphilis is an infection with spirochete bacteria called *Treponema pallidum* that can cause chronic cardiovascular and nervous system impairments. Untreated syphilis progresses through three clinical stages. Primary syphilis presents as a painless skin lesion called a chancre. The second stage is characterized by a rash on the palms of the hands and the soles of the feet as well as symptoms such as swollen lymph nodes and fatigue. Late stage syphilis may persist for years and cause weakened arterial walls and nervous system impairment.[59] When pregnant women have syphilis, there is a high rate of stillbirth, neonatal mortality, and birth defects.[60] About 5.6 million people contract syphilis each year, and the global prevalence is estimated to be nearly 20 million because many people with syphilis have not been treated for it.[57] Untreated maternal syphilis causes more than 140,000 fetal deaths and stillbirths and more than 100,000 clinical cases of congenital syphilis each year.[61] Screening all pregnant women for syphilis so that infected women can receive treatment early in pregnancy reduces the risk of complications.[62]

Several STIs are caused by viruses, including HIV, herpes, and HPV. **Herpes** is an infection with a herpesvirus that can cause painful ulcers. Genital herpes is usually caused by herpes simplex virus type 2 (HSV-2). A related virus, HSV-1, causes lesions on the mouth that are often called "cold sores." More than 400 million people worldwide have HSV-2 infections.[63] There is no cure for herpes infections, but antiviral medications (such as acyclovir, faciclovir, and valaciclovir) can reduce the severity and frequency of flareups.[64] Human papillomavirus (HPV) causes genital warts and is associated with a significant increase in the risk of cervical cancer and cancers of the oropharynx, especially the throat.[65] A vaccine for HPV is now available in some countries,[66] but no effective vaccine has been developed for HIV or herpes.

A few parasites can also be transmitted through sexual contact. **Trichomoniasis** is a protozoal sexually transmitted infection caused by *Trichomonas vaginalis*. More than 150 million people become infected with this parasite every year.[57] Pubic lice (*Pthirus pubis*), also called crabs or pediculosis pubis, are ectoparasites that cling to human hair, feed on human blood, and cause intense itching.[67]

STIs can be prevented by abstinence from sexual activity, the use of barriers such as condoms that limit direct contact with body fluids (although some infections may occur even with condom use), and treatment of infected individuals so that they do not transmit the infection to sexual partners. Public health interventions to reduce the population-level burden from STIs include sex education, risk reduction counseling, condom distribution, HPV vaccination, screening for asymptomatic infections, treatment or management of diagnosed cases, and testing and treating sexual partners of known cases.[68] **Partner notification** is the process of a patient diagnosed with an STI communicating with his or her sexual partners (or a public health official communicating with the partners of the diagnosed individual) about their need to be tested so that they can receive appropriate treatment, if necessary, and they can take steps to protect the health of future partners.[69]

8.7 Tuberculosis

Tuberculosis (TB) is the disease caused by infection with *Mycobacterium tuberculosis* bacteria, which are spread through airborne droplets.[70] TB can affect any part of the body, but it usually occurs in the lungs. TB affecting the lungs is called pulmonary TB. TB outside of the lungs is called extrapulmonary TB. Pulmonary TB used to be called consumption because people with the disease were "consumed" by it as they developed a bloody cough, persistent fever, wasting, and pale skin. Anyone can become infected with TB, but the rate of infection is higher among individuals who are undernourished, have other health conditions that are not being medically managed, smoke tobacco, and live or work in crowded facilities that have poor ventilation and high levels of indoor air pollution.[71]

A distinction is made between having TB infection and having TB disease. An **infection** occurs when an infectious agent is reproducing inside a person. This usually causes an immunological response specific to the pathogen, and that response can often be detected through laboratory testing. **Disease** is the presence of signs or symptoms of poor health. **TB disease** (or **active TB**) is the symptomatic, contagious

form of tuberculosis. Some people who contract TB infection quickly develop TB disease, and some instead develop a chronic infection that is neither symptomatic nor contagious.[72] All people with TB disease have TB infection, but most people with TB infection will never develop TB disease.

The **incubation period** for an infectious disease is the time between exposure to a pathogen and onset of symptoms. The **latent period** for an infection is the time between exposure to a pathogen and onset of contagious disease. The latent period may be shorter or longer than the incubation period. **Latent TB infection (LTBI)** is present when tuberculosis bacteria are reproducing within a person's body without causing the individual to feel sick or be contagious. LTBI occurs when the body's immune system forms a granuloma by deploying cells to surround the bacteria and contain them within one part of the lung.[73] LTBI may persist for decades without progressing into a symptomatic illness, but about 5%–15% of people with LTBI who do not have HIV infection will develop TB disease during their lifetimes.[74] People with HIV infection are about 20 times more likely to develop active TB disease than people without HIV infection.[75] The risk of infection is also higher among people who are undernourished, have diabetes, smoke tobacco, or consume large quantities of alcohol.[76]

TB disease occurs when someone with a new TB infection or someone with LTBI develops symptoms and becomes ill (**Figure 8.19**). The symptoms of TB disease include fevers, weight loss, night sweats, and a cough that may produce bloody sputum (phlegm from the lungs). Some people with active TB may develop a disseminated form of TB in which the bacteria spread from the lungs into other parts of the body. Active TB is a contagious form of TB infection. People with TB disease may infect several other people each year, especially if they have frequent and prolonged interactions with susceptible individuals.[77]

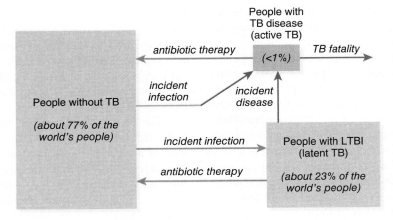

Figure 8.19 TB infection, latent TB infection (LTBI), and TB disease.

Laboratory tests for TB are used as part of routine screening for people who have elevated risk for TB, such as people with HIV infection and those who have occupational exposure to silica[78]; for clinically diagnosing people with symptoms of TB disease; and as part of outbreak responses that test contacts of TB cases so that treatment can be initiated before infected contacts develop TB disease.[79] Two types of screening tests are used to detect possible cases of TB.[80] One is the purified protein derivative (PPD) skin test, also called the Mantoux tuberculin skin test (TST), in which a small amount of TB bacterial protein is injected under the skin and the reaction is monitored. A person with TB infection will have an immune response and develop a rash at the injection site. The other is the interferon-gamma release assay (IGRA) blood test. If a person has a positive skin or blood test, a chest X-ray will be taken to look for lesions that might be pockets of TB infection. If pulmonary TB is suspected, a sputum smear test is conducted on the phlegm produced by deep coughs. A microscope is used to check the stained specimen for the presence of acid-fast bacilli (AFB). The diagnosis can be confirmed with a positive culture grown in a laboratory for several days.

The standard treatment regimen for TB requires patients to take several different types of antibiotics daily for six months or longer.[81] First-time TB patients typically start with two months

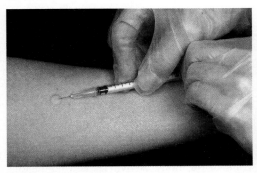

Tuberculin skin test.

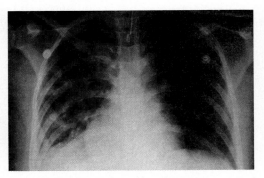

Chest X-ray of a person with pulmonary tuberculosis.

of intensive therapy in which they take isoniazid, rifampicin, pyrazinamide, and ethambutol daily, and then they continue to take at least isoniazid and rifampicin for an additional four months of continuation therapy. Most symptoms of TB disease resolve after the first two months, but completing the full course of treatment is essential for ensuring that even the hardiest bacteria are killed. The Global TB Drug Facility, founded in 2011, provides medications for a standard six-month course of treatment for about $40 per patient.[82] Complicated cases require more expensive antibiotics and longer durations of treatment.

8.8 TB Epidemiology

About 1.7 billion people worldwide—about 23% of the global population—are currently infected with the TB bacillus.[83] Almost all of these individuals have latent TB infection rather than active TB disease. Some of these individuals will convert from LTBI to active TB disease each year, and many people with new TB infections will also develop TB disease. The total number of people with TB disease in a calendar year includes people experiencing TB disease for the first time plus individuals with TB disease that has persisted for longer than one year and those with recurrent infections due to relapse or reinfection. A relapse occurs when someone who has tested negative for TB during treatment has a reactivation of the infection and tests positive again after completing the full course of prescribed antibiotics. A reinfection occurs when someone who has been successfully treated for TB in the past becomes infected with a new strain.

In a typical recent year, an estimated 10 million people developed new cases of TB disease.[82] About 93% of those incident cases were new TB disease and about 7% were relapses.[74] However, there is considerable uncertainty about the incidence and prevalence of TB disease because of underdiagnosis and underreporting.[84] The **case detection rate** (CDR) is the proportion of people with a disease who are diagnosed as having that disease and, if the condition is a notifiable disease,

have that case reported to government health agencies. The CDR for TB disease is low in many countries. In a typical recent year, about 30% of cases of new TB disease are estimated not to have been diagnosed or reported, which means that nearly one in three people with TB disease was not accessing TB care.[74] Expanded access to diagnosis and treatment would reduce the incidence of new infections by decreasing the prevalence of contagious infections in the population and would lower the case fatality rate by enabling more people with active TB to start treatment before they are critically ill.

The number of deaths from TB each year has decreased substantially since 2000, but tuberculosis remains the leading cause of infectious disease mortality in a typical year. By the start of 2020, about 1.4 million TB deaths were occurring annually, including about 1.2 million among people without HIV and 200,000 among people with HIV.[74] (Because the COVID-19 pandemic reduced access to diagnosis and treatment, the number of deaths among people without HIV increased to about 1.3 million in 2020.[82])

In recent years, about 10% of new cases of TB disease worldwide and about 15% of TB deaths have occurred in people with HIV infection (**Figure 8.20**).[25] TB is the leading immediate cause of death among people with HIV, although TB dropped from causing about 35% of AIDS mortality in 2000 to about 25% of all AIDS deaths in 2020 as more people with HIV received ART and treatment for LTBI before it became active TB.[25] Because TB fatalities among people with HIV are usually classified as HIV deaths rather than as TB deaths, statistics for TB are typically reported separately by HIV status. Communities with the highest HIV prevalence and mortality rates have the highest burden from HIV-associated TB (**Figure 8.21**).[25]

Males bear a disproportionate burden from TB, accounting for at least 55% of incident cases and about 63% of deaths (**Figure 8.22**).[25] The reasons for the observed sex differences are not well understood, but they may be a function of both socio-behavioral and biological factors.[85] Men are more likely than women

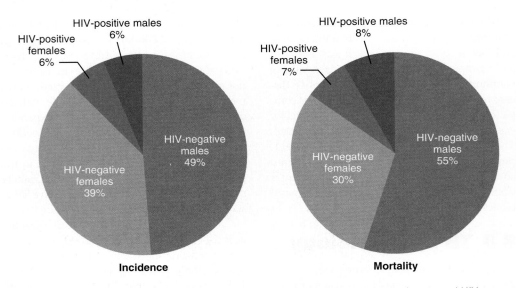

Figure 8.20 Incidence of and mortality from TB disease in a typical recent year, by sex and HIV status.

Data from GBD 2019 Diseases and Injuries Collaborators. Global burden of 369 diseases and injuries in 204 countries and territories, 1990–2019: a systematic analysis for the Global Burden of Disease Study 2019. *Lancet*. 2020;396:1204–1222.

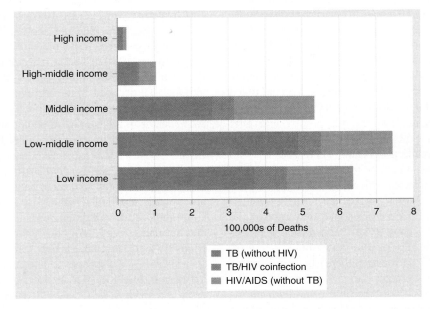

Figure 8.21 Number of deaths from TB, TB/HIV-coinfection, and HIV/AIDS in a typical (nonpandemic) year, by country sociodemographic group.

Data from GBD 2019 Diseases and Injuries Collaborators. Global burden of 369 diseases and injuries in 204 countries and territories, 1990–2019: a systematic analysis for the Global Burden of Disease Study 2019. *Lancet*. 2020;396:1204–1222.

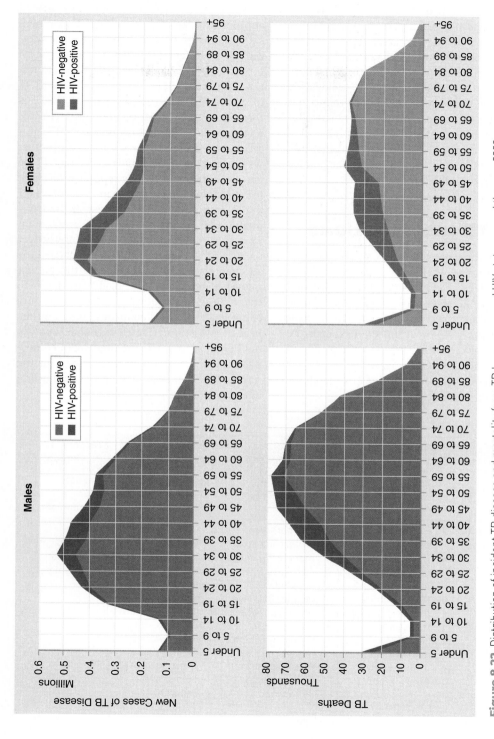

Figure 8.22 Distribution of incident TB disease and mortality from TB by sex, age, and HIV status around the year 2020.

Data from GBD 2019 Diseases and Injuries Collaborators. Global burden of 369 diseases and injuries in 204 countries and territories, 1990–2019: a systematic analysis for the Global Burden of Disease Study 2019. *Lancet.* 2020;396:1204–1222.

to experience lung damage due to tobacco use, work-related hazardous substances, and other exposures that may increase vulnerability to tuberculosis infection and disease. Males may also have immune system and inflammatory responses that make them more biologically vulnerable than females to *M. tuberculosis* and other respiratory pathogens. There are also geographic disparities in TB status. TB occurs in every country worldwide, but the vast majority of people with TB infections and TB disease live in LMICs.[82]

8.9 TB Interventions

Global partnerships have worked for decades to reduce the worldwide burden from TB. Interventions that improve TB diagnosis and treatment success rates reduce population incidence, prevalence, and mortality rates (**Figure 8.23**).[86] New TB infections can also be prevented by isolating people with suspected or confirmed TB disease, teaching TB patients to practice cough etiquette, and ensuring good ventilation of indoor spaces.[87]

Completion of full courses of prescribed antibiotic therapy are critical for TB treatment success. In 1994, the WHO began promoting TB treatment using **DOTS**, an acronym for **d**irectly **o**bserved **t**herapy, **s**hort-course. (DOTS is sometimes shortened to just DOT to emphasize that the key part of DOTS is the directly observed component.) Patients receiving TB treatment under a DOTS protocol are required to have a trained observer watch them take their pills every day. If the patient is hospitalized or reports to a clinic for his or her daily treatment, the observer might be a nurse or pharmacist. If the treatment is community based, the observer might be a shopkeeper or other community leader or a family member who is supervised by another community member. If the patient misses a dose, a public health worker will track the patient down and try to ensure compliance. Some countries have public health laws stipulating that people who are not compliant with TB treatment can be hospitalized under guard or imprisoned for the duration of their treatment, although most do not enforce these regulations.

Level of Prevention	Primordial Prevention	Primary Prevention	Secondary Prevention	Tertiary Prevention
Goal	Prevent risk factors for TB	Mitigate risk factors in people without TB	Detect TB before it becomes symptomatic	Manage TB after it becomes symptomatic
Examples of interventions	▪ Reduce residential crowding ▪ Have good ventilation systems in buildings ▪ Make cough etiquette (covering mouth and nose when coughing or sneezing) a community expectation	▪ Use personal protective equipment (PPE) such as masks when working with people who have active TB disease ▪ Treat people with active TB to reduce the risk of transmission to susceptible individuals	▪ Detect and treat latent TB infection (LTBI) before it converts to active TB, if appropriate ▪ Use the Bacillus Calmette-Guérin (BCG) vaccine to reduce the risk of severe active TB disease in children	▪ Take combination antibiotic therapy

Figure 8.23 Examples of interventions for TB.

HIV treatment programs are important contributors to TB control. HIV-negative people who develop TB disease and are not treated for it have about a 45% case fatality rate; HIV-positive people who develop TB disease and do not receive treatment have a nearly 100% case fatality rate.[74] However, people with HIV infection can be successfully treated for TB if they are strong enough to survive several months of antibiotic treatment. In typical recent years, the treatment success rate among people receiving combination antibiotic therapy was about 85% for people without HIV and about 75% for people with HIV who were taking both HIV and TB medications.[74]

BCG (Bacillus Calmette-Guérin) is a vaccine that confers some protection against TB disease in children. BCG is not effective at preventing TB infection, but BCG reduces the risk of TB disease and related complications in countries where children often contract TB infection.[88] (Several new TB vaccines that might prevent infection or prevent disease in adults are being developed and tested, but they are not yet ready for widespread use.[89]) TB disease can also be prevented by treating LTBI before it advances to TB disease. People with a high likelihood of developing active TB, including individuals with HIV, are a priority for LTBI treatment programs.[90] For example, the WHO recommends that adolescents and adults with HIV who live in places where there is a high rate of TB transmission take isoniazid preventive treatment (IPT) daily for three years or longer to reduce TB disease incidence and mortality.[91]

Controlling the spread of TB requires local and national structures to be in place to support diagnosis and treatment, including a supply chain that provides consistent access to all essential TB medications and a reporting system that allows governments to track their progress toward improved prevention, diagnosis, and treatment. Clinicians, public health workers, and members of communities with a high prevalence of TB play critical roles in local and national TB control by diagnosing, treating, and supporting individuals with TB disease. At the global level, UN organizations, national and subnational governmental agencies, public–private partnerships, foundations, charities (including patient support networks), pharmaceutical companies, research institutions, and other groups are working together to develop and operationalize action plans for reducing the global burden from TB. The **Stop TB Partnership**, founded in 2000 and led by the WHO, is an international network that coordinates the efforts of hundreds of organizations working on tuberculosis control.

The Stop TB Strategy (2006–2015) led by the WHO spelled out a plan for reducing the prevalence of TB disease, reducing the number of deaths each year from TB, and expanding access to a variety of diagnostic and treatment services so that the proportion of TB disease cases diagnosed and treated under a DOTS protocol would increase.[92] Good progress toward reducing the global burden from TB was made under the Stop TB Strategy. The target was to achieve a 50% reduction in TB disease prevalence and TB mortality between 2000 and 2015, and prevalence decreased by 42% and mortality by 47% during those years.[93]

The follow-up to the Stop TB Strategy is the End TB Strategy (2016–2035). The Stop TB Strategy targeted prevalence and mortality; the End TB Strategy targets incidence and mortality. End TB aims to reduce new and relapse cases of TB by 20% of 2015 levels by 2020, 50% by 2025, 80% by 2030, and 90% by 2035.[94] This will require reducing the global incidence of TB disease from about 142 per 100,000 people in 2015 to about 10 per 100,000 in 2035 (**Figure 8.24**).[82] End TB aims to reduce deaths from TB more quickly than the reduction in incidence, by reducing deaths by 35% of 2015 levels by 2020, 75% by 2025, 90% by 2030, and 95% by 2035; the plan also calls for universal health coverage so that no households affected by TB suffer from catastrophic medical costs.[82]

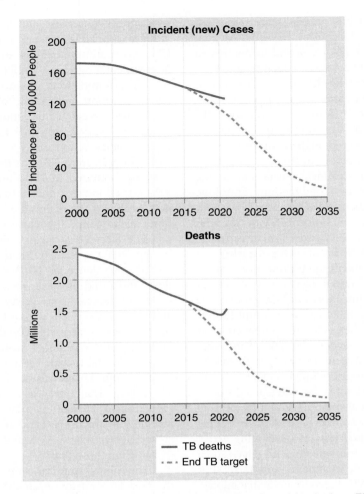

Figure 8.24 Incidence of TB disease per 100,000 people and number of deaths from TB (including people with and without HIV infection).

Data from *Global Tuberculosis Report 2021*. Geneva: World Health Organization; 2021; *Global Tuberculosis Report 2020*. Geneva: World Health Organization; 2020; and *Global Tuberculosis Report 2016*. Geneva: World Health Organization; 2016.

Unfortunately, none of the End TB milestones for 2020 were achieved. TB incidence was reduced by 11% rather than 20% between 2015 and 2020, TB deaths decreased by 9% rather than 35%, and 47% rather than 0% of TB patients faced catastrophic costs.[82] Even before the pandemic setbacks, the world was not on track to achieve the End TB targets.

Eliminating TB as a global public health problem will be impossible without increased funding from domestic and international sources. Fully funding the End TB Strategy, which directs most resources toward prevention and control activities in the populous LMICs that have the greatest TB burden, would require an annual budget of about $13 billion by 2022, but by the start of 2020 only half this amount was being funded.[74] In a typical recent year, about $11 billion total was spent on TB prevention, diagnosis, treatment, and other activities in LMICs.[95] About 65% of the funds were provided by the governments of LMICs, about 15% was DAH from high-income countries, and about 20%

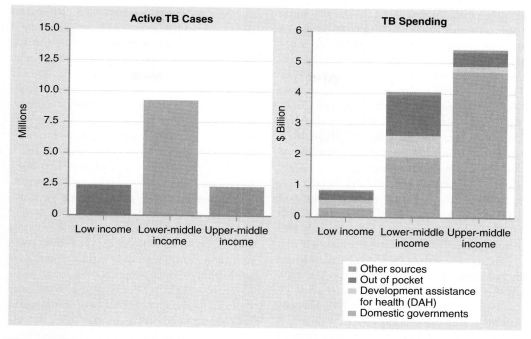

Figure 8.25 Health spending on tuberculosis in low- and middle-income countries (left) and the distribution of prevalent active TB cases (right) in a typical recent year, by country income level.

Data from *Financing Global Health 2019: Tracking Health Spending in a Time of Crisis.* Seattle: Institute for Health Metrics and Evaluation; 2020; GBD 2019 Diseases and Injuries Collaborators. Global burden of 369 diseases and injuries in 204 countries and territories, 1990–2019: a systematic analysis for the Global Burden of Disease Study 2019. *Lancet.* 2020;396:1204–1222.

was out-of-pocket spending by households affected by TB.[51] Total spending on TB control in low- and lower-middle-income countries was less than $5 billion, and the amount of money spent per TB case in these lower-income countries was only about one-fifth the amount spent per case in upper-middle-income countries (**Figure 8.25**).[51] The world's ability to achieve the End TB Strategy will be dependent on additional international funding being directed toward TB control programs in low- and lower-middle-income countries.

8.10 Antimicrobial Resistance

A pathogen is sensitive or susceptible to a medication if it is vulnerable to it. A pathogen is resistant to a medication if it can withstand treatment with it. **Antimicrobial resistance**

(AMR), or drug resistance, occurs when a pathogen that used to be susceptible to a therapeutic agent mutates in a way that makes that medication ineffective.[96] Bacteria are usually susceptible to certain types of antibiotics, and they will be killed when they are exposed to correct doses of the right classes of these medications. However, a growing number of pathogenic bacteria have developed resistance to at least some of the antibiotics that were once effective against them.[97] Other types of disease-causing agents are also developing resistance, making antivirals, antiparasitic drugs, and antifungal medications less effective. For example, some strains of HIV have developed resistance to first-line antiretroviral drugs, and many strains of malaria are resistant to antiparasitic medications.

Drug-resistant TB (DR-TB) is a growing global health problem.[98] **MDR-TB** is multidrug-resistant tuberculosis that does not respond to two of the standard antibiotic therapies, rifampicin and isoniazid.[99] **XDR-TB** is extensively drug-resistant tuberculosis that does not respond to rifampicin, isoniazid, fluoroquinolones, and at least one second-line injectable TB drug.[100] A few strains of *M. tuberculosis* have been deemed to be totally drug resistant (TDR-TB) and are incurable with currently available antibiotics. Drug susceptibility testing can determine whether an infectious agent is sensitive or resistant to an antimicrobial agent. In 2020, about 3% of new cases of TB and 18% of previously treated cases were rifampicin-resistant TB (RR-TB) or MDR-TB.[74] (About 80% of RR/MDR-TB cases were MDR-TB.) The nearly half a million new cases of drug-resistant TB that occur each year are not evenly distributed across the locations with high TB burdens. The rates of DR-TB are especially high in Eastern Europe and Central Asia, but XDR-TB or TDR-TB cases anywhere are a threat to people everywhere.

The **default rate** is the proportion of people who are diagnosed with an infectious disease and begin treatment but do not complete the full course of prescribed antimicrobials. The default rate for TB is high in some places. People with TB disease who interrupt their treatment regimens or do not complete the full duration of prescribed antibiotic therapy may develop DR-TB. The treatment success rate for RR/MDR-TB is currently below 60%, which is much lower than the 85% success rate for drug-susceptible TB.[74] The antibiotics used to treat MDR-TB are more expensive than first-line therapy, and the course of treatment is much longer, taking up to two years rather than six months.[101] About 45% of people with drug-susceptible TB disease spend more than 20% of their annual household income on TB-related costs; among people with DR-TB, about 80% experience this catastrophic financial burden.[74] People who develop DR-TB as a result of defaulting on their treatment put their own lives at risk, but they are not the only individuals who are harmed. Everyone they infect will have a first case of TB disease that is drug resistant.

A **healthcare-associated infection** (HAI), also called a hospital-acquired infection or a **nosocomial infection**, is an infection that is contracted while receiving care in a hospital, nursing or rehabilitation center, or another medical facility. HAIs include central line–associated bloodstream infections, catheter-associated urinary tract infections, surgical site infections, ventilator-associated pneumonia, *Clostridium difficile* infections, and others.[102] While most HAIs are not drug-resistant ones, some are. **MRSA**, or methicillin-resistant *Staphylococcus aureus*, infections are very difficult to treat, and MRSA can cause severe "flesh-eating" infections (necrotizing fasciitis) and bloodstream infections. The first cases of MRSA were reported within months of methicillin being released for use as an antibiotic in 1960.[103] MRSA is now frequently transmitted within hospitals (where it is called hospital-acquired MRSA), but the bacteria can also be transmitted through unsterilized sports equipment and other everyday items that cause community-acquired MRSA.[104] Handwashing (by healthcare workers, patients, and visitors), the use of personal protective equipment, clean laundry, sterilized equipment, environmental sanitation, and waste management help prevent the spread of HAIs.[105] Patient risk is also reduced by avoiding unnecessary medical procedures and minimizing the use of invasive medical devices.

The misuse of antibiotics is driving the development of many forms of AMR.[106] Biologists use the term **selection** to describe the preferential survival and reproduction of advantaged organisms. If someone who has a mild bacterial infection, such as an uncomplicated case of bronchitis or an ear infection, takes antibiotics for only a few days rather than finishing the entire prescription, the antibiotics will have killed the bacteria that are most susceptible to the drugs, but the hardier bacteria may have survived. Those bacteria may develop resistance to the antibiotics that were originally used against the infection, and that resistant strain may be passed to others. In addition to selective pressure, AMR also develops due to random mutations in the genetic code of pathogens and through gene transfers between bacteria.[107]

Overuse of antimicrobials also contributes to AMR. Viral infections like the common cold do not respond to antibiotics, and people who take antibiotics when they have a viral infection may kill off the helpful bacteria in their bodies and enable harmful bacteria to become drug resistant. Prescribing the wrong type of antibiotic for a bacterial infection may similarly enable bacteria that are not causing illness to develop drug resistance. Antibiotics are also frequently overused in cattle, pigs, poultry, and other animal populations raised for food production.[108] Misuse of antimicrobials in human or animal populations creates AMR risks that could become threats to public health.

Inappropriate access to and use of medications in one nation can rapidly cause a global antimicrobial resistance problem.[109] Public health threats from drug resistance come from DR-TB, MRSA, drug-resistant types of Enterobacteriaceae (such as cephalosporin- and fluoroquinolone-resistant *E. coli* and cephalosporin- and carbapenem-resistant *Klebsiella pneumoniae*), penicillin-resistant *Streptococcus pneumoniae*, fluoroquinolone-resistant *Salmonella* and *Shigella*, and cephalosporin-resistant *N. gonorrhoeae*.[110] They also come from numerous other agents, including multidrug-resistant *Acinetobacter*, drug-resistant *Campylobacter*, vancomycin-resistant *Enterococcus* (VRE), multidrug-resistant *Pseudomonas aeruginosa*, and others.[102] AMR prevention strategies include preventing infections so that antibiotics are not needed, expanding the use of diagnostic tests to ensure that appropriate antibiotics are prescribed, reducing the overuse of antibiotics to treat diseases in humans and livestock, and developing new types of antibiotics.[111] Antimicrobial stewardship programs that ensure that patients are prescribed the right medications at the right doses for the right durations and through the right routes help reduce the risk of adverse outcomes from HAIs and drug-resistant infections.[112]

More than 1 million people may already die from AMR bacterial infections each year.[113] Antibiotic medications that cure bacterial infections are a core part of many infectious disease control programs, and AMR may reduce the effectiveness of those programs at preventing new infections and treating existing ones. A new "superbug" that evolves anywhere in the world poses a threat to the whole world, so all countries must be committed to taking steps to prevent pathogens from developing resistance to new antibiotic medications and to contain the AMR strains already in circulation.[114] This will require a multisectoral response that includes policy and practice solutions in the health, agriculture, and environmental sectors.[115]

References

1. Brandt AM. How AIDS invented global health. *N Engl J Med*. 2013;368:2149–2152.
2. Global Burden of Disease Health Financing Collaborator Network. Health sector spending and spending on HIV/AIDS, tuberculosis, and malaria, and development assistance for health: progress towards Sustainable Development Goal 3. *Lancet*. 2020;396:693–724.
3. *Results Report 2020*. Geneva: The Global Fund; 2020.
4. Horton R, Lo S. Investing in health: why, what, and three reflections. *Lancet*. 2013;382:1859–1861.
5. Gottlieb GS, Raugi DN, Smith RA. 90–90–90 for HIV-2? Ending the HIV-2 epidemic by enhancing care and clinical management of patients infected with HIV-2. *Lancet HIV*. 2018;5:e390–e399.
6. Maartens G, Celum C, Lewin SR. HIV infection: epidemiology, pathogenesis, treatment, and prevention. *Lancet*. 2014;384:258–271.
7. Mocroft A, Furrer HJ, Miro JM, et al. The incidence of AIDS-defining illnesses at a current CD4 count ≥200 cells/μL in the post-combination antiretroviral therapy era. *Clin Infect Dis*. 2013;57:1038–1047.

8. *WHO Case Definitions of HIV for Surveillance and Revised Clinical Staging and Immunological Classification of HIV-Related Disease in Adults and Children.* Geneva: World Health Organization; 2007.

9. *Update of Recommendations on First- and Second-Line Antiretroviral Regimens.* Geneva: World Health Organization; 2019.

10. Jaffar S, Grant AD, Whitworth J, Smith PG, Whittle H. The natural history of HIV-1 and HIV-2 infections in adults in Africa: a literature review. *Bull World Health Organ.* 2004;82:462–469.

11. Holmes C, Hallett T, Walensky R, Bärnighausen T, Pillay Y, Cohen M. Effectiveness and cost-effectiveness of treatment as prevention for HIV (chapter 5). In: Holmes KK, Bertozzi S, Bloom BR, Jha P, eds. *Disease Control Priorities: Major Infectious Diseases.* Vol. 6. 3rd ed. Washington DC: IBRD/World Bank; 2017:91–112.

12. *Consolidated Guidelines on the Use of Antiretroviral Drugs for Treating and Preventing HIV Infection: Recommendations for a Public Health Approach.* 2nd ed. Geneva: World Health Organization; 2016.

13. Chaiyachati KH, Ogbuoji O, Price M, Suthar AB, Negussie EK, Bärnighausen T. Interventions to improve adherence to antiretroviral therapy: a rapid systematic review. *AIDS.* 2014;28(Suppl 2): S187–S204.

14. Stöhr W, Fidler S, McClure M, et al. Duration of HIV-1 viral suppression on cessation of antiretroviral therapy in primary infection correlates with time on therapy. *PLoS One.* 2013;8:e78287.

15. Pitisuttithum P, Marovich MA. Prophylactic HIV vaccine: vaccine regimens in clinical trials and potential challenges. *Expert Rev Vacc.* 2020;19:133–142.

16. Gray GE, Laher F, Doherty T, et al. Which new health technologies do we need to achieve an end to HIV/AIDS? *PLoS Biol.* 2016;14:e1002372.

17. Faria NR, Rambaut A, Suchard MA, et al. The early spread and epidemic ignition of HIV-1 in human populations. *Science.* 2014;346:56–61.

18. Pneumocystis pneumonia—Los Angeles, 1981. *MMWR Morb Mortal Wkly Rep.* 1981;30:250–252.

19. Jaffe HW, Bregman DJ, Selik RM. Acquired immune deficiency syndrome in the United States: the first 1000 cases. *J Infect Dis.* 1983;148:339–345.

20. Gallo RC, Montagnier L. The discovery of HIV as the cause of AIDS. *N Engl J Med.* 2003;349:2283–2285.

21. *UNAIDS Data 2021.* Geneva: UNAIDS; 2021.

22. *Global AIDS Update 2020: Seizing the Moment: Tackling Entrenched Inequalities to End Epidemics.* Geneva: UNAIDS; 2020.

23. *Fast-Track: Ending the AIDS Epidemic by 2030.* Geneva: UNAIDS; 2014.

24. *Political Declaration on HIV and AIDS: On the Fast Track to Accelerating the Fight Against HIV and to Ending the AIDS Epidemic by 2030.* Geneva: World Health Organization; 2016.

25. GBD 2019 Diseases and Injuries Collaborators. Global burden of 369 diseases and injuries in 204 countries and territories, 1990–2019: a systematic analysis for the Global Burden of Disease Study 2019. *Lancet.* 2020;396:1204–1222.

26. *Consolidated HIV Strategic Information Guidelines: Driving Impact Through Programme Monitoring and Management.* Geneva: World Health Organization; 2020.

27. *UNAIDS World AIDS Day Report 2011: How to Get to Zero: Faster. Smarter. Better.* Geneva: UNAIDS; 2011.

28. *AIDS by the Numbers 2016.* Geneva: UNAIDS; 2016.

29. *Global Health Sector Response to HIV, 2000–2015: Focus on Innovations in Africa.* Geneva: World Health Organization; 2015.

30. Andrews G, Skinner D, Zuma K. Epidemiology of health and vulnerability among children orphaned and made vulnerable by HIV/AIDS in sub-Saharan Africa. *AIDS Care.* 2006;18:269–276.

31. GBD 2019 HIV Collaborators. Global, regional, and national sex-specific burden and control of the HIV epidemic, 1990–2019, for 204 countries and territories: the Global Burden of Diseases Study 2019. *Lancet HIV.* 2021;8:e633–e651.

32. Quinn TC, Overbaugh J. HIV/AIDS in women: an expanding epidemic. *Science.* 2005;308:1582–1583.

33. Higgins JA, Hoffman S, Dworkin SL. Rethinking gender, heterosexual men, and women's vulnerability to HIV/AIDS. *Am J Public Health.* 2010;100:435–445.

34. *Integrating Gender into HIV/AIDS Programmers in the Health Sector: Tools to Improve Responsiveness to Women's Needs.* Geneva: World Health Organization; 2009.

35. *Consolidated Guidelines on HIV Prevention, Diagnosis, Treatment and Care for Key Populations.* Geneva: World Health Organization; 2016.

36. *"15 by 15": A Global Target Achieved.* Geneva: UNAIDS; 2015.

37. *90–90–90: An Ambitious Treatment Target to Help End the AIDS Epidemic.* Geneva: UNAIDS; 2014.

38. Denison JA, O'Reilly KR, Schmid GP, Kennedy CE, Sweat MD. HIV voluntary counseling and testing and behavioral risk reduction in developing countries: a meta-analysis, 1990–2005. *AIDS Behav.* 2008;12:363–373.

39. *Consolidated Guidelines on HIV Testing Services—5 Cs: Consent, Confidentiality, Counselling, Correct Results and Connection.* Geneva: World Health Organization; 2015.

40. De Cock KM, Fowler MG, Mercier E, et al. Prevention of mother-to-child HIV transmission in resource-poor countries: translating research into policy and practice. *JAMA.* 2000;283:1175–1182.

41. Siegfried NL, van der Merwe L, Brocklehurst P, Sint TT. Antiretrovirals for reducing the risk of mother-to-child transmission of HIV infection. *Cochrane Database Syst Rev.* 2011;7:CD003510.

42. *Guideline: Updates on HIV and Infant Feeding: The Duration of Breastfeeding, and Support from Health Services to Improve Feeding Practices Among Mothers Living with HIV.* Geneva: World Health Organization/UNICEF; 2016.

43. *WHO Technical Update on Pre-Exposure Prophylaxis (PrEP).* Geneva: World Health Organization; 2015.

44. *Guidelines on Post-Exposure Prophylaxis for HIV and the Use of Co-Trimoxazole Prophylaxis for HIV-Related Infections Among Adults, Adolescents and Children: Recommendations for a Public Health Approach.* Geneva: World Health Organization; 2014.

45. Murphy EM, Greene ME, Mihailovic A, Olupot-Olupot P. Was the "ABC" approach (abstinence, being faithful, using condoms) responsible for Uganda's decline in HIV? *PLoS Med.* 2006;3:e379.

46. Boily MC, Baggaley RF, Wang L, et al. Heterosexual risk of HIV-1 infection per sexual act: a systematic review and meta-analysis of observational studies. *Lancet Infect Dis.* 2009;9:118–129.

47. Hayes RJ, Watson-Jones D, Celum C, van de Wijgert J, Wasserheit J. Treatment of sexually transmitted infections for HIV prevention: end of the road or new beginning? *AIDS.* 2010;24:S15–S26.

48. *Preventing HIV Through Safe Voluntary Medical Male Circumcision for Adolescent Boys and Men in Generalized HIV Epidemics: Recommendations and Key Considerations.* Geneva: World Health Organization; 2020.

49. Abdul-Quader AS, Feelemyer J, Modi S, et al. Effectiveness of structural-level needle/syringe programs to reduce HCV and HIV infection among people who inject drugs: a systematic review. *AIDS Behav.* 2013;17:2878–2892.

50. Khan JG, Bollinger L, Stover J, Marseille E. Improving the efficiency of the HIV/AIDS policy response: a guide to resource allocation modeling (chapter 9). In: Holmes KK, Bertozzi S, Bloom BR, Jha P, eds. *Disease Control Priorities: Major Infectious Diseases.* Vol. 6. 3rd ed. Washington DC: IBRD/World Bank; 2017:179–202.

51. *Financing Global Health 2019: Tracking Health Spending in a Time of Crisis.* Seattle: Institute for Health Metrics and Evaluation; 2020.

52. *PEPFAR 2020 Annual Report to Congress.* Washington DC: U.S. Department of State; 2020.

53. *Global Health Sector Strategy on Sexually Transmitted Infections 2016–2021: Towards Ending STIs.* Geneva: World Health Organization; 2016.

54. *WHO Guidelines for the Treatment of* Chlamydia trachomatis. Geneva: World Health Organization; 2016.

55. *WHO Guidelines for the Treatment of* Neisseria gonorrhoeae. Geneva: World Health Organization; 2016.

56. *WHO Guidelines for the Treatment of* Treponema pallidum *(Syphilis).* Geneva: World Health Organization; 2016.

57. Rowley J, Vander Hoorn S, Korenromp E, et al. Chlamydia, gonorrhea, trichomoniasis and syphilis: global prevalence and incidence estimates, 2016. *Bull World Health Organ.* 2019;97:548–562.

58. Unemo M, Nicholas RA. Emergence of multidrug-resistant, extensively drug-resistant and untreatable gonorrhea. *Future Microbiol.* 2012;7:1401–1422.

59. Hook EW III. Syphilis. *Lancet.* 2017;389:1550–1557.

60. Newman L, Kamb M, Hawkes S, et al. Global estimates of syphilis in pregnancy and associated adverse outcomes: analysis of multinational antenatal surveillance data. *PLoS Med.* 2013;10:e1001396.

61. Korenromp EL, Rowley J, Alonso M, et al. Global burden of maternal and congenital syphilis and associated adverse birth outcomes: estimates for 2016 and progress since 2012. *PLoS One.* 2019;14:e0211720.

62. *WHO Guideline on Syphilis Screening and Treatment for Pregnant Women.* Geneva: World Health Organization; 2017.

63. Looker KJ, Magaret AS, Turner KME, Vickerman P, Gottlieb SL, Newman LM. Global estimates of prevalent and incident herpes simplex virus type 2 infections in 2012. *PLoS One.* 2015;10:e114989.

64. *WHO Guidelines for the Treatment of Genital Herpes Simplex Virus.* Geneva: World Health Organization; 2016.

65. Muñoz N, Castellsagué X, de González AB, Gissmann L. HPV in the etiology of human cancer. *Vaccine.* 2006;24(Suppl 3):1–10.

66. Bruni L, Diaz M, Barrionuevo-Rosas L, et al. Global estimates of human papillomavirus vaccination coverage by region and income level: a pooled analysis. *Lancet Glob Health.* 2016;4:e453–e463.

67. Orion E, Matz H, Wolf R. Ectoparasitic sexually transmitted diseases: scabies and pediculosis. *Clin Dermatol.* 2004;22:513–519.

68. Unemo M, Bradshaw CS, Hocking JS. Sexually transmitted infections: challenges ahead. *Lancet Infect Dis.* 2017;17:e235–e279.

69. Ferreira A, Young T, Mathews C, Zunza M, Low N. Strategies for partner notification for sexually transmitted infections, including HIV. *Cochrane Database Syst Rev.* 2013;2013:CD002843.

70. Dheda K, Barry CE III, Maartens G. Tuberculosis. *Lancet.* 2015;387:1211–1226.

71. Lönnroth K, Jaramillo E, Williams BG, Dye C, Raviglione M. Drivers of tuberculosis epidemics: the role of risk factors and social determinants. *Soc Sci Med.* 2009;68:2240–2246.

72. Lin PL, Flynn JL. Understanding latent tuberculosis: a moving target. *J Immunol.* 2010;185:15–22.

73. Gideon HP, Flynn JL. Latent tuberculosis: what the host "sees"? *Immunol Res.* 2011;50:202–212.

74. *Global Tuberculosis Report 2020.* Geneva: World Health Organization; 2020.

75. *Tuberculosis and HIV: Progress Toward the 2020 Target.* Geneva: UNAIDS; 2019.

76. Patra J, Jha P, Rehm J, Suraweera W. Tobacco smoking, alcohol drinking, diabetes, low body mass index and the risk of self-reported symptoms of active tuberculosis: individual participant data (IPD) meta-analyses of 72,684 individuals in 14 high tuberculosis burden countries. *PLoS One*. 2014;9:e96433.

77. Sepkowitz KA. How contagious is tuberculosis. *Clin Infect Dis*. 1996;23:954–962.

78. *Systematic Screening for Active Tuberculosis: An Operational Guide*. Geneva: World Health Organization; 2015.

79. *Implementing the End TB Strategy: The Essentials*. Geneva: World Health Organization; 2015.

80. *Implementing Tuberculosis Diagnostics: Policy Framework*. Geneva: World Health Organization; 2015.

81. *Treatment of Tuberculosis: Guidelines for Treatment of Drug-Susceptible Tuberculosis and Patient Care (2017 Update)*. Geneva: World Health Organization; 2017.

82. *Global Tuberculosis Report 2021*. Geneva: World Health Organization; 2021.

83. Houben RMGJ, Dodd PJ. The global burden of latent tuberculosis infection: a re-estimation using mathematical modeling. *PLoS Med*. 2016;13:e1002152.

84. Bloom BR, Atun R, Cohen T, et al. Tuberculosis (chapter 11). In: Holmes KK, Bertozzi S, Bloom BR, Jha P, eds. *Disease Control Priorities: Major Infectious Diseases*. Vol. 6. 3rd ed. Washington DC: IBRD/World Bank; 2017:233–312.

85. Hertz D, Schneider B. Sex differences in tuberculosis. *Semin Immunopathol*. 2019;41:225–237.

86. Reid MJA, Arinaminpathy N, Bloom A, et al. Building a tuberculosis-free world: the Lancet Commission on tuberculosis. *Lancet*. 2019;393:1331–1384.

87. *WHO Guidelines on Tuberculosis Infection Prevention and Control 2019 Update*. Geneva: World Health Organization; 2019.

88. BCG vaccine: WHO position paper – February 2018. *Wkly Epidemiol Rec*. 2018;93:73–96.

89. Evans TG, Schrager L, Thole J. Status of vaccine research and development of vaccines for tuberculosis. *Vaccine*. 2016;34:2911–2914.

90. *Guidelines on the Management of Latent Tuberculosis Infection*. Geneva: World Health Organization; 2015.

91. *WHO Consolidated Guidelines on Tuberculosis. Module 1: Prevention – Tuberculosis Preventive Treatment*. Geneva: World Health Organization; 2020.

92. *The Stop TB Strategy: Building On and Enhancing DOTS to Meet the TB-Related Millennium Development Goals*. Geneva: World Health Organization; 2006.

93. *Global Tuberculosis Report 2015*. Geneva: World Health Organization; 2015.

94. *The End TB Strategy: Global Strategy and Targets for Tuberculosis Prevention, Care and Control after 2015*. Geneva: World Health Organization; 2014.

95. Su Y, Baena IG, Harle AC, et al. Tracking total spending on tuberculosis by source and function in 135 low-income and middle-income countries, 2000–17: a financially modelling study. *Lancet Infect Dis*. 2020;20:929–942.

96. Marston HD, Dixon DM, Knisely JM, Palmore TN, Fauci AS. Antimicrobial resistance. *JAMA*. 2016;316:1193–1204.

97. Goldbert DE, Siliciano RF, Jacobs WR. Outwitting evolution: fighting drug-resistant TB, malaria, and HIV. *Cell*. 2012;148:1271–1283.

98. Dheda K, Gumbo T, Maartens G, et al. The epidemiology, pathogenesis, transmission, diagnosis, and management of multidrug-resistant, extensively drug-resistant, and incurable tuberculosis. *Lancet Respir Med*. 2017;5:291–360.

99. *Guidelines for the Programmatic Management of Drug-Resistant Tuberculosis 2016 Update*. Geneva: World Health Organization; 2016.

100. Matteelli A, Roggi A, Carvalho ACC. Extensively drug-resistant tuberculosis: epidemiology and management. *Clin Epidemiol*. 2014;6:111–118.

101. *Companion Handbook to the WHO Guidelines for the Programmatic Management of Drug-Resistant Tuberculosis*. Geneva: World Health Organization; 2014.

102. *Antibiotic Resistance Threats in the United States 2019*. Atlanta GA: Centers for Disease Control and Prevention; 2019.

103. Grundmann H, Aires-de-Sousa M, Boyce J, Tiemersma E. Emergence and resurgence of meticillin-resistant *Staphylococcus aureus* as a public-health threat. *Lancet*. 2006; 368:874–885.

104. Kluytmans S, Harbath S. MRSA transmission in the community: emerging from under the radar. *Lancet Infect Dis*. 2020;20:147–149.

105. *Guidelines on Core Components of Infection Prevention and Control Programmes at the National and Acute Health Care Facility Level*. Geneva: World Health Organization; 2016.

106. *Global Action Plan on Antimicrobial Resistance*. Geneva: World Health Organization; 2015.

107. Tenover FC. Mechanisms of antimicrobial resistance in bacteria. *Am J Med*. 2006;119:S3–S10.

108. *The OIE Strategy on Antimicrobial Resistance and the Prudent Use of Antimicrobials*. Paris: World Organisation for Animal Health; 2016.

109. Miller-Petrie M, Pant S, Laxminarayan R. Drug resistant infections (chapter 18). In: Holmes KK, Bertozzi S, Bloom BR, Jha P, eds. *Disease Control Priorities: Major Infectious Diseases*. Vol. 6. 3rd ed. Washington DC: IBRD/World Bank; 2017:433–448.

110. *Antimicrobial Resistance: Global Report on Surveillance*. Geneva: World Health Organization; 2014.

111. Laxminarayan R, Duse A, Wattal C, et al. Antibiotic resistance: the need for global solutions. *Lancet Infect Dis.* 2013;13:1057–1098.

112. Dyar OJ, Huttner B, Schouten J, Pulcini C. What is antimicrobial stewardship? *Clin Microbiol Infect.* 2017;23:793–798.

113. Antimicrobial Resistance Collaborators. Global burden of bacterial antimicrobial resistance in 2019: a systematic analysis. *Lancet.* 2022;399:629–655.

114. Laxminarayan R, Sridhar D, Blaser M, Wang M, Woolhouse M. Achieving global targets for antimicrobial resistance. *Science.* 2016;353:874–875.

115. Holmes AH, Moore LSP, Sundsfjord A, et al. Understanding the mechanisms and drivers of antimicrobial resistance. *Lancet.* 2016;387:176–187.

Diarrheal, Respiratory, and Other Infections

Children in lower-income countries experience a disproportionate burden of preventable illnesses and deaths from diarrheal diseases and pneumonia, but everyone is at risk of foodborne infections, influenza, coronavirus, viral hepatitis, and other infectious diseases. Global cooperation is critical for containing emerging infectious diseases with pandemic potential and enabling every child to receive recommended vaccines.

9.1 Infectious Diseases and Global Health

Infectious diseases caused by bacteria, viruses, and parasites cause millions of deaths every year. In the early and middle decades of the 20th century, new laboratory techniques led to the identification of many disease-causing microbes and the development of vaccines and antibiotics like penicillin. These discoveries generated a great deal of optimism and confidence about the ability of humans to control and eradicate communicable diseases. Yet even though modern science has provided a good understanding of the infectious disease process and allowed for the development of therapies and cures for many types of infectious diseases, microbes continue to adapt and

emerge. Pandemics still happen. Even with improved preventive and therapeutic techniques, infectious diseases continue to be a health risk in all populations in every part of the world. The development of new interventions for preventing, diagnosing, and treating infectious diseases remains a global health priority.

Most people who live in high-income countries would correctly consider heart disease, cancer, or diabetes to be their number one health concern. Few high-income country residents would mention infectious diseases as a top threat to their own health, except when a major infectious disease outbreak is getting a lot of media attention. This happens occasionally when there are new fears about the emergence of a particularly bad influenza strain—or when there is a once-in-a-century threat to public health like the coronavirus pandemic. These worries usually fade quickly among people who live in high-income countries. In low-income countries, by contrast, infectious diseases are a constant risk, and they remain responsible for a significant proportion of the burden of disease (**Figure 9.1**).[1]

Children bear a heavy burden from both fatal and nonfatal infectious diseases. In a typical (nonpandemic) recent year, about one in three people who died from an infectious disease was an infant, child, or adolescent (**Figure 9.2**).[1] Most infants and children who died between one month and nine years of age succumbed to infections (**Figure 9.3**).[1] These losses were not equally distributed (**Figure 9.4**); most infectious disease deaths among infants and children occurred in low- or lower-middle-income countries (**Figure 9.5**).[1] The vast majority of fatal childhood infections could have been prevented with inexpensive interventions like vaccinations, reliable access to clean drinking water, and bednets to block mosquito bites.[2] When prevention methods failed to stop the occurrence of an infection,

the majority of deaths from these infectious diseases could still have been averted with antibiotics and other types of basic medical care.

The unnecessary burden of infectious diseases on children in low-income countries is more than sufficient reason for infectious disease prevention and control to remain a global health priority. One of the eight Millennium Development Goals was to reduce the mortality rate among children between birth and their fifth birthdays (under-5 children) by two-thirds between 2000 and 2015 (MDG 4). The mortality rate dropped by more than half during that 15-year period, and infectious disease programs were critical contributors to the good progress made toward achieving this goal.[3] This trajectory will need to continue in order to make progress toward achieving the Sustainable Development Goals (SDGs) target of ending preventable deaths of young children by 2030 (SDG 3.2).[4]

But infectious diseases are not just about children. Many pathogens can kill or

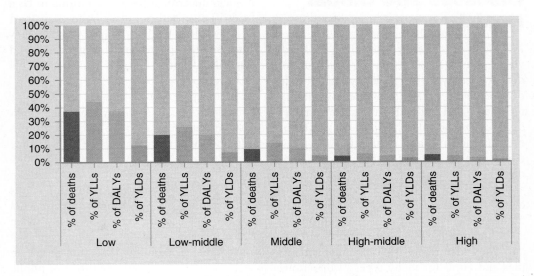

Figure 9.1 Proportional all-ages burden of disease from infectious diseases in a typical (nonpandemic) year, by country sociodemographic group.

Data from GBD 2019 Diseases and Injuries Collaborators. Global burden of 369 diseases and injuries in 204 countries and territories, 1990–2019: a systematic analysis for the Global Burden of Disease Study 2019. *Lancet*. 2020;396:1204–1222.

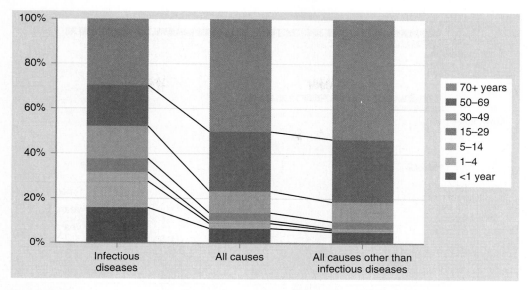

Figure 9.2 Percentage of deaths from infectious diseases and other causes, by age group.

Data from GBD 2019 Diseases and Injuries Collaborators. Global burden of 369 diseases and injuries in 204 countries and territories, 1990–2019: a systematic analysis for the Global Burden of Disease Study 2019. *Lancet.* 2020;396:1204–1222.

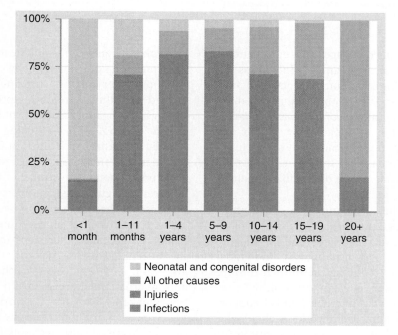

Figure 9.3 Proportionate mortality rates, by cause and age group.

Data from GBD 2019 Diseases and Injuries Collaborators. Global burden of 369 diseases and injuries in 204 countries and territories, 1990–2019: a systematic analysis for the Global Burden of Disease Study 2019. *Lancet.* 2020;396:1204–1222.

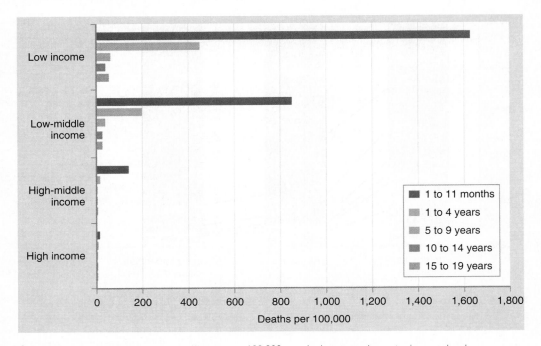

Figure 9.4 Infectious disease mortality rate per 100,000 people, by age and country income level.

Data from GBD 2019 Diseases and Injuries Collaborators. Global burden of 369 diseases and injuries in 204 countries and territories, 1990–2019: a systematic analysis for the Global Burden of Disease Study 2019. *Lancet.* 2020;396:1204–1222.

disable people of all ages, all socioeconomic levels, and all geographies. Infectious diseases are spread through social and trade networks, and the web of human contacts is becoming more complex as globalized transportation systems allow people and products to travel almost anywhere in the world within a day. Infectious agents can adapt, mutate, and be disseminated quickly. Everyone is at risk.

Individuals, communities, governmental agencies, and health organizations all have a role to play in the control and prevention of infectious diseases. Individuals contribute to reducing the burden of infectious disease by engaging in healthy behaviors, such as washing their hands frequently and staying home from work or school when they are sick so they do not continue the chain of transmission. Communities play

key roles in environmental health, reducing infection transmission by increasing drinking water quality, ensuring access to sanitation facilities, promoting proper waste management, implementing policies that reduce air pollution, reducing mosquito populations through water drainage and insecticides, and controlling rodent and snail populations. Governments implement food safety regulations, enforce zoning laws that restrict the number of individuals who can share a dwelling unit, require pet vaccination, and take other steps to minimize the infectious disease risks in the natural and built environments. At the national and international levels, health scientists, policymakers, and others work together to create and distribute vaccines, diagnostics, and other health technologies and to monitor and respond to emerging infectious

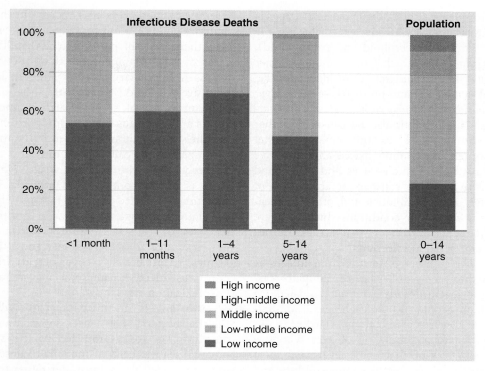

Figure 9.5 Distribution of infectious disease deaths by country sociodemographic group compared to the distribution of the world's child population.

Data from GBD 2019 Diseases and Injuries Collaborators. Global burden of 369 diseases and injuries in 204 countries and territories, 1990–2019: a systematic analysis for the Global Burden of Disease Study 2019. *Lancet.* 2020;396:1204–1222.

disease concerns. One country alone cannot stop a pandemic. Infectious disease control requires international cooperation.

9.2 Diarrheal Diseases

An **enteric infection** is an infection of the intestinal tract. **Gastroenteritis** is infection-induced inflammation of the inner lining of the stomach (gastro-) and/or intestines (entero-) that causes diarrhea, nausea, vomiting, cramps, and fever. **Diarrhea** is characterized by loose or liquid feces and an increased frequency of defecation. Severe diarrhea can lead to **dehydration**, the excessive loss of water from the body. Fluid loss decreases blood volume and causes low blood pressure, a fast and weak pulse, rapid breathing (but insufficient oxygen intake), sunken dry eyes, loss of skin elasticity, muscle contractions, convulsions, and delirium. Dehydration-induced imbalances of sodium, potassium, bicarbonate, and other electrolytes can cause kidney and heart failure, and then death.

Each year, there are more than 6 billion incident (new) cases of infectious diarrheal disease worldwide, and that number is increasing as the global human population increases.[1] The pathogens that are the most frequent causes of gastroenteritis include rotaviruses, noroviruses, caliciviruses, astroviruses, and adenoviruses[5]; bacteria such as *Salmonella* species (including the ones that cause typhoid and paratyphoid), *Shigella*, *Vibrio cholerae*, *Campylobacter jejuni*, *Escherichia coli*, *Clostridium difficile*, and *Aeromonas*; and protozoa, such as *Cryptosporidium*, *Entamoeba histolytica*, and *Giardia*.[6] Diarrhea can also be caused by other conditions, such as inflammatory bowel disorders like Crohn's disease and ulcerative colitis, lactose intolerances and other food sensitivities that cause poor absorption of water, some antibiotics and other medications, and other conditions, but those are infrequent contributors to diarrhea mortality compared to infections.[7]

The number of deaths from infectious diarrhea each year has been steadily decreasing in recent decades, but an estimated 1.5 million people still die each year from diarrheal diseases.[1] Infectious diarrhea cases occur among people of all ages who live in countries of all income levels, but most fatalities occur among young children and older adults who live in low- or lower-middle-income countries (**Figure 9.6**).[1] (By comparison, pneumonia deaths occur in countries of all income levels.) For children less than five years old, the most frequent causes of death from enteric infections in recent years have been rotavirus and *Shigella*, with adenovirus, *Campylobacter*, cholera, and *Cryptosporidium* also major contributors; by contrast, the most frequent causes among adults aged 70 years or older have been norovirus and *Campylobacter*, with rotavirus, *Cryptosporidium*, and many other agents also contributing to diarrhea-related mortality.[6]

Diarrhea is the most frequent cause of infectious disease death among children who are more than one year old (**Figure 9.7**).[1] **Rotavirus** is the most frequent cause of severe diarrhea among infants and young children. The numbers of hospitalizations and deaths from rotavirus in pediatric populations have decreased substantially as more

countries include rotavirus vaccine in their national immunization programs,[8] but each year there are still more than 200 million cases of rotavirus and more than 100,000 deaths from rotavirus among children less than five years old.[9] **Norovirus** is the most frequent cause of severe diarrhea among adults and also causes a large proportion of diarrhea cases among children.[10] (Norovirus is part of the calicivirus family and was formerly called Norwalk-like virus.) Norovirus is highly contagious. Outbreaks are sometimes reported by cruise ships when the majority of passengers become ill within just a few days at sea.[11] Outbreaks also occur in restaurants, daycare centers, and other venues.[12] Most people recover quickly from norovirus infection, but some may require hospitalization for dehydration.

Cholera is an infection with *Vibrio cholerae* bacteria that causes severe watery diarrhea. The toxin produced by the bacteria causes the cells of the small intestine to secrete electrolytes and water rather than absorbing nutrients.[13] The severe dehydration caused by cholera can quickly become fatal if the body's electrolyte balance cannot be maintained through fluid replacement.[14] A cholera cot is a simple bed with a hole cut in the center so that a bucket can be placed below the bed to capture the liquid being expelled from the intestines. Being able to quantify the amount of fluid lost allows an appropriate amount of water to be replaced through drinking or intravenous drips. Up to 3 million cases of cholera have occurred annually in recent years.[15] Some countries in sub-Saharan Africa and Asia have endemic cholera, and some countries in those and other regions experience cholera epidemics.[16] An epidemic in Haiti after the devastating earthquake in 2010 was notable because the origin of the outbreak was traced back to United Nations (UN) peacekeepers from Nepal who were participating in the international response to the disaster. This unfortunate event led to changes in the protocols

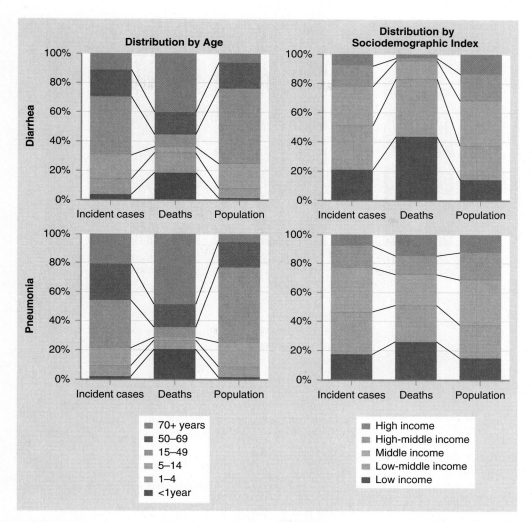

Figure 9.6 Enteric infection (diarrheal disease) and lower respiratory infection (pneumonia) cases and deaths compared to the distribution of the total population, by age and country sociodemographic group.

Data from GBD 2019 Diseases and Injuries Collaborators. Global burden of 369 diseases and injuries in 204 countries and territories, 1990–2019: a systematic analysis for the Global Burden of Disease Study 2019. *Lancet.* 2020;396:1204–1222; and GBD 2019 Demographics Collaborators. Global age-sex-specific fertility, mortality, health life expectancy (HALE), and population estimates in 204 countries and territories, 1950–2019: a comprehensive demographic analysis for the Global Burden of Disease Study 2019. *Lancet.* 2020;396:1160–1203.

for UN deployments, including mandatory cholera vaccinations and higher standards for sanitation.[17] The Global Task Force on Cholera Control aims to eliminate cholera as a public health threat by 2030 through improved prevention interventions, early warning surveillance systems, and better responses to outbreaks.[18]

Escherichia coli bacteria are very common, with *E. coli* present in the intestines of most humans. Most types of *E. coli* are non-pathogenic, which means that they are not harmful and do not cause disease. However, some strains produce pathogenic toxins. These types of *E. coli* are described by the damage they cause, such as enterotoxigenic

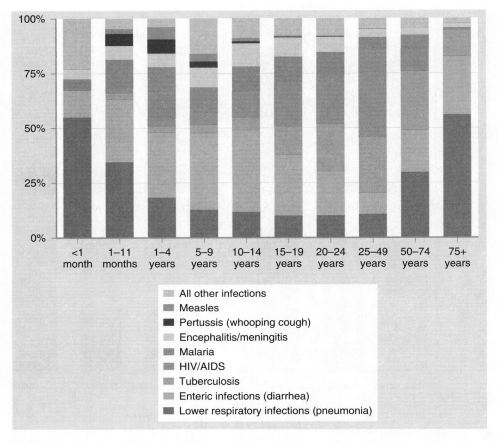

Figure 9.7 Distribution of infectious disease deaths by cause in a typical (nonpandemic) recent year, by age group.

Data from GBD 2019 Diseases and Injuries Collaborators. Global burden of 369 diseases and injuries in 204 countries and territories, 1990–2019: a systematic analysis for the Global Burden of Disease Study 2019. *Lancet.* 2020;396:1204–1222.

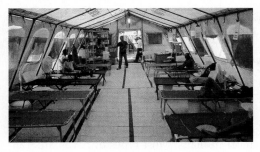

Cholera cots in a cholera treatment center in Haiti in 2010.

CDC Centers for Disease Control and Prevention. https://phil.cdc.gov/Details.aspx?pid=19812. Reference to specific commercial products, manufacturers, companies, or trademarks does not constitute its endorsement or recommendation by the U.S. Government, Department of Health and Human Services, or Centers for Disease Control and Prevention.

E. coli (ETEC), which is a frequent cause of diarrhea in children and travelers, and enteropathogenic *E. coli* (EPEC), which can be fatal in infants.[19] *E. coli* O157:H7, a Shiga toxin-producing *E. coli* (STEC), can cause hemolytic uremic syndrome, which is characterized by bloody diarrhea and kidney failure.[20] *E. coli* O157:H7 bacteria are spread via fecal contamination of food (such as produce or undercooked beef) and water (including swimming pools that are not properly maintained) and by person-to-person contact (typically in a daycare or other institutional setting).[21] **Food intoxication,** illness caused when ingested bacteria produce toxins in the body, is also caused by some other types of bacteria, including *Bacillus cereus*, *Clostridium perfringens*, and *Staphylococcus aureus*.[22]

Campylobacter, *Salmonella*, and *Shigella* are Gram-negative bacteria that are frequent causes of diarrhea. Campylobacteriosis, a disease of the small intestines caused by infection with *Campylobacter jejuni* and other species, is usually acquired through undercooked poultry and meat products.[23] There are more than 2,600 serotypes of *Salmonella*, and they affect both the large and small intestines.[24] *Salmonella* infections are divided into two main categories, typhoid fever and nontyphoidal *Salmonella*. Typhoid (*Salmonella* Typhi, also called *Salmonella enterica* serotype Typhi) infections are often mild, but typhoid sometimes causes a high fever and weeks of severe diarrhea.[25] A **carrier** is a person with a persistent contagious infection who does not have symptoms of the disease but can pass the infectious agent on to others. A small percentage of people infected with typhoid bacteria become chronic carriers of the pathogen. Carriers play a major role in sustaining typhoid transmission in communities because typhoid does not have an animal or environmental reservoir.[26]

Dysentery is bloody diarrhea, with the blood often mixed with mucus, and it can be caused by several different types of bacteria and parasites.[27] Bacillary dysentery is caused by *Shigella* bacteria, which typically affect the colon. Amoebic dysentery is caused by *Entamoeba histolytica*, a protozoan. Other protozoa can also cause diarrheal disease. Cryptosporidiosis is a waterborne protozoal disease (typically caused by *Cryptosporidium hominis* or *C. parvum*) that can be fatal in infants and immunocompromised adults.[28] The parasites are often found in livestock, and outbreaks in humans can occur when drinking water supplies become contaminated with the feces of infected animals. A 1993 outbreak of cryptosporidiosis in Wisconsin, in the United States, which was caused by a failure of the water treatment system, made more than 400,000 people in Milwaukee sick and caused more than 100 deaths.[29]

While most diarrheal infections resolve after a few days, some bacterial and parasitic infections can become chronic diseases. **Giardiasis** is a protozoal disease that can cause persistent diarrhea. Infection with *Giardia duodenalis* (also called *G. intestinalis* and *G. lamblia*) usually lasts for two to six weeks, but some infected individuals experience watery diarrhea and greasy stools for several months or longer.[30] Other chronic foodborne infections include brucellosis and *Helicobacter pylori*. Neither of these diseases has diarrhea as a primary symptom. Brucellosis is caused by bacteria (*Brucella abortus*, *B. melitensis*, and other *Brucella* species) that are transmitted to humans through unpasteurized dairy products and contact with livestock. If untreated, the infection may cause chronic undulant (cyclic) fevers and damage the valves of the heart.[31] Untreated *H. pylori* infection is associated with stomach ulcers.[32] Other foodborne diseases that typically do not cause diarrhea include listeriosis and botulism. *Listeria monocytogenes*, which can be acquired from processed meats and other foods, is of public health concern because pregnant women who contract the bacterium have an increased risk of miscarriages, stillbirths, and preterm delivery.[33] Botulism is a rare disease caused by ingesting toxins from *Clostridium botulinum* bacteria, usually in meals containing honey or improperly canned goods, and it causes cranial nerve palsies, descending paralysis, and the risk of respiratory failure and death.[34]

9.3 Diarrhea Interventions

Two key sets of interventions decrease the mortality rate from diarrhea: primary prevention actions that reduce the incidence of new disease and tertiary prevention actions that reduce the risk of death after onset of diarrhea (**Figure 9.8**). For children, vaccinations against rotavirus, measles, and (where available) cholera and typhoid are important primary prevention methods. People of all ages benefit from water, sanitation, and hygiene (WASH) interventions, which reduce **fecal-oral transmission**, the acquisition of an infectious agent by eating or drinking products contaminated with fecal matter from animals or humans.

Fecal-oral transmission is often described as being a function of the "5 Fs": fluids, fields, fingers, flies, and food.[35] When feces are not properly disposed of, they can contaminate drinking water (fluids) and soil (fields). The fecal matter can then get onto hands (fingers), especially the hands of young children who frequently touch the ground. Hands can transport the fecal matter to food when people do not wash their hands before preparing food or before eating. Insects (flies) can also spread feces to food and water, and flies thrive where fecal matter is in the open. The 5 Fs are sometimes expanded to a set of 6 Fs by adding fomites to the list. A **fomite** is an inanimate object or surface that has been contaminated with infectious agents, such as a doorknob, handrail, light switch, faucet handle, kitchen sponge, stethoscope, or other item that has become coated in pathogenic microbes.

Environmental interventions to reduce the incidence of infections with fecal-oral transmission modes include improvements in access to reliable sources of safe drinking water (fluids), community-wide sanitation facilities for safely disposing of feces (fields), soap for hand hygiene (fingers) plus surface disinfection (fomites), insect control (flies), and food safety (food).[36] Food producers, processors, distributors, and retailers all play critical roles in ensuring the safety of foods and beverages.[37] For consumers, the key food safety practices include maintaining a clean kitchen area and practicing good hand hygiene, separating raw

Level of Prevention	Primordial Prevention	Primary Prevention	Secondary Prevention	Tertiary Prevention
Goal	Prevent risk factors for diarrheal disease or severe diarrhea	Mitigate risk factors in people without diarrheal disease	Detect diarrheal disease before it becomes severe	Manage diarrheal disease after it becomes symptomatic
Examples of interventions	■ Community-led total sanitation ■ Good nutritional practices, such as exclusive breastfeeding of infants for six months followed by complementary feeding ■ Vitamin A supplementation if needed	■ Rotavirus and other vaccines ■ Clean drinking water ■ Hand hygiene with soap ■ Food safety practices	■ Educate parents about early signs of dehydration and when to seek medical care	■ Low-osmolarity oral rehydration therapy (ORT) ■ Continued feeding ■ Zinc supplementation if needed

Figure 9.8 Examples of interventions for diarrheal diseases.

and cooked food, cooking food thoroughly, keeping food at safe hot or cold temperatures, and using safe water and food products.[38]

Once someone has severe infectious diarrhea, the most important action for preventing death is **oral rehydration therapy (ORT)**, drinking enough water to prevent or treat the dehydration caused by diarrhea.[39] **Oral rehydration salts (ORS)**, also called oral rehydration solution, are a mixture of sugar, salt, and other chemicals that restores the balance of electrolytes in the blood when they are mixed with clean drinking water and consumed to replace lost fluids. ORS packets are sometimes distributed at clinics, usually in a low osmolarity formula that contains sodium, chloride, glucose, potassium, and citrate.[40] People can also make their own ORS solution by mixing 8 teaspoons of sugar and one-half teaspoon of salt into 1 liter of boiled water.[41] Potassium can be added to the solution through fruit juice, coconut water, or mashed bananas. Individuals with diarrhea need to drink ORT every time they pass watery stool for a total of at least 1 liter each day. If they also have vomiting, they need to drink more ORT to replace those lost fluids.

Continued feeding is the process of encouraging individuals with diarrhea to eat the same foods that they typically consume if they are not vomiting too much to keep food down. Continued feeding includes breastfeeding infants and young children as usual during their illness. ORT combined with continued feeding, zinc supplementation, and antibiotics for dysentery leads to the best health outcomes for children with diarrhea.[42] After children recover from diarrhea, they should be encouraged to eat more food than usual to regain lost weight and lost nutrients.[43] Children who have vitamin A deficiency, zinc deficiency, or other forms of undernutrition have a higher risk of diarrhea

mortality.[44] Improved nutrition during the recovery period after an illness protects children from the adverse outcomes of their next bout with an infectious disease.[45]

The Global Action Plan for Pneumonia and Diarrhea (GAPPD), initiated by the World Health Organization (WHO), the United Nations Children's Fund (UNICEF), and dozens of partner groups in 2013, set a goal of reducing the diarrhea mortality rate among children less than five years old to less than 1 per 1,000 live births by 2025.[46] The number of diarrheal disease deaths of children younger than five years old decreased from about 1.2 million in 2000 to less than half that number by 2020,[1] even as the number of children worldwide increased, but many lower-income countries are not on track to achieve the GAPPD target rate even if they have made significant progress in reducing death rates from diarrhea (**Figure 9.9**).[1] Although the benefits of ORT for childhood diarrhea have been known for decades,[47] less than half of under-5 children who live in low- or middle-income countries (LMICs) receive ORT when they have diarrhea.[48] To achieve global child survival goals, every young child with diarrhea needs to be treated with ORT.[49]

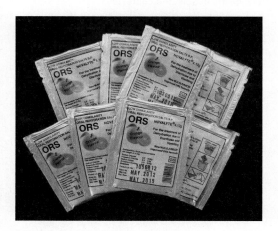

Packets of oral rehydration salts.

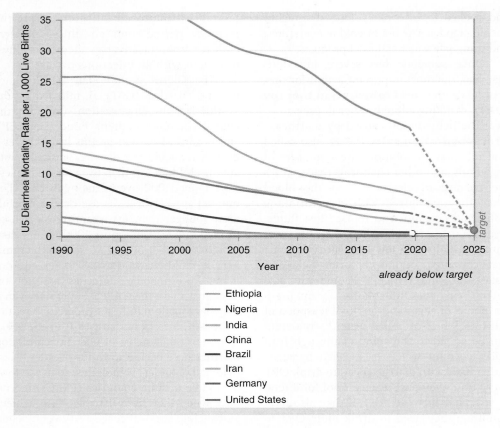

Figure 9.9 Diarrhea disease mortality among children less than five years old (under-5s) per 1,000 live births in selected countries.

Data from GBD 2019 Diseases and Injuries Collaborators. Global burden of 369 diseases and injuries in 204 countries and territories, 1990–2019: a systematic analysis for the Global Burden of Disease Study 2019. *Lancet.* 2020;396:1204–1222; and GBD 2019 Demographics Collaborators. Global age-sex-specific fertility, mortality, health life expectancy (HALE), and population estimates in 204 countries and territories, 1950–2019: a comprehensive demographic analysis for the Global Burden of Disease Study 2019. *Lancet.* 2020;396:1160–1203.

9.4 Acute Respiratory Infections

In health, an **acute** condition is one that has a rapid onset and typically resolves within a few days or weeks. An **acute respiratory infection** (ARI) is an infection of the respiratory tract characterized by rapid onset of symptoms and a relatively short duration of illness. For example, rhinovirus infections can induce the symptoms of a common cold within a few hours after infection, but the symptoms rarely persist for more than two weeks.[50] By contrast, a **chronic** condition develops slowly and may worsen over months or years. Tuberculosis is a chronic infection of the lungs that may last for months or years, and it is not classified as an ARI because it is not an acute infection.

ARIs are divided into two categories based on whether they occur in the upper or lower respiratory tract. An **upper respiratory infection**, or upper respiratory tract infection, is an acute infection of the nose, sinuses, pharynx, larynx (voice box), or trachea. Most upper respiratory infections cause a few days of mild or moderate symptoms, but some can cause long-term damage. **Strep throat** is a Group A *Streptococcus* infection of the pharynx that if left untreated can lead to complications such as rheumatic fever, a condition that may permanently damage the valves of the heart.[51] A **lower respiratory infection** (LRI) is an acute infection of the bronchi, bronchioles, or lungs.

The main function of the body's respiratory system is the exchange of gases, including taking in oxygen and getting rid of carbon dioxide (**Figure 9.10**). When a person takes a breath, the inhaled air enters the lungs and fills tiny air sacs called alveoli. Each alveolus is wrapped in tiny blood vessels called capillaries. Because alveoli and capillaries have very thin walls, small molecules can pass between the air sacs and the bloodstream. After blood is oxygenated within the capillaries in the lungs, it is pumped into the heart and then through arteries to the rest of the body so that all of the body's cells can receive the oxygen they need to function properly. As those cells absorb oxygen from nearby capillaries, they release carbon dioxide and other waste products into the bloodstream. The deoxygenated blood is returned through veins to the heart and then pumped into the lungs, where carbon dioxide passes from the bloodstream into the alveoli and is then exhaled out of the body.

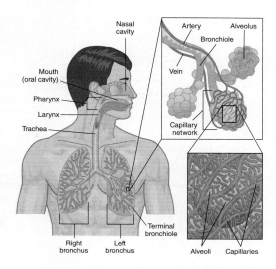

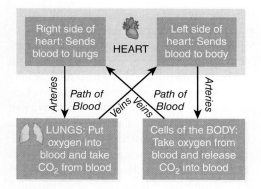

Figure 9.10 Path of blood through the heart, lungs, and body.

Pneumonia is an infection-induced inflammation that causes the air sacs of the lungs to fill with fluid. When the alveoli are filled with fluid, they cannot efficiently exchange oxygen and carbon dioxide. The symptoms of pneumonia usually include a cough accompanied by difficult rapid breathing. People with pneumonia can feel like they are drowning as fluid fills their lungs and they develop **hypoxia**, an inadequate supply of oxygen in body tissues. A child with severe pneumonia may even turn bluish in color due to hypoxia.

Pneumonia cases occur across all age groups, but most fatalities occur among infants and older adults.[52] More precisely, the rate of pneumonia mortality is high among infants in lower-income countries and among older adults in countries of all income levels (**Figure 9.11**).[1] Since high-income countries have older populations than middle-income countries, the crude mortality rate from LRIs is higher in high-income and low-income countries than in middle-income countries. Age-standardized mortality rates that adjust for the different age structures in low-, middle-, and high-income countries show that low- and middle-income countries would have higher rates of LRI mortality if they had populations as old as the global

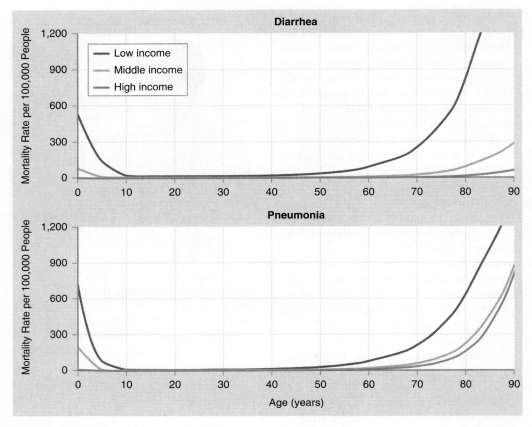

Figure 9.11 Enteric infection (diarrheal disease) and lower respiratory infection (pneumonia) mortality rate per 100,000 people, by age and country sociodemographic group.

Data from GBD 2019 Diseases and Injuries Collaborators. Global burden of 369 diseases and injuries in 204 countries and territories, 1990–2019: a systematic analysis for the Global Burden of Disease Study 2019. Lancet. 2020;396:1204–1222.

average, while high-income countries would have much lower rates of LRI mortality if they had populations as young as the global average (**Figure 9.12**).[1]

A variety of bacteria, viruses, and fungi can cause respiratory illnesses in children and adults. Rapid onset pneumonias accompanied by fever and rapid breathing are usually bacterial in origin.[53] The most frequent cause of pneumonia among both children and adults is *Streptococcus pneumoniae*.[54] **Pneumococcus**

is a synonym for *S. pneumoniae* infection, and pneumococcal disease refers to symptomatic diseases caused by pneumococcus. Many people carry *S. pneumoniae* bacteria in their upper airways without developing symptoms. Some individuals with *S. pneumoniae* infections develop noninvasive pneumococcal diseases like otitis media (ear infections), sinusitis, and bronchitis, and some develop invasive pneumococcal diseases, such as sepsis (blood poisoning) and meningitis (infections of the brain and

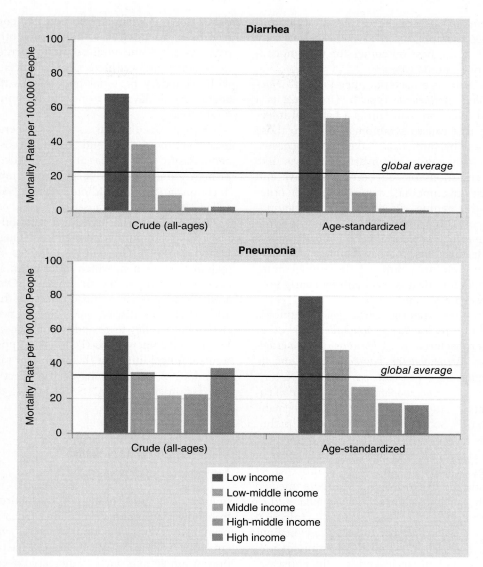

Figure 9.12 Crude and age-standardized all-cause mortality rates from enteric infections (diarrheal diseases) and lower respiratory infections (pneumonia) per 100,000 people, by country sociodemographic group.

Data from GBD 2019 Diseases and Injuries Collaborators. Global burden of 369 diseases and injuries in 204 countries and territories, 1990–2019: a systematic analysis for the Global Burden of Disease Study 2019. *Lancet.* 2020;396:1204–1222.

spinal cord).[55] If the bacteria proliferate and invade the lower respiratory tract, they can cause pneumococcal pneumonia.[56] Pneumococcal conjugate vaccines help prevent pneumonia in young children, and pneumococcal polysaccharide vaccines help prevent pneumonia in older adults, but these vaccines do not work against all strains of pneumococcus.[57] Antibiotics and other therapies used in combination may lead to the best outcomes for pneumococcal pneumonia cases.[56]

"**Hib**" is a bacterial infection with *Haemophilus influenzae* type **b**. (Influenza is a viral infection, and Hib is a bacterial infection that causes symptoms similar to those caused by influenza.) Like pneumococcus, Hib can cause noninvasive diseases like ear infections or can become invasive and cause pneumonia, meningitis, and other life-threatening diseases; unlike pneumococcus, Hib primarily affects young children rather than affecting people of all ages.[58] Widespread use of Hib conjugate vaccine among children reduced the annual number of child deaths from Hib by nearly 90% between 2000 and 2015.[59]

Other bacterial causes of pneumonia include *Klebsiella pneumoniae* and other Enterobacteriaceae, *Pseudomonas aeruginosa*, *Acinetobacter baumannii*, *Chlamydia pneumoniae*, *Coxiella burnetii* (Q fever), *Legionella pneumophila*, *Mycoplasma pneumoniae*, *Staphylococcus aureus*, and many others.[60] Some of these respiratory pathogens have been linked to special modes of transmission. Psittacosis, also called parrot fever, can be acquired when bird owners inhale the dried droppings of pets infected with the bacterium *Chlamydophila psittaci* (formerly *Chlamydia psittaci*).[61] Infection with *Legionellae* bacteria, called Legionnaires' disease when the symptoms are severe or Pontiac fever for milder disease, is acquired through the inhalation of moistened water from air conditioners, hot tubs, and humidifiers.[62]

Viral pneumonias occur most often among young children.[53] **Respiratory syncytial virus (RSV)** is a frequent cause of severe pneumonia among neonates and other young infants.[63] Other causes of viral pneumonia include rhinovirus, influenza viruses, human metapneumovirus,

parainfluenza viruses, bocavirus, coronaviruses, adenoviruses, and many other pathogens.[53] Some viral respiratory infections, including influenza, are associated with secondary bacterial pneumonias that occur several days after onset of the initial viral disease.[53]

Fungal pneumonias (such as aspergillosis, blastomycosis, and cryptococcosis) and parasitic pneumonias are rare and occur primarily among individuals who are immunocompromised. Coccidioidomycosis, also called Valley fever, is caused by *Coccidioides immitis*, a fungus that lives in desert soil in places like the southwestern United States.[64] Histoplasmosis is caused by the fungus *Histoplasma capsulatum*, which is found in soil containing bird or bat droppings.[65] Older adults who take immunosuppressive therapy for chronic diseases have an increased risk of both Valley fever and histoplasmosis. *Pneumocystis* pneumonia (PCP) is an opportunistic fungal infection that occurs primarily among people who have HIV infection that has progressed to AIDS.[66]

9.5 Pneumonia Interventions

Interventions for reducing the burden from lower respiratory infections focus on primary prevention actions such as vaccinations and air quality and on tertiary prevention actions such as increased access to medical services after onset of pneumonia (**Figure 9.13**). Some pneumonia-preventing vaccines are specifically for children, such as Hib and RSV. Some are recommended for both children and at-risk adults, including vaccines for influenza, pertussis (whooping cough), and pneumococcus. Primary prevention also includes reducing exposure to indoor air pollution and smoke, since polluted air damages the

Level of Prevention	Primordial Prevention	Primary Prevention	Secondary Prevention	Tertiary Prevention
Goal	Prevent risk factors for pneumonia	Mitigate risk factors in people without pneumonia	Detect pneumonia before it becomes severe	Manage pneumonia after it becomes symptomatic
Examples of interventions	■ Reduce household air pollution ■ Ensure adequate nutrition ■ Practice good hygiene	■ Vaccinate against pneumococcus, Hib, RSV, influenza, pertussis, measles, and other infections ■ Use personal protective equipment such as face coverings or face masks	■ Educate caregivers about early signs of pneumonia and when to seek medical care	■ Antibiotics ■ Oxygen therapy if needed

Figure 9.13 Examples of interventions for acute lower respiratory infections.

respiratory tract and increases susceptibility to respiratory diseases.

Most respiratory pathogens enter the environment when infected people exhale, speak, sing, cough, or sneeze. Exhaled air contains small water and mucus particles that may carry pathogens from the respiratory tract.[67] Larger, heavier particles usually quickly land on surfaces within a few feet of the mouth and nose. Those surfaces may become fomites that host viable pathogens for minutes to days.[68] Smaller, lighter particles usually evaporate quickly, leaving the carried pathogens suspended in the air as aerosols for minutes or even hours and traveling much farther than a few feet. Larger particles are often called "droplets" and smaller particles "droplet nuclei."

Contamination of air and surfaces generates four different pathways for transmission of respiratory pathogens.[69] **Direct transmission** occurs when an infected person transfers a pathogen to a susceptible person by touching that person or breathing directly onto that person's face. **Indirect transmission** occurs when an infected person transfers a pathogen to a surface or other item that is subsequently touched (or otherwise encountered) by a susceptible host. Droplet spread occurs when a susceptible individual in close proximity to an infected person breathes in some of the droplets that the infected person breathes out. **Airborne transmission** occurs when a susceptible individual breathes in pathogens that have become aerosolized and are suspended as small droplet nuclei in the air.

The risk of all of these forms of transmission can be reduced when infected individuals practice cough hygiene (covering the mouth and nose when coughing or sneezing). Isolating infected persons and having them wear face coverings while they are receiving medical treatment can also help reduce transmission of respiratory

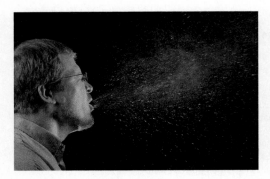

Droplets expelled by a sneeze.

© CDC/James Gathany. https://phil.cdc.gov/Details.aspx?pid=11162. Reference to specific commercial products, manufacturers, companies, or trademarks does not constitute its endorsement or recommendation by the U.S. Government, Department of Health and Human Services, or Centers for Disease Control and Prevention.

pathogens. Susceptible individuals can lower their risk of direct and indirect transmission with frequent handwashing and use of personal protective equipment, such as masks, gloves, and face shields or goggles that protect the eyes. The risk of airborne transmission can be mitigated with good indoor ventilation and reduced crowding.

Some airborne pathogens are acquired from environmental sources rather than from infected humans.[70] For example, some hantaviruses are acquired by inhaling aerosolized rat urine or feces that are lifted into the air when sweeping or cleaning.[71] These risks can be reduced by mitigating environmental hazards and using protective equipment like respirators in locations where exposure to respiratory pathogens is likely.

Tertiary prevention focuses on treating people who are ill from lower respiratory infections. Bacterial pneumonia can often be cured by inexpensive oral antibiotics if treatment is initiated soon after the onset of symptoms.[72] Antibiotics will not speed recovery from colds and other respiratory infections that are caused by viruses, but they are usually effective against early-stage bacterial pneumonia. Oxygen therapy may also help prevent cases of severe pneumonia from becoming fatal.[73]

The estimated annual number of pneumonia deaths among children less than five years old decreased from more than 1.5 million in 2000 to less than half that number by 2020 (**Figure 9.14**),[1] even as the child population increased, but more than half a million children still die each year from LRIs. The number of infant deaths from pneumonia is so high that it is a more frequent cause of death than diarrhea in the under-5 population even though diarrhea causes more deaths than pneumonia after infancy.[74] The Global Action Plan for Pneumonia and Diarrhea (GAPPD) aims to reduce the under-5 pneumonia mortality rate to less than 3 per 1,000 live births by 2025.[46] Many lower-income countries are not on track to reach this rate in the near future (**Figure 9.15**).[1]

An important component of improving child survival is educating caregivers to seek medical care as soon as the symptoms of pneumonia appear so that a course of antibiotics can be initiated. In typical recent years, less than 70% of under-5 children with symptoms of an ARI who live in an LMIC were taken to a healthcare provider,[48] so millions of children with pneumonia did not receive the recommended antibiotic therapy. Increased rates of hospitalization for childhood pneumonia in lower-income countries are associated with decreased case fatality rates because children with severe pneumonia are much more likely to survive if they are treated at hospitals rather than at home.[75]

9.6 Influenza

Influenza is a highly contagious respiratory infection caused by an orthomyxovirus. Influenza viruses cause fevers and respiratory disease and can exacerbate existing medical conditions, especially lung and heart diseases, and lead to potentially fatal secondary infection

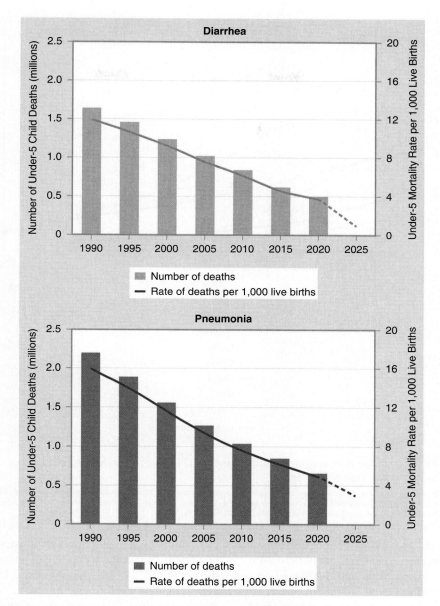

Figure 9.14 Global mortality from diarrheal diseases and lower respiratory infections (pneumonia) among children less than five years old (under-5s) per 1,000 live births, and target for 2025.

Data from GBD 2019 Diseases and Injuries Collaborators. Global burden of 369 diseases and injuries in 204 countries and territories, 1990–2019: a systematic analysis for the Global Burden of Disease Study 2019. *Lancet.* 2020;396:1204–1222; and GBD 2019 Demographics Collaborators. Global age-sex-specific fertility, mortality, health life expectancy (HALE), and population estimates in 204 countries and territories, 1950–2019: a comprehensive demographic analysis for the Global Burden of Disease Study 2019. *Lancet.* 2020;396:1160–1203.

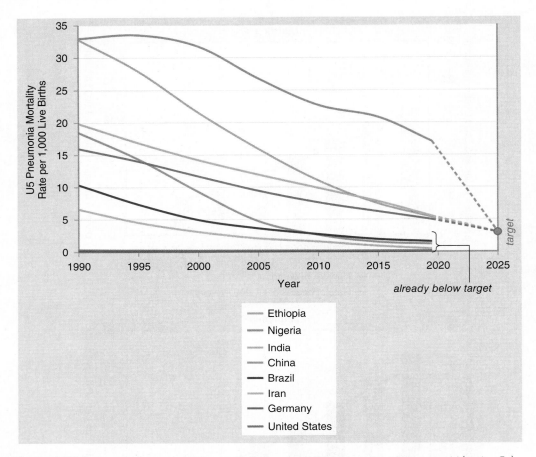

Figure 9.15 Lower respiratory infection mortality among children less than five years old (under-5s) per 1,000 live births in selected countries.

Data from GBD 2019 Diseases and Injuries Collaborators. Global burden of 369 diseases and injuries in 204 countries and territories, 1990–2019: a systematic analysis for the Global Burden of Disease Study 2019. *Lancet.* 2020;396:1204–1222; and GBD 2019 Demographics Collaborators. Global age-sex-specific fertility, mortality, health life expectancy (HALE), and population estimates in 204 countries and territories, 1950–2019: a comprehensive demographic analysis for the Global Burden of Disease Study 2019. *Lancet.* 2020;396:1160–1203.

with bacterial pneumonia.[76] ("Stomach flu" and other types of gastroenteritis are not caused by influenza viruses.) Although the highest fatality rates from influenza are usually among the elderly and immunocompromised individuals, anyone who contracts influenza can die from it.

Seasonal influenza outbreaks occur almost every year, and the viruses that cause these epidemics are constantly mutating. When a novel strain of influenza emerges, it can cause pandemic influenza, sometimes shortened to just "pan flu."[77] The first influenza pandemic likely occurred in 1510,

soon after the global shipping industry was launched, and other pandemics occurred in the 1730s, 1760s, 1780s, 1830s, 1840s, 1890s, and several times thereafter.[78] Pandemic describes the geographic dispersion of a pathogen and is not necessarily an indicator of the severity of the infection,[79] but pandemic influenza strains can be dangerous. The most serious influenza pandemic in the 20th century began in 1918 during World War I.[80] That strain killed a disproportionate number of young adults as it spread through populations across the globe.[81] The emergence of a new strain of influenza today could rapidly spark a global health crisis.[82]

Two types of influenza viruses cause epidemics in human populations, influenza A and influenza B. Influenza A viruses are classified by their surface antigens. An **antigen** is a substance that originates outside the body and triggers an immune response once inside the body. The two key surface antigens for influenza A are hemagglutinin (H) and neuraminidase (N). Influenza A strains are named using abbreviations like H3N2 and H1N1 that are derived from the viruses' hemagglutinin and neuraminidase types. The dominant strain circulating in human populations changes over time. H1N1 was the dominant strain of human influenza from 1918 until it was displaced by H2N2 in the late 1950s; then H2N2 was displaced by H3N2 in the late 1960s.[83]

Influenza viruses affect humans and also many types of animals, including chickens, ducks, pigs, horses, and even dogs, whales, and bats.[84] An **anthroponosis** is an infectious disease that usually occurs only in humans. A **zoonosis** is an infectious disease that usually occurs in animals and only occasionally infects humans. Some strains of influenza circulate in human populations and some strains are zoonoses, but the virus strains can mutate in ways that enable them to cause severe disease in other species. Most strains of influenza that affect humans originate in bird or mammal populations. A total of 17 types of influenza hemagglutinin types and 10 influenza neuraminidase types have been found in animals, but only a few of these have been found in humans.

If a human's immune system has previously been exposed to an antigen, it is often able to quickly recognize and neutralize new pathogens that have that antigen on their surfaces. Influenza viruses evade the immune systems of their hosts by changing their surface antigens so that the hosts' immune systems cannot recognize them. There are two processes by which surface antigens change: antigenic drift and antigenic shift.[85] **Antigenic drift** is a minor genetic mutation of an influenza virus that

causes a small change in the virus's surface antigens. The changes from antigenic drift make it necessary for scientists to develop new seasonal influenza vaccines every year.

Antigenic shift is a major change in the genome of an influenza virus that occurs when the genetic material from two very different types of influenza A viruses recombine to form a new strain.[86] Antigenic shift led to the emergence in 1997 of an H5N1 strain of avian influenza ("bird flu") that spread rapidly through the bird populations in parts of Southeast Asia, affecting both domestic birds (such as ducks and chickens) and wild migrating fowl. The H5N1 strain of influenza was deemed to be a **highly pathogenic avian influenza** (HPAI), a strain of influenza that causes serious disease and high case fatality rates among infected birds.[87]

When a virus circulating in animal populations mutates in a way that allows it to pass easily between humans and make humans severely ill and subsequently becomes established in human populations, that new strain is no longer a zoonosis.[88] For example, when a type of H1N1 "swine flu" began circulating widely in human populations in 2009, it ceased being an influenza of pigs and became a disease of humans.[89] Within months, human cases had been reported in 200 countries.[90] In 2013, an H7N9 influenza that primarily affects poultry caused several humans to become severely ill.[91] Within a few years, several other HPAI H7N9 strains had infected human poultry workers in Asia.[92] Sporadic human infections with H5N6, H5N8, and

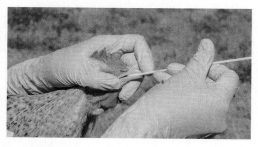

H9N2 viruses that were circulating in bird populations had also been detected.[93] When H5N1, H7N9, another strain of "bird flu," or another type of influenza not currently circulating in human populations further mutates in a way that allows it to be easily transmitted between humans, a pandemic may result.

The term **influenza-like illness** (ILI) is used to describe the status of people with an acute illness who have fever and a cough but have not tested positive for influenza or another pathogen that causes similar symptoms. Rapid laboratory tests are available to confirm the presence of influenza A or B viral antigens in the body fluids of people suspected to have influenza infections. People who test positive for influenza can be prescribed antiviral medications that reduce the severity of symptoms from some strains of influenza. However, these medications do not cure the infection, and they do not work against strains that have developed resistance to antivirals.[94]

Several public health methods have been used since before the modern medical era to contain outbreaks of influenza and other contagious diseases.[95] **Isolation** is the physical separation of people who have a contagious infection from people who are susceptible to the infection. Caregivers of people in isolation take precautions to protect themselves from infection with careful hygiene and **personal protective equipment** (PPE), which includes gowns, gloves, face masks, eye protection, and other barriers that prevent infection. People who have mild illnesses may be able to isolate at home. People who require hospitalization may be placed in rooms where the air that leaves the room is filtered and vented away from other patients. **Quarantine** is the restriction of freedom of movement of healthy contacts of people with an infectious disease as part of a strategy to contain the spread of a contagious disease. Quarantine is applied to people who have no signs of infection at the time they are quarantined. Isolation is for sick people; quarantine is for healthy contacts of

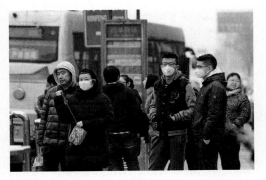

© Testing/Shutterstock

sick people. **Contact tracing** is the process of identifying the primary contacts of infected individuals (and sometimes also the contacts of those primary contacts, who are called secondary contacts) so that they can be tested, monitored, and possibly quarantined.

Influenza is a prime example of how global travel contributes to the rapid spread of newly mutated infectious agents. An infected person can fly to any part of the world in a day or two and spark an outbreak in a new location.[96] Because globalization processes cause pandemics, global communication is a necessary part of the response to pandemics. During the 2009 H1N1 influenza pandemic, countries across the globe reported cases of H1N1 to the WHO, and the WHO used its Pandemic Alert System to keep member nations and the public informed about the spread of the epidemic.[97] Coordinated capacity-building efforts initiated before the pandemic enabled pharmaceutical companies around the globe to expedite the development, testing, and manufacturing of H1N1 diagnostics and vaccines.[90] The lessons learned from H1N1 were then integrated into refined local, national, and global preparedness plans that were ready for implementation when the next major respiratory pandemic emerged.

9.7 Coronaviruses

Most coronavirus infections in humans are mild, such as the approximately 15% of common colds caused by coronaviruses,[98] but some cause severe disease and have the potential to cause pandemics.[99] **SARS** is an abbreviation for the severe acute respiratory syndrome caused by the SARS-CoV-1 virus. The first cases of SARS were identified in Guangdong, in southern China, in November 2002.[100] In March 2003, SARS spread to Hong Kong and a secondary outbreak occurred in Toronto, Canada. Several other countries also reported cases in international travelers and some of their contacts. The affected countries contained their SARS epidemics by isolating patients and carefully observing the people they had contact with so that anyone who developed symptoms could be isolated immediately and treated under strict infection control protocols.[101] In July 2003, the WHO announced that the global outbreak had been contained and travel alerts were lifted. In total, about 8,000 cases were diagnosed, and about 10% of those individuals died from SARS.[102] Although SARS did not cause a widespread pandemic or become an endemic disease, the outbreak raised alarms about gaps in global health communication, surveillance, and response capacity.[103] The International Health Regulations were significantly revised in 2005 to improve responses to future emerging disease events.

Middle East respiratory syndrome (MERS) is the human disease caused by the MERS-CoV virus. The first case of MERS was identified in Saudi Arabia in 2012, and subsequent studies determined that the virus was enzootic in dromedary camel populations across the Arabian Peninsula.[104] An **enzootic** is an adverse health condition that is always present in an animal population (just like an endemic condition is one that is constantly present in human populations). Genetic studies of MERS-CoV suggested that bats were the natural reservoir for the virus and camels were an intermediate host.[105] The findings were consistent with analyses of SARS-CoV-1, which pointed toward bats being the natural reservoir for that virus and civets and raccoon dogs serving as intermediate hosts in China.[106] Although MERS had a high case fatality rate among the early cases

that were identified, it did not demonstrate high contagiousness. Only a few thousand cases total were identified worldwide in the decade after MERS was first identified, and the only significant outbreak outside of the Middle East occurred in South Korea in 2015 and included less than 200 cases.[107]

COVID-19 (derived from **co**rona**vi**rus **di**sease originating in 20**19**) is the disease caused by the SARS-CoV-2 virus. The disease was first identified in late 2019 in Wuhan, China. The typical symptoms of COVID-19 included a cough, fever, anosmia (loss of the sense of smell), and ageusia (loss of taste),[108] but some people with SARS-CoV-2 infection developed respiratory distress and other severe symptoms. On January 30, 2020, the WHO declared the novel coronavirus to be a public health emergency of international concern (PHEIC). On March 11, 2020, the WHO characterized the spread of COVID-19 as a pandemic. Public health measures like travel bans, school and workplace closures, and other nonpharmaceutical interventions (NPIs) were used in many countries to try to slow the spread of the virus and prevent hospitals from being overwhelmed by more critically ill patients than they could care for, but by October 2020 more than 1 million people had died from COVID-19.[109] The development, testing, and approval of several coronavirus vaccines before the end of 2020 provided new tools for infection control,[110] but millions of additional COVID deaths occurred in subsequent years as new variants sparked waves of epidemics.

9.8 Immunization

Vaccination is the intentional delivery of a substance into the body in order to stimulate development of immunity against a particular disease. **Immunization** is the process of a person's immune system developing immunity against a particular infection after receipt of a vaccine. Vaccination is the action of delivering a vaccine to an individual; immunization is what happens in the body after a vaccine is injected or otherwise dispensed. A vaccine prompts the body's immune system to create antibodies specific to the antigens contained in the vaccine. An **antibody** is a protein produced by the human body (by B lymphocytes) in response to the presence of antigens. Antibodies can bind to antigens and destroy them. If person who has been vaccinated with a particular antigen is exposed later on to the same antigen when it is part of an infectious agent, the body's immune system will be able to quickly recognize the agent and destroy it.

Active immunity is protection against infectious diseases that occurs when the body's immune system produces antibodies against a specific infectious agent. This long-lasting protection against an infectious disease can be conferred by both infection and vaccination. By contrast, **passive immunity** is temporary protection against infectious diseases that is conferred by antibodies produced by another human or an animal.[111] Newborns and infants have some protection from maternal antibodies acquired transplacentally. For older children and adults, some protection can be conferred for a few weeks or months through blood products or immunoglobulin shots containing high concentrations of antibodies.

There are several different types of vaccines.[112] A **live attenuated vaccine** is a vaccine that contains a pathogen that has been intentionally weakened. A single dose of a live attenuated vaccine may be sufficient to confer lifelong immunity. However, live attenuated vaccines are not safe for some people with compromised immune systems, and they must be maintained at precise temperatures to maintain their effectiveness. If the cold chain is interrupted, as often occurs in places with unreliable electrical systems, the vaccine will be useless to the recipient. An **inactivated vaccine** is a vaccine that contains a killed bacterium or an inactive virus that has been rendered harmless by heat, chemicals, or radiation. Inactivated vaccines are safer and more stable than live attenuated vaccines, but they are not

as effective at stimulating an immune response. Multiple doses of inactivated vaccines may be required to confer and maintain immunity.

Some inactivated vaccines are whole-virus vaccines, and some are fractional vaccines that contain parts of a pathogen rather than the entire microbe. Fractional vaccines may be protein or polysaccharide based. Protein-based fractional vaccines include toxoid vaccines and subunit vaccines. A toxoid vaccine protects recipients from the toxins released by some bacteria, like the ones that cause diphtheria and tetanus. Subunit vaccines against bacteria and viruses have strong safety profiles, but they are a challenge to create. An adjuvant is an ingredient added to some subunit vaccines to boost the body's immune response to the vaccine. Polysaccharide-based fractional vaccines may be pure or conjugate vaccines. A conjugate vaccine has additional ingredients added to it to help infants' immune systems develop immunity against bacterial infections.

Other types of vaccines created through more complex laboratory methods are also available or in development. An mRNA (messenger ribonucleic acid) vaccine uses genetic material that codes for a pathogen-specific antigen.[113] After the mRNA from a vaccine enters human cells, the genetic strands prompt the cells to produce the antigen. The body's immune system will then produce antibodies specific to that antigen. The mRNA does not change the DNA of the human host, and the strands quickly degrade after the antigen proteins are made. Because mRNA vaccines are not made from pathogens, they cannot cause the infection they seek to protect against. Two of the earliest COVID-19 vaccines were mRNA vaccines: one from Pfizer-BioNTech and one from Moderna.[114]

New vaccines are often developed through partnerships of governments, pharmaceutical companies, scientists, clinicians, nonprofit health organizations, and other groups that work together to fund vaccine research, create and test new vaccine candidates, identify and educate the populations that would most benefit from the vaccine, and manufacture and deliver the vaccines to those populations. A new vaccine undergoes multiple rounds of testing before approval to confirm that the product is safe and effective at conferring immunity against the targeted disease.[115] Most products go through three stages of pre-licensure clinical trials in humans.[116] Phase 1 trials typically enroll 20–100 healthy volunteers to test safety and dosage. Phase 2 trials enroll several hundred volunteers to further examine safety, dosage, and the timing of initial and follow-up shots. Phase 3 trials expand the number of participants to several thousand people. After a vaccine is approved, post-licensure studies continue to monitor safety and effectiveness.[117]

Licensed vaccines have undergone extensive testing to prove that they safe for most people, but a small number of individuals will have allergic reactions to vaccines or experience other problems after vaccine administration.[112] An **adverse reaction** is a negative side effect of a medication, vaccination, medical device, or other medical exposure. The most typical adverse reactions to vaccines are redness at the injection site, some local pain or swelling, and mild fevers or general achiness. Severe adverse reactions are extremely rare.[118] An **adverse event** is a negative outcome that may be the result of a medication, vaccination, or other medical exposure or may be a coincidental occurrence that is not directly related to the exposure. Adverse events encompass both adverse reactions and other negative events that occur after vaccination but appear to be coincidental rather than being a result of the vaccine.[119]

Based on reports of adverse reactions and other types of post-licensure health surveillance data, some individuals who are members of populations approved to receive a vaccine will be advised to postpone or avoid a particular vaccine. A **precaution** is a condition that might make a vaccine ineffective at producing immunity or might increase the likelihood of an adverse reaction in a particular individual. For example, the best option for people with acute illnesses may be to wait until they have recovered before they receive a new vaccine. A **contraindication** is a condition that makes it unsafe for an individual to receive a particular vaccine, medication, device, procedure, or other medical intervention. For example, a severe allergic reaction like anaphylaxis after a first dose of a vaccine is a contraindication for a second dose of that particular vaccine. Most individuals who have a contraindication for one vaccine are able to safely receive other vaccines. Pregnancy is a contraindication for some types of attenuated virus vaccines, but once the pregnancy is over the contraindication no longer applies.

When individuals receive a vaccination, they are not just protecting themselves from disease. They are also protecting the people around them who are unable to be vaccinated because of contraindications and those who are among the small percentage of vaccine recipients who do not develop immunity after vaccination. The theory of **herd immunity**, or community immunity, says that when a high proportion of a population is immune to a specific infectious disease, the entire community is protected, including those who are unable to receive vaccines.[120] Suppose that during an outbreak, each infected person exposes about 10 other people to the infection. In a completely susceptible population, all 10 of the exposed people might become infected, and each of those 10 people could spread the infection to many others. But if 80% of the members of the population have been vaccinated, only 2 of the initial 10 contacts are likely to result in infection, and those 2 newly infected people will not be able to spread the infection to many others. Community immunity requires a large proportion of a population to contract and recover from an infectious disease or to be immunized against it.

One challenge for achieving high levels of vaccination in a population is **vaccine hesitancy**, the decision to delay receiving recommended vaccines or to refuse offered vaccines.[121] Almost all countries report at least some vaccine

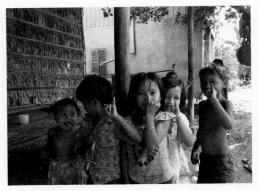

Ink marks the fingers of children vaccinated during an immunization campaign event.

CDC/Sue Chu. https://phil.cdc.gov/Details.aspx?pid=16724. Reference to specific commercial products, manufacturers, companies, or trademarks does not constitute its endorsement or recommendation by the U.S. Government, Department of Health and Human Services, or Centers for Disease Control and Prevention.

hesitancy among their residents.[122] The most frequent reasons for vaccine hesitancy include limited knowledge about the adverse outcomes associated with vaccine-preventable diseases, fear of possible side effects from vaccination, skepticism about the effectiveness of vaccines, a belief that only one vaccine should be received at a time even if a childhood vaccination schedule recommends receipt of several vaccines at one clinic visit, and various social and cultural factors (such as religious beliefs).[123] Vaccine confidence is highest in places where consumers have access to high-quality health information, communities and trusted leaders support vaccination as a local norm, and healthcare providers reliably provide high-quality vaccination services.[124]

9.9 Vaccine-Preventable Infections

Vaccination programs are a key component of many infectious disease prevention and control strategies. The **Expanded Program on Immunization (EPI)** was established by the WHO in 1974 to ensure universal child access to critical vaccines. EPI initially focused on expanding access to vaccines for six preventable infectious diseases: diphtheria, measles, pertussis, polio,

tetanus, and tuberculosis (BCG).[125] (BCG is the only one of these vaccines that is not recommended for all children. The tuberculosis vaccine Bacillus Calmette-Guérin protects against serious tuberculosis disease but is of limited value in preventing colonization with the bacteria that cause tuberculosis,[126] so BCG is not used in countries where the risk of tuberculosis infection is very low.) Today, about a dozen vaccines are routinely recommended for children, including hepatitis B, Hib, pneumococcus, rotavirus, and rubella (**Figure 9.16**).

Measles is a very contagious viral infection that infects immune system cells and causes several months of immunosuppression.[127] The initial symptoms of measles are a fever, cough, a runny nose (coryza), and watery eyes. A few days later, small white spots (Koplik spots) appear on the inside of the mouth, then red spots show up on the face and the maculopapular rash progresses down the trunk and extremities.[128] Young children who have vitamin A deficiency or other comorbidities may experience serious complications, such as severe diarrhea, pneumonia, encephalitis, deafness, blindness, brain damage, and death.[129] A single measles infection confers lifelong immunity against the measles virus, but it can cause "immune amnesia" in which the body's immune system "forgets" many of the pathogen-specific antibodies the body created in response to past infections with other infectious diseases.[130] This leaves survivors more susceptible to infectious diseases for several years after they recover from measles.

Measles-containing vaccine (MCV) is part of the routine childhood vaccination schedule in all countries.[131] The number of cases and deaths from primary measles infection decreased by nearly 90% between 2000 and 2016 as the global vaccination rate increased, but then cases began to resurge as vaccination rates plateaued and some countries with low vaccination rates experienced large outbreaks (**Figure 9.17**).[132] Most measles cases occur in lower-income countries, but all countries are at risk. The United States was declared to

Vaccine	Type of Agent	Agent
Diphtheria	Bacterium	*Corynebacterium diphtheriae*
Hepatitis B	Virus	Hepatitis B virus (hepadnavirus family)
Hib	Bacterium	*Haemophilus influenzae* type b
Measles (rubeola)	Virus	Measles morbillivirus (paramyxovirus family)
Pertussis (whooping cough)	Bacterium	*Bordetella pertussis*
Pneumococcal disease (pneumococcus)	Bacterium	*Streptococcus pneumoniae*
Polio	Virus	Poliovirus (picornavirus)
Rotavirus	Virus	Rotavirus (reovirus family)
Rubella (German measles)	Virus	Rubella virus (matonavirus family)
Tetanus	Bacterium	*Clostridium tetani*

Figure 9.16 World Health Organization recommended routine vaccinations for all children.

Data from *WHO Recommendations for Routine Immunization.* Geneva: World Health Organization; 2020.

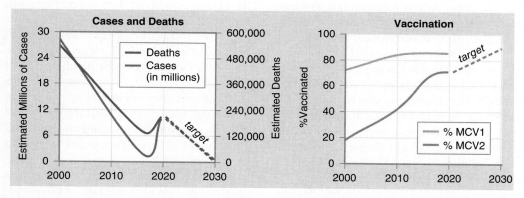

Figure 9.17 Estimated measles cases and deaths and the percentage of young children receiving one dose (MCV1) or two doses (MCV2) of measles-containing vaccine, 2000–2019, with targets for 2030.

Data from Patel MK, Goodson JL, Alexander JP Jr, et al. Progress toward regional measles elimination—worldwide, 2000–2019. *MMWR Morb Mort Wkly Rep.* 2020;69:1700–1705; and *Implementing the Immunization Agenda 2030: A Framework for Action through Coordinated Planning, Monitoring & Evaluation, Ownership & Accountability, and Communications & Advocacy.* Geneva: World Health Organization; 2021.

have eliminated measles in 2000 because there was no sustained endemic transmission even though some cases among international travelers and their contacts were still occurring each year.[133] In recent years, the number of case clusters and the total number of people infected with measles each year in the United States has risen,[134] with many of the outbreaks occurring in cultural communities with low rates of vaccination.[135] While waning immunity after vaccination allows some vaccinated individuals to contract the virus,[136] most measles cases occur among unvaccinated children and adults.

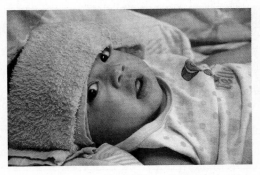

A child with a maculopapular measles rash.

CDC/Jim Goodson, M.P.H. https://phil.cdc.gov/Details.aspx?pid=19433. Reference to specific commercial products, manufacturers, companies, or trademarks does not constitute its endorsement or recommendation by the U.S. Government, Department of Health and Human Services, or Centers for Disease Control and Prevention.

The measles vaccine is often distributed as part of a combination MMR (measles, mumps, and rubella) vaccine.[137] **Mumps** is a viral infection that causes the parotid salivary glands in the cheeks to swell.[138] Mumps can also cause serious complications, including encephalitis, meningitis, deafness, and, in adolescent and adult males, testicular inflammation (orchitis) that may cause infertility.[139] **Rubella**, also called German measles, is a viral infection that can cause miscarriage and birth defects when contracted early in pregnancy.[140] Most individuals who contract rubella experience only a mild rash, but babies born with congenital rubella syndrome often have cataracts, congenital heart disease, deafness, and other health problems.[141] The Measles & Rubella Initiative is a global partnership founded in 2001 that aims to eliminate both measles and congenital rubella through scaled-up access to infant and child vaccination.[142]

A combination vaccine is also usually used to confer protection against diphtheria, tetanus, and pertussis. **Diphtheria** is a membranous inflammation of the airway caused by a toxin produced by *Corynebacterium*. In severe cases, pseudomembranous pharyngitis can cause fatal airway obstruction.[143] The toxin can also cause heart arrhythmias, kidney failure, and neuropathy.[144] Tetanus, also called lockjaw, causes painful muscle spasms throughout the body, starting in the muscles of the lower face.[145] **Pertussis**, also known as whooping cough, is a bacterial infection that causes violent fits of coughing (paroxysms) punctuated by a "whoop" sound when inhaling.[146] Periodic coughing fits may persist for 10 weeks or longer and may be so vigorous that they cause rib fractures. **Apnea** describes long pauses in breathing, especially during sleep. Infants who contract pertussis often do not cough but instead suffer from bouts of apnea that may result in brain damage or death.[147]

Hib[148] and pneumococcus[149] vaccines protect against respiratory infections, and rotavirus vaccines protect infants and young children from a type of severe gastroenteritis.[150] Access to Hib, pneumococcus, and rotavirus vaccines is increasing, but the distribution of these newer vaccines lags behind the rates of more established vaccines (**Figure 9.18**).[151] By 2019, only about 70% of infants received three doses of Hib vaccine, less than 50% received three doses of pneumococcal conjugate vaccine (PCV), and only about 35% received rotavirus vaccine.[151] The cost per dose of these newer products is substantially greater than the cost of older vaccines. Hepatitis B, measles, oral polio, and tetanus vaccines cost the health systems of LMICs much less than $1 per dose, while Hib, PCV, and rotavirus vaccines often cost several dollars per dose.[152] Even with the support of global health partnerships, some countries cannot afford to include higher-priced vaccines in their routine childhood vaccination schedules.

Polio is a viral infection that causes paralysis in a small percentage of the people who contract it, and because it is the focus of a massive global eradication campaign, it is strongly recommended for all children.[153] The human papillomavirus (HPV) vaccine is recommended for adolescent females.[154] Other available vaccines that are recommended in some regions of the world and for some populations with high risk include cholera,[155] dengue,[156] hepatitis A,[157] Japanese encephalitis,[158] meningococcal disease,[159] rabies,[160] tick-borne encephalitis,[161] typhoid fever,[162] varicella (chickenpox and shingles),[163] and yellow fever[164] (**Figure 9.19**). Vaccination is an important tool for

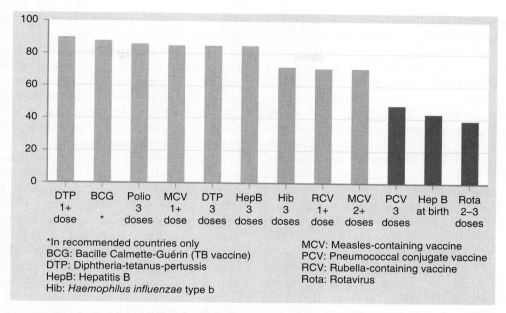

Figure 9.18 Percentage of infants receiving the recommended doses of vaccines in 2019.

Data from Chard AN, Gacic-Dobo M, Diallo MS, Sodha SV, Wallace AS. Routine vaccination coverage – worldwide, 2019. *MMWR Morb Mortal Wkly Rep.* 2020;69:1706–1710.

Vaccine	Type of Agent	Agent
Cholera	Bacterium	*Vibrio cholerae*
Coronavirus	Virus	SARS-CoV-2 (coronavirus family)
Dengue	Virus	Dengue virus (flavivirus family)
Hepatitis A	Virus	Hepatitis A virus (picornavirus family)
HPV	Virus	Human papillomavirus (papillomavirus family)
Influenza	Virus	Influenza virus (orthomyxovirus family)
Japanese encephalitis	Virus	Japanese encephalitis virus (flavivirus family)
Meningococcal disease (meningococcus)	Bacterium	*Neisseria meningitidis*
Mumps	Virus	Mumps rubulavirus (paramyxovirus family)
Rabies	Virus	Rabies lyssavirus (rhabdovirus family)
Tick-borne encephalitis (TBE)	Virus	Tick-borne encephalitis virus (flavivirus family)
Typhoid fever	Bacterium	*Salmonella enterica* Typhi
Varicella (chickenpox/shingles)	Virus	Varicella-zoster virus/human herpesvirus 3 (herpesvirus family)
Yellow fever	Virus	Yellow fever virus (flavivirus family)

Figure 9.19 Examples of other available vaccinations.

Data from *WHO Recommendations for Routine Immunization*. Geneva: World Health Organization; 2020.

reducing the burden from influenza,[165] but seasonal influenza vaccines are not consistently effective at protecting people from the circulating strains.[166] Starting in January 2021, the WHO recommended that coronavirus vaccines be made available to populations in which clinical trials demonstrated a strong safety profile and good protection against COVID.[167] Additionally, several vaccines have been licensed for use in at least one country, such as ones for anthrax and hepatitis E,[168] and others are in advanced clinical trials. These and other vaccines may become more widely available after additional data demonstrate the safety and efficacy of the products.

Vaccines have played a key role in the significant reductions in mortality from childhood infectious diseases that have occurred in the 21st century.[169] EPI and global health partnerships such as Gavi, the Vaccine Alliance, are facilitating continued progress on access to vaccines in LMICs. However, the child vaccination rates in many low-income countries continue to lag behind the rates in higher-income countries

(**Figure 9.20**).[48] Immunization Agenda 2030 (IA2030) aims to increase vaccination coverage through improvements in primary healthcare services (including strengthening vaccine supply chains, vaccine safety monitoring, and surveillance for outbreaks of vaccine-preventable diseases), greater public confidence in vaccines, and people-centered approaches to enabling all people of all ages in all communities to access recommended vaccines.[170] Most countries experienced decreased childhood vaccination rates in 2020 due to supply chain issues, closed clinics, stay-at-home orders, and other pandemic-related challenges.[171] IA2030 aims to overcome those setbacks so that at least 90% of children will be receiving globally recommended vaccines by 2030.[172]

9.10 Viral Hepatitis

Hepatitis is inflammation of the liver. Several types of viral hepatitis caused by pathogens from different viral families are global public health concerns (**Figure 9.21**). **Hepatitis A** is a vaccine-preventable picornavirus infection

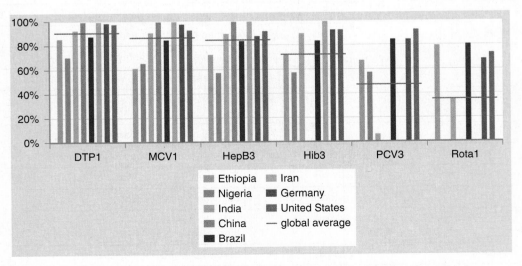

Figure 9.20 Percentage of infants receiving the recommended doses of childhood vaccines in selected countries in 2019.

Data from *State of the World's Children 2019*. New York: UNICEF; 2019.

Disease	Viral Family	Primary Mode of Transmission	Risk of Persistent Infection?	Vaccine Preventable?	Curative Treatment Available?
Hepatitis A	Picornavirus	Fecal-oral (contaminated food and water)	No	Yes	No
Hepatitis B	Hepadnavirus	Contact with blood or body fluids	Yes	Yes	Antivirals can manage but not cure chronic infection
Hepatitis C	Flavivirus	Contact with blood	Yes	No	Yes
Hepatitis E	Hepevirus	Fecal-oral (contaminated food and water)	Rarely	A vaccine is available in a few countries	No

Figure 9.21 Major types of viral hepatitis.

that is spread through contaminated food and water and can cause acute liver inflammation.[173] Chronic hepatitis A virus (HAV) infection does not occur. Young children who contract HAV typically have no symptoms. **Jaundice** is a yellowing of the skin and sclera (the whites of the eyes) due to the buildup of bilirubin levels in the blood. Older children and adults who contract HAV usually experience jaundice, nausea, and fatigue for several weeks, and a small proportion of people with HAV infections develop life-threatening fulminant hepatitis that causes acute liver failure. Lifelong protection from the virus is conferred by infection and by vaccination. Most children in low-income countries contract HAV in very early childhood and develop immunity to the virus, but a large proportion of adults in high-income countries remain vulnerable to the infection.[174]

Hepatitis B is a vaccine-preventable hepadnavirus infection that is spread through blood and other body fluids and can cause chronic liver disease. A **parenteral infection** is an infection that enters the body through a route other than the digestive tract. Hepatitis B virus (HBV) can be transmitted through parenteral contact with blood or other body fluids as a result of a needle stick, an open wound (such as a cut or abrasion), or another tear in the skin or mucous membranes; through sexual activity; and through perinatal transmission in which the virus is passed from the mother to the neonate during delivery.[175] Most people with acute HBV infections have no symptoms, although some adults develop fatigue, nausea, and jaundice.[176] While most adults clear the infection within a few months, about 90% of neonates, 30% of children, and 5% of adults who contract HBV become chronic carriers.[177] Chronic HBV infection increases the risk of cirrhosis (scarring of the liver) and hepatocellular carcinoma (a type of liver cancer). Receiving a first dose of hepatitis B vaccine within 24 hours after birth helps protect newborns exposed to HBV during the birth process.[178] Completing a series of hepatitis B vaccines in infancy provides young children with further protection from chronic HBV infections.[179] For individuals who develop chronic hepatitis B, antiviral therapy can suppress the virus but does not cure the infection.[180] Vaccination is contributing to a decrease in the incidence of HBV infection among young people, but the prevalence of chronic HBV infection among adults born before hepatitis B vaccines were available remains high in some parts of Africa and Asia.[181]

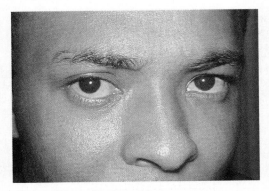

Jaundice caused by hepatitis A.

CDC/Dr. Thomas F. Sellers; Emory University. https://phil.cdc.gov/Details.aspx?pid=2860. Reference to specific commercial products, manufacturers, companies, or trademarks does not constitute its endorsement or recommendation by the U.S. Government, Department of Health and Human Services, or Centers for Disease Control and Prevention.

Hepatitis C is a chronic flavivirus infection that is now transmitted primarily through injecting drug use.[182] Hepatitis C virus (HCV) can also be transmitted sexually and, rarely, from mother to child during birth. There is no vaccine against HCV. More than half of people who contract HCV develop a chronic infection, and chronic infection substantially increases the risk of cirrhosis and hepatocellular carcinoma.[183] Several antiviral medications can completely eliminate the virus from most people who complete a course of treatment.[184] However, these medications are too expensive to be widely available in low-income countries or universally available in middle-income countries.[185] HCV occurs in every world region, with considerable variation in prevalence by country.[186]

Hepatitis E is a waterborne hepevirus infection that can cause acute liver failure and death in pregnant women.[187] There are four known genotypes of hepatitis E virus (HEV). Genotypes 1 and 2 cause occasional outbreaks in some lower-income countries. Pregnant women who contract one of these genotypes have a significantly elevated risk of acute liver failure, especially if they are in the third trimester of pregnancy, and the case fatality rate among those women might be as high as 15% or 20%.[188] Genotypes 3 and 4 mostly affect swine, and humans are accidental hosts.

Immunocompromised people who contract genotype 3 may develop chronic infection and experience neurological complications.[189] A hepatitis E vaccine has been available in China since 2012, but few other countries have sought licensure for hepatitis E vaccines.[168]

More than 250 million people contract viral hepatitis infections each year, and HAV is the causative agent for the majority of these cases.[1] Acute viral hepatitis can cause several weeks of illness and may require hospitalization, but the case fatality rate is very low. Fewer than 100,000 deaths from acute viral hepatitis have occurred annually in typical recent years.[1] However, an estimated 6 to 10 million of the individuals who contract HBV or HCV each year fail to clear the infection and become chronic carriers who may develop severe liver disease 30 or more years later.[190] Chronic viral hepatitis infections currently contribute to more than 1 million deaths each year from cirrhosis, liver cancer, and other complications of chronic HBV and HCV infections.[1]

The WHO estimated that in 2015 about 260 million people were living with chronic HBV infection and about 70 million were living with chronic HCV infection.[191] Two sets of interventions will help reduce the prevalence rate: preventing new infections (through hepatitis B vaccination, safe blood products, and safe injections) and treating existing cases of HBV and HCV with direct-acting antiviral (DAA) medications. The WHO, in partnership with the World Hepatitis Alliance, aims between 2015 and 2030 to decrease the incidence of chronic HBV infections by 95%, decrease the incidence of chronic HCV infections by 80%, increase the diagnosis rate for chronic viral hepatitis from less than 5% to 90%, and increase treatment of viral hepatitis B and C from less than 1% of infected people to 80%.[190] Achieving those targets would require several billion dollars to be invested each year in increasing access to diagnostics and medicines.[192] If greater funding enables the targets to be reached, the annual number of deaths from chronic viral hepatitis could decrease by 65%, from about 1.4 million in 2015 to less than 500,000 cases per year by 2030.[190]

9.11 Meningitis

Meningitis is an inflammation of the meninges, the membranes that cover the brain and spinal cord. Meningitis causes a severe headache and stiff neck along with confusion, nausea, sensitivity to light, and possibly sepsis (commonly called blood poisoning). **Encephalitis** is an acute inflammation of the brain. The symptoms of encephalitis are similar to those of meningitis and include headaches, confusion, drowsiness, hallucinations, and seizures. When both meningitis and encephalitis occur in the same person, it is called meningoencephalitis.

Meningitis can be caused by a variety of infectious agents, including fungi and parasites. Viral infections are the most frequent cause of meningitis, but bacterial meningitis is of greater concern because it has a higher case fatality rate.[193] The four main causes of bacterial meningitis are *Neisseria meningitidis* (meningococcus), *Streptococcus pneumoniae* (pneumococcus), *Haemophilus influenzae*, and *Streptococcus agalactiae* (group B *Streptococcus*).[194] Vaccines are available to prevent the diseases caused by three of those four agents: meningococcus, pneumococcus, and Hib.

Meningococcus is a synonym for infection with the bacterium *Neisseria meningitidis*, and meningococcal disease refers to any disease caused by meningococcus.[195] Meningococcal disease occurs worldwide, but rates of disease have been especially high in the "meningitis belt," an area that extends across the northern countries of sub-Saharan Africa from Senegal in the west to Ethiopia in the east.[196] Large outbreaks of meningococcus historically occurred in the meningitis belt every few years during the dry season,[197] but the incidence of meningitis decreased rapidly after the introduction of meningococcus vaccine to the region in 2010.[198] It is not possible with current technology to eradicate bacterial meningitis, but epidemics could be eliminated through improved surveillance that detects outbreaks early so that vaccination campaigns and other medical and public health control measures can be implemented before cases become widespread.[199]

References

1. GBD 2019 Diseases and Injuries Collaborators. Global burden of 369 diseases and injuries in 204 countries and territories, 1990–2019: a systematic analysis for the Global Burden of Disease Study 2019. *Lancet.* 2020;396:1204–1222.
2. Babigumira J, Gelband H, Garrison LP Jr. Cost-effectiveness of strategies for the diagnosis and treatment of febrile illness in children (chapter 15). In: Holmes KK, Bertozzi S, Bloom BR, Jha P, eds. *Disease Control Priorities: Major Infectious Diseases.* Vol. 6. 3rd ed. Washington DC: IBRD/World Bank; 2017:385–400.
3. *The Millennium Development Goals Report 2015.* New York: United Nations; 2015.
4. *Transforming Our World: The 2030 Agenda for Sustainable Development.* New York: United Nations; 2015.
5. Bányai K, Estes MK, Martella V, Parashar U. Viral gastroenteritis. *Lancet.* 2018;392:175–186.
6. GBD 2016 Diarrhoeal Disease Collaborators. Estimates of the global, regional, and national morbidity, mortality, and aetiologies of diarrhoea in 195 countries: a systematic analysis for the Global Burden of Disease Study 2016. *Lancet Infect Dis.* 2018;18:1211–1228.
7. Juckett G, Trivedi R. Evaluation of chronic diarrhea. *Am Fam Physician.* 2011;84:1119–1126.
8. Burnett E, Parashar UD, Tate JE. Global impact of rotavirus vaccination on diarrheal hospitalizations and deaths among children <5 years old: 2006–2019. *J Infect Dis.* 2020;222:1731–1739.
9. Troeger C, Khalil IA, Rao PC, et al. Rotavirus vaccination and the global burden of rotavirus diarrhea among children younger than 5 years. *JAMA Pediatr.* 2018;172:958–965.
10. Lopman BA, Steele D, Kirkwood CD, Parashar UD. The vast and varied global burden of norovirus: prospects for prevention and control. *PLoS Med.* 2016;13:e1001999.

11. Bert F, Scaioli G, Gualano MR, et al. Norovirus outbreaks on commercial cruise ships: a systematic review and new targets for the public health agenda. *Food Environ Virol.* 2014;6:67–74.

12. Robilotti E, Deresinski S, Pinsky BA. Norovirus. *Clin Microbiol Rev.* 2015;28:134–164.

13. Sack DA, Sack RB, Nair GB, Siddique AK. Cholera. *Lancet.* 2004;363:223–233.

14. Butler T. Treatment of severe cholera: a review of strategies to reduce stool output and volumes of rehydration fluid. *Trans R Soc Trop Med Hyg.* 2017;111:204–210.

15. Legros D. Global cholera epidemiology: opportunities to reduce the burden of cholera by 2030. *J Infect Dis.* 2018;218(Suppl 3):S137–S140.

16. Azman AS, Moore SM, Lessler J. Surveillance and the global fight against cholera: setting priorities and tracking progress. *Vaccine.* 2020;38(Suppl 1): A28–A30.

17. Piarroux R, Frerichs RR. Cholera and blame in Haiti. *Lancet Infect Dis.* 2015;15:1380–1381.

18. Global Task Force on Cholera Control. *Ending Cholera: A Global Roadmap to 2030.* Geneva: World Health Organization; 2017.

19. *Bad Bug Book: Foodborne Pathogenic Microorganisms and Natural Toxins Handbook.* 2nd ed. Silver Spring MD: FDA Center for Food Safety and Applied Nutrition; 2014.

20. Tarr PI, Gordon CA, Chandler WL. Shiga-toxin-producing *Escherichia coli* and haemolytic uraemic syndrome. *Lancet.* 2005;365:1073–1086.

21. Pennington H. *Escherichia coli* O157. *Lancet.* 2010;376:1428–1435.

22. Bennett SD, Walsh KA, Gould LH. Foodborne disease outbreaks caused by *Bacillus cereus, Clostridium perfringens,* and *Staphylococcus aureus*: United States, 1998–2008. *Clin Infect Dis.* 2013;57:425–433.

23. Kaakoush NO, Castaño-Rodríguez N, Mitchell HM, Man SM. Global epidemiology of *Campylobacter* infection. *Clin Microbiol Rev.* 2015;28:687–720.

24. Gal-Mor O, Boyle EC, Grassl GA. Same species, different diseases: how and why typhoidal and non-typhoidal *Salmonella enterica* serovars differ. *Front Microbiol.* 2014;5:391.

25. Wain J, Hendriksen RS, Mikoleit ML, Keddy KH, Ochiai RL. Typhoid fever. *Lancet.* 2015;385:1136–1145.

26. Parry CM, Hien TT, Dougan G, White NJ, Farrar JJ. Typhoid fever. *N Engl J Med.* 2002;347:1770–1782.

27. Pfeiffer ML, DuPont HL, Ochoa TJ. The patient presenting with acute dysentery: a systematic review. *J Infect.* 2012;64:374–386.

28. Innes EA, Chalmers RM, Wells B, Pawlowic MC. A One Health approach to tackle cryptosporidiosis. *Trends Parasitol.* 2020;36:290–303.

29. Mac Kenzie WR, Hoxie NJ, Proctor ME, et al. A massive outbreak in Milwaukee of *Cryptosporidium* infection transmitted through the public water supply. *N Engl J Med.* 1994;331:161–167.

30. Einarsson E, Ma'ayeh S, Svärd SG. An up-date on *Giardia* and giardiasis. *Curr Opin Microbiol.* 2016;34:47–52.

31. Hull NC, Schumaker BA. Comparisons of brucellosis between human and veterinary medicine. *Infect Ecol Epidemiol.* 2018;8:1500846.

32. Kuipers EJ, Thijs JC, Festen HP. The prevalence of *Helicobacter pylori* in peptic ulcer disease. *Aliment Pharmacol Ther.* 1995;9(Suppl 2):59–69.

33. Madjunkov M, Chaudhry S, Ito S. Listeriosis during pregnancy. *Arch Gynecol Obstet.* 2017;296:143–152.

34. Sobel J. Botulism. *Clin Infect Dis.* 2005;41:1167–1173.

35. Conant J, Fadem P. *Community Guide to Environmental Health.* Berkeley CA: Hesperian Foundation; 2008.

36. Julian TR. Environmental transmission of diarrheal pathogens in low and middle income countries. *Environ Sci Process Impacts.* 2016;18:944–955.

37. Codex Alimentarius Commission. *Food Hygiene: Basic Texts.* 4th ed. Rome: World Health Organization/Food and Agriculture Organization of the United Nations; 2009.

38. *Five Keys to Safer Food Manual.* Geneva: World Health Organization; 2006.

39. Wolfheim C, Fontaine O, Merson M. Evolution of the World Health Organization's programmatic actions to control diarrheal diseases. *J Glob Health.* 2019;9:020802.

40. *Oral Rehydration Salts: Production of the New ORS.* Geneva: World Health Organization/UNICEF; 2006.

41. *Where There Is No Doctor.* Berkeley CA: Hesperian Health Guides; 2017.

42. Black R, Fontaine O, Lamberti L, et al. Drivers of the reduction in childhood diarrhea mortality 1980–2015 and interventions to eliminate preventable diarrhea deaths by 2030. *J Glob Health.* 2019;9:020810.

43. Bhutta ZA, Das JK, Walker N, et al. The Lancet Diarrhoea and Pneumonia Interventions Study Group. Interventions to address deaths from childhood pneumonia and diarrhea equitably: what works and at what cost? *Lancet.* 2013;381:1417–1429.

44. Fischer-Walker CL, Rudan I, Liu L, et al. Global burden of childhood pneumonia and diarrhoea. *Lancet.* 2013;381:1405–1416.

45. Chopra M, Mason E, Borrazzo J, et al. Ending of preventable deaths from pneumonia and diarrhoea: an achievable goal. *Lancet.* 2013;381:1499–1506.

46. *Ending Preventable Child Deaths from Pneumonia and Diarrhoea by 2025: The Integrated Global Action Plan for Pneumonia and Diarrhoea (GAPPD).* New York: UNICEF/World Health Organization; 2013.

47. Local Burden of Disease Diarrhoea Collaborators. Mapping geographical inequalities in oral rehydration therapy coverage in low-income and middle-income countries, 2000–17. *Lancet Glob Health.* 2020;8:e1038–e1060.

48. *State of the World's Children 2019.* New York: UNICEF; 2019.

49. *One Is Too Many: Ending Child Deaths from Pneumonia and Diarrhoea.* New York: UNICEF; 2016.

50. Heikkinen T, Järvinen A. The common cold. *Lancet.* 2003;361:51–59.

51. Gerber MA, Baltimore RS, Eaton CB, et al. Prevention of rheumatic fever and diagnosis and treatment of acute Streptococcal pharyngitis: a scientific statement from the American Heart Association Rheumatic Fever, Endocarditis, and Kawasaki Disease Committee of the Council on Cardiovascular Disease in the Young, the Interdisciplinary Council on Functional Genomics and Translational Biology, and the Interdisciplinary Council on Quality of Care and Outcomes Research: endorsed by the American Academy of Pediatrics. *Circulation.* 2019;119:1541–1551.

52. GBD 2016 Lower Respiratory Infections Collaborators. Estimates of the global, regional, and national morbidity, mortality, and aetiologies of lower respiratory infections in 195 countries, 1990–2016: a systematic analysis for the Global Burden of Disease Study 2016. *Lancet Infect Dis.* 2016;18:1191–1210.

53. Ruuskanen O, Lahti E, Jennings LC, Murdoch DR. Viral pneumonia. *Lancet.* 2011;377:1264–1275.

54. Prina E, Ranzani OT, Torres A. Community-acquired pneumonia. *Lancet.* 2015;386:1097–1108.

55. Randle E, Ninis N, Inwald D. Invasive pneumococcal disease. *Arch Dis Child Educ Pract Ed.* 2011;96:183–190.

56. van der Poll T, Opal SM. Pathogenesis, treatment, and prevention of pneumococcal pneumonia. *Lancet.* 2009;374:1543–1556.

57. Van Werkhoven CH, Huijts SM. Vaccines to prevent pneumococcal community-acquired pneumonia. *Clin Chest Med.* 2018;39:733–752.

58. Slack M, Esposito S, Haas H, et al. *Haemophilus influenzae* type b disease in the era of conjugate vaccines: critical factors for successful eradication. *Expert Rev Vaccines.* 2020;19:903–917.

59. Wahl B, O'Brien KL, Greenbaum A, et al. Burden of *Streptococcus pneumoniae* and *Haemophilus influenzae* type b disease in children in the era of conjugate vaccines: global, regional, and national estimates for 2000–15. *Lancet Glob Health.* 2018;6:e744–e757.

60. Cilloniz C, Martin-Loeches I, Garcia-Vidal C, San Jose A, Torres A. Microbial etiology of pneumonia: epidemiology, diagnosis and resistance patterns. *Int J Mol Sci.* 2016;17:2120.

61. Stewardson AJ, Grayson ML. Psittacosis. *Infect Dis Clin North Am.* 2010;24:7–25.

62. Cunha BA, Burillo A, Bouza E. Legionnaires' disease. *Lancet.* 2015;387:376–385.

63. The Pneumonia Etiology Research for Child Health (PERCH) Study Group. Causes of severe pneumonia requiring hospital admission in children without HIV infection from Africa and Asia: the PERCH multi-country case-control study. *Lancet.* 2019;394:757–779.

64. Odio CD, Marciano BE, Galgiani JN, Holland SM. Risk factors for disseminated coccidioidomycosis, United States. *Emerg Infect Dis.* 2017;23:308–311.

65. Rodrigues AM, Beale MA, Hagen F, et al. The global epidemiology of emerging *Histoplasma* species in recent years. *Stud Mycol.* 2020;97:100095.

66. Shibata S, Kikuchi T. *Pneumocystis* pneumonia in HIV-1 infected patients. *Respir Investig.* 2019;57:213–219.

67. Drossinos Y, Stilianakis NI. What aerosol physics tells us about airborne pathogen transmission. *Aerosol Sci Tech.* 2020;54:639–643.

68. Hall CB. The spread of influenza and other respiratory viruses: complexities and conjectures. *Clin Infect Dis.* 2007;45:353–359.

69. Shiu EYC, Leung NHL, Cowling BJ. Controversy around airborne versus droplet transmission of respiratory viruses: implication for infection prevention. *Curr Opin Infect Dis.* 2019;32:372–379.

70. Tang JW. The effect of environmental parameters on the survival of airborne infectious agents. *J R Soc Interface.* 2009;6(Suppl 6):S737–S746.

71. Jonsson BC, Figueiredo LTM, Vapalahti O. A global perspective on hantavirus ecology, epidemiology, and disease. *Clin Microbiol Rev.* 2010;23:412–441.

72. *Revised WHO Classification and Treatment of Childhood Pneumonia at Health Facilities: Evidence Summaries.* Geneva: World Health Organization; 2014.

73. *Oxygen Therapy for Children: A Manual for Health Workers.* Geneva: World Health Organization; 2016.

74. *Fighting for Breath Call to Action: End Childhood Pneumonia.* New York: Every Breath Counts Coalition; 2019.

75. McAllister DA, Liu L, Shi T, et al. Global, regional, and national estimates of pneumonia morbidity and mortality in children younger than 5 years between 2000 and 2015: a systematic analysis. *Lancet Glob Health.* 2019;7:e47–e57.

76. Gupta RK, George R, Nguyen-Van-Tam JS. Bacterial pneumonia and pandemic influenza planning. *Emerg Infect Dis.* 2008;14:1187–1192.

77. Doshi P. The elusive definition of pandemic influenza. *Bull World Health Organ.* 2011;89:532–538.

78. Morens DM, Fauci AS. The 1918 influenza pandemic: insights for the 21st century. *J Infect Dis.* 2007;195:1018–1028.

79. Card AJ. Pandemicity and severity are separate constructs. *Am J Public Health.* 2012;102:e12.

80. Brundage JF, Shanks G. Deaths from bacterial pneumonia during the 1918–19 influenza pandemic. *Emerg Infect Dis.* 2008;14:1193–1199.

81. Murray CJL, Lopez AD, Chin B, Feehan D, Hill KH. Estimation of potential global pandemic influenza mortality on the basis of vital registry data from the 1918–20 pandemic: a quantitative analysis. *Lancet.* 2006;368:2211–2218.

82. *Global Influenza Strategy* 2019–2030. Geneva: World Health Organization; 2019.

83. Glezen WP. Emerging infections: Pandemic influenza. *Epidemiol Rev.* 1996;18:64–76.

84. Yoon SW, Webby RJ, Webster RG. Evolution and ecology of influenza A viruses. *Curr Top Microbiol Immunol.* 2014;385:359–375.

85. Bouvier NM, Palese P. The biology of influenza viruses. *Vaccine.* 2008;26(Suppl 4):D49–D53.

86. Webster RG, Govorkova EA. Continuing challenges in influenza. *Ann N Y Acad Sci.* 2014;1323:115–139.

87. Kalthoff D, Globig A, Beer M. (Highly pathogenic) avian influenza as a zoonotic agent. *Vet Microbiol.* 2010;140:237–245.

88. Reperant LA, Kuiken T, Osterhaus AD. Adaptive pathways of zoonotic influenza viruses: from exposure to establishment in humans. *Vaccine.* 2012;30:4419–4434.

89. Novel Swine-Origin Influenza A (H1N1) Virus Investigation Team, Dawood FS, Jain S, Finelli L, et al. Emergence of a novel swine-origin influenza A (H1N1) virus in humans. *N Engl J Med.* 2009;360:2605–2615.

90. Girard MP, Tam JS, Assossou OM, Kieny MP. The 2009 A (H1N1) influenza virus pandemic: a review. *Vaccine.* 2010;28:4895–4902.

91. Gao R, Cao B, Hu Y, et al. Human infection with a novel avian-origin influenza A (H7N9) virus. *N Engl J Med.* 2013;368:1888–1897.

92. Ma MJ, Yang Y, Fang LQ. Highly pathogenic avian H7N9 influenza viruses: recent challenges. *Trends Microbiol.* 2019;27:93–95.

93. Adlhoch C, Fusaro A, Gonzales JL, et al. Avian influenza overview December 2020–February 2021. *EFSA J.* 2021;19:e06497.

94. Hayden FG, de Jong MD. Emerging influenza antiviral resistance threats. *J Infect Dis.* 2011;203:6–10.

95. Ferguson NM, Cummings DAT, Fraser C, Cajka JC, Cooley PC, Burke DS. Strategies for mitigating an influenza pandemic. *Nature.* 2006;442:448–452.

96. Viboud C, Bjørnstad ON, Smith DL, Simonsen L, Miller MA, Grenfell BT. Synchrony, waves, and spatial hierarchies in the spread of influenza. *Science.* 2006;312:447–451.

97. Gostin LO. Influenza A (H1N1) and pandemic preparedness under the rule of international law. *JAMA.* 2009;301:2376–2378.

98. Greenberg SB. Update on human rhinovirus and coronavirus infections. *Semin Respir Crit Care Med.* 2016;37:555–571.

99. Yang Y, Peng F, Wang R, et al. The deadly coronaviruses: the 2003 SARS pandemic and the 2020 novel coronavirus epidemic in China. *J Autoimmun.* 2020;109:102434.

100. Peiris JSM, Yuen KY, Osterhaus ADME, Stöhr K. The severe acute respiratory syndrome. *N Engl J Med.* 2003;349:2431–2441.

101. Lipsitch M, Cohen T, Cooper B, et al. Transmission dynamics and control of severe acute respiratory syndrome. *Science.* 2003;300:1966–1970.

102. Cherry JD. The chronology of the 2002–2003 SARS mini pandemic. *Pediatr Respir Rev.* 2004;5:262–269.

103. Heymann DL. The international response to the outbreak of SARS in 2003. *Philos Trans R Soc Lond B Biol Sci.* 2004;359:1227–1229.

104. Mackay IM, Arden KE. MERS coronavirus: diagnostics, epidemiology and transmission. *Virol J.* 2015;12:222.

105. Lu G, Wang Q, Gao GF. Bat-to-human: spike features determining 'host jump' of coronavirus SARS-CoV, MERS-CoV, and beyond. *Trends Microbiol.* 2015;23:468–478.

106. Shi Z, Hu Z. A review of studies on animal reservoirs of the SARS coronavirus. *Virus Res.* 2008;133;74–87.

107. Chen X, Chughtai AA, Dyda A, MacIntyre CR. Comparative epidemiology of Middle East respiratory syndrome coronavirus (MERS-CoV) in Saudi Arabia and South Korea. *Emerg Microbes Infect.* 2017;6:e51.

108. Struyf T, Deeks JJ, Dinnes J, et al. Signs and symptoms to determine if a patient presenting in primary care or hospital outpatient settings has COVID-19. *Cochrane Database Syst Rev.* 2021;2:CD013665.

109. Ioannidis JPA. Global perspective of COVID-19 epidemiology for a full-cycle pandemic. *Eur J Clin Invest.* 2020;50:e13423.

110. COVID-19 vaccines: no time for complacency. *Lancet.* 2020;396:1607.

111. Keller MA, Stiehm ER. Passive immunity in prevention and treatment of infectious diseases. *Clin Microbiol Rev.* 2000;13:602–614.

112. *Epidemiology and Prevention of Vaccine-Preventable Diseases.* 14th ed. Atlanta GA: Centers for Disease Control and Prevention; 2021.

113. Pardi N, Hogan MJ, Porter FW, Weissman D. mRNA vaccines: a new era in vaccinology. *Nat Rev Drug Discov.* 2018;17:261–279.

114. Meo SA, Bukhari IA, Akram J, Meo AS, Klonoff DC. COVID-19 vaccines: comparison of biological, pharmacological characteristics and adverse effects of Pfizer/BioNTech and Moderna vaccines. *Eur Rev Med Pharmacol Sci.* 2021;25:1663–1669.

115. Chen RT, Orenstein WA. Epidemiologic methods in immunization programs. *Epidemiol Rev.* 1996;18:99–117.

116. Pickering LK, Orenstein WA. Development of pediatric vaccine recommendations and policies. *Semin Pediatr Infect Dis.* 2002;13:148–154.

117. Hanquet G, Valenciano M, Simondon F, Moren A. Vaccine effects and impact of vaccination programmes in post-licensure studies. *Vaccine.* 2013;31:5634–5642.

118. Miller ER, Moro PL, Cano M, Schimabukuro T. Deaths following vaccination: what does the evidence show? *Vaccine.* 2015;33:3288–3292.

119. Ellenberg SS, Chen RT. The complicated task of monitoring vaccine safety. *Public Health Rep.* 1997;112:10–21.

120. Fine PE. Herd immunity: history, theory, practice. *Epidemiol Rev.* 1993;15:265–302.

121. MacDonald NE, the SAGE Working Group on Vaccine Hesitancy. Vaccine hesitancy: definition, scope and determinants. *Vaccine.* 2015;33:4161–4164.

122. Lane S, MacDonald NE, Marti M, Dumolard L. Vaccine hesitancy around the globe: analysis of three years of WHO/UNICEF Joint Reporting Form data 2015–2017. *Vaccine.* 2018;36:3861–3867.

123. Kulkarni S, Harvey B, Prybylski D, Jalloh MF. Trends in classifying vaccine hesitancy reasons reported in the WHO/UNICEF Joint Reporting Form, 2014–2017: Use and comparability of the Vaccine Hesitancy Matrix. *Hum Vaccin Immunother.* 2021;17:2001–2007.

124. Hickler B, MacDonald NE, Senouci K, et al. Efforts to monitor global progress on individual and community demand for immunization: development of definitions and indicators for the Global Vaccine Action Plan strategic objective 2. *Vaccine.* 2017;35:3515–3519.

125. Casey RM, Dumolard L, Danovaro C, et al. Global routine vaccination coverage, 2015. *Wkly Epidemiol Rec.* 2016;91:537–543.

126. BCG vaccine: WHO position paper – February 2018. *Wkly Epidemiol Rec.* 2018;93:73–96.

127. Mina MJ, Metcalf CJE, de Swart RL, Osterhaus ADME, Grenfell BT. Long-term measles-induced immunomodulation increases overall childhood infectious disease mortality. *Science.* 2015;348:694–699.

128. Bester JC. Measles and measles vaccination: a review. *JAMA Pediatr.* 2016;170:1209–1215.

129. Moss WJ. Measles. *Lancet.* 2017;390:2490–2502.

130. Mina MJ, Kula T, Leng Y, et al. Measles virus infection diminishes preexisting antibodies that offer protection from other pathogens. *Science.* 2019;366:599–606.

131. Orenstein WA, Cairns L, Hinman A, Nkowane B, Olivé JM, Reingold AL. Measles and Rubella Global Strategic Plan 2012–2020 midterm review report: background and summary. *Vaccine.* 2018;36(Suppl 1):A35–A42.

132. Patel MK, Goodson JL, Alexander JP Jr, et al. Progress toward regional measles elimination—worldwide, 2000–2019. *MMWR Morb Mort Wkly Rep.* 2020;69:1700–1705.

133. Papania MJ, Wallace GS, Rota PA, et al. Elimination of endemic measles, rubella, and congenital rubella syndrome from the Western hemisphere: the US experience. *JAMA Pediatr.* 2014;168:148–155.

134. Dimala CA, Kadia BM, Nji MAM, Bechem NN. Factors associated with measles resurgence in the United States in the post-elimination era. *Sci Rep.* 2021;11:51.

135. Sundaram ME, Guterman LB, Omer SB. The true cost of measles outbreaks during the postelimination era. *JAMA.* 2019;321:1155–1156.

136. Moss M. Measles in vaccinated individuals and the future of measles elimination. *Clin Infect Dis.* 2018;67:1320–1321.

137. Measles vaccines: WHO position paper – April 2017. *Wkly Epidemiol Rec.* 2017;92:205–228.

138. Hviid A, Rubin S, Mühlemann K. Mumps. *Lancet.* 2008;371:932–944.

139. Mumps virus vaccines: WHO position paper. *Wkly Epidemiol Rec.* 2007;82:51–60.

140. Lambert N, Strebel P, Orenstein W, Icenogle J, Poland GA. Rubella. *Lancet.* 2015;385:2297–2307.

141. Rubella vaccines: WHO position paper – July 2020. *Wkly Epidemiol Rec.* 2020;95:306–324.

142. Grant GB, Masresha BG, Moss WJ, et al. Accelerating measles and rubella elimination through research and innovation: findings from the Measles & Rubella Initiative research prioritization process, 2016. *Vaccine.* 2019;37:5754–5761.

143. Clarke KEN, MacNeil A, Hadler S, Scott C, Tiwari TSP, Cherian T. Global epidemiology of diphtheria, 2000–2017. *Emerg Infect Dis.* 2019;25:1834–1842.

144. Diphtheria vaccine: WHO position paper – August 2017. *Wkly Epidemiol Rec.* 2017;92:417–436.

145. Tetanus vaccine: WHO position paper – February 2017. *Wkly Epidemiol Rec.* 2017;92:53–76.

146. Pertussis vaccines: WHO position paper – August 2015. *Wkly Epidemiol Rec.* 2015;90:433–460.

147. Cherry JD, Tan T, Wirsing von König CH. Global definitions of pertussis: summary of a Global Pertussis Initiative roundtable meeting, February 2011. *Clin Infect Dis.* 2012;54:1756–1764.

148. *Haemophilus influenzae* type b (Hib) vaccination position paper – September 2013. *Wkly Epidemiol Rec.* 2013;88:413–428.

149. Pneumococcal conjugate vaccines in infants and children under 5 years of age: WHO position paper – February 2019. *Wkly Epidemiol Rec.* 2019;94:85–104.

150. Rotavirus vaccines: WHO position paper – January 2013. *Wkly Epidemiol Rec.* 2013;88:49–64.

151. Chard AN, Gacic-Dobo M, Diallo MS, Sodha SV, Wallace AS. Routine vaccination coverage – worldwide, 2019. *MMWR Morb Mortal Wkly Rep.* 2020;69:1706–1710.

152. Portnoy A, Ozawa S, Grewal S, et al. Costs of vaccine programs across 94 low- and middle-income countries. *Vaccine.* 2015;33(Suppl 1):A99–A108.

153. Polio vaccines: WHO position paper – March 2016. *Wkly Epidemiol Rec.* 2016;91:145–168.

154. Human papillomavirus vaccines: WHO position paper, May 2017. *Wkly Epidemiol Rec.* 2017;92:241–268.

155. Cholera vaccines: WHO position paper – August 2017. *Wkly Epidemiol Rec.* 2017;92:477–500.

156. Dengue vaccine: WHO position paper – September 2018. *Wkly Epidemiol Rec.* 2018;93:457–476.

157. WHO position paper on hepatitis A vaccines – June 2012. *Wkly Epidemiol Rec.* 2012;87:261–276.

158. Japanese encephalitis vaccines: WHO position paper – February 2015. *Wkly Epidemiol Rec.* 2015;90:69–88.

159. Meningococcal A conjugate vaccine: updated guidance, February 2015. *Wkly Epidemiol Rec.* 2015;90:57–62.

160. Rabies vaccines: WHO position paper – April 2018. *Wkly Epidemiol Rec.* 2018;93:201–220.

161. Vaccines against tick-borne encephalitis: WHO position paper. *Wkly Epidemiol Rec.* 2011;86:241–256.

162. Typhoid vaccines: WHO position paper – March 2018. *Wkly Epidemiol Rec.* 2018;93:153–172.

163. Varicella and herpes zoster vaccines: WHO position paper, June 2014. *Wkly Epidemiol Rec.* 2014;89:265–288.

164. Vaccines and vaccination against yellow fever: WHO position paper – June 2013. *Wkly Epidemiol Rec.* 2013;88:269–284.

165. Vaccines against influenza: WHO position paper – November 2012. *Wkly Epidemiol Rec.* 2012;87: 461–476.

166. Osterholm MT, Kelley NS, Sommer A, Belongia EA. Efficacy and effectiveness of influenza vaccines: a systematic review and meta-analysis. *Lancet Infect Dis.* 2012;12:36–44.

167. *Interim Recommendations for Use of the Pfizer–Biontech COVID-19 Vaccine, BNT162b2, Under Emergency Use Listing: Interim Guidance 8 January 2021.* Geneva: World Health Organization; 2021.

168. Hepatitis E vaccine: WHO position paper, May 2015. *Wkly Epidemiol Rec.* 2015;90:185–200.

169. Li X, Mukandavire C, Cucunubá ZM, et al. Estimating the health impact of vaccination against ten pathogens in 98 low-income and middle-income countries from 2000 to 2030: a modelling study. *Lancet.* 2021;397:398–408.

170. *Immunization Agenda 2030: A Global Strategy to Leave No One Behind.* Geneva: World Health Organization; 2020.

171. *State of the World's Children 2021.* New York: UNICEF; 2021.

172. *Implementing the Immunization Agenda 2030: A Framework for Action through Coordinated Planning, Monitoring & Evaluation, Ownership & Accountability, and Communications & Advocacy.* Geneva: World Health Organization; 2021.

173. Jacobsen KH, Koopman JS. Declining hepatitis A seroprevalence: a global review and analysis. *Epidemiol Infect.* 2004;133:1005–1022.

174. Jacobsen KH. Globalization and the changing epidemiology of hepatitis A virus. *Cold Spring Harbor Perspect Med.* 2018;8:a031716.

175. Trépo C, Chan HLY, Lok A. Hepatitis B virus infection. *Lancet.* 2014;384:2053–2063.

176. Liang TJ. Hepatitis B: the virus and the disease. *Hepatology.* 2009;49(5 Suppl):S13–S21.

177. Hyams KC. Risks of chronicity following acute hepatitis B virus infection: a review. *Clin Infect Dis.* 1995;20:992–1000.

178. *Prevention of Mother-to-Child Transmission of Hepatitis B Virus: Guidelines on Antiviral Prophylaxis in Pregnancy.* Geneva: World Health Organization; 2020.

179. Hepatitis B vaccines: WHO position paper – July 2017. *Wkly Epidemiol Rec.* 2017;92:369–392.

180. *Guidelines for the Prevention, Care and Treatment of Persons with Chronic Hepatitis B Infection.* Geneva: World Health Organization; 2015.

181. Schweitzer A, Horn J, Mikolajczyk RT, Krause G, Ott JJ. Estimations of worldwide prevalence of chronic hepatitis B virus infection: a systematic review of data published between 1965 and 2013. *Lancet.* 2015;386:1546–1555.

182. Webster DP, Klenerman P, Dusheiko GM. Hepatitis C. *Lancet.* 2015;385:1124–1135.

183. Manns MP, Buti M, Gane E, et al. Hepatitis C virus infection. *Nat Rev Dis Primers.* 2017;3:17006.

184. *Guidelines for the Care and Treatment of Persons Diagnosed with Hepatitis C Virus Infection.* Geneva: World Health Organization; 2018.

185. *Accelerating Access to Hepatitis C Diagnostics and Treatment: Overcoming Barriers in Low- and Middle-Income Countries: Global Progress Report 2020.* Geneva: World Health Organization; 2021.

186. Petruzziello A, Marigliano S, Loquercio G, Cozzolino A, Cacciapuoti C. Global epidemiology of hepatitis C virus infection: an up-date of the distribution and circulation of hepatitis C virus genotypes. *World J Gastroenterol.* 2016;22:7824–7840.

187. Kamar N, Bendall R, Legrand-Abravanel F, et al. Hepatitis E. *Lancet.* 2012;379:2477–2488.

188. Pérez-Gracia MT, Suay-García B, Mateos-Lindemann ML. Hepatitis E and pregnancy: current state. *Rev Med Virol.* 2017;27:e1929.

189. Hoofnagle JH, Nelson KE, Purcell RH. Hepatitis E. *N Engl J Med.* 2012;367:1237–1244.

190. *Global Health Sector Strategy on Viral Hepatitis 2016–2021.* Geneva: World Health Organization; 2016.

191. *Global Hepatitis Report, 2017.* Geneva: World Health Organization; 2017.

192. Tordrup D, Hutin Y, Stenberg K, et al. Additional resource needs for viral hepatitis elimination through universal health coverage: projections in 67 low-income and middle-income countries, 2016–30. *Lancet Glob Health.* 2019;7:e1180–e1188.

193. McGill F, Heyderman RS, Panagiotou S, Tunkel AR, Solomon T. Acute bacterial meningitis in adults. *Lancet.* 2016;388:3036–3047.

194. *Defeating Meningitis by 2030: A Global Road Map.* Geneva: World Health Organization; 2020.

195. Stephens DS, Greenwood B, Brandtzaeg P. Epidemic meningitis, meningococcaemia, and *Neisseria meningitidis. Lancet.* 2007;369:2196–2210.

196. Molesworth AM, Thomson MC, Connor SJ, et al. Where is the meningitis belt? Defining an area at risk of epidemic meningitis in Africa. *Trans R Soc Trop Med Hyg.* 2002;96:242–249.

197. Agier L, Martiny N, Thiongane O, et al. Towards understanding the epidemiology of *Neisseria meningitidis* in the African meningitis belt: a multi-disciplinary overview. *Int J Infect Dis.* 2017;54:103–112.

198. Lingani C, Bergeron-Caron C, Stuart JM, et al. Meningococcal meningitis surveillance in the African meningitis belt, 2004–2013. *Clin Infect Dis.* 2015;61(Suppl 5):S410–S415.

199. Control of epidemic meningitis in countries in the African meningitis belt, 2019. *Wkly Epidemiol Rec.* 2020;95:133–144.

CHAPTER 10

Malaria and Neglected Tropical Diseases

Parasitic diseases like malaria, other vector-borne infections, and helminth (worm) diseases are rare in high-income countries, but they cause significant disability in low-income countries. Investments in preventing and treating neglected tropical diseases (NTDs), supporting eradication campaigns, and detecting and containing emerging infectious diseases yield economic and security benefits for all partners.

10.1 Malaria, NTDs, and Global Health

Malaria has been the target of international public health efforts since the late 1800s, when scientists first discovered that the malaria parasite was transmitted to humans through the bites of infected mosquitoes. Initial research and development (R&D) investments by high-income countries focused on protecting military personnel and business interests in the tropics and on eliminating domestic threats posed by malaria.[1] (CDC, the U.S. Centers for Disease Control and Prevention, is headquartered in Atlanta because the agency evolved from the national malaria control program.[2]) Today, a diversity of governmental, charitable, and corporate partners are involved in developing and implementing control and elimination strategies for malaria and other debilitating infections.

Most countries where malaria still occurs are places where other dreadful tropical and parasitic diseases are also common. Many of these diseases are unimaginable to the typical person living in a high-income country, including parasites that cause body parts to swell to many times their typical size or leave their victims scarred and blind; disfiguring bacterial and protozoal infections that eat through skin, muscle, and even bones, causing permanent disability; and intestinal worms that can proliferate to completely block the digestive tract. A single photograph of any of these conditions would likely be enough to convince most people that these diseases deserve to be added to the list of priorities for global health funding. The need for prioritization becomes even clearer after seeing the epidemiological statistics showing that these conditions are far from rare.[3] More than 1 billion people from the world's lowest-income households have at least one of the bacterial, viral, or parasitic conditions that are classified by the World Health Organization (WHO) as prioritized neglected tropical diseases (**Figure 10.1**).[4]

Neglected tropical diseases (NTDs) are infectious diseases that primarily occur in the poorest regions of the world and have not historically been a priority for global policymakers, funding agencies, or pharmaceutical companies.[5] The "big three" infectious diseases—HIV, tuberculosis, and malaria—have received the bulk of global infectious disease attention and financing in recent decades. The NTD designation is intended to call attention to infectious diseases that have been relatively invisible to the major players in global health even though they affect millions of people in the lowest-income countries and contribute to

Disease	Pathogen/Toxin	Section of This Chapter
Dengue	Virus	10.6
Chikungunya	Virus	10.7
Lymphatic filariasis	Helminth	10.8
Onchocerciasis (river blindness)	Helminth	10.9
Schistosomiasis	Helminth	10.10
Soil-transmitted helminthiases	Helminth	10.11
Chagas disease	Protozoan	10.12
Human African trypanosomiasis (sleeping sickness)	Protozoan	10.12
Leishmaniasis	Protozoan	10.13
Leprosy	Bacterium	10.14
Buruli ulcer	Bacterium	10.14
Trachoma	Bacterium	10.14
Yaws and other endemic treponematoses	Bacterium	10.15
Mycetoma, chromoblastomycosis, and other deep mycoses	Bacterium/fungus	10.15
Scabies and other ectoparasites	Mites	10.15
Taeniasis and neurocysticercosis	Helminth	10.16
Echinococcosis	Helminth	10.16
Foodborne trematodiases (clonorchiasis, opisthorchiasis, fascioliasis, and paragonimiasis)	Helminth	10.16
Rabies	Virus	10.17
Snakebite envenoming	Snake venom	10.17
Dracunculiasis (guinea worm disease)	Helminth	10.19

Figure 10.1 Neglected tropical diseases prioritized by the World Health Organization.

Data from *Ending the Neglect to Attain the Sustainable Development Goals: A Road Map for Neglected Tropical Diseases 2021–2030*. Geneva: World Health Organization; 2020.

the cycle of poverty by causing long-term illnesses and disabilities.[6] Neglected does not mean infrequent; NTDs affect about one in six of the world's people.[7] Neglected describes conditions that were overlooked as the field of global health emerged in the early 21st century.[8]

During the Millennium Development Goals (MDG) era (2000–2015), the world worked to "combat HIV/AIDS, malaria, and other diseases" (MDG 6). This priority area was expanded in the Sustainable Development Goals (SDGs) to call for commitments to "end the epidemics of AIDS, TB, malaria, and neglected tropical diseases" by 2030 and "combat hepatitis, waterborne diseases, and other communicable diseases" (SDG 3.3) (**Figure 10.2**).[9] Donors have answered this call by increasing their support for malaria and NTD control. For example, the London Declaration on Neglected Tropical Diseases, an ambitious plan to control 10 NTDs by 2020, was launched in 2012 by the WHO, the Bill & Melinda Gates Foundation, several multinational pharmaceutical companies, and other partners.[10] The participants donated billions of doses of existing NTD treatments to control initiatives in endemic areas, and many major drug companies contributed to R&D through product development partnerships like the Drugs for Neglected Diseases initiative (DNDi).[11] These actions to recognize and reduce the population health burden from NTDs are a sign that NTDs are no longer being neglected. However, it will take continued commitments from global partnerships to alleviate the preventable physical, mental, social, and economic burden that malaria and NTDs impose on the world's poorest children and families.[12]

10.2 Protozoa and Helminths

Many of the most burdensome tropical diseases, including malaria, are parasitic diseases. A **parasite** is an organism that survives by living in or on a host organism. Parasites are eukaryotes that consist of a complex cell or cells that have a membrane-bound nucleus. (Animals, plants, and fungi are eukaryotes; bacteria and viruses are not.) Some parasites have complex life cycles and undergo life stages in several different animal hosts and in the environment. An **intermediate host** is an animal host in which an immature parasite develops but does not reach sexual maturity. Some parasites have one intermediate host, and some have two different

3.3.1	Number of new HIV infections per 1,000 uninfected population
3.3.2	Tuberculosis incidence per 100,000 population
3.3.3	Malaria incidence per 1,000 population
3.3.4	Hepatitis B incidence per 100,000 population
3.3.5	Number of people requiring interventions against neglected tropical diseases
3.8.1	Coverage of essential health services, including access to safe, effective, quality, and affordable essential medicines and vaccines for all
3.b.1	Proportion of the target population covered by all vaccines included in their national program
3.b.3	Proportion of health facilities that have a core set of relevant essential medicines available and affordable on a sustainable basis
3.d.2	Percentage of bloodstream infections due to selected antimicrobial-resistant organisms

Figure 10.2 Examples of Sustainable Development Goal indicators focused on infectious diseases.

Data from United Nations Economic and Social Council. *Report of the Inter-Agency and Expert Group on Sustainable Development Goal Indicators* (E/CN.3/2021/2). New York: United Nations; 2021.

intermediate hosts. A **definitive host** is the animal host in which a parasite reaches sexual maturity and reproduces.

Parasites can be acquired when a host walks barefoot in contaminated soil, wades in contaminated water, ingests contaminated food or water, is bitten by parasite-infested insects, or experiences another species-specific mode of transmission. Once inside the human body, some parasites only minimally affect their hosts, but others can cause severe illness and disability. Antiparasitic medications will kill some parasites, but most medicines are not effective against all life stages of the parasites. For some parasitic infections, drug resistance means that medications that previously were effective treatments no longer work.

There are two main types of parasites that live inside the human body and adversely affect human health: protozoa and helminths. A **protozoan** is a single-celled organism that has animal-like characteristics. Some protozoa are free living, and some are parasitic. Protozoa are classified based on how they move and on the characteristics of their life cycles. Most protozoa have life cycles that involve a dormant cyst stage and an active trophozoite stage, but some are more complex; most protozoa reproduce asexually, but some use both asexual and sexual reproduction.

- Amoebas use pseudopods ("false feet") to move. They reproduce using binary fission in which the organism makes copies of its organelles and then divides into two complete organisms. *Entamoeba histolytica*, which causes bloody diarrhea (dysentery), is an example of an amoeba infection.
- Ciliates have rows of hairlike projections (cilia) that help the organisms move, and they reproduce using transverse binary fission. *Balantidium coli* is a ciliate that can cause dysentery in humans.
- Flagellates have a "tail" that assists with motion, and they reproduce using longitudinal binary fission. Examples of disease-causing flagellates include *Giardia*

intestinalis (which causes chronic diarrhea), *Leishmania* (which is transmitted by sand flies), *Trichomonas vaginalis* (a sexually transmitted infection), and *Trypanosoma cruzi* (which causes Chagas disease).
- Apicomplexans (or sporozoans) have no specialized structures for locomotion. They often have complex life cycles involving multiple hosts, and they go through multiple life stages, such as a sporozoite stage and a merozoite stage. *Cryptosporidium* (which causes diarrhea) and *Plasmodium* (which causes malaria) are examples of human diseases caused by apicomplexans.

A **helminth** is a multicellular parasitic worm. Some helminths that live inside the human body are microscopic, but others grow to be several inches long or even several feet in length as they mature in the human body. Helminths usually produce eggs or offspring that are expelled from the body of the host (typically through the intestinal tract) so that they will infect other hosts rather than competing with the parent for resources. Helminths are classified by their shapes and life cycles. There are three main types of helminths that are human parasites: nematodes, cestodes, and trematodes. (Nematodes are in the Nematoda phylum. Both cestodes and trematodes are flatworms in the Platyhelminth phylum.)

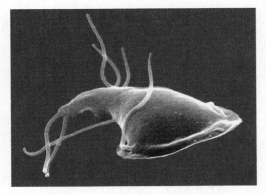

A *Giardia* protozoan is a flagellate.

CDC/Dr. Stan Erlandsen; Dr. Dennis Feely. https://phil.cdc.gov/Details.aspx?pid=11649. Reference to specific commercial products, manufacturers, companies, or trademarks does not constitute its endorsement or recommendation by the U.S. Government, Department of Health and Human Services, or Centers for Disease Control and Prevention.

- A **nematode**, or roundworm, is a cylindrically shaped (tubelike) worm with a simple digestive system that extends the full length of the worm from the mouth to the anus. Nematodes usually have two sexes and reproduce sexually, with adults producing eggs that mature into larvae and then adult worms. There are many types of nematodes that have humans as hosts, including filarial worms, guinea worms, hookworms, pinworms, roundworms, threadworms, and whipworms.
- A **cestode**, or tapeworm, is a ribbonlike worm consisting of a mouthpiece (scolex) and numerous flat segments. Cestodes have no mouth or gut. They absorb nutrients from their hosts through a body-covering tissue called tegument. Each segment contains both male and female organs, and the worms reproduce hermaphroditically. Eggs mature into metacestodes and then adults. Most tapeworms in humans prefer to live in the human digestive tract, and some of these tapeworms can grow to be many feet long.
- A **trematode**, or fluke, is a flat, unsegmented worm that typically has a complex life cycle involving two different animal hosts. Trematodes have oral and ventral suckers but only a blind gut and not a full

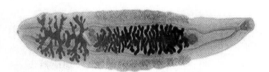

Adult liver fluke *(Clonorchis sinensis)*.

digestive system. They absorb nutrients from their hosts through their tegument. Most trematodes are hermaphroditic, but some have two sexes. An egg matures into a miracidium, then a sporocyst, redia, cercaria, metacercaria, and finally an adult. In humans, trematodes infect a variety of body systems. For example, there are blood flukes (such as *Schistosoma*), liver flukes (such as *Clonorchis*), and lung flukes (such as *Paragonimus*).

10.3 Malaria

Malaria is a mosquito-borne parasitic infection with *Plasmodium* protozoa that can cause cyclic fevers, anemia, neurological complications, and death. Protozoans in the ***Plasmodium*** genus cause malaria, and they have complex life cycles involving both sexual and asexual reproduction within the red blood cells of human hosts. Five *Plasmodium* species are known to cause human infection: *P. falciparum*, *P. vivax*, *P. malariae*, *P. ovale*, and *P. knowlesi*. **Falciparum malaria** is an infection with the species of *Plasmodium* that is most likely to cause life-threatening disease.[13] Almost 99% of malaria cases in sub-Saharan Africa are caused by *P. falciparum*; in other endemic areas, about half of malaria cases are caused by *P. falciparum* and half by *P. vivax*.[14]

A **vector** is an organism (usually a nonvertebrate, such as an insect) that transmits a pathogen to another organism.[15] ***Anopheles* mosquitoes** are the vector that transmits malaria-causing parasites to humans. *Plasmodia* undergo developmental stages in both humans and mosquitoes (**Figure 10.3**).

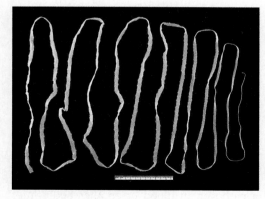

13-foot-long adult *Taenia saginata* tapeworm.

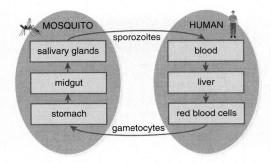

Figure 10.3 Life cycle of the *Plasmodium* parasites that cause malaria.

Most mosquitoes need a bloodmeal from a bird or mammal in order to produce and lay eggs. If a female *Anopheles* mosquito takes a bloodmeal from an infected human, the mosquito can become infected with *Plasmodium*. After the malaria parasites undergo several stages of development in the gut of the mosquito, they travel to the salivary gland of the mosquito and are injected into a human during a subsequent bloodmeal.[16] Once the parasites enter the bloodstream of the human, they move to the liver and reproduce rapidly. After several days of maturation, the parasites enter the bloodstream and invade the red blood cells that carry oxygen throughout the body. The parasites grow and divide inside the red blood cells. Every two to three days (depending on the species of *Plasmodium*), the red blood cells rupture, releasing parasites and toxins into the bloodstream and causing fever, chills, and anemia. The cycle continues for 10 to 14 days and may persist longer if untreated.

Malaria usually causes cyclic fevers, headaches, and joint pain, but it can cause organ failure and death. Although anyone can contract malaria, children and pregnant women have an especially high risk of severe and fatal complications.[17] Two frequent complications of malaria are anemia and cerebral malaria. **Malarial anemia** is the destruction of so many red blood cells by malaria-causing parasites that the body cannot adequately transport oxygen through the bloodstream.[18] Since growing children and pregnant women are often anemic even before a bout of malaria, the loss of additional red blood cells from malaria can be dangerous. Another complication in children is **cerebral malaria**, a neurological complication of *Plasmodium* infection that is characterized by seizures and coma (impaired consciousness).[19] If children survive cerebral malaria, they may have permanent brain damage and learning disabilities.[20]

For decades, the drug of choice for treating malaria was chloroquine, but drug resistance has made the medication ineffective in most parts of the world. The parasites that cause malaria are also becoming resistant to other pharmaceutical treatments, such as sulfadoxone/pyrimethamine (SP).[21] Widespread drug resistance means that there are few antimalarial medications that work today, and the complexity of the organisms that cause malaria makes it scientifically challenging to develop new therapeutic agents.[22] **Artemisinin-based combination therapy (ACT)** is malaria treatment that combines at least two different antimalarial drugs, one of which is an artemisinin-based drug. For example, ACT could be in the form of artemether plus lumefantrine, artesunate plus amodiaquine, or dihydroartemisinin plus piperaquine. Malaria control experts strongly urge the use of ACT because combination medications slow the emergence of further drug resistance.[23]

For most malaria control programs, the best option is to prescribe antimalarial medications only to people with laboratory-confirmed malaria. Exceptions may be made in places where there is such a high prevalence of malaria that it is safe and cost effective to prescribe treatment based on a presumptive diagnosis. **Parasitemia** is the presence of parasites in the blood. A **rapid diagnostic test** (RDT) is a test that can quickly detect the presence of a pathogen or markers for a pathogen in blood or another body fluid. A malaria RDT can detect the presence of specific antigens produced by malaria parasites in a small drop of blood within 15 to

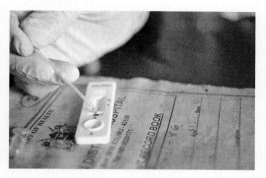

Rapid diagnostic test.
Courtesy of USAID

30 minutes.[24] If an RDT is positive for malaria, ACT can be prescribed. Prompt treatment of confirmed malaria reduces the likelihood of severe disease and death. If an RDT is negative for malaria, the febrile individual can be referred for additional clinical laboratory testing to determine the actual cause of the illness so that appropriate treatment can be prescribed.

Adults who grew up in malaria-endemic areas usually have some degree of protection from severe malaria because their immune systems have responded to prior infections.[25] However, susceptibility to malaria increases during pregnancy, and complications occur often because pregnant women are typically anemic even before additional red blood cells are destroyed by *Plasmodium*; babies born to mothers with malaria are at increased risk of low birthweight and other birth complications.[26] **Intermittent preventive treatment (IPT)** is the routine distribution of anti-infective medications to vulnerable people so that they maintain therapeutic drug levels in their blood during times of high risk for disease. IPT in pregnancy (IPTp) is the routine distribution of antimalarial medications to all pregnant women who live in malaria-endemic countries, even if the women do not have symptoms of malaria at the time of treatment.[27] IPTp medications are typically dispensed at two to four antenatal care visits during the second and third trimesters

of pregnancy.[28] Presumptive treatment for malaria with IPTp is effective at increasing the average birthweight and survival rates of babies born to women in endemic areas who receive the recommended doses.[29] In very high-transmission areas, IPT of infants (IPTi) may also be a cost-effective intervention for reducing the burden from malaria.[30]

10.4 Malaria Epidemiology

About 94% of malaria cases and deaths in recent years occurred in sub-Saharan Africa, and children bore a disproportionate share of that burden.[14] The WHO estimates that the percentage of people who die from malaria who are less than five years old decreased from 84% of fatalities in 2000 to 67% by 2020, but young children still account for two-thirds of malaria deaths.[14] Children and adults with malaria can usually be treated successfully with inexpensive antimalarial tablets, but malaria can cause weeks or even months of illness due to relapses and fatigue. Reinfection with malaria occurs often, and children who live in endemic areas may have several bouts of malaria each year.

Each bout of malaria causes several days or weeks of absence from work or school for the infected individual (and often also a caregiver) and the inability to be productive at home. Infection rates are highest during the seasons when subsistence farmers grow and harvest their crops. When malaria (or caring for people with malaria) keeps family members from being in the fields at this crucial time, it can result in chronic food insecurity for all members of the household.[31] The cost of lost productivity due to malaria extends to entire countries as well. Malaria-endemic countries have lower rates of economic growth than countries without malaria.[32]

Most cases of malaria occur in the tropics, where mosquitoes survive year-round.

Anopheles mosquitoes deposit their eggs in relatively still but well-oxygenated water, so any places where water collects (like ponds, lakes, and puddles) can serve as mosquito habitats, especially during rainy seasons. Environmental changes related to road building, mining, logging, agriculture, and irrigation may also create breeding sites, further increasing the mosquito population.[33] These factors can make the environmental control of insect populations through land and water management prohibitively expensive.

Cases of malaria or other infectious diseases that are locally acquired rather than imported are called **autochthonous** cases. Until the middle of the 20th century, malaria was endemic across much of the globe, with autochthonous cases reported as far north as Canada and Siberia. The Global Malaria Eradication Programme, which was implemented between 1955 and 1969, was a massive WHO-led insecticide spraying program that eliminated malaria from dozens of countries.[34] One contributor to malaria elimination was the spraying of DDT in large quantities over cities and crops to kill mosquitoes.[35] A **persistent organic pollutant** (POP) is an organic compound that does not degrade easily. **DDT** (dichloro-diphenyl-trichloroethane) is a POP that used to be widely used as an agricultural pesticide. DDT bioaccumulates in the fatty tissues of animals. The highest concentrations of DDT occur in animals higher up in the food chain, such as fish and birds. The United States banned DDT in 1972 in large part because of the uproar caused by Rachel Carson's book *Silent Spring*, which had been published in 1962, and many other countries across the income spectrum also enacted DDT bans.[36] DDT bans led to a drastic increase in the incidence of malaria in many countries.[37] In 2001, a global treaty sponsored by the UN Environment Programme and many private environmental organizations banned 11 POPs, but the treaty made a special exemption for the indoor use of DDT for public health purposes.[38] Use of the chemical is now limited but not banned. DDT is not approved for widespread application as an outdoor pesticide, but it can be used indoors when an equally effective and cost-effective product is not available.[23]

Indoor residual spraying (IRS) is the application of long-lasting insecticides to walls and other surfaces where mosquitoes might rest. The insecticides used for IRS stick to the walls so that the pesticide only needs to be applied once or twice a year. Small amounts of the approved chemicals seem to be harmless to humans and household animals, but when mosquitoes land on IRS-treated surfaces anytime during the six months (or longer) after IRS has been applied, they absorb a lethal dose of the insecticidal chemical.[39] The insecticides used for IRS protect people from bites only while they are indoors, and some mosquitoes are resistant to the effects of these chemicals. Still, the WHO now endorses the use of IRS for mosquito control in areas that have endemic or epidemic malaria transmission, and DDT could contribute, if used correctly, to preventing millions of malaria deaths.[40] Although still controversial, the policy changes that have enabled the reintroduction of DDT for home protection may end up being an example of how people with different views on the risks and benefits of an environmental intervention can find a middle ground that is acceptable to most parties involved.

10.5 Malaria Interventions

The only way that humans contract malaria is by being bit by an infected mosquito, and the only way that mosquitoes become infected is by biting an infected human.[41] Malaria control interventions interrupt the mosquito–human–mosquito transmission cycle (**Figure 10.4**). Some malaria control interventions use antiparasitic medications to treat

Level of Prevention	Primordial Prevention	Primary Prevention	Secondary Prevention	Tertiary Prevention
Goal	Prevent risk factors for malaria or malaria complications	Mitigate risk factors in people without malaria	Detect and treat malaria before it becomes symptomatic	Manage malaria after it becomes symptomatic
Examples of interventions	■ Environmental management of water resources ■ Treat anemia, intestinal worms, and other infections ■ Good nutritional practices	■ Control mosquito populations using indoor residual spraying (IRS) and other tools ■ Avoid mosquito bites, such as by sleeping under insecticide-treated nets (ITNs) and wearing protective clothing	■ Use presumptive intermittent preventive therapy (IPT) of malaria for pregnant women (IPTp) and infants (IPTi) in high-risk areas	■ Take combination antimalarial medication ■ Access advanced therapies when needed

Figure 10.4 Examples of interventions for malaria.

people who have malaria in order to reduce the risk of mosquitoes getting *Plasmodium* from a bloodmeal. Some use environmental actions like IRS to limit the number of mosquitoes that live in proximity to human populations. Some promote human behavior change to reduce the likelihood of humans being bit by infected mosquitoes.

Because *Anopeheles* typically bite at dusk, dawn, and night, one of the most effective ways to prevent new malaria infections is the use of bednets. An **insecticide-treated net (ITN)** is a mesh sheet dipped in insecticides and then hung over a bed so that it provides a barrier between sleeping humans and mosquitoes while also killing any mosquitoes that land on it. Most ITNs need to be re-dipped in a pyrethroid insecticide every six months or so in order to maintain their effectiveness. A **long-lasting insecticidal net (LLIN)** is an ITN that has been impregnated with a pesticide that remains effective for two years or longer before requiring retreatment.[42]

ITNs protect humans from mosquito bites. When they are used consistently, they significantly reduce child mortality in malaria-endemic areas.[43] ITNs also reduce the risk of mosquitoes biting humans with *Plasmodium* infections and becoming carriers of the parasites. People with current malaria symptoms can infect mosquitoes, and so can adults who grew up in malaria-endemic areas and continue to have low-level parasitemia even when they are asymptomatic.[44] It is therefore advisable for all children and adults who live in at-risk areas to consistently use ITNs, to protect themselves and others.

Rates of ITN use in sub-Saharan Africa increased significantly as the percentage of households owning bednets rose from less than 5% of households in 2000 to more than 65% by 2020 (**Figure 10.5**).[14] About two-thirds of the reduction in malaria cases achieved during the MDG era (2000–2015) was attributed to the scaled-up use of ITNs.[45] Most children and adults in at-risk areas of sub-Saharan Africa now sleep under bednets. However, there is growing

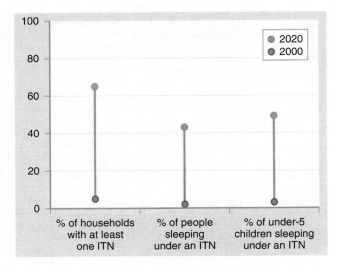

Figure 10.5 Use of insecticide-treated nets (ITNs) in sub-Saharan Africa.
Data from *World Malaria Report 2021*. Geneva: World Health Organization; 2021.

concern about the percentage of mosquitoes in malaria-endemic areas that have become resistant to the pyrethroid insecticides that are most often used to treat ITNs.[14] Because ITNs protect the same indoor spaces that IRS protects, IRS use in at-risk parts of sub-Saharan Africa decreased from about 10% of households in 2000 to about 6% as use of ITNs expanded. IRS may need to be scaled up again if pyrethroid-impregnated ITNs stop being effective at killing mosquitoes.

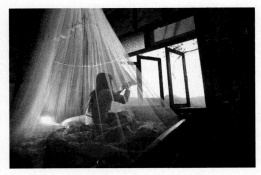

A bednet hung from the ceiling of a room and tucked under a mattress.

© Tuttoo/Shutterstock.

Other barrier methods for insect bite protection include wearing clothes that cover the arms and legs during the times of the day when mosquitoes are most likely to bite and having screens or curtains cover the windows and doors of houses when the structure of the building allows for this. Insect repellents like bug sprays, especially those that contain DEET (N,N-diethyl-m-toluamide), can also be helpful when they are affordable and used appropriately.[46] (DEET is a very different chemical than DDT. **DEET** is an effective insect repellent, but it does not kill mosquitoes.)

Although travelers from nonendemic areas to places where malaria is endemic generally take prophylactic (preventive) antimalarial drugs, these are not fully effective in preventing the disease. More importantly, it is not realistic or healthy to encourage prophylactic use among people who live in highly endemic areas. The financial cost would be high, long-term drug use could be detrimental to users' health, and the widespread use of anti-parasitic agents would contribute to the development of more drug-resistant *Plasmodium* at a time when many species are no longer susceptible to existing antimalarial medications. Barrier methods are a safer long-term option for reducing malaria risk.

While individuals and households bear much of the responsibility for implementing malaria control strategies, they are supported by national and global initiatives to develop, promote, and finance strategies for malaria prevention, diagnosis, treatment, and control. The RBM Partnership to End Malaria (RBM is short for "Roll Back Malaria," a previous initiative to reduce the global burden from the disease) provides a platform for the WHO, UNICEF, other multilateral organizations; national governments from malaria-endemic countries and donor countries; researchers; and representatives from foundations, nongovernmental organizations, academia, and the private sector to work together to increase and sustain access to effective malaria prevention and treatment technologies.[47]

Other partnerships are focused on creating new preventive, diagnostic, and treatment tools, such as the Medicines for Malaria Venture and the Malaria Vaccine Initiative.[48] The RTS,S (or RTS,S/AS01) malaria vaccine, known by the trade name Mosquirix, was first developed in 1987, demonstrated modest efficacy over many rounds of clinical testing, and beginning in 2019 was made available to young children in a few malaria-endemic countries as part of a pilot implementation study.[49] In October 2021, the WHO recommended that RTS,S be approved for widespread use among children living in endemic countries in sub-Saharan Africa even though four doses of the vaccine confer only about a 30% reduction in the risk of severe malaria in children.[50] Several other malaria vaccine candidates are in development and being tested,[51] but rollout is expected to take many more years.[52]

The global malaria burden was significantly reduced during the MDG era, with the incidence rate decreasing by about 37% and the mortality rate by about 60% between 2000 and 2015.[53] These improvements were attributed to expanded access to malaria prevention and treatment interventions. The WHO's current global technical strategy (GTS) for malaria aims to further reduce malaria incidence and malaria mortality rates in affected areas by 90% between 2016 and 2030, eliminating malaria in at least 35 countries and preventing resurgences in countries that have reached malaria-free status.[54]

The WHO estimates that the incidence rate decreased from about 81 per 1,000 people at risk in 2000 to about 59 per 1,000 in 2015 and then plateaued (**Figure 10.6**).[14] Global population growth kept the case counts nearly steady for the past 20 years, at over 200 million per year, even as the rate of new cases decreased (**Figure 10.7**).[14] The WHO estimates that the mortality rate decreased from about 30 per 100,000 people at risk in 2000 to about 15 per 100,000 in 2015 and then plateaued; the number of deaths per year decreased from nearly 900,000 in 2000 to 560,000 in 2015 and then increased during the COVID-19 pandemic due to reduced access to prevention tools and clinical treatment.[14] The GTS milestones called for at least a 40% reduction in both incidence and mortality between 2015 and 2020, but these numbers remained almost unchanged over that five-year period.[55] The world is not on track to achieve the GTS targets.

In a typical recent year, about $5 billion total was spent on malaria prevention, control, treatment, and other activities in malaria-endemic countries; about 50% of that funding came from development assistance for health from high-income countries and other external donors, about 30%

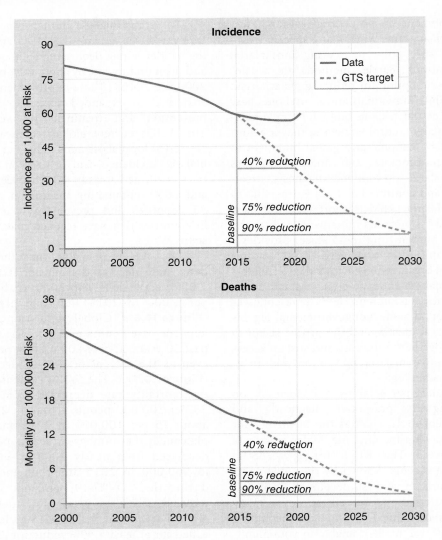

Figure 10.6 Progress toward achieving the malaria global technical strategy (GTS) goals by 2030.

Data from *World Malaria Report 2021.* Geneva: World Health Organization; 2021.

from the governments of malaria-endemic countries, and about 20% from patients and their families.[56] More than $3 billion is spent each year specifically on malaria control and elimination programs, but that is only about half of what is required to meet the GTS milestones.[14] Expanded financial, scientific, and social support for malaria elimination efforts will be necessary to accelerate progress toward achieving the SDG goal of ending malaria.[57]

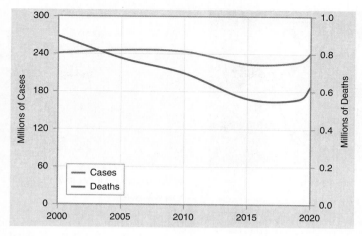

Figure 10.7 Number of cases and deaths worldwide per year from malaria.

Data from *World Malaria Report 2021*. Geneva: World Health Organization; 2021.

10.6 Dengue

Dengue is a mosquito-borne viral infection that is sometimes called breakbone fever because it can cause severe joint and muscle pain. There are four distinct serotypes of dengue virus. Infection with any one strain of this flavivirus confers protection against future infections with that strain, but it does not protect against the other three dengue virus strains. People who live in places where multiple strains are co-endemic can have dengue up to four times, once with each strain. Infection with a first strain is often asymptomatic, but it may cause a high sudden-onset fever, a severe headache, retroorbital (behind the eyes) pain, musculoskeletal pain, nausea, and a rash.[58] Infection with a second strain can lead to severe dengue, which can include symptoms such as hemorrhagic fever and shock.[59]

About 50 to 100 million people are expected to have symptomatic dengue infections this year, and many millions more will have asymptomatic infections that may increase their risk of severe dengue if they contract a different strain of the virus later in their lives.[60] The geographic range of places where dengue occurs has expanded significantly over the past several decades.[61] Dengue is now endemic across South Asia, Southeast Asia, tropical South America, and some parts of tropical sub-Saharan Africa.[62] Local transmission of the virus is also occurring in subtropical areas, such as the southeastern United States and coastal southern China, which are likely to experience intensified disease burden in the coming decades.[61] About 4 billion people today live in a dengue-endemic area, and that number may rise to closer to 6 billion by 2050.[61]

Dengue virus is transmitted to humans by the bites of infected **Aedes mosquitoes**, a genus of mosquito that has black and white stripes on its body and legs, thrives in urban areas, and can be an aggressive day biter. (*Aedes aegypti* are the main vector for dengue, but *Ae. albopictus* and other species within the *Aedes* genus can also serve as vectors.) **Vector control** interventions reduce the size and density of arthropod populations. Dengue vector control programs prevent mosquitoes from breeding by using insecticides and eliminating the standing water where the mosquitoes that

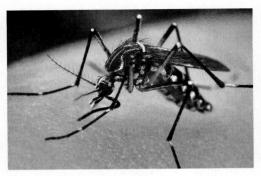

Adult *Aedes aegypti* mosquito.

CDC/Prof. Frank Hadley Collins, Dir., Cntr. for Global Health and Infectious Diseases, Univ. of Notre Dame/James Gathany. https://phil.cdc.gov/Details.aspx?pid=9252. Reference to specific commercial products, manufacturers, companies, or trademarks does not constitute its endorsement or recommendation by the U.S. Government, Department of Health and Human Services, or Centers for Disease Control and Prevention.

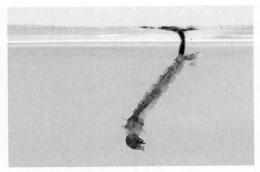

Aedes mosquito larva in water.

© Amir Ridhwan/Shutterstock

transmit the virus breed.[63] Any small body of standing water, such as the water that collects in old cans and discarded tires, can become a breeding ground for *Aedes*. Since one household that does not clean up its yard can put a whole neighborhood at risk, health education and community engagement are critical components for the success of these programs.

Dengue control programs also promote appropriate disposal of waste, use of barriers and repellents to reduce exposure to mosquitoes, and scaled-up use of insecticides in places where dengue epidemics are occurring. New technologies, such as the release of mosquitoes that have been genetically modified to be sterile or have been intentionally infected with *Wolbachia* bacteria strains that inhibit mosquito reproduction, must be used with caution because of ethical and environmental concerns.[64]

Scientists have worked for decades to develop a tetravalent vaccine that is effective against all four serotypes of dengue virus.[65] A dengue vaccine (CYD-TDV, or Dengvaxia®) was licensed for the first time at the end of 2015, but safety concerns limited its suitability for widespread use.[66] The vaccine was effective at preventing severe disease among adults and older children with prior dengue infections, but it increased the risk of people with no history of dengue having severe disease if they contracted

their first strain of dengue virus after being vaccinated.[67] Because of this risk, the WHO recommended this vaccine only for people with serological evidence of prior dengue infection.[68] Dengue vaccines that might be safe for people who have no history of dengue infection are being tested in clinical trials but are not yet approved for use.[69]

10.7 Other Arboviruses

An **arthropod** is an insect (like a mosquito, fly, or flea) or an arachnid (like a tick, louse, or mite). An insect has six legs, an external covering made of chitin, a pair of antennae, and three body sections (a head, a thorax, and an abdomen). An arachnid has eight legs, an exoskeleton, compound eyes, and two body sections (a cephalothorax and an abdomen). A **vector-borne infection** is one in which the pathogen is transmitted to humans via an arthropod. The **cycle of transmission** describes how an infectious agent passes between different species. Some infections have a human–human–human cycle, like measles and sexually transmitted infections. Some have a vertebrate–vertebrate–vertebrate cycle and only occasionally affect humans, like rabies. A vector-borne infection has a human–arthropod–human cycle or an animal–arthropod–animal cycle that occasionally affects a human. A variety of arthropod vectors can transmit infectious agents to humans (**Figure 10.8**).

Disease	Name of Pathogen	Type of Pathogen	Primary Vector (*Genus*)
African trypanosomiasis (sleeping sickness)	*Trypanosoma brucei*	Protozoan (flagellate)	Tsetse flies (*Glossina*)
Chagas disease	*Trypanosoma cruzi*	Protozoan (flagellate)	Reduviid bugs (*Triatominae*)
Leishmaniasis	*Leishmania*	Protozoan (flagellate)	Sand flies (*Lutzomyia* and *Phlebotomus*)
Loiasis (African eye worm)	*Loa loa*	Helminth (filarial nematode)	Deer flies (*Chrysops*)
Lyme disease (borreliosis)	*Borrelia burgdorferi*	Bacterium	Ticks (*Ixodes*)
Lymphatic filariasis	*Wuchereria bancrofti, Brugia malayi, Brugia timori*	Helminth (filarial nematode)	Mosquitoes
Malaria	*Plasmodium*	Protozoan (sporozoan)	Mosquitoes (*Anopheles*)
Onchocerciasis (river blindness)	*Onchocerca volvulus*	Helminth (filarial nematode)	Blackflies (*Simulium*)
Plague	*Yersinia pestis*	Bacterium	Fleas (*Xenopsylla*)
Rocky Mountain spotted fever	*Rickettsia rickettsii*	Bacterium (rickettsia)	Ticks (*Dermacentor*)
Tularemia	*Francisella tularensis*	Bacterium	Ticks
Typhus fever	*Rickettsia prowazekii*	Bacterium (rickettsia)	Body lice (*Pediculus*)

Figure 10.8 Examples of bacterial and parasitic vector-borne diseases.

An **arbovirus**, short for **ar**thropod-**bo**rne virus, is a virus transmitted to humans by an arthropod. All arboviruses are viral infections (**Figure 10.9**); bacterial and parasitic infections are not arboviruses because they are not viral. Dengue is an arboviral infection because it is caused by a mosquito-borne virus. Malaria is caused by a parasite, so it is not an arboviral disease. Most arboviruses are spread by mosquitoes. **Chikungunya** is an *Aedes*-transmitted arbovirus that can cause long-term disability from joint pain. Unlike many arbovirus diseases, most cases of chikungunya are symptomatic. Many infected people suffer from weeks of severe pain in the joints of their arms and legs. For some people, the arthralgia and arthritis persist for

months or even years.[70] Chikungunya was first identified in Africa and southeast Asia in the 1950s, and the virus continues to circulate in those regions. The first cases in Europe were detected in 2007 and the first cases in the Americas were identified in 2013.[71] The number of places where endemic and epidemic chikungunya occur is expanding, and chikungunya could become an expensive public health problem because of the chronic disability associated with the disease. Several vaccine candidates are in development,[72] but at present vector control is the only available preventive measure.

Yellow fever is a vaccine-preventable mosquito-borne viral infection that causes the skin and eyes of infected people to become

Disease	Viral Family	Primary Vector (*Genus*)
Chikungunya	Togavirus	Mosquitoes (*Aedes*)
Crimean-Congo hemorrhagic fever	Bunyavirus	Ticks (*Hyalomma*)
Dengue fever	Flavivirus	Mosquitoes (*Aedes*)
Japanese encephalitis	Flavivirus	Mosquitoes (*Culex*)
Rift Valley fever	Bunyavirus	Mosquitoes (*Aedes*)
Tick-borne encephalitis	Flavivirus	Ticks (*Ixodes*)
West Nile virus	Flavivirus	Mosquitoes (*Culex*)
Yellow fever	Flavivirus	Mosquitoes (*Aedes*)
Zika	Flavivirus	Mosquitoes (*Aedes*)

Figure 10.9 Examples of arboviral diseases.

yellow due to jaundice. About 15% to 20% of people who contract the yellow fever virus develop a severe hemorrhagic fever, and 20% to 60% of those individuals die from complications of the disease.[73] Historical accounts of yellow fever show the devastation that can be caused by outbreaks. In 1793, an outbreak in Philadelphia, Pennsylvania, which was then serving as the capital city of the United States, shut down the federal government and may have killed 10% of the city's residents.[74] The initial attempt to construct the Panama Canal in the 1880s failed after thousands of workers died of yellow fever.[75] Today, epidemics of yellow fever occur primarily in tropical areas of South America and Africa where the *Aedes* mosquitoes that transmit the yellow fever virus to humans thrive, but outbreaks have occurred in other regions.[76] In between outbreaks in human populations, the virus is maintained through a sylvatic (wild animal) transmission cycle involving mosquitoes and nonhuman primates that live in forests. A yellow fever vaccine first became available in the 1930s, and modern vaccines are critical tools for controlling outbreaks today.[77] The global infectious disease control protocols spelled out in the International Health Regulations mandate vaccination for travelers to and from places where outbreaks are occurring.[78]

West Nile virus is an arbovirus that has become endemic to the United States and can cause encephalitis. The virus typically cycles between mosquitoes and birds, but it occasionally affects humans.[79] The primary vectors for human infection are **Culex mosquitoes**, a genus of mosquito that deposits rafts of 100 or more eggs on water rather than laying eggs singly. Most people who become infected with West Nile virus have no symptoms or only mild symptoms, but a small percentage (<1%) develop severe neurological complications.[80] West Nile virus was first identified in Africa, but outbreaks have occurred in many world regions. The virus started circulating in the New York City metropolitan area in 1999,[81] and within just a few years local transmission of the virus was occurring across the continental United States.[82] There is not yet a West Nile virus vaccine.

Japanese encephalitis virus is closely related to West Nile virus and is also transmitted by *Culex* mosquitoes. Like West Nile virus, most people who contract Japanese encephalitis virus experience no symptoms, but a small proportion develop a severe neurological disease that can cause permanent disability or result in death. Outbreaks of Japanese encephalitis occur regularly in Asia and Oceania even though the infection is vaccine preventable.[83] There are concerns that Japanese encephalitis could become endemic in new world regions, similar to the way that West Nile virus became endemic in North America.[84]

Zika virus is a mosquito-borne viral infection that is usually asymptomatic but has been linked to an increased risk of microcephaly in babies born to women who contract the virus during the pregnancy. Until recently, infection with Zika virus was considered to be such an inconsequential threat to human health that it was rarely tested for and only a few research papers had been published about it.[85] That perception changed dramatically in 2015, when the virus spread to the Americas for the first time and an outbreak in Brazil was linked to a possible increase in the incidence of **microcephaly**, an abnormally small head that is a sign of aberrant brain development.[86] Concerns about Zika's emergence were exacerbated by the discovery that Zika virus could be transmitted not only through the bites of infected mosquitoes but also through sexual contact.[87]

The dengue, yellow fever, West Nile, Japanese encephalitis, and Zika viruses are all in the flavivirus genus of the *Flaviviridae* family, but disease-causing viruses from other viral families are also spread by insects. For example, chikungunya virus is in the alphavirus genus of the togavirus family, and Rift Valley fever virus is in the phlebovirus genus of the bunyavirus family. **Rift Valley fever** is a zoonotic arbovirus infection that can cause outbreaks of pregnancy loss in livestock herds. Most humans who contract Rift Valley fever virus have a mild infection, but a small percentage develop vision loss, meningoencephalitis, or hemorrhagic fever.[88]

Arbovirus epidemics are occurring more frequently as urbanization, international travel, and other globalization processes enable pathogens to be introduced to and then spread through susceptible populations.[89] Widespread epidemics of mosquito-borne arboviruses have occurred recently, including outbreaks of dengue, chikungunya, yellow fever, and Zika. Tick-borne arboviruses like the ones that cause Crimean-Congo hemorrhagic fever and tick-borne encephalitis occur less often, but they

can also cause outbreaks. The WHO aims to reduce the incidence of vector-borne diseases by at least 60% between 2016 and 2030 and reduce mortality from vector-borne diseases by at least 75% during that time period.[90] This will be a challenge to achieve, especially since climate change is expanding the range of *Aedes* mosquitoes and some other types of vectors and enabling outbreaks in new cities and regions.[91]

10.8 Lymphatic Filariasis

Lymphatic filariasis (LF) is a mosquito-borne helminth infection that can block lymph nodes and cause fluid buildup in affected legs and other body parts. LF is caused by three types of filarial nematodes—*Wuchereria bancrofti*, *Brugia malayi*, and *B. timori*—that are transmitted by several different types of mosquito vectors.[92] Mosquitoes become infected by taking blood-meals from humans who have microfilariae circulating in their blood. After the microfilariae mature into larvae within the mosquito, the larvae can be deposited in the skin of the humans they bite during subsequent bloodmeals. The larvae mature into adults within the human lymphatic system, and adult female worms then produce microfilariae that can infect other mosquitoes and launch new infection cycles.

The lymphatic system is a network of lymph nodes, lymphatic vessels, and other tissues that produce, store, and transport white blood cells throughout the body and move interstitial fluid (fluid between cells) from body tissues toward the heart. **Lymphedema** is the swelling of body parts due to retained lymph fluid in the tissues. When worms block the flow of lymph, it can cause lymphedema of the legs. Chronic lymphedema and poor hygiene can cause **elephantiasis**, in which the skin of an affected limb thickens and develops a coarse texture similar to that of an elephant's leg. (Elephantiasis can also be caused by podoconiosis, which is thought to result from a genetic

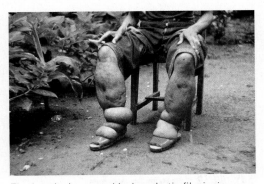

Elephantiasis caused by lymphatic filariasis.

CDC/Amanda Moore, MT; Todd Parker, PhD; Audra Marsh. https://phil.cdc.gov/Details.aspx?pid=373. Reference to specific commercial products, manufacturers, companies, or trademarks does not constitute its endorsement or recommendation by the U.S. Government, Department of Health and Human Services, or Centers for Disease Control and Prevention.

predisposition to have an inflammatory reaction when bare feet are chronically exposed to the volcanic minerals in red clay.[93]) Males with lymphatic filariasis may develop **hydrocele**, lymphedema of the scrotum. More than 1 million people are living with LF-associated lymphedema, and more than 500,000 men have hydrocele.[94] Many of these individuals will have permanent disfigurement and disability due to prolonged severe swelling. Antihelminthic medications kill microfilariae in the blood, but they are ineffective in killing the adult worms that cause LF.[95]

Treatment of infected people is important for interrupting the cycle of infection by preventing new infections in mosquitoes. **Preventive chemotherapy** (PC) is the use of a safe medicine as part of a public health strategy to prevent and control an infectious disease. **Mass drug administration** (MDA) is the distribution of preventive chemotherapy to large population groups at regular time intervals as part of strategies for preventing and controlling infectious diseases. MDA is used as part of the control strategy for several NTDs: albendazole and ivermectin are used for LF, ivermectin for onchocerciasis, praziquantel for schistosomiasis, albendazole for soil-transmitted helminths, azithromycin for trachoma and yaws, and praziquantel and triclabendazole for foodborne trematodiases.[4] In a typical year, more than 1 billion people

receive preventive chemotherapy for at least one NTD.[96] In total, about 60% of people for whom MDA for NTDs is recommended by the WHO currently receive it.[96] The WHO aims to increase coverage to at least 75% by 2030.[4]

The WHO Global Programme to Eliminate Lymphatic Filariasis (GPELF) was launched in 2000. GPELF uses widespread distribution of antihelminthic medications in endemic places to reduce transmission rates.[97] In 2000, up to 200 million people had the microfilariae that cause LF circulating in their blood; 20 years later, that number had been reduced to about 50 million, with most cases occurring in south or southeast Asia or in west or central Africa.[98] That reduction in the prevalence of infection represents significant progress toward elimination. However, an estimated 850 million people live in places that are still endemic for LF and therefore remain at risk of contracting LF-causing parasites.[94]

One limitation of MDA is that recipients are often susceptible to reinfection almost immediately after taking the medication. To be effective, MDA must be repeated for many years in endemic areas and must be accompanied by health education and environmental health programs that reduce the reinfection rate. For LF, that means that both MDA and vector control are part of control and elimination strategies.[99]

10.9 Onchocerciasis

Onchocerciasis, also known as river blindness, is a fly-borne helminth infection that can cause blindness. Onchocerciasis is caused by a filarial helminth called *Onchocerca volvulus*, which is transmitted to humans by the bites of infected black flies from the *Simulium* genus.[92] Adult worms form nodules in the subcutaneous tissue under the skin and release microfilariae into surrounding tissues. This causes a skin rash and intense itching, and it may also change the skin appearance, such as causing depigmentation of skin on the shins (a condition colloquially called leopard skin). If the

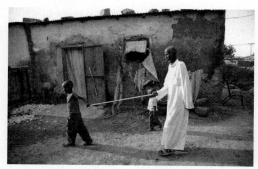

An adult blinded by onchocerciasis (river blindness) being guided by a child.

Copyright © E. Aegler/The End Fund

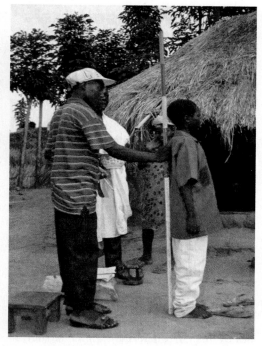

A community health center staff member shows village health workers how to determine the right dosage for ivermectin delivered as part of an MDA campaign. Colored bands on the stick show the doses appropriate for people of various heights.

© WHO/TDR/Andy Craggs

microfilariae enter the eyes, they can scar the corneas and cause the host to become permanently blind.

Preventive chemotherapy with an antiparasitic medication called ivermectin is used to kill microfilariae in people who live in onchocerciasis-endemic areas. Ivermectin is typically distributed to entire communities once or twice a year. MDA for onchocerciasis has been used since the 1970s by a variety of national, regional, and global elimination initiatives.[100] One challenge for onchocerciasis control programs is that ivermectin is dangerous to use in people who are infected with large numbers of *Loa loa* parasites.[101] Loiasis, also known as African eye worm, is caused by a filarial helminth that is transmitted by deer flies from the *Cyrsops* genus. Loiasis does not cause blindness, but people with high *Loa loa* parasite loads who take ivermectin are at risk of severe adverse events such as fatal brain inflammation (encephalopathy).[102] Testing for loiasis prior to PC for onchocerciasis enables evidence-based decisions to be made about when ivermectin can be used for local control efforts, but it can be expensive and time consuming to conduct these screening and diagnostic tests.

The Onchocerciasis Elimination Program for the Americas, launched in 1993, was so successful that cases in the Americas are now limited to a small rural area at the border between Brazil and Venezuela.[103] However, the disease remains endemic in many countries in sub-Saharan Africa even though the African Programme for Onchocerciasis Control, which launched in 1995 (and built on the work done by the Onchocerciasis Control Program, which started in West Africa in 1974), has significantly lowered prevalence rates across the region.[104] About 200 million Africans still live in places that have endemic onchocerciasis, and about 70% of those individuals live in districts that deliver MDA with the support of international partnerships.[105] New cases of blindness from onchocerciasis are becoming rare, but there are emerging concerns that onchocerciasis infections may increase the risk of epilepsy in children.[106]

10.10 Schistosomiasis

Schistosomiasis is a blood fluke disease that can increase the risk of bladder cancer among people with chronic infection. *Schistosoma* are trematodes that cycle between snails and humans. Snails are the intermediate host for *Schistosoma*, which means that snails are hosts to immature parasites. Humans are the definitive host in which the parasites reach sexual maturity. Humans become infected by wading in fresh water infested with parasite-infected snails while fishing, washing clothes, bathing, or doing other activities.

Immature schistosomes are called cercariae, the name for the free-swimming larvae of trematodes. Schistosome cercariae penetrate through human skin, enter the blood supply, and then eventually travel to the veins of the intestines or bladder, where male–female pairs lay thousands of eggs. Some of those eggs become trapped in nearby tissues, where they trigger an inflammatory response that causes scarring.[107] Some of the eggs pass through the abdominal tissues and enter the bladder or intestines. Infected humans who urinate or defecate in water release those eggs into the environment, where the eggs hatch and release larvae called miracidia. The larvae penetrate the snails that live in the water, and then the miracidia mature within the snails and produce cercariae. When cercariae leave the snails, they seek out a new human host and restart the cycle of infection.

Schistosomiasis, sometimes called bilharzia, is the disease caused by the presence of *Schistosoma* blood flukes in the body. There are several types of schistosomiasis.[108] *S. haematobium* occurs primarily in parts of Africa and the Middle East, and it causes urogenital schistosomiasis. Urogenital schistosomiasis instigates bloody urine (hematuria) and anemia in its early stages. If untreated, the resulting fibrous scarring of the bladder can lead to bladder cancer.[109] Chronic infection can also cause kidney damage. *S. mansoni*, which occurs in parts of South America and the Caribbean as well as in Africa and the Middle East, and *S. japonicum*, which occurs primarily in Asia, cause intestinal schistosomiasis. Intestinal schistosomiasis induces abdominal pain, diarrhea, and bloody stool and can also cause enlargement of the liver and spleen (hepatosplenomegaly).

A medication called praziquantel kills the parasites that cause schistosomiasis. At least 140 million people worldwide are thought to have schistosomiasis.[110] At least 230 million children and adults live in districts where preventive chemotherapy for schistosomiasis is recommended, and about 60% of those individuals are able to access MDA sponsored by international partnerships, most of which is distributed through school-based programs.[111] However, people who

A *Schistosoma mansoni* cercaria (larva).

CDC/Dr. D.S. Martin. https://phil.cdc.gov/Details.aspx?pid=21586. Reference to specific commercial products, manufacturers, companies, or trademarks does not constitute its endorsement or recommendation by the U.S. Government, Department of Health and Human Services, or Centers for Disease Control and Prevention.

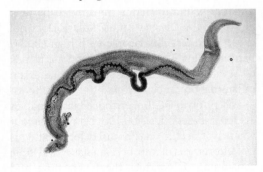

A pair of mating adult *Schistosoma mansoni* trematodes.

CDC/Dr. Shirley Maddison. https://phil.cdc.gov/Details.aspx?pid=11194. Reference to specific commercial products, manufacturers, companies, or trademarks does not constitute its endorsement or recommendation by the U.S. Government, Department of Health and Human Services, or Centers for Disease Control and Prevention.

are treated for schistosomiasis are almost immediately susceptible to new infection when they
come into contact with contaminated water.

Each host in the cycle of infection must be
considered for inclusion in an infection control
plan. Molluscicides are sometimes used to kill the
snails that live in infested waters, but snails may
repopulate these waterbodies. New snail habitats
are created when dams and irrigation systems are
built. The prevalence of schistosomiasis increased
significantly when the Aswan Dam was built on
the Nile River in Egypt, when dams were built on
the Senegal and Volta Rivers and in other locations
in West Africa, and when small dams and irrigation projects have been introduced into rural communities in many parts of the world.[112] A comprehensive schistosomiasis control plan includes snail
control, treatment of existing cases with praziquantel, and a community-led total sanitation program that includes health education.[113] If people
with schistosomiasis consistently use toilets, snails
will not become infected with the parasites, and
the cycle of infection will be interrupted.

10.11 Soil-Transmitted Helminths

A **reservoir** is the environmental home for
an infectious agent. Some agents have an environmental reservoir and live in soil or water.
A **soil-transmitted helminth** (STH), also
called a geohelminth, is a nematode infection contracted through contact with soil
that contains feces mixed with worm eggs or
larvae.[114] Once the worms mature inside a
human host, most STHs are intestinal parasites. They increase the risk of malnutrition
because nutrients from food go to the worms
instead of the human host. The parasites are
also associated with stunted growth, low energy
levels, reduced cognitive performance, school
absences, and other adverse health and development outcomes.[115] Four highly prevalent
STHs in humans are WHO priorities: ascariasis,
trichuriasis, hookworm, and strongyloidiasis.
Pinworm (*Enterobius vermicularis*), toxocariasis

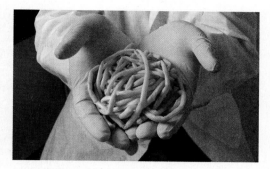

Ascaris lumbricoides passed from the intestines
of a young child.

CDC/James Gathany. https://phil.cdc.gov/Details.aspx?pid=9813. Reference to specific commercial
products, manufacturers, companies, or trademarks does not constitute its endorsement or
recommendation by the U.S. Government, Department of Health and Human Services, or Centers for
Disease Control and Prevention.

(*Toxocara* species), and other intestinal worms
are also prevalent in humans.

Ascariasis is the most prevalent intestinal
helminth infection, and people with the condition have long worms dwelling in their small
intestines. After a human swallows eggs from
Ascaris lumbricoides, the ingested larvae hatch
in the small intestine; penetrate the intestinal
wall; travel through the blood to the lungs,
where they may be coughed up and swallowed;
and then develop into mature, egg-producing
worms in the small intestine. Adult worms in
the intestine grow, on average, to about a foot
(30 centimeters) in length, and eggs passed in
the stool may lead to infection in others if open
defecation is practiced. Children with ascariasis can host hundreds of intestinal worms.
That can cause distension of the abdomen and
sometimes leads to obstruction of the intestines
and subsequent peritonitis.[116] The number of
people worldwide with ascariasis is estimated
to have decreased from more than 700 million
in 2000 to about 460 million in 2020.[117]

Trichuriasis, also known as whipworm,
occurs when *Trichuris trichiura* are residing in
the large intestine. When the eggs that cause
trichuriasis are swallowed, the eggs hatch
in the small intestine. The released larvae
mature in the colon into adults that are about
1.5 inches (4 centimeters) long. Trichuriasis
can cause chronic digestive system symptoms

associated with colitis, including bloody diarrhea (dysentery) and rectal prolapse.[118] The number of cases of trichuriasis worldwide may have decreased from about 460 million in 2000 to 360 million in 2020.[117]

Hookworm is a helminth that latches onto the walls of the intestine. Both *Necator americanus* and *Ancylostoma duodenale* cause hookworm, and they are most often acquired by walking barefoot through contaminated soil. After the larvae penetrate human skin and pass through the bloodstream, heart, and lungs, they move up the respiratory tract, are coughed up into the throat, are swallowed, pass through the stomach, hook into the wall of the small intestine, and mature into adults that are about 0.4 inches (1 centimeter) long. Because they are attached to the intestinal wall, hookworms cause the host to constantly lose small amounts of blood.[119] This blood loss significantly increases the risk of anemia, especially in children and pregnant women. The number of people with hookworm is thought to have decreased significantly with sanitation improvements from an estimated 450 million in 1990 to 350 million in 2000, 270 million in 2010, and 170 million in 2020.[117]

Strongyloidiasis, sometimes called threadworm, is usually soil transmitted but has the capacity to reproduce entirely within a human host. *Strongyloides stercoralis* larvae are acquired by walking barefoot in contaminated soil. The larvae travel to the small intestine and mature into egg-producing adults. The eggs mature into larvae within the gut. Most of the larvae are evacuated from the human hosts in stool, but some remain inside the human body, where they cause autoinfection by completing an entire life cycle within the human host. The larvae that are expelled mature into free-living male and female adult worms that produce eggs that hatch and mature into larvae in soil. Both dogs and humans can serve as definitive hosts. While most cases of human strongyloidiasis are asymptomatic, people who have immune deficiencies can experience hyperinfection from a large number of worms autoinfecting within the body.[120] Hyperinfection can be fatal for the host.

Preventive chemotherapy, typically albendazole or mebendazole distributed to schoolchildren in endemic areas once or twice per year, is the primary current approach to STH prevention and control.[121] About 300 million preschool-aged children and more than 700 million school-aged children live in areas where MDA for soil-transmitted helminthiases is recommended; prior to the COVID pandemic, the percentage of children receiving treatment through global initiatives had increased to about 50% of preschoolers and 60% of primary school students, but these proportions decreased during the pandemic.[122] Reinfection after deworming can occur quickly when eggs from the worms remain in the local environment, so improved sanitation is a necessary component of STH interventions.[123] Community-led total sanitation programs are helpful for reducing the disease burden from STHs because fewer helminth eggs will be in the soil if everyone consistently uses a toilet. However, sanitation facilities do not remove the eggs that are passed into the environment by infected livestock and other animals.

10.12 Chagas Disease and Trypanosomiasis

Two of the NTDs prioritized by the WHO and partner groups are caused by arthropod-borne protozoa from the *Trypanosoma* genus: Chagas disease and trypanosomiasis. **Chagas disease** is a trypanosome infection that can cause chronic heart and intestinal damage. Chagas disease is caused by *T. cruzi* parasites, which are spread by triatomines (also called reduviids, cone-nosed bugs, or "kissing bugs") that live in the cracks of walls and roofs of low-quality houses in Central and South America. The insects emerge at night to take bloodmeals from sleeping people. The feces of infected insects contain *T. cruzi* protozoa, which can enter the human bloodstream through the wound left after the bloodmeal. Within a few days, a sore may develop at the site of the bite. This wound is often near the eye, where it may cause Romaña's sign, a swollen

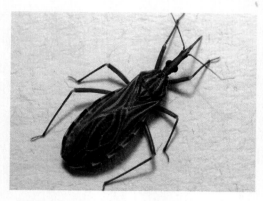

A triatomine bug, the vector for Chagas disease.

Erwin Huebner, University Of Manitoba, Winnipeg, Canada

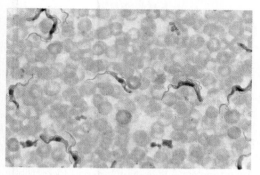

Trypanosoma brucei in the blood of a person with human African trypanosomiasis (HAT).

CDC/Dr. Mae Melvin. https://phil.cdc.gov/Details.aspx?pid=10167. Reference to specific commercial products, manufacturers, companies, or trademarks does not constitute its endorsement or recommendation by the U.S. Government, Department of Health and Human Services, or Centers for Disease Control and Prevention.

eyelid characteristic of acute *T. cruzi* infection.[124] About 30% of people who are infected with *T. cruzi* develop a chronic infection that damages the heart (Chagas cardiomyopathy) in ways that can cause heart failure and possibly fatal arrhythmias decades after the initial infection.[125] Up to 10% of people who contract *T. cruzi* infection develop chronic problems of the digestive tract (gastrointestinal Chagas).[126]

There is no vaccine against *T. cruzi*, and because wildlife and domestic animals serve as reservoirs for the parasite, it is not possible to eliminate the disease. Vector control programs, improved housing construction, food safety measures, blood donor screening, and treatment of acute infections with antiparasitic medications have reduced the incidence of new infections, but millions of people are already living with the damage caused by long-term *T. cruzi* infection.[127] Because many of those adults are people who have emigrated from endemic areas of the Americas and now live in North America, Europe, Japan, Australia, and other locations, the need for improved Chagas disease care is a global one.[128]

Human African **trypanosomiasis** (HAT) is commonly called African sleeping sickness because it causes infected humans to fall into comas (deep sleeps) and die. HAT is caused by *Trypanosoma brucei*, which is transmitted to animals and humans by the bites of infected tsetse flies (biting flies from the *Glossina* genus).[129] Two subspecies of the protozoan can cause human disease. *T. b. rhodesiense* is found in eastern and southern Africa and is primarily a zoonotic infection. Animal African trypanosomiasis, or nagana, causes chronic anemia and wasting of infected cattle and other animals. Farmers in endemic areas may be unable to raise livestock if they do not have the financial resources to invest in resistant breeds of animals, insecticides to protect them, and medications and veterinary care if they become infected. *T. b. gambiense* is found in western and central Africa and is primarily a human disease that affects rural populations.

People who become infected with *T. brucei* experience chronic fevers and headaches in an initial hemolymphatic stage, and then the disease progresses to a meningoencephalitic stage, which leads to coma and death if not treated. Without treatment, HAT is fatal within a few weeks or months for *T. b. rhodesiense* and about three years for *T. b. gambiense*.[130] The available treatments have limited efficacy and are often toxic, causing pain and dangerous side effects.[131] In the early 2000s, more than 25,000 cases of HAT were reported annually; today, fewer than 1,000 cases are diagnosed each year.[132] However, millions of people live in at-risk places where HAT could resurge if vector control and surveillance interventions stopped. The high case fatality rate makes HAT a continuing public health concern in those locations.[129]

10.13 Leishmaniasis

Leishmaniasis is a sand fly–transmitted protozoal disease that can cause disfigurement and death. The disease can be caused by protozoa from a variety of species of the *Leishmania* genus. (Some people with infection never develop symptoms, and they are not considered to have leishmaniasis disease.) The parasites are transmitted to humans by female phlebotomine sand flies, which need blood from a mammal in order to develop their eggs. Leishmaniasis occurs across parts of Asia (including India), North Africa and the Middle East, Africa (including Ethiopia), and South America (including Brazil).[133]

There are three main presentations of leishmaniasis disease. Cutaneous leishmaniasis causes skin lesions that can lead to permanent disfigurement, but it does not cause life-threatening infections because the lesions can be treated with medications and wound care methods. Mucocutaneous leishmaniasis is rare but can be debilitating because it destroys the mucous membranes in the nose, mouth, and throat. Visceral leishmaniasis, also known as kala-azar, causes chronic fevers, weight loss, anemia, and swelling of the spleen and liver. Without treatment, visceral leishmaniasis is fatal within a few years. People who are diagnosed as having visceral leishmaniasis are typically treated

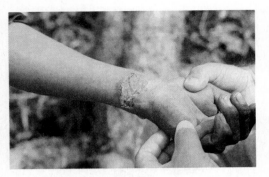

A cutaneous leishmaniasis lesion.

CDC/Dr. A.J. Sulzer. https://phil.cdc.gov/Details.aspx?pid=14971. Reference to specific commercial products, manufacturers, companies, or trademarks does not constitute its endorsement or recommendation by the U.S. Government, Department of Health and Human Services, or Centers for Disease Control and Prevention.

with combination drug therapy.[134] Some people who recover from visceral leishmaniasis develop post-kala-azar dermal leishmaniasis that can take more than a year to heal.

Each year, about 1 million people develop cutaneous leishmaniasis.[135] The incidence of visceral leishmaniasis has decreased significantly in recent years to less than 100,000 new cases per year.[136] Prevention and control strategies must be targeted to the particular types of *Leishmania*, vectors, and animals that are involved in transmission in each affected country.[134] *L. donovani* is the primary cause of visceral leishmaniasis and has humans as the primary reservoir, but nearly 20 different species with animal hosts (such as dogs and rodents) cause cutaneous leishmaniasis. Increased diagnosis rates will enable more cases to be successfully treated.

10.14 Leprosy, Buruli Ulcer, and Trachoma

Several bacterial diseases that have been recognized as problems for a long time but have not been public health priorities are receiving new attention because of their designation as NTDs. These chronic infections affect the skin (leprosy and Buruli ulcer) and eyes (leprosy and trachoma).

Leprosy, now more commonly called **Hansen's disease**, is a chronic

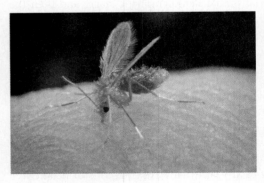

A phlebotomine sand fly, the vector for *Leishmania*.

CDC/James Gathany. https://phil.cdc.gov/Details.aspx?pid=10275. Reference to specific commercial products, manufacturers, companies, or trademarks does not constitute its endorsement or recommendation by the U.S. Government, Department of Health and Human Services, or Centers for Disease Control and Prevention.

mycobacterium infection that can cause nerve damage that leads to amputations. Leprosy was first described in ancient times as a disfiguring disease that caused its victims to be ostracized from their communities, and it still exists as a public health concern.[137] *Mycobacterium leprae* infection initially causes skin lesions, after which about one in three people suffers peripheral nerve damage.[138] When people have numb hands and feet, it is easy for them to accidentally burn or otherwise injure themselves. Those wounds may become infected, and those secondary bacterial infections may cause amputation of the digits. Additionally, many people with leprosy develop vision impairment due to nerve damage, infections, and other ocular complications.[139] Although *M. leprae* infection can be treated with long-term courses of multiple types of antibiotics, the nerve damage and scarring are not reversible.[140] In the mid-1980s, more than 5 million cases of leprosy still occurred annually.[141] Today, about 200,000 cases of leprosy are diagnosed in a typical year, including about 115,000 cases in India; 25,000 in Brazil; 3,000 each in Ethiopia and Nigeria; and additional cases from other countries across the globe.[142] The Global Partnership for Zero Leprosy aims to expand access to diagnosis and treatment with multidrug therapy as part of its ultimate goal of ending new cases of leprosy.[143]

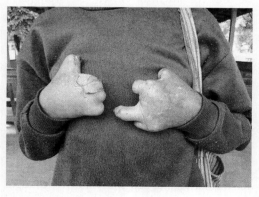

Amputations due to leprosy.

© NikomMaelao Production/Shutterstock

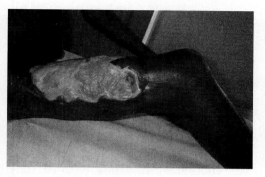

A severe Buruli ulcer.

Marion, E, Carolan, K, Adeye, A, Kempf, M, Chauty, A, Marsollier, L. Buruli ulcer in South Western Nigeria: a retrospective cohort study of patients treated in Benin. *PLoS Negl Trop Dis.* 2015;9(1):e3443.

Buruli ulcer is a mycobacterial infection that causes painless lesions that can become so deep that they extend from the skin to the underlying tendons and bones of the arms or legs. The wounds caused by *Mycobacterium ulcerans* infection are often painless, even when the ulcer is large, because the bacteria release a necrotizing toxin called mycolactone, which has analgesic effects. Advanced cases may progress to osteomyelitis, contractures, and even amputation. Cases are found primarily in Central and West Africa and in Australia, but the full geographic range is not known.[144] The mode of transmission for the bacterium is suspected to be an insect, but until a specific vector is identified it will not be possible to develop a prevention strategy.[145] Early infection can be treated with wound care and antibiotics, but later stages of the disease require surgery to remove dead tissue, cover open wounds, and correct deformities.[146]

Trachoma is a bacterial eye infection that can lead to blindness in people who do not practice good facial hygiene. *Chlamydia trachomatis* bacteria are spread when eye and nose secretions are passed between people by person-to-person contact, shared clothes, and flies.[147] Chronic infection scars the inside of the eyelids, and the inward turning of the eyelids caused by that scar tissue makes the eyelashes curl inward (a condition called trichiasis), scratch the surface of the eye, and scar the cornea. Trachoma is a direct result of poor facial hygiene, so face washing is a core part of trachoma prevention. The WHO-recommended trachoma control plan is the **SAFE strategy**, which combines **s**urgery to treat trichiasis, **a**ntibiotics to kill the bacteria, **f**acial cleanliness encouraged by hygiene education, and **e**nvironmental improvements to ensure reliable access to water and sanitation.[148] In 2000, nearly 8 million people were living with trachoma trichiasis, and about 1.5 billion people lived in areas that were endemic for trachoma; by 2020, those numbers had dropped to about 2 million and 140 million, respectively.[149] However, the goal of eliminating trachoma as a public health problem by 2020 was not met, and new cases continue to occur across much of Africa, the Middle East, and some countries in other world regions.

Yaws lesions before treatment (left) and three weeks after treatment (right) with a single dose of azithromycin.

Asiedu K, Fitzpatrick C, Jannin J. Eradication of yaws: historical efforts and achieving WHO's 2020 target. *PLoS Negl Trop Dis.* 2014;8(9):e3016. Figure 6. Photo by Mr. Lam Duc Hien and MSF-Epicentre, Paris, France.

10.15 Skin NTDs

Eight sets of NTDs currently prioritized by the WHO are classified as skin diseases. In addition to lymphatic filariasis, onchocerciasis, cutaneous leishmaniasis, leprosy, and Buruli ulcer, these include yaws and other endemic treponematoses, mycetoma and other deep mycoses, and scabies and other ectoparasites.[4]

A treponematosis is an infection with bacteria from the *Treponema* genus. Three endemic treponematoses are on the NTD priority list: bejel (*Treponema pallidum* subspecies endemicum), which occurs in parts of Africa and the Middle East; pinta (*T. carateum*), which occurs in the Americas; and yaws (*T. pallidum* subspecies pertenue), which occurs in sub-Saharan Africa, southeast Asia (primarily Indonesia), and some Pacific Island nations.[150] **Yaws** is the most prevalent endemic treponematosis, and it causes disfiguring skin lesions. If untreated, the infection can cause permanent disability by spreading to bone and cartilage. A single dose of an antibiotic can cure yaws, which is transmitted from person to person. The Global Yaws Control Programme, which was implemented between 1952 and 1964, reduced the number of cases worldwide by 95% through mass treatment with penicillin injections.[151] After a resurgence of yaws in the early 21st century, the WHO approved a plan in 2013 to attempt to eradicate yaws by 2020 by using mass administration of oral azithromycin in endemic areas followed by targeted treatment of remaining patients.[152] Drug-resistant strains of the bacterium were discovered in Papua New Guinea in 2018, raising concerns that eradication efforts would be unsuccessful with current medications.[153] The 2020 eradication goal was not met, but efforts to end the disease continue.

Mycetoma (also called Madura foot) is a chronic granulomatous inflammatory disease of the subcutaneous tissue of the foot (or other body part). People with mycetoma have swollen, disfigured feet that ooze pus. Mycetoma is caused by a diversity of fungi (which cause eumycetoma) and by bacteria in the *Actinomycetes* order (which cause actinomycetoma).[154] Soil is thought to be the reservoir for the pathogens, and skin trauma is thought to provide a portal of entry.[155] The number of

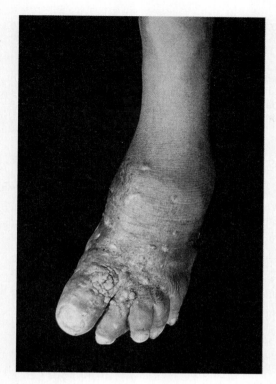

Mycetoma.

CDC/Dr. Victoria (Mexico); Dr. Lucille K. Georg. https://phil.cdc.gov/Details.aspx?pid=14816. Reference to specific commercial products, manufacturers, companies, or trademarks does not constitute its endorsement or recommendation by the U.S. Government, Department of Health and Human Services, or Centers for Disease Control and Prevention.

cases worldwide has not yet been determined, but most victims are young men.[156] Treatment options include antibiotics and surgery. More research is required to understand the epidemiology of mycetoma and the options for prevention and control. Mycetoma is grouped with chromoblastomycosis (also called chromomycosis) and other deep mycoses (such as sporotrichosis and paracoccidioidomycosis) on the WHO list of NTDs. Chromoblastomycosis is a chronic fungal infection that can affect limbs after skin trauma creates a portal of entry.[157]

An **endoparasite**, such as a protozoan or helminth, lives inside the body of its host. An **ectoparasite**, such as a louse or a scabies-causing mite, lives on the exterior surface of its host's body. **Scabies** occurs when tiny mites (*Sarcoptes scabiei* var. *hominis*) burrow into the

outer layer of human skin between fingers, at the wrists, and in other locations (such as the elbows, back, and groin), living and laying eggs at those sites. The immune response to this infestation causes intense itchiness, and the wounds created by the mites and scratching at the skin can lead to severe secondary bacterial infections.[158] More than 200 million people may have scabies at any given time.[159] The mites are transmitted between people in crowded places where close body contact occurs often. Individuals can be treated with topical (skin) antiparasitic medications.[160] Washing the bedding, clothes, and towels of recently treated individuals in very hot water can help reduce the risk of reinfection of the treated individual and household contacts. MDA of ivermectin can help reduce the population burden from scabies.[161] Infestation with lice (pediculosis) and other ectoparasites can also cause discomfort.

Early efforts to control NTDs tended to be disease-specific (vertical or siloed) programs that were driven by donor agendas and had their success measured by inputs like the processes that were implemented and other actions that were taken; current efforts seek to be multisectoral and more integrated into health systems (horizontal), operate as partnerships between countries and donors, and measure success based on impacts and outcomes.[4] The WHO's recent addition of new items like mycetoma and scabies to its list of prioritized NTDs shows a responsiveness to health concerns that are local priorities in endemic areas even if they are not prevalent or deadly enough to be considered global burdens.[162]

10.16 Foodborne NTDs

Several NTDs are caused by foodborne parasites that thrive in tropical areas but can occur across a diversity of climates. These tapeworms, flukes, and other parasites often have complex life cycles that involve two or more different host organisms (**Figure 10.10**).

Disease	Type of Parasite	Animal Host	Food Products That Can Cause Infection If Raw or Undercooked	Control Interventions
Cysticercosis (taeniasis)	Tapeworm (*Taenia solium*)	Pigs (intermediate hosts) → humans (definitive host)	Pork	Vaccinate and deworm pigs; improved sanitation to prevent pigs from contact with human feces
Cystic echinococcosis (hydatid disease)	Tapeworm (*Echinococcus granulosus*)	Sheep and other ungulates (intermediate hosts) → dogs and other canids (definitive hosts)	Food contaminated with tapeworm eggs	Deworm dogs; safe food practices
Alveolar echinococcosis	Tapeworm (*Echinococcus multilocularis*)	Rodents (intermediate hosts) → red foxes and other canids (definitive hosts)	Food contaminated with tapeworm eggs	Safe food practices
Clonorchiasis	Liver fluke (*Clonorchis sinensis*)	Snails (first intermediate hosts) → fish and crustaceans (second intermediate hosts) → dogs and other mammals (definitive hosts)	Freshwater fish	Safe food practices
Opisthorchiasis	Liver fluke (*Opisthorchis* spp.)	Snails (first intermediate hosts) → fish (second intermediate hosts) → cats and other mammals (definitive hosts)	Freshwater fish	Safe food practices
Fascioliasis	Liver fluke (*Fasciola* spp.)	Snails (intermediate hosts) → ruminants (like sheep and cattle) and other mammals (definitive hosts)	Freshwater plants	Safe food practices
Paragonimiasis	Lung fluke (*Paragonimus* spp.)	Snails (first intermediate hosts) → crustaceans (second intermediate hosts) → cats, dogs, and other mammals (definitive hosts)	Crabs and crayfish	Safe food practices

Figure 10.10 Foodborne NTDs.

Taeniasis occurs when tapeworms that cycle between pigs or cattle and humans are living in human intestines. Pigs are the intermediate host for *T. solium*, and humans are the definitive host for the worm. *Taenia solium* undergo early development in the muscle tissue of pigs and then mature in the intestines of humans who consume undercooked pork containing *T. solium* larvae. *T. saginata* has a similar life cycle but has cattle rather than swine as the intermediate host. Livestock become infected with *Taenia* by ingesting human feces containing tapeworm eggs. Taeniasis caused by beef tapeworm and pork tapeworm usually causes no symptoms in humans, but pork tapeworms can cause serious problems if they invade the human nervous system.[163]

Cysticercosis is the disease caused by *Taenia solium* forming cysts in muscle tissue or in other parts of the body. **Neurocysticercosis** occurs when *T. solium* larvae, called cysticerci, trigger epileptic seizures and other problems associated with brain lesions.[164] About 1 in 25 people living in tropical countries of the Americas, sub-Saharan Africa, and southern and eastern Asia have taeniasis, and about 15% have serological evidence of past infection, with considerable variation in levels between and within countries.[165] About one in three people with epilepsy in endemic areas has seizures that are caused by neurocysticercosis.[166] The interventions for preventing and controlling cysticercosis include treatment of already infected pigs and humans with antihelminthic medications along with improved sanitation, vaccination of pigs, and meat inspection and other food safety practices.[167]

Echinococcosis is the disease caused when humans become the accidental host for a cyst-inducing tapeworm that usually matures in dogs. Two types of human disease are caused by *Echinococcus*: cystic echinococcosis and alveolar echinococcosis. Cystic echinococcosis is caused by *E. granulosus*, which has a life cycle that requires an early developmental stage in sheep or other hoofed animals (the intermediate host) followed by maturation in dogs (the definitive host). Most human infections with *E. granulosus* are asymptomatic, but some infected individuals develop a disabling condition called **hydatid disease** (also called hydatid cyst disease), which occurs when the larvae cause cysts to form in the liver and lungs. Alveolar echinococcosis is caused by *E. multilocularis*, which has a life cycle in which rodents are the intermediate host and foxes, coyotes, and dogs are the definitive hosts. *E. multilocularis* is rare but can cause invasive parasitic tumors to grow in the liver or other organs over several years, and that condition is fatal if it is not treated with surgery and antiparasitic medications.[168] The cycling of the cestodes between animals can be slowed with sheep vaccination and by responsible care of pets and stray dogs, but echinococcosis remains an expensive zoonotic disease that occurs in nearly every world region.[169]

Four foodborne trematodiases that have snails as intermediate hosts are included on the WHO list of NTDs: clonorchiasis, opisthorchiasis, fascioliasis, and paragonimiasis.[170] Clonorchiasis (*Clonorchis sinensis*),[171] which occurs in many Asian countries, and opisthorchiasis (*Ophithorchis viverini* and *O. felineus*),[172] which is found in countries in Asia and Europe, are caused by ingesting the larvae of liver flukes found in raw or undercooked fish. Fascioliasis (*Fasciola hepatica* and *F. gigantica*) is a liver fluke disease that is present in nearly every world region and is spread through consumption of uncooked freshwater plants.[173] Paragonimiasis (various species of *Paragonimus*) is caused by a lung fluke acquired by eating raw or undercooked freshwater crabs and crayfish, and it occurs in parts of Africa, Asia, and the Americas.[174] These fluke infections affect millions of people.[175] Control strategies include preventive chemotherapy and environmental management of snail populations and other risks.

A diversity of other helminth diseases that have not been designated as prioritized NTDs affect large numbers of people and cause health problems in humans. Some can be acquired by consuming contaminated food products, such as angiostrongyliasis (a roundworm of mollusks), diphyllobothriasis (a tapeworm of fish), fasciolopsiasis (liver flukes from aquatic plants), and trichinosis or trichinellosis (a tapeworm of pork and other meats). Contact with contaminated feces transmits worms that cause enterobiasis (pinworm), hymenolepiasis (a tapeworm), and toxocariasis (a roundworm). Some protozoa can also be transmitted through food. For example, toxoplasmosis (*Toxoplasma gondii*) is a sporozoan infection that can harm fetuses if a woman becomes infected while pregnant.[176] Most of these infections can be treated with antiparasitic drugs, but these medications are not always available to the populations that need them.

10.17 Rabies and Snakebite Envenoming

Two NTDs occur after animal bites. **Rabies** is a lethal zoonotic virus infection transmitted through the bites of infected mammals. Any mammal can contract rabies, including bats, and the virus circulates in wild animal populations on every continent except Antarctica. Dogs are responsible for more than 95% of rabies cases in humans because dogs usually live in proximity to people.[177] Humans contract the rabies virus when they are bitten by infected animals that are shedding the virus in their saliva. The rabies virus, which is in the lyssavirus genus of the rhabdovirus family, then attacks the central nervous system. Rabies disease in humans presents as either furious rabies, which is characterized by psychosis and cardiac arrest, or as paralytic rabies, which progresses through stages of ascending paralysis, coma, and death.

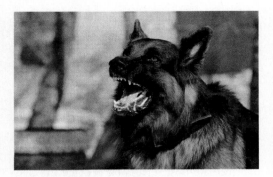

Most human cases of rabies are acquired through dog bites.
© Victoria Antonova/Shutterstock

No one who is bitten by a rabid animal survives without post-bite vaccination, a type of post-exposure prophylaxis (PEP). Each year, about 20 million people receive rabies PEP within a few days after an animal attack.[178] Not all animals that bite humans are rabid, but PEP after animal bites likely prevents hundreds of thousands of rabies deaths. Most of the 60,000 rabies deaths among humans worldwide each year occur in lower-income countries in Africa and Asia where access to PEP is limited.[179] Rabies cannot be eradicated because it circulates in wild animal populations. However, it is possible to prevent all human rabies deaths through expanded use of dog vaccinations, education promoting responsible pet ownership and bite prevention, and universal access to post-bite rabies treatment for humans.[180] Pre-exposure prophylaxis of humans is recommended for veterinarians, animal handlers, and others who know they will have occupational exposure to animals that might have rabies.[181]

Snakebites were added to the WHO's NTD priority list because of the large burden of psychological and physical disability caused by snakebites each year.[182] Most venomous snakes, such as vipers, cobras, mambas, and asps, live in warm-weather tropical climates, and most people who are bitten by snakes are farmers, people who live in poorly constructed homes, and other low-income residents of lower-income countries.

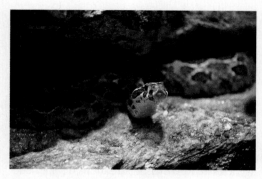

Snakebite envenoming can be fatal.
Image by gautherottiphaine from Pixabay

Venom is a toxic secretion that is injected into a victim through the fangs of a biting snake. Some venom has cytotoxic (cell-killing) or myotoxic (muscle-killing) effects that cause local tissue damage that may be so severe that it requires amputation of the limb that was bitten. Some venom has systemic effects, such as neurotoxicity, which can paralyze muscles and impair the ability to swallow and breathe. Some venom causes coagulopathies (blood clotting disorders) that lead to hemorrhage and related cardiovascular problems. Extreme pain and swelling, acute kidney injury, reduced liver function, hypotension (low blood pressure), and shock are frequent occurrences after envenoming.[183]

More than 2 million people are bitten by venomous snakes every year, and an estimated 100,000 people die from snakebites.[183] The only antidotes that counteract venom are antivenom immunoglobulin therapies, which usually must be administered intravenously within several hours of a bite. Fluid management, ventilators for patients with impaired breathing, and other supportive therapies can improve the chances of survival and recovery. Access to wound care and surgery (to amputate necrotic tissue or repair contractures) can enhance quality of life among snakebite survivors. A global consortium aims to reduce deaths and disability from snakebites by 50% between 2019 and 2030 by increasing access to antivenom treatments and improved post-bite clinical care.[184]

Snakebite prevention options include reducing contact with snakes by wearing shoes, using a flashlight when walking at night, clearing vegetation from around the home, and sleeping on an elevated platform (or under a bed net) instead of the floor if local venomous snakes typically bite at night while people are sleeping. Widespread killing of snakes is usually not recommended because it may cause rodent populations to increase, which may decrease agricultural productivity and increase the risk of diseases associated with vermin living near homes.[185]

10.18 Eradication

Control is the process of using public health interventions to reduce the incidence or prevalence of an adverse health condition to a substantially lower level within a community or a larger geopolitical area. Infection control measures like behavior change, environmental and vector control, vaccination, and preventive chemotherapy can be used to limit the morbidity, disability, and mortality caused by an infectious disease in a local area. Control is achieved when incidence or prevalence rates have dropped below a target threshold defined by the community but a resurgence of the disease would likely occur if disease control measures ceased.[186]

Elimination is the process of removing all risk of new infection in a defined geopolitical area. Elimination uses control measures to reduce the incidence of a disease to zero in selected locations. For NTDs, the WHO promotes two stages of elimination.[187] The first step is the elimination of both infection and disease as a public health problem, even though case counts would resurge in the absence of continued prevention and control interventions. The second step is the interruption of transmission by reducing the incidence of new infections to zero in a defined geographic area. At this stage, there is minimal risk of reintroduction of the pathogen to the population, but there is still a need for efforts to monitor the situation and prevent transmission cycles from being reestablished.

For some infectious diseases, it is possible, at least in theory, to completely eradicate the infectious agent. **Eradication** is the process of eliminating an infectious disease globally. Eradication is achieved when there is no risk of infection or disease anywhere in the world, even in the absence of immunization and other control measures. Eradication requires complete global elimination, and the term should not be used to describe the elimination of a disease within a country or region when cases are still occurring in other places. The WHO uses the term validation to describe the documentation of the elimination of the infection and disease as a public health problem, verification to describe the documentation of interruption of transmission, and certification to describe the achievement of eradication (**Figure 10.11**).

To be a candidate for eradication, an infectious disease must meet several scientific criteria.[186] There must be an intervention that is highly effective at interrupting the chain of transmission. There should be clinical and laboratory tools that make it relatively easy to diagnose the infection so that outbreaks can be identified and contained. Also, eradication is more likely to be achievable when the infection occurs only in humans since it might be impossible to monitor and contain cases among wild animals that serve as hosts for an infectious agent.

Candidates for eradication must also meet several economic and political criteria. Eradication campaigns require funding and administrative support for years of intensive interventions followed by years of continued surveillance. A disease being considered for eradication must be costly enough in terms of health and economics to justify the significant financial investment that an eradication campaign would demand. Eradication campaigns fail when governmental agencies and partner organizations do not make long-term commitments to fund them.[188]

Only two infectious diseases have been eradicated thus far: smallpox and rinderpest. **Rinderpest** was a zoonotic disease that decimated cattle herds. The virus that caused the disease, a paramyxovirus related to the one that causes measles in humans, spread easily when animals had physical contact with one another. An **epizootic** is an outbreak in an animal population; epidemics occur among humans and epizootics occur among animals. Epizootics of rinderpest sometimes killed entire herds, leaving affected communities with devastating economic losses and prolonged food insecurity due to not having cattle to assist with plowing fields and providing fertilizer for crops.[189] The primary intervention for the eradication campaign was cattle vaccination delivered by community-based animal health workers in rural areas of the countries in Africa and Asia where rinderpest was endemic.[190] Rinderpest was declared to be eradicated in 2011, making it the first and thus far only zoonotic infectious disease to be eradicated.

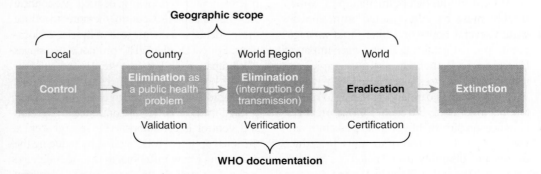

Figure 10.11 The eradication process.

Smallpox was a viral disease of humans that caused blisters to form all over the body and could cause death or permanent disability. The blisters first appeared on the face, then spread to the extremities and then the trunk.[191] (This is different from the pattern for chickenpox blisters, which typically first appear on the torso.) There were two strains of the smallpox virus, which was in the poxvirus family of the orthopoxvirus genus. Variola major was the most frequently occurring variant, and one in three people who contracted it died. Variola minor had only a 1% case fatality rate, but it was the less common strain. Nearly all smallpox survivors had severe scarring, and some were blind from corneal ulceration or had disabilities from skeletal complications.[192] An aggressive worldwide immunization campaign, which included re-vaccination in areas where any new case of smallpox occurred, led to the successful eradication of the disease in the late 1970s.[193]

There is some limited concern that viable smallpox virus could be obtained from a laboratory or long-deceased corpse and used as a bioweapon.[194] Eradication is achieved when an infectious agent is no longer circulating in human or animal populations. **Extinction** is the process of destroying all laboratory specimens of an eradicated pathogen so that there is no possibility of the pathogen reentering the human population. Extinction is complete when an agent no longer exists in nature or in a laboratory. Because several laboratories have retained samples of smallpox virus, the disease is considered to be eradicated but not extinct.

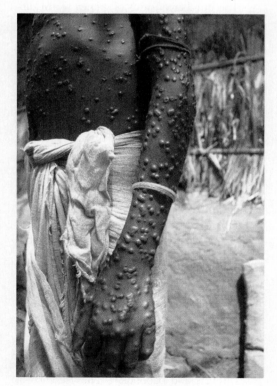

Smallpox.

CDC/Jean Roy. https://phil.cdc.gov/Details.aspx?pid=10661. Reference to specific commercial products, manufacturers, companies, or trademarks does not constitute its endorsement or recommendation by the U.S. Government, Department of Health and Human Services, or Centers for Disease Control and Prevention.

10.19 Guinea Worm Disease

Two diseases are far along in the process toward eradication: dracunculiasis and polio. **Dracunculiasis**, also known as **guinea worm disease**, is a painful condition in which a long filarial helminth takes weeks to slowly emerge from its human host.[195] People contract the guinea worm (*Dracunculus medinensis*) by drinking water that contains water fleas called copepods that are infected with worm larvae. Stomach acids kill ingested copepods and release guinea worm larvae, which migrate into the abdominal cavity of the human and then into the subcutaneous tissues, where they mature and reproduce. An adult female guinea worm may grow to nearly 3 feet (1 meter) in length. Once the worm is fertilized, about a year after ingestion of the infected copepod, the worm forms a painful blister on the skin of its host. When the cyst ruptures, the worm begins to emerge from the human host's body. The blister is often near the foot, but the worm can also emerge from a wrist or another body part.

It takes weeks for the worm to be extracted from the body, and a person with an emerging guinea worm is usually unable to work or go

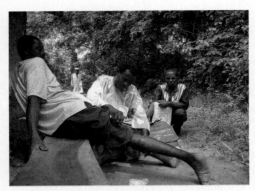

© CDC/E. Staub. https://phil.cdc.gov/Details.aspx?pid=8227. Reference to specific commercial products, manufacturers, companies, or trademarks does not constitute its endorsement or recommendation by the U.S. Government, Department of Health and Human Services, or Centers for Disease Control and Prevention.

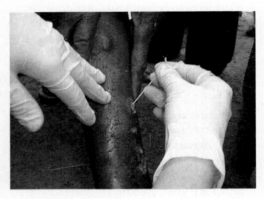

Guinea worm extraction.

© CDC/E. Wolfe. https://phil.cdc.gov/Details.aspx?pid=8210. Reference to specific commercial products, manufacturers, companies, or trademarks does not constitute its endorsement or recommendation by the U.S. Government, Department of Health and Human Services, or Centers for Disease Control and Prevention.

to school during this time because of the pain. The worm cannot simply be pulled out of the body because if it breaks and part of the worm is left inside the body, serious infections like cellulitis and abscesses can result. Instead, the worm is often tied to a stick, and the live guinea worm is coiled around the stick as the worm slowly makes its way out of the human's body, at a rate of an inch or so per day. Many people with an emerging worm feel relief from the pain only by putting their feet in cool water, but this causes the worm to release thousands of eggs. Those eggs can contaminate drinking water supplies and restart the cycle of infection.

There is no medication for dracunculiasis and no vaccine, and humans who have had guinea worm in the past do not develop immunity against the disease. Even so, the disease is nearing eradication thanks to a campaign, led by The Carter Center, which emphasizes health education over technology. Guinea worm education programs promote filtering of drinking water to remove the copepods that host the worm larvae and teach infected people to stay out of water so they will not pass worm eggs to susceptible copepods. Some stagnant sources of drinking water are treated with Abate® (the trade name for the organophosphate temephos) or other larvicides that kill copepods but are safe for human and animal consumption. Every case of the disease is tracked as part of monitoring progress toward eradication.

The number of cases of guinea worm disease diagnosed each year has dropped from an estimated 3.5 million cases in 1986, when The Carter Center began leading global eradication efforts, to less than 100,000 per year by 1997 to less than 100 per year since 2015 (**Figure 10.12**).[196] The disease has been eliminated from many countries in Africa and Asia where it used to be endemic. However, as of 2020, cases were still occurring in Angola, Chad, Ethiopia, Mali, and South Sudan.[197] Those countries are located in eastern, western, and southern Africa, so despite the low case counts the helminth had not yet been contained to a small geographic area.

Scientists perplexed about why sporadic cases of guinea worm could occur in places that had not had any cases for years discovered that domestic dogs appeared to be playing a role in transmission.[198] Dogs and some other animals can become guinea worm hosts if they eat fish entrails or raw aquatic animals. Once scientists began looking for animal cases, hundreds of cases in dogs were identified, along with some cases in cats and baboons.[199] The presence of animal hosts complicates eradication efforts.[200] The new interventions being used to prevent animal cases include encouraging households in endemic areas to tether dogs and bury fish

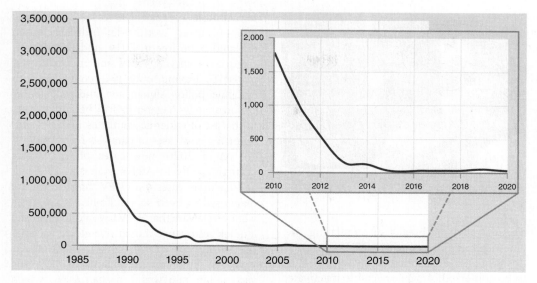

Figure 10.12 Number of cases of guinea worm globally each year.

Data from Hopkins DR, Ruiz-Tiben E, Eberhard ML, et al. Dracunculiasis eradication: are we there yet? *Am J Trop Med Hyg.* 2018;99:388–395.

entrails, improving veterinary care, and providing cash rewards for any human or animal cases that are reported to the Guinea Worm Eradication Programme so that surveillance reports will be as complete as possible.[199]

10.20 Polio

Polio, also called poliomyelitis or infantile paralysis, is a viral infection that can attack the spinal cord and cause permanent paralysis. Poliovirus, which is in the enterovirus genus, is typically transmitted through fecal-oral transmission, such as when infants and children with dirty hands touch their mouths. About 1 in 200 people who contract poliovirus develop a condition called acute flaccid paralysis, which is a sudden onset of weakness of the legs or a more widespread paralysis that might include weakness of the diaphragm, a muscle essential for breathing.[201] Some people who develop polio-related paralysis recover, but some die, some are left with permanent disabilities, and some who appear to recover develop post-polio syndrome years after their infection and have a recurrence of their muscle weakness.[202]

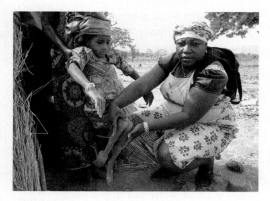

A child paralyzed by polio.

CDC/Dr. Mariam Florence Ogo, Nigeria. https://phil.cdc.gov/Details.aspx?pid=19658. Reference to specific commercial products, manufacturers, companies, or trademarks does not constitute its endorsement or recommendation by the U.S. Government, Department of Health and Human Services, or Centers for Disease Control and Prevention.

There is no cure for polio, but it is vaccine preventable.[203] Oral polio vaccine (OPV) is a live attenuated virus administered by placing a drop of vaccine in the mouth. In very rare cases, an OPV recipient can develop vaccine-associated paralytic poliomyelitis (VAPP) or the virus in the vaccine may mutate and become transmissible,

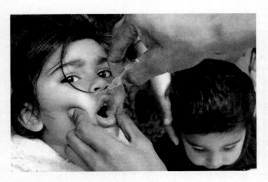

Oral polio vaccine.
© Asianet-Pakistan/Shutterstock

causing small outbreaks of circulating vaccine-derived poliovirus (cVDPV).[204] Several doses of OPV are required for full protection to be conferred. A safe injectable inactivated polio virus (IPV) that carries no risk of VAPP is available, but IPV is not as effective as OPV in inducing immunity.

The term wild poliovirus (WPV) is used to distinguish naturally acquired cases of polio from vaccine-derived poliovirus cases. There used to be three strains of WPV, called WPV1, WPV2, and WPV3. The last known case of WPV2 occurred in 1999, and that strain was declared eradicated in 2015.[205] Trivalent (three-strain) oral polio vaccines were replaced by bivalent (two-strain) OPV formulations that contained only WPV1 and WPV3.[206] The last known case of WPV3 occurred in 2012, and that strain was declared eradicated in 2019.[207] The only remaining strain in circulation is WPV1. However, these successes do not necessarily mean that polio is on the verge of eradication.

The Global Polio Eradication Initiative (GPEI) was launched in 1988 by the WHO, The Rotary Foundation, U.S. CDC, and UNICEF, along with other collaborators. The initial goal was to eradicate polio by 2000.[208] Before the launch of the GPEI, more than 350,000 children in more than 125 countries were paralyzed by polio every year; in 2000, about 3,000 cases of WPV paralysis occurred in 20 countries.[209] That represented good progress, but GPEI was far from achieving eradication.

In 2015, fewer than 100 cases of paralytic polio occurred worldwide; India had been declared polio free in 2014, and Nigeria was removed from the list of endemic countries in 2015, leaving only two countries with endemic polio, Afghanistan and Pakistan.[210] Unfortunately, Nigeria had to be added back to the list of endemic countries in 2016 after reporting new cases of paralysis from WPV.[211]

As of 2020, new cases of WPV were occurring only in Afghanistan and Pakistan, and far more cases of cVDPV than WPV were diagnosed.[207] Even so, public health scientists were very aware that WPV1 would likely make a quick resurgence if intensive global vaccination efforts ceased.[209] Polio vaccination rates were alarmingly low in Nigeria. In India, the vaccination rate was less than 90%, which was especially concerning since India had an elevated risk for flare-ups because polio was still occurring in neighboring countries (**Figure 10.13**).[212] Sustained effort for many more years will be required to eradicate polio and permanently protect children from the risk of polio-induced disability.[213]

10.21 Emerging Infectious Diseases

All infectious agents, whether newly emerging or long established in a population, are continually adapting and changing in ways that can make them more or less transmissible, infective, pathogenic, and virulent.[214] **Transmissibility** is the ease with which an infectious agent is passed from an infected host to another individual. **Infectivity** is the capacity of an infectious agent to cause infection when a susceptible host without immunity to the infection acquired from prior infection or vaccination is exposed to the agent. **Pathogenicity** is the capacity of an infectious agent to cause disease (symptomatic illness) in an infected host. **Virulence** is the ability of an infectious agent to cause severe disease or death in a host. A virulent infection often has a

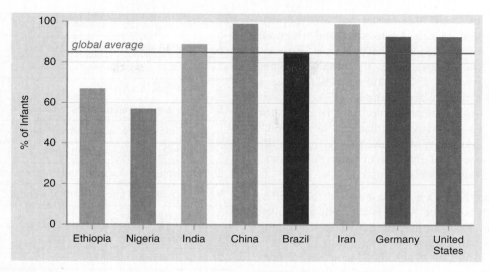

Figure 10.13 Percentage of infants receiving three doses of polio vaccine in 2019.
Data from *State of the World's Children 2019*. New York: UNICEF; 2019.

high case fatality rate because a sizable proportion of people who become ill from the infection will die. A mutation that causes greater transmissibility, infectivity, pathogenicity, or virulence in an influenza strain or another pathogen can pose a major threat to human populations globally.

Even as modern science has allowed the control, elimination, and even eradication of some diseases, other infectious diseases are becoming larger threats to human and animal health. An **emerging infectious disease** (EID) is caused by an infection with a pathogen that has not previously caused severe disease in humans or is affecting human populations in new ways. (Reemerging infectious diseases are ones that were controlled at some point in the past but are becoming problematic again.[215]) Most EID events are due to zoonotic pathogens mutating in a way that enables an infectious agent that previously affected only nonhuman hosts to be transmitted to and between humans and cause illness.

Many EID events have occurred in recent years. Several of these events were international news items when they happened, such as:

- Nipah virus, which causes encephalitis, was first identified in human populations in 1999 when cases occurred in people in Malaysia and Singapore. Outbreaks of Nipah and Hendra henipaviruses have since occurred in Bangladesh, Indonesia, and other countries.[216]

- In 2009, a strain of H1N1 influenza that had affected swine mutated in a way that allowed it to cause disease in humans and spread between them. The new strain was first detected in Mexico in February, and by May of that year it had spread to dozens of countries.[217]

- **Ebola virus disease** is a viral hemorrhagic fever caused by a filovirus that is transmitted through the body fluids of infected individuals. A large outbreak of Ebola caused thousands of deaths in Guinea, Liberia, and Sierra Leone when the viral disease first occurred in West Africa in 2014.[218]

- A novel coronavirus that emerged in China in late 2019 sparked a global pandemic of coronavirus disease (COVID) in 2020. A **syndemic** occurs when two or more diseases cluster within a population, in part due to social and structural conditions, and the interaction between the diseases makes the health outcomes worse.[219] COVID-19 was described as a syndemic between the SARS-CoV-2 virus and noncommunicable diseases such as hypertension, diabetes, and chronic respiratory diseases, which significantly increased the risk of severe illness and death from the virus.[220]

Some NTDs are also considered to be EIDs, such as dengue, which is occurring more often than it did in the past and has an expanding geographic range.[221]

The U.S. Institute of Medicine has concluded that these new health threats derive from a complex interaction of genetic, biological, environmental, ecological, social, political, and economic factors (**Figure 10.14**).[222] As the world population increases (#6), humans and domestic animals move into previously uninhabited natural environments (#5) and are exposed to new plants, animals, and microbes. Alteration of the environment (#4), such as deforestation, dam building, and manipulation of wetlands, creates new environmental reservoirs for infectious agents and their hosts, and natural disasters (#3) like floods and droughts can alter the landscape and introduce new infectious agents to a region. Changes in dietary and other behaviors (#6) that become trendy and spread globally may also facilitate transmission. Urbanization facilitates emergence as people with different strains of infections interact with one another (#2) and create new habitats for vectors (#5). Technology is also speeding up the rate of emergence. Modern transportation (#8) has made it possible for a person with a contagious disease to travel nearly anywhere in the world within hours. Healthcare innovations (#7) have created new risks and risk groups.

1	Microbial adaptation and change
2	Human susceptibility to infection
3	Climate and weather
4	Changing ecosystems
5	Economic development and land use
6	Human demographics and behavior
7	Technology and industry
8	International travel and commerce
9	Breakdown of public health measures
10	Poverty and social inequality
11	War and famine
12	Lack of political will
13	Intent to harm

Figure 10.14 Risk factors for emerging infectious diseases identified by the U.S. Institute of Medicine.

Data from Smolinski MS, Hamburg MA, Lederberg J, eds. *Microbial Threats to Health: Emergence, Detection, and Response.* Washington DC: National Academies Press; 2003.

Advanced medical therapies like the immunosuppressive drugs used by people who have had organ transplants and the technology for keeping premature infants alive have created new populations of highly susceptible people (#2). Healthcare-associated infections may be very hardy and difficult to treat, and antimicrobial resistance is increasing (#1). Other technological advances have created new places for infectious agents to grow and new methods of dispersion.

New infectious diseases can emerge anywhere in the world and spread quickly, so the distinction between local public health problems and global ones is increasingly limited. Systems for identifying and controlling emerging threats to human health no matter where they first occur are an important part of protecting the health of all the world's people.

References

1. Keusch GT, Kilama WL, Moon S, Szlezák NA, Michaud CM. The global health system: linking knowledge with action—learning from malaria. *PLoS Med.* 2010;7:e100179.
2. Parascandola J. From MCWA to CDC: origins of the Centers for Disease Control and Prevention. *Public Health Rep.* 1996;111:549–551.
3. Hotez PJ, Fenwick A, Savioli L, Molyneux DH. Rescuing the bottom billion through control of neglected tropical diseases. *Lancet.* 2009;373:1570–1575.
4. *Ending the Neglect to Attain the Sustainable Development Goals: A Road Map for Neglected Tropical Diseases 2021–2030.* Geneva: World Health Organization; 2020.
5. Feasey N, Wansbrough-Jones M, Mabey DCW, Solomon AW. Neglected tropical diseases. *Br Med Bull.* 2010;93:179–200.
6. Bhutta ZA, Sommerfeld J, Lassi ZS, Salam RA, Das JK. Global burden, distribution, and interventions for infectious diseases of poverty. *Infect Dis Poverty.* 2014;3:21.
7. *Reaching a Billion: Fifth Progress Report of the London Declaration on NTDs.* London: Uniting to Combat Neglected Tropical Diseases; 2017.
8. Fitzpatrick C, Nwankwo U, Lenk E, de Vlas SJ, Bundy D. An investment case for ending neglected tropical diseases (chapter 17). In: Holmes KK, Bertozzi S, Bloom BR, Jha P, eds. *Disease Control Priorities: Major Infectious Diseases.* Vol. 6. 3rd ed. Washington DC: IBRD/World Bank; 2017:411–432.
9. Fitzpatrick C, Engels D. Leaving no one behind: a neglected tropical disease indicator and tracers for the Sustainable Development Goals. *Int Health.* 2016;8(Suppl 1):i15–i18.
10. Molyneux DH. The 'neglected tropical diseases': now a brand identity; responsibilities, context and promise. *Parasit Vectors.* 2012;5:23.
11. *An Innovative Approach to R&D for Neglected Patients: Ten Years of Experience & Lessons Learned by DNDi.* Geneva: Drugs for Neglected Diseases Initiative; 2014.
12. Hamill LC, Haslam D, Abrahamsson S, et al. People are neglected, not diseases: the relationship between disability and neglected tropical diseases. *Trans R Soc Trop Med Hyg.* 2019;113:829–834.
13. Severe malaria. *Trop Med Int Health.* 2014;19(Suppl 1):7–131.
14. *World Malaria Report 2021.* Geneva: World Health Organization; 2021.
15. Wilson AJ, Morgan ER, Booth M, et al. What is a vector? *Philos Trans R Soc Lond B Biol Sci.* 2017;372:20160085.
16. Aly ASI, Vaughan AM, Kappe SHI. Malaria parasite development in the mosquito and infection of the mammalian host. *Annu Rev Microbiol.* 2009;63:195–221.
17. *Management of Severe Malaria: A Practical Handbook.* 3rd ed. Geneva: World Health Organization; 2013.
18. Ghosh K, Ghosh K. Pathogenesis of anaemia in malaria: a concise review. *Parasitol Res.* 2007;101:1463–1469.
19. Idro R, Marsh K, John CC, Newton CR. Cerebral malaria: mechanisms of brain injury and strategies for improved neurocognitive outcomes. *Pediatr Res.* 2010;68:267–274.
20. Idro R, Jenkins NE, Newton CR. Pathogenesis, clinical features, and neurological outcomes of cerebral malaria. *Lancet Neuro.* 2005;4:827–840.
21. Plowe CV. The evolution of drug-resistant malaria. *Trans R Soc Trop Med Hyg.* 2009;103(Suppl 10):S11–S14.
22. Hemingway J, Shretta R, Wells TNC, et al. Tools and strategies for malaria control and elimination: what do we need to achieve a grand convergence in malaria. *PLoS Biol.* 2016;14:e1002380.
23. *WHO Guidelines for Malaria.* Geneva: World Health Organization; 2021.
24. *Universal Access to Malaria Diagnostic Testing: An Operational Manual.* Geneva: World Health Organization; 2011.
25. Doolan DL, Dobaño C, Baird JK. Acquired immunity to malaria. *Clin Microbiol Rev.* 2009;22:13–36.
26. Fried M, Duffy PD. Malaria during pregnancy. *Cold Spring Harb Perspect Med.* 2017;7:a025551.
27. Desai M, Hill J, Fernandes S, et al. Prevention of malaria in pregnancy. *Lancet Infect Dis.* 2018;18:e119–e132.
28. *WHO Policy Brief for the Implementation of Intermittent Preventive Treatment of Malaria in Pregnancy Using Sulfadoxine-Pyrimethamine (IPTp-SP).* Geneva: World Health Organization; 2013.
29. Eisele TP, Larsen DA, Anglewicz PA, et al. Malaria prevention in pregnancy, birthweight, and neonatal mortality: a meta-analysis of 32 national cross-sectional datasets in Africa. *Lancet Infect Dis.* 2012;12:942–949.
30. Conteh L, Sicuri E, Manzi F, et al. The cost-effectiveness of intermittent preventive treatment for malaria in infants in sub-Saharan Africa. *PLoS One.* 2010;5:e10313.
31. Asenso-Okyere K, Asante FA, Tarekegn J, Andam KS. A review of the economic impact of malaria in agricultural development. *Agric Econ.* 2011;42:293–304.
32. Sarma N, Patouillard E, Cibulskis RE, Arcand JL. The economic burden of malaria: revisiting the evidence. *Am J Trop Med Hyg.* 2019;101:1405–1415.
33. Yasuoka J, Levins R. Impact of deforestation and agricultural development on anopheline ecology and malaria epidemiology. *Am J Trop Med Hyg.* 2007;76:450–460.
34. Nájera JA, González-Silva M, Alonso PL. Some lessons for the future from the Global Malaria Eradication Programme (1955–1969). *PLoS Med.* 2011;8:e1000412.

35. Mendis K, Rietveld A, Warsame M, Bosman A, Greenwood B, Wernsdorfer WH. From malaria control to eradication: the WHO perspective. *Trop Med Int Health.* 2009;14:802–809.

36. Dunn R. In retrospect: Silent Spring. *Nature.* 2012;485:578–579.

37. Attaran A, Roberst DR, Curtis CF, Kilama WL. Balancing risks on the backs of the poor. *Nat Med.* 2000;6:729–731.

38. Sadasivaiah S, Tozan Y, Breman JG. Dichloro-diphenyltrichloroethane (DDT) for indoor residual spraying in Africa: how can it be used for malaria control? *Am J Trop Med Hyg.* 2007;77(Suppl 6): 249–263.

39. *Indoor Residual Spraying: An Operational Manual for Indoor Residual Spraying (IRS) for Malaria Transmission Control and Elimination.* 2nd ed. Geneva: World Health Organization; 2015.

40. *The Use of DDT in Malaria Vector Control: WHO Position Statement.* Geneva: World Health Organization; 2011.

41. Shretta R, Liu J, Cotter C, et al. Malaria elimination and eradication (chapter 12). In: Holmes KK, Bertozzi S, Bloom BR, Jha P, eds. *Disease Control Priorities: Major Infectious Diseases.* Vol. 6. 3rd ed. Washington DC: IBRD/World Bank; 2017:315–346.

42. WHO Global Malaria Program. *Insecticide-Treated Mosquito Nets: A WHO Position Statement.* Geneva: World Health Organization; 2007.

43. Pryce J, Richardson M, Lengeler C. Insecticide-treated nets for preventing malaria. *Cochrane Database Syst Rev.* 2018;11:CD000363.

44. Bousema T, Okell L, Felger I, Drakeley C. Asymptomatic malaria infections: detectability, transmissibility and public health relevance. *Nat Rev Microbiol.* 2014;12:833–840.

45. Bhatt S, Weiss DJ, Cameron E, et al. The effect of malaria control on *Plasmodium falciparum* in Africa between 2000 and 2015. *Nature.* 2015;526:207–211.

46. Chen-Hussey V, Behrens R, Logan JG. Assessment of methods used to determine the safety of the topical insect repellent N,N-diethyl-m-toluamide (DEET). *Parasit Vectors.* 2014;7:173.

47. *RBM Partnership to End Malaria Annual Report 2019.* Geneva: RBM Partnership; 2020.

48. Berdud M, Towse A, Kettler H. Fostering incentives for research, development, and delivery of interventions for neglected tropical diseases: lessons from malaria. *Oxford Rev Econ Pol.* 2016;32:64–87.

49. Laurens MB. RTS,S/AS01 vaccine (Mosquirix™): an overview. *Hum Vaccin Immunother.* 2020;16:480–489.

50. Meeting of Strategic Advisory Group of Experts on Immunization, October 2021: conclusions and recommendations. *Wkly Epidemiol Rec.* 2021;50: 613–632.

51. Birkett AJ. Status of vaccine research and development of vaccines for malaria. *Vaccine.* 2016;34:2915–2920.

52. Malaria vaccine: WHO position paper – January 2016. *Wkly Epidemiol Rec.* 2016;91:33–52.

53. *Achieving the Malaria MDG Target: Reversing the Incidence of Malaria 2000–2015.* Geneva: World Health Organization/UNICEF; 2015.

54. *Global Technical Strategy for Malaria 2016–2030.* Geneva: World Health Organization; 2015.

55. *Global Technical Strategy for Malaria 2016–2030, 2021 Update.* Geneva: World Health Organization; 2021.

56. *Financing Global Health 2019: Tracking Health Spending in a Time of Crisis.* Seattle: Institute for Health Metrics and Evaluation; 2020.

57. Feachem RGA, Chen I, Akbari O, et al. Malaria eradication within a generation: ambitious, achievable, and necessary. *Lancet.* 2019;394:1056–1112.

58. Wilder-Smith A, Ooi EE, Horstick O, Wills B. Dengue. *Lancet.* 2019;393:350–363.

59. Katzelnick LC, Gresh L, Halloran ME, et al. Antibody-dependent enhancement of severe dengue disease in humans. *Science.* 2017;358:929–932.

60. Castro MC, Wilson ME, Bloom DC. Disease and economic burdens of dengue. *Lancet Infect Dis.* 2017;17:e70–e78.

61. Messina JP, Brady OJ, Scott TW, et al. Global spread of dengue virus types: mapping the 70 year history. *Trends Microbiol.* 2014;22:138–146.

62. Bhatt S, Gething PW, Brady OJ, et al. The global distribution and burden of dengue. *Nature.* 2013; 496:504–507.

63. *Global Strategy for Dengue Prevention and Control 2012–2020.* Geneva: World Health Organization; 2012.

64. *WHO Guidance: Ethics and Vector-Borne Diseases.* Geneva: World Health Organization; 2020.

65. Schwartz LM, Halloran ME, Durbin AP, Longini IM Jr. The dengue vaccine pipeline: implications for the future of dengue control. *Vaccine.* 2015;33:3293–3298.

66. Vannice KS, Durbin A, Hombach J. Status of vaccine research and development of vaccines for dengue. *Vaccine.* 2016;34:2934–2938.

67. Normile D. Safety concerns derail dengue vaccination program. *Science.* 2017;358:1114–1115.

68. Dengue vaccine: WHO position paper – September 2018. *Wkly Epidemiol Rec.* 2018;93:457–476.

69. Prompetchara E, Ketloy C, Thomas SJ, Ruxrungtham K. Dengue vaccine: global development update. *Asian Pac J Allergy Immunol.* 2020;38:178–185.

70. Paixão ES, Rodrigues LC, Costa MCN, et al. Chikungunya chronic disease: a systematic review and meta-analysis. *Trans R Soc Trop Med Hyg.* 2018;112:301–316.

71. Weaver SC, Lecuit M. Chikungunya virus and the global spread of a mosquito-borne disease. *N Engl J Med.* 2015;372:1231–1239.

72. Rezza G, Weaver SC. Chikungunya as a paradigm for emerging viral diseases: evaluating disease impact and hurdles to vaccine development. *PLoS Negl Trop Dis.* 2019;13:e0006919.

73. Paules CI, Fauci AS. Yellow fever – once again on the radar screen in the Americas. *N Engl J Med.* 2017;376:1397–1399.

74. Foster KR, Jenkins MF, Toogood AC. The Philadelphia yellow fever epidemic of 1793. *Sci Am.* 1998;279:88–93.

75. Brès PL. A century of progress in combatting yellow fever. *Bull World Health Organ.* 1986;64:775–786.

76. Monath TP, Vasconcelos PF. Yellow fever. *J Clin Virol.* 2015;64:160–173.

77. Frierson JG. The yellow fever vaccine: a history. *Yale J Biol Med.* 2010;83:77–85.

78. Simons H, Patel D. International Health Regulations in practice: focus on yellow fever and poliomyelitis. *Hum Vaccin Immunother.* 2016;12:2690–2693.

79. Hayes EB, Komar N, Nasci RS, Montgomery SP, O'Leary DR, Campbell GL. Epidemiology and transmission dynamics of West Nile virus disease. *Emerg Infect Dis.* 2005;11:1167–1173.

80. Petersen LR, Brault AC, Nasci RS. West Nile virus: review of the literature. *JAMA.* 2013;310:308–315.

81. Lindsey NP, Staples JE, Lehman JA, Fischer M, CDC. Surveillance for human West Nile Virus disease— United States, 1999–2008. *MMWR Surveill Summ.* 2010;59:1–17.

82. Kilpatrick AM. Globalization, land use and the invasion of West Nile virus. *Science.* 2011;334:323–327.

83. Turtle L, Solomon T. Japanese encephalitis: the prospects for new treatments. *Nat Rev Neurol.* 2018;14:298–313.

84. Pearce JC, Learoyd TP, Langendorf BJ, Logan JG. Japanese encephalitis: the vectors, ecology and potential for expansion. *J Travel Med.* 2018;25(Suppl 1):S16–S26.

85. Hayes EB. Zika virus outside Africa. *Emerg Infect Dis.* 2009;15:1347–1350.

86. Mlakar J, Korva M, Tul N, et al. Zika virus associated with microcephaly. *N Engl J Med.* 2016;374:951–958.

87. D'Ortenzio E, Matheron S, Yazdanpana Y, et al. Evidence of sexual transmission of Zika virus. *N Engl J Med.* 2016;374:2195–2198.

88. Hartman A. Rift Valley fever. *Clin Lab Med.* 2017;37:285–301.

89. Wilder-Smith A, Gubler DJ, Weaver SC, Monath TP, Heymann DL, Scott TW. Epidemic arboviral diseases: priorities for research and public health. *Lancet Infect Dis.* 2017;17:e101–e106.

90. *Global Vector Control Response 2017–2030.* Geneva: World Health Organization; 2017.

91. Mordecai EA, Ryan SJ, Caldwell JM, Shah MM, LaBeaud AD. Climate change could shift disease burden from malaria to arboviruses in Africa. *Lancet Planetary Health.* 2020;4:e416–e423.

92. Taylor MJ, Hoerauf A, Bockarie M. Lymphatic filariasis and onchocerciasis. *Lancet.* 2010;376:1175–1185.

93. Davey G, Tekola F, Newport MJ. Podoconiosis: non-infectious geochemical elephantiasis. *Trans R Soc Trop Med Hyg.* 2007;101:1175–1180.

94. Global programme to eliminate lymphatic filariasis: progress report, 2019. *Wkly Epidemiol Rec.* 2020;95:509–524.

95. *Lymphatic Filariasis: Managing Morbidity and Preventing Disability: An Aide-Mémoire for National Programme Managers.* Geneva: World Health Organization; 2013.

96. Summary of global update on implementation of preventive chemotherapy against neglected tropical diseases in 2019. *Wkly Epidemiol Rec.* 2020;95:469–474.

97. Ramaiah KD, Ottesen EA. Progress and impact of 13 years of the Global Programme to Eliminate Lymphatic Filariasis on reducing the burden of filarial disease. *PLoS Negl Trop Dis.* 2014;8:e3319.

98. Local Burden of Disease 2019 Neglected Tropical Diseases Collaborators. The global distribution of lymphatic filariasis, 2000–18: a geospatial analysis. *Lancet Glob Health.* 2020;8:e1186–e1194.

99. Bockarie MJ, Pedersen EM, White GB, Michael E. Role of vector control in the global program to eliminate lymphatic filariasis. *Annu Rev Entomol.* 2009;54:469–487.

100. Boatin B. The Onchocerciasis Control Programme in West Africa (OCP). *Ann Trop Med Parasitol.* 2008;102(Suppl 1):13–17.

101. Padgett JJ, Jacobsen KH. Loiasis: African eye worm. *Trans R Soc Trop Med Hyg.* 2008;102:983–989.

102. Chesnais CB, Pion SD, Boullé C, et al. Individual risk of post-ivermectin serious adverse events in subjects infected with Loa loa. *EClinicalMedicine.* 2020;28:100582.

103. Sauerbrey M, Rakers JL, Richards FO Jr. Progress toward elimination of onchocerciasis in the Americas. *Int Health.* 2018;10:i71–i78.

104. Tekle AH, Zouré HGM, Noma M, et al. Progress toward onchocerciasis elimination in the participating countries of the African Programme for Onchocerciasis Control: epidemiological evaluation results. *Infect Dis Poverty.* 2016;5:66.

105. Progress report on the elimination of human onchocerciasis, 2019–2020. *Wkly Epidemiol Rec.* 2020;95:545–554.

106. Colebunders R, Siewe FJN, Hotterbeekx A. Onchocerciasis-associated epilepsy, an additional reason for strengthening onchocerciasis elimination programs. *Trends Parasitol.* 2018;34:208–216.

107. King CH. Toward the elimination of schistosomiasis. *N Engl J Med.* 2009;360:106–109.

108. Colley DG, Bustinduy AL, Secor WE, King CH. Human schistosomiasis. *Lancet.* 2014;383:2253–2264.

109. Honeycutt J, Hammam O, Fu CL, Hsieh MH. Controversies and challenges in research on urogenital schistosomiasis-associated bladder cancer. *Trends Parasitol.* 2014;30:324–332.

110. Deol AK, Fleming FM, Calvo-Urbano B, et al. Schistosomiasis: assessing progress toward the

2020 and 2015 global goals. *N Engl J Med.* 2019;381:2519–2528.

111. Schistosomiasis and soil-transmitted helminthiases: numbers of people treated in 2018. *Wkly Epidemiol Rec.* 2019;94:601–612.

112. Steinmann P, Keiser J, Bos R, Tanner M, Utzinger J. Schistosomiasis and water resources development: systematic review, meta-analysis, and estimates of people at risk. *Lancet.* 2006;6:411–425.

113. Rollinson D, Knopp S, Levitz S, et al. Time to set the agenda for schistosomiasis elimination. *Acta Trop.* 2013;128:423–440.

114. Jourdan PM, Lamberton PHL, Fenwick A, Addiss DG. Soil-transmitted helminth infections. *Lancet.* 2017;391:252–265.

115. Bundy DA, Walson JL, Watkins KL. Worms, wisdom, and wealth: why deworming can make economic sense. *Trends Parasitol.* 2013;29:142–148.

116. Dold C, Holland CV. Ascaris and ascariasis. *Microbes Infect.* 2011;13:632–637.

117. GBD 2019 Diseases and Injuries Collaborators. Global burden of 369 diseases and injuries in 204 countries and territories, 1990–2019: a systematic analysis for the Global Burden of Disease Study 2019. *Lancet.* 2020;396:1204–1222.

118. Hechenbleikner EM, McQuade JM. Parasitic colitis. *Clin Colon Rectal Surg.* 2015;28:79–86.

119. Loukas A, Hotez PJ, Diemart D, et al. Hookworm infection. *Nat Rev Dis Primers.* 2016;2:16088.

120. Nutman TB. Human infection with *Strongyloides stercoralis* and other related *Strongyloides* species. *Parasitology.* 2017;144:263–273.

121. *Guideline: Preventive Chemotherapy to Control Soil-Transmitted Helminth Infections in At-Risk Population Groups.* Geneva: World Health Organization; 2017.

122. Schistosomiasis and soil-transmitted helminthiases: progress report, 2020. *Wkly Epidemiol Rec.* 2021;96:585–595.

123. Weatherhead JE, Hotez PJ, Mejia R. The global state of helminth control and elimination in children. *Pediatr Clin North Am.* 2017;64:867–877.

124. Bern C. Chagas' disease. *N Engl J Med.* 2015;373:456–466.

125. Pereira Nunes MC, Beaton A, Acquatella H, et al. Chagas cardiomyopathy: an update of current clinical knowledge and management: a scientific statement from the American Heart Association. *Circulation.* 2018;138:e169–e209.

126. Pérez-Molina JA, Molina I. Chagas disease. *Lancet.* 2018;391:82–94.

127. Stanaway JD, Roth G. The burden of Chagas disease: estimates and challenges. *Glob Heart.* 2015;10:139–144.

128. Schmunis GA, Yadon YE. Chagas disease: a Latin American health problem becoming a world health problem. *Acta Trop.* 2010;115:14–21.

129. Franco JR, Simarro PP, Diarra A, Jannin JG. Epidemiology of human African trypanosomiasis. *Clin Epidemiol.* 2014;6:257–275.

130. Büscher P, Cecchi G, Jamonneau V, Priotto G. Human African trypanosomiasis. *Lancet.* 2017;390:2397–2409.

131. Lutje V, Seixas J, Kennedy A. Chemotherapy for second-stage human African trypanosomiasis. *Cochrane Database Syst Rev.* 2013;2013:CD006201.

132. *Report of the Third WHO Stakeholders Meeting on Gambiense Human African Trypanosomiasis Elimination.* Geneva: World Health Organization; 2018.

133. Leishmaniasis in high-burden countries: an epidemiological update based on data reported in 2014. *Wkly Epidemiol Rec.* 2016;91:287–296.

134. *Control of the Leishmaniases: Report of a Meeting of the WHO Expert Committee on the Control of Leishmaniases, Geneva, 22–26 March 2010.* Geneva: World Health Organization Technical Report Series; 2010.

135. Alvar J, Vélez ID, Bern C, et al. Leishmaniasis worldwide and global estimates of its incidence. *PLoS One.* 2012;7:e35671.

136. Burza S, Croft SL, Boelaert M. Leishmaniasis. *Lancet.* 2018;392:951–970.

137. *WHO Expert Committee on Leprosy: Eighth Report.* Geneva: World Health Organization; 2012.

138. Rodrigues LC, Lockwood DNJ. Leprosy now: epidemiology, progress, challenges, and research gaps. *Lancet Infect Dis.* 2011;11:464–470.

139. Grzybowski A, Nita M, Virmond M. Ocular leprosy. *Clin Dermatol.* 2015;33:79–89.

140. Suzuki K, Akama T, Kawashima A, Yoshihara A, Yotsu RR, Ishii N. Current status of leprosy: epidemiology, basic science and clinical perspectives. *J Dermatol.* 2012;39:121–129.

141. Schreuder PAM, Noto S, Richardus JH. Epidemiologic trends of leprosy for the 21st century. *Clin Dermatol.* 2016;34:24–31.

142. Global leprosy (Hansen disease) update, 2019: time to step-up prevention initiatives. *Wkly Epidemiol Rec.* 2020;95:417–440.

143. Steinmann P, Dusenbury C, Addiss D, Mirza F, Smith WCS. A comprehensive research agenda for zero leprosy. *Infect Dis Poverty.* 2020;9:156.

144. Simpson H, Deribe K, Tabah EN, et al. Mapping the global distribution of Buruli ulcer: a systematic review with evidence consensus. *Lancet Glob Health.* 2019;7:e912–e922.

145. Guarner J. Buruli ulcer: review of a neglected skin mycobacterial disease. *J Clin Microbiol.* 2018;56:e01507–e01517.

146. *Treatment of Mycobacterium Ulcerans Disease (Buruli Ulcer): Guidance for Health Workers.* Geneva: World Health Organization; 2012.

147. *Trachoma Control: A Guide for Programme Managers.* Geneva: World Health Organization; 2006.

148. Emerson P, Frost L, Bailey R, Mabey D. *Implementing the SAFE Strategy for Trachoma Control: A Toolbox of Interventions for Promoting Facial Cleanliness and Environmental Improvement.* Atlanta GA: The Carter Center/International Trachoma Initiative; 2006.

149. WHO Alliance for the Global Elimination of Trachoma by 2020: progress report, 2019. *Wkly Epidemiol Rec.* 2020;95:349–360.

150. Marks M, Solomon AW, Mabey DC. Endemic *Treponema* diseases. *Trans R Soc Trop Med Hyg.* 2014;108:601–607.

151. Mitjà O, Asiedu K, Mabey D. Yaws. *Lancet.* 2013; 381:763–773.

152. Mitjà O, Marks M, Donan DJ, et al. Global epidemiology of yaws: a systematic review. *Lancet Glob Health.* 2015;3:e324–e331.

153. Mitjà O, Godornes C, Houinei W, et al. Re-emergence of yaws after single mass azithromycin treatment followed by targeted treatment: a longitudinal study. *Lancet.* 2018;391:1599–1607.

154. Ziljstra E, van de Sande WW, Welsh O, Mahgoub ES, Goodfellow M, Fahal AH. Mycetoma: a unique neglected tropical disease. *Lancet Infect Dis.* 2016;16:100–112.

155. Van de Sande WWJ, Fahal AH, Ahmed SA, et al. Closing the mycetoma knowledge gap. *Med Mycol.* 2018;51(Suppl 1):S153–S164.

156. Van de Sande WW. Global burden of human mycetoma: a systematic review and meta-analysis. *PLoS Negl Trop Dis.* 2013;7:e2550.

157. Queiroz-Telles F, de Hoog S, Santos DWCL, et al. Chromoblastomycosis. *Clin Rev Microbiol.* 2017;30:233–276.

158. Romani L, Steer AC, Whitfield MJ, Kaldor JM. Prevalence of scabies and impetigo worldwide: a systematic review. *Lancet Infect Dis.* 2015;15:960–967.

159. Karimkhani C, Colombara DV, Drucker AM, et al. The global burden of scabies: a cross-sectional analysis from the Global Burden of Disease Study 2015. *Lancet Infect Dis.* 2017;17:1247–1254.

160. Stamm LV, Strowd LC. Ignoring the "itch": the global health problem of scabies. *Am J Trop Med Hyg.* 2017;97:1647–1649.

161. Engelman D, Cantey PT, Marks M, et al. The public health control of scabies: priorities for research and action. *Lancet.* 2019;394:81–92.

162. Engels D, Zhou XN. Neglected tropical diseases: an effective global response to local poverty-related disease priorities. *Infect Dis Poverty.* 2020;9:10.

163. *Preventable Epilepsy:* Taenia Solium *Infection Burdens Economies, Societies and Individuals: A Rationale for Investment and Action.* Geneva: World Health Organization; 2016.

164. Gripper LB, Welburn SC. Neurocysticercosis infection and disease: a review. *Acta Trop.* 2017;166:218–224.

165. Coral-Almeida M, Gabriël S, Abatih EN, Praet N, Benitez W, Dorny P. *Taenia solium* human cysticercosis: a systematic review of sero-epidemiological data from endemic zones around the world. *PLoS Negl Trop Dis.* 2015;9:e0003919.

166. Ndimubanzi PC, Carabin H, Budke CM, et al. A systematic review of the frequency of neuro-cysticercosis with a focus on people with epilepsy. *PLoS Negl Trop Dis.* 2010;4:e870.

167. Thomas LF. *Landscape Analysis: Control of Taenia solium.* Geneva: World Health Organization; 2015.

168. Budke CM, Casulli A, Kern P, Vuitton DA. Cystic and alveolar echinococcosis: successes and continuing challenges. *PLoS Negl Trop Dis.* 2017;11:e0005477.

169. Craig PS, McManus DP, Lightowlers MW, et al. Prevention and control of cystic echinococcosis. *Lancet Infect Dis.* 2007;7:385–394.

170. Keiser J, Utzinger J. Emerging foodborne trematodiasis. *Emerg Infect Dis.* 2005;11:1507–1514.

171. Qian MB, Utzinger J, Keiser J, Zhou XN. Clonorchiasis. *Lancet.* 2016;387:800–810.

172. Ogorodova LM, Fedorova OS, Sripa B, et al. Opisthorchiasis: an overlooked danger. *PLoS Negl Trop Dis.* 2015;9:e0003563.

173. Mas-Coma S, Valero MA, Bargues MD. Fascioliasis. *Adv Exp Med Biol.* 2014;766:77–114.

174. Blair D. Paragonimiasis. *Adv Exp Med Biol.* 2014;766:115–152.

175. Fürst T, Keiser J, Utzinger J. Global burden of human food-borne trematodiases: a systematic review and meta-analysis. *Lancet Infect Dis.* 2012;12:210–221.

176. Torgerson PR, Mastroiacovo P. The global burden of congenital toxoplasmosis: a systematic review. *Bull World Health Organ.* 2013;91:501–508.

177. Fahrion AS, Mikhailov A, Abela-Ridder B, Giacinti J, Harries J. Human rabies transmitted by dogs: current status of global data, 2015. *Wkly Epidemiol Rec.* 2016;91:13–20.

178. *WHO Expert Consultation on Rabies: Third Report.* Geneva: World Health Organization Technical Report Series; 2018.

179. Hampson K, Coudeville L, Lembo T, et al. Estimating the global burden of endemic canine rabies. *PLoS Negl Trop Dis.* 2015;9:e0003709.

180. Global Alliance for Rabies Control. *Zero by 30: The Global Strategic Plan to End Human Deaths from Dog-Mediated Rabies by 2030.* Geneva: World Health Organization/Food and Agriculture Organization of the United Nations/World Organization for Animal Health; 2018.

181. Rabies vaccines: WHO position paper – April 2018. *Wkly Epidemiol Rec.* 2018;93:201–220.

182. Williams DJ, Faiz MA, Abela-Ridder B, et al. Strategy for a globally coordinated response to a priority neglected tropical disease: snakebite envenoming. *PLoS Negl Trop Dis.* 2019;13:e0007059.

183. Gutiérrez JM, Calvete JJ, Habib AG, Harrison RA, Williams DJ, Warrell DA. Snakebite envenoming. *Nat Rev Dis Primers.* 2017;3:17063.

184. *Snakebite Envenoming: A Strategy for Prevention and Control.* Geneva: World Health Organization; 2019.

185. Warrell DA. Snake bite. *Lancet.* 2010;375:77–88.

186. Dowdle WR. The principles of disease elimination and eradication. *Bull World Health Organ.* 1998; 76(Suppl 2):22–25.

187. *Generic Framework for Control, Elimination and Eradication of Neglected Tropical Diseases.* Geneva: World Health Organization; 2015.

188. Hopkins DR. Disease eradication. *N Engl J Med.* 2013;368:54–63.

189. Morens DM, Holmes EC, Davis AS, Taubenberger JK. Global rinderpest eradication: lessons learned and why humans should celebrate too. *J Infect Dis.* 2011;204:502–505.

190. Roeder P, Mariner J, Kock R. Rinderpest: the veterinary perspective on eradication. *Philos Trans R Soc Lond B Biol Sci.* 2013;368:20120139.

191. Moore ZS, Seward JF, Lane JM. Smallpox. *Lancet.* 2006;367:425–435.

192. Breman JG, Henderson DA. Diagnosis and management of smallpox. *N Engl J Med.* 346:1300–1308.

193. Henderson DA. Principles and lessons from the smallpox eradication programme. *Bull World Health Organ.* 1987;65:535–546.

194. Henderson DA, Inglesby TV, Bartlett JG, et al. Smallpox as a biological weapon: medical and public health management: Working Group on Civilian Biodefense. *JAMA.* 1999;281:2127–2137.

195. Cairncross S, Muller R, Zagaria N. Dracunculiasis (guinea worm disease) and the eradication initiative. *Clin Microbiol Rev.* 2002;15:223–246.

196. Hopkins DR, Ruiz-Tiben E, Eberhard ML, et al. Dracunculiasis eradication: are we there yet? *Am J Trop Med Hyg.* 2018;99:388–395.

197. *Eradication of Guinea Worm Disease: Case Statement.* Atlanta GA: The Carter Center/World Health Organization; 2020.

198. Molyneux D, Sankara DP. Guinea worm eradication: progress and challenges: should we beware of the dog? *PLoS Negl Trop Dis.* 2017;11:e0005495.

199. Hopkins DR, Weiss AJ, Roy SL, Yerian S, Sapp SGH. Progress toward global eradication of dracunculiasis, January 2019–June 2020. *MMWR Morb Mortal Wkly Rep.* 2020;69:1563–1568.

200. Molyneux DH, Eberhard ML, Cleaveland S, et al. Certifying guinea worm eradication: current challenges. *Lancet.* 2020;396:1857–1860.

201. Hinman AR, Foege WH, de Quadros CA, Patriarca PA, Orenstein WA, Brink EW. The case for global eradication of poliomyelitis. *Bull World Health Organ.* 1987;65:835–840.

202. Howard RS. Poliomyelitis and the postpolio syndrome. *BMJ.* 2005;330:1314–1318.

203. Polio vaccines: WHO position paper – March, 2016. *Wkly Epidemiol Rec.* 2016;91:145–168.

204. Minor P. Vaccine-derived poliovirus (VDPV): impact on poliomyelitis eradication. *Vaccine.* 2009;27: 2649–2652.

205. Apparent global interruption of wild poliovirus type 2 transmission. *MMWR Morb Mortal Wkly Rep.* 2001;50:222–224.

206. Patel M, Orenstein W. A world free of polio: the final steps. *N Engl J Med.* 2016;374:501–503.

207. Chard AN, Datta SD, Tallis G, et al. Progress toward polio eradication – worldwide, January 2018–March 2020. *Wkly Epidemiol Rec.* 2020;95:283–290.

208. Blume S, Geesink I. A brief history of polio vaccines. *Science.* 2000;288:1593–1594.

209. *Global Polio Eradication Initiative Investment Case 2019–2023.* Geneva: World Health Organization; 2019.

210. *Polio Global Eradication Initiative: Annual Report 2015.* Geneva: World Health Organization; 2016.

211. Roberts L. New polio cases in Nigeria spur massive response. *Science.* 2016;353:738.

212. *State of the World's Children 2019.* New York: UNICEF; 2019.

213. *Polio Eradication Strategy 2022–2026: Delivering on a Promise.* Geneva: World Health Organization; 2021.

214. Barreto ML, Teixeira MG, Carmo EH. Infectious disease epidemiology. *J Epidemiol Community Health.* 2006;60:192–195.

215. Morens DM, Folkers GK, Fauci AS. The challenge of emerging and re-emerging infectious diseases. *Nature.* 2004;430:242–249.

216. Aditi, Shariff M. Nipah virus infection: a review. *Epidemiol Infect.* 2019;147:e95.

217. Neumann G, Noda T, Kawaoka Y. Emergence and pandemic potential of swine-origin H1N1 influenza virus. *Nature.* 2009;459:931–939.

218. WHO Ebola Response Team. Ebola virus disease in West Africa – the first 9 months of the epidemic and forward projections. *N Engl J Med.* 2014;317:1481–1495.

219. Singer M, Bulled N, Ostrach B, Mendenhall E. Syndemics and the biosocial conception of health. *Lancet.* 2017;389:941–950.

220. Horton R. COVID-19 is not a pandemic. *Lancet.* 2020;396:874.

221. Mackey TK, Liang BA, Cuomo R, Hafen R, Brouwer KC, Lee DE. Emerging and reemerging neglected tropical diseases: a review of key characteristics, risk factors, and the policy and innovation environment. *Clin Microbiol Rev.* 2014;27:949–979.

222. Smolinski, MS, Hamburg MA, Lederberg J, eds. *Microbial Threats to Health: Emergence, Detection, and Response.* Washington DC: National Academies Press; 2003.

CHAPTER 11

Reproductive Health

Most international support for reproductive health focuses on slowing global population growth through increased access to contraceptives and reducing maternal and neonatal mortality through improved medical care of pregnant women and babies. A more comprehensive set of interventions supports family planning and sexual healthcare services for adolescents and adults of all genders.

11.1 Reproductive Health and Global Health

Sustainable Development Goal (SDG) 3 focuses on health, and one of its targets is to "ensure universal access to sexual and reproductive health-care services, including for family planning, information, and education, and the integration of reproductive health into national strategies and programs" (SDG 3.7) (**Figure 11.1**).[1] **Sexual health** is the enjoyment of safe, voluntary, and nonviolent sexual experiences. **Reproductive health** encompasses issues related to fertility and infertility, pregnancy and childbirth, contraception, the prevention and treatment of sexually transmitted infections, and other aspects of gynecological and urological health. Reproductive health is about more than pregnancy, and it is relevant to adolescents and adults of all genders and ages.

SDG 5 focuses on gender equality, and one of its targets is to "ensure universal access to sexual and reproductive health and reproductive rights as agreed in accordance with the Programme of Action of the ICPD and the Beijing Platform for Action and the outcome documents of their review conferences" (SDG 5.6).[1] **Reproductive rights** describe the freedom for women and their partners to decide how many children they want without interference from governments or other organizations. Although there is consensus on the merit of improving the health of mothers, infants, and children, reproductive rights continue to be a controversial global health topic because they require frank discussions about sexual behaviors and gender inequities.

The International Conference on Population and Development (ICPD) was a United Nations (UN) meeting held in Cairo, Egypt, in 1994.[2] The Cairo Conference program of action emphasized reproductive rights.[3] This agenda raised concerns among a diversity of religious and social

3.1.1	Maternal mortality ratio (maternal deaths per 100,000 live births)
3.1.2	Proportion of births attended by skilled health personnel
3.7.1	Percentage of women of reproductive age (aged 15–49) who have their need for family planning satisfied with modern methods
3.7.2	Adolescent birth rate (aged 10–19) per 1,000 women in that age group
5.2.1	Proportion of ever-partnered women and girls aged 15 years and older subjected to physical, sexual, or psychological violence by a current or former intimate partner in the past 12 months
5.2.2	Proportion of women and girls aged 15 years and older subjected to sexual violence by persons other than an intimate partner in the past 12 months
5.3.1	Percentage of women aged 20–24 years who were married or in a union before age 15 and before age 18
5.3.2	Percentage of girls and women aged 15–49 years who have undergone female genital mutilation/cutting
5.6.1	Proportion of women aged 15–49 years who make their own informed decisions regarding sexual relations, contraceptive use, and reproductive health care
5.6.2	Number of countries with laws and regulations that guarantee full and equal access to women and men aged 15 years and older to sexual and reproductive health care, information, and education
11.7.2	Proportion of persons who were victims of physical or sexual harassment in the previous 12 months
16.1.3	Proportion of population subjected to physical violence, psychological violence, and sexual violence in the previous 12 months
16.2.2	Number of victims of human trafficking per 100,000 population
16.2.3	Percentage of young women and men aged 18–29 years who experienced sexual violence by age 18

Figure 11.1 Examples of Sustainable Development Goal indicators related to reproductive and sexual health.

Data from United Nations Economic and Social Council. *Report of the Inter-Agency and Expert Group on Sustainable Development Goal Indicators* (E/CN.3/2021/2). New York: United Nations; 2021.

groups, with the Roman Catholic Church especially vocal about its concerns related to the promotion of contraception and possible increases in the number of abortions.[4] The Beijing Platform for Action was the result of the UN Fourth World Conference on Women, held in China in 1995.[5] The Beijing Conference vigorously advocated for gender equality and women's empowerment.[6] The religious and political implications of linking reproductive health with women's rights made the action plans from both conferences contentious.[7] In the generation since those landmark UN conferences, significant progress has been made toward reducing the number of women who die in childbirth each year, increasing access to the tools for family planning, and protecting the rights of women. However, reproductive health remains a hot topic in global health because of the lack of unanimity about the promotion of contraceptive use, reproductive rights, and gender equity.

Maternal health programs support the health of women and adolescents during pregnancy, childbirth, and the weeks after delivery. **Maternal and child health** (MCH) is an area of public health practice that focuses on the health of mothers, infants, and children who are less than five years old. The primary goal of most MCH programs is helping babies and young children get their healthiest start in life. The maternal health components of MCH programs emphasize that the healthiest babies are born to women who were healthy before they conceived their offspring, had access to health services during pregnancy, and had skilled clinicians provide care during delivery and the postnatal period. Increased access to quality health services for pregnant people, new parents, and their babies has contributed to significant decreases in maternal, infant, and child mortality in recent years.

While some MCH programs are integrated with programs that equip women and their partners with the tools to prevent pregnancy,[8] few MCH programs and family planning clinics are designed to provide services related to infertility, gynecological and urological disorders, sexual dysfunction, prevention and treatment of sexually transmitted infections, reproductive cancers, prevention of gender-based violence, and other aspects of sexual and reproductive health.[9] Universal access to sexual and reproductive health will require comprehensive, affordable, culturally acceptable, high-quality services to become available to all adolescents and adults.[10] Increased funding will be required to meet the SDG targets for universal access to reproductive health care and reproductive rights by 2030.[11]

11.2 The Fertility Transition

Demography is the study of the size and composition of human populations. The **demographic transition** is a health transition characterized by changes in population size and composition that accompany a shift toward lower birth and death rates (**Figure 11.2**).[12]

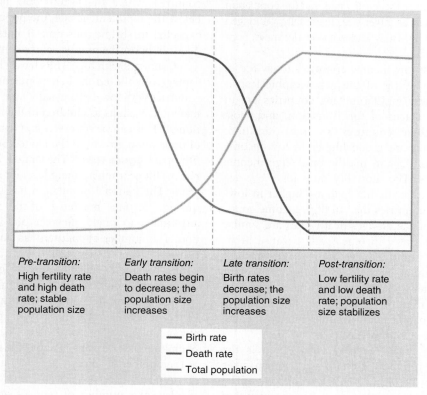

Pre-transition:
High fertility rate and high death rate; stable population size

Early transition:
Death rates begin to decrease; the population size increases

Late transition:
Birth rates decrease; the population size increases

Post-transition:
Low fertility rate and low death rate; population size stabilizes

—— Birth rate
—— Death rate
—— Total population

Figure 11.2 The fertility, mortality, and demographic transitions.

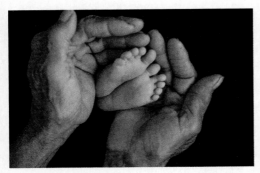

© DONOT6_STUDIO/Shutterstock

Pre-transition populations have high birth rates and high mortality rates, so they maintain stable but relatively small numbers of people. During the early stages of the demographic transition, the death rate decreases because of improvements in nutritional and health status, and the population size increases because the birth rate remains high. In later stages of the demographic transition, education, technology, economic growth, and other factors reduce the fertility rate, and the population stabilizes at its larger size. Eventually, prolonged low birth rates may lead to a slow decline in population size.

Most low-income countries today are in the early stages of the demographic transition, many middle-income countries are in the late stages of the transition, and most high-income countries are post-transition. Birth rates are much higher in low-income countries than in middle- and high-income countries. The mortality rates for every age group across the life span are higher in low-income countries than in high-income countries, but the all-ages death rates are similar across country income levels because high-income countries have a large percentage of older adults in their populations. Different birth rates and similar death rates mean that the rate of population growth is much higher in low-income countries than in high-income countries (**Figure 11.3**).[13]

The **total fertility rate** (TFR) is the average number of children a woman gives birth to during her childbearing years. The **fertility transition** is a health transition characterized by a reduction in the number of children born to the typical woman. The TFR has decreased significantly in recent decades in most countries, but TFRs remain higher in low-income countries than in high-income countries (**Figure 11.4**).[13]

A **replacement population** is a demographic pattern in which the average woman gives birth to two children, one to "replace" her in the next generation and one to "replace" her partner. (The replacement-level fertility rate is often considered to be a TFR of 2.1 rather than 2.0 to account for infant mortality.[14]) In populations with TFRs near 2, the population size will remain about the same from generation to generation if most children survive to adulthood. If the TFR is greater than 2, then the size of the population will increase over time. If the TFR is less than 2, the number of people in the total population will begin to decrease. In the upper-middle-income and high-income countries where the fertility rate has fallen below the replacement rate, the population is expected to shrink over time if immigration does not boost the number of residents.

Countries with high TFRs have a high percentage of children in their populations, and countries with low TFRs usually have about as many older adults as children in their populations.[13] This can be observed in a comparison of population growth in the United States and Ethiopia (**Figure 11.5**).[13] The United States has had a TFR near replacement level for about 50 years. The national population has increased during that time, but much of the growth is attributable to longer life spans and immigration. The number of children has stayed relatively stable over time, while the number of adults has increased substantially, especially the number of older adults. By contrast, Ethiopia's population has increased dramatically in recent decades, and most of this growth is attributable to a high birth rate. The number of children is increasing at about the same rate as the number of adults.

A **population pyramid** is a graphic that displays the number of females and males

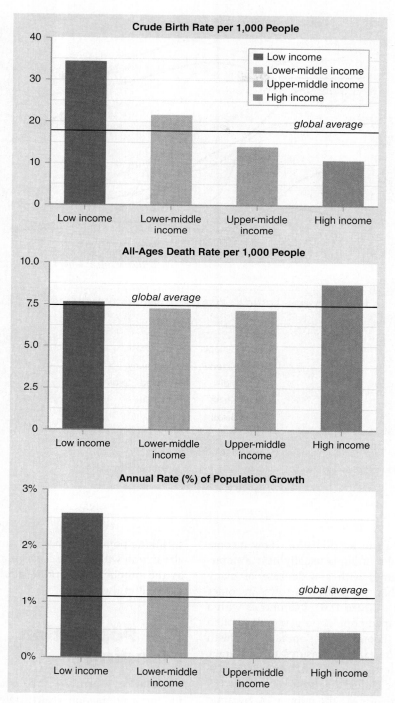

Figure 11.3 Birth rate per 1,000 people, crude (all-ages) death rate per 1,000 people, and annual rate of population growth in a typical recent year, by country income level.

Data from United Nations Department of Economic and Social Affairs. *World Population Prospects: The 2019 Revision.* New York: United Nations; 2019.

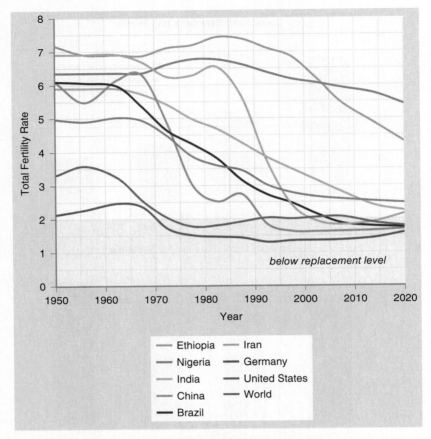

Figure 11.4 Total fertility rates over time in selected countries.

Data from United Nations Department of Economic and Social Affairs. *World Population Prospects: The 2019 Revision.* New York: United Nations; 2019.

by age group in a population. Low-income countries like Ethiopia usually have a population pyramid with a wide base of many children that gradually narrows in older age groups (**Figure 11.6**).[13] Countries with a triangle-shaped population pyramid are often concerned about high population growth rates and are taking measures to encourage decreased fertility rates. High-income countries like the United States often have low fertility rates that make the population pyramid look more like a cube. Some of these countries with narrow bases of few children face a

shrinking population size and are concerned about who will care for the aging population as the number of working adults for each older adult dwindles.

11.3 Population Planning

Population planning is the practice of promoting a population growth rate that aligns with a country's demographic goals. National population planning policies are intended to

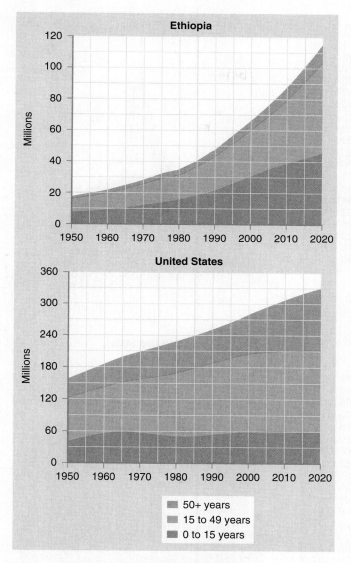

Figure 11.5 Population by age in Ethiopia and the United States, 1950–2020.

Data from United Nations Department of Economic and Social Affairs. *World Population Prospects: The 2019 Revision.* New York: United Nations; 2019.

enhance a country's future socioeconomic pro-file. Ideally, these governmental policies also help improve the health status of current and future infants and children, reproductive-age adults, older adults, families, and communi-ties.[15] Some nonprofit organizations and other groups that are concerned about how the growth of the global population may adversely affect planetary health, sustainable develop-ment, and women's rights also work to pro-mote lower fertility rates.[16]

The populations of most low- and lower-middle-income countries are expected to grow considerably during the next several

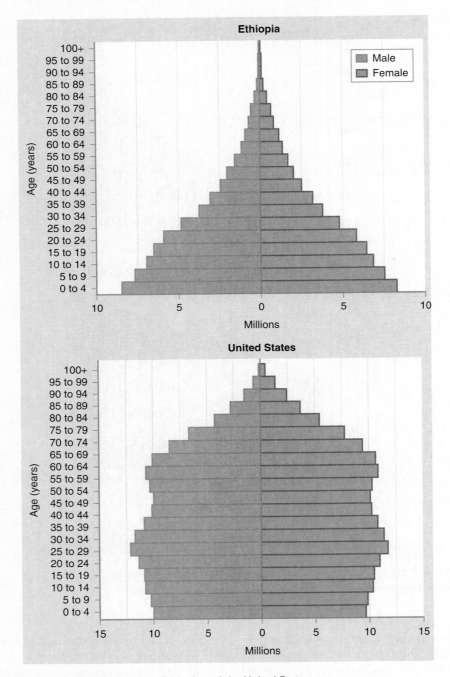

Figure 11.6 Population pyramids for Ethiopia and the United States.

Data from United Nations Department of Economic and Social Affairs. *World Population Prospects: The 2019 Revision.* New York: United Nations; 2019.

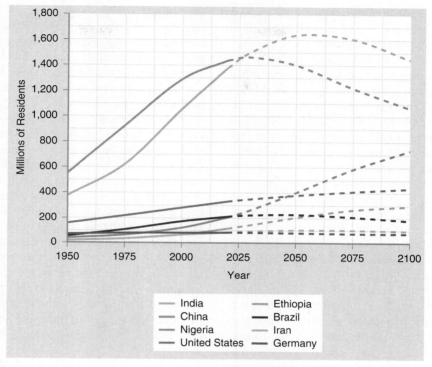

Figure 11.7 Projections of population growth in selected countries.

Data from United Nations Department of Economic and Social Affairs. *World Population Prospects: The 2019 Revision.* New York: United Nations; 2019.

decades (**Figure 11.7**).[13] Countries with high fertility rates usually provide direct government support for the distribution of family planning information and contraceptives.[17] Many high-fertility countries also promote female education as part of their population policies because women who complete more years of school typically have smaller families due to delayed marriage and first pregnancy; a desire to participate in the paid workforce; and the ability to read and act on information about health, nutrition, and child development.[18] Reductions in TFR in places where the fertility rate is well above the replacement level are usually associated with economic growth.[19]

Most upper-middle-income countries experienced significant population growth over the past few decades but have now transitioned to having fertility rates near replacement level. There is considerable diversity in how population policies in upper-middle-income countries are framed and implemented.[17] These are obvious in a comparison of Brazil, Iran, and China. Brazil has experienced a significant decrease in fertility rates with minimal governmental intervention.[20] Iran's aging population has led to the government's adoption of a pro-natalist agenda that actively promotes higher fertility rates through support for marriage at younger ages, financial incentives to have more children, and access to treatment for infertility.[21] By contrast, China has had very active government involvement in limiting population growth.

China's "late, long, few" policy in the 1970s encouraged delayed childbearing, longer spacing between children, and fewer children, and it cut the TFR in half.[22] China's one-child policy, adopted in 1979, used economic and educational incentives to promote one-child families, especially in urban areas. Because there were exemptions to the policy for rural residents, highly educated and wealthy parents, parents who were both only children, and some minority groups, the TFR by the mid-1990s was closer to 1.8 children rather than 1 child per couple, but this was sufficient to significantly slow population growth.[23] The program was controversial because of reports of forced abortions and sterilizations, infanticide (especially of females in rural areas), and other human rights abuses, even though these actions were contrary to the official policy.[24] Another concern was that the preference for sons over daughters and the availability of sex-selective abortions skewed male–female birth ratios.[25] The natural sex ratio at birth is about 1.05 males per female, but it was as high as 1.18 in China under the one-child policy.[26] By 2015, China had achieved what it deemed to be satisfactory population growth and fertility rates, and the one-child policy was replaced with a much less restrictive policy.[27] Within China, some concern has been expressed about the many families with a "one-two-four" structure, meaning only one young person to support two parents and four grandparents.[28] However, most young adults living in China today have a desire for small families, so the fertility rate is expected to remain below the replacement rate.[29]

Fertility rates in most high-income countries have remained below replacement level for more than a generation.[30] Countries with low fertility rates often promote fertility by covering the full medical costs of pregnancy, supporting lengthy paid leaves from work for new parents, offering tax incentives that encourage childbearing, and providing subsidies to offset childcare costs.[31] In countries that are concerned about the future economic burden of caring for aged populations, policies that promote increased fertility are often complemented by policies supporting increased immigration and older ages at retirement from the workforce.[32]

11.4 Family Planning

Family planning is a process by which adults make informed decisions about how many children they want to have, how many years apart they want those pregnancies to be, and the actions they will take to achieve these goals. Family planning programs target both women and men because household reproductive decisions should involve both partners and increased access to information about reproduction and contraception helps prevent unplanned pregnancies, unsafe abortions, and sexually transmitted infections (STIs).

Women and their babies are usually healthier when women have fewer pregnancies. Parents, babies, and children also benefit from **birth spacing**, waiting until at least two years after the birth of one child before conceiving the next child.[33] When the time between the birth of one baby and

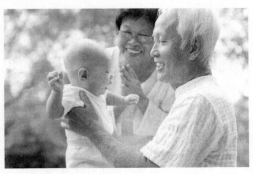

© Szefei/Shutterstock

the conception of the next one is short, the older baby is at risk of malnutrition because of being weaned from breast milk at a young age, and the younger baby has an increased risk of low birthweight and preterm birth.[34] Family planning also has social and economic benefits because the adults in families with fewer children have more years of productivity in the workforce and more resources available to invest in each child.[11]

There are several ways to report female reproductive history. **Gravidity** refers to the total number of times a woman has been pregnant, including miscarriages, abortions, stillbirths, and live births. A primigravida is a woman who is pregnant for the first time. A multigravida is a pregnant woman who has been pregnant before. **Fertility** is the total number of births, including live births and stillbirths. **Parity** refers

to the total number of live births. A nulliparous woman has had no previous live births. Because few miscarriages and abortions are reported to healthcare professionals, most global health reports use fertility to measure pregnancies in populations. The goal of family planning is to minimize unplanned pregnancies and maximize the health of babies from pregnancies that do occur so that parity is as close as possible to gravidity.[35]

Fertility rates are highest among women who are in their 20s and early 30s (**Figure 11.8**).[13] Adolescent fertility rates have been decreasing in most countries in recent decades, but they remain high in many low-income countries.[36] Adolescents who become pregnant have a higher risk than young adults of experiencing preterm delivery, low birthweight, and other

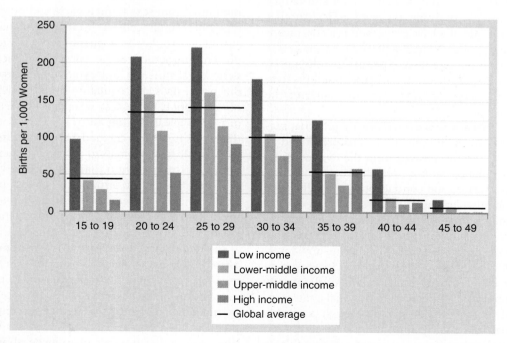

Figure 11.8 Age-specific fertility rates (births per 1,000 women per year) in typical recent years, by country income level.

Data from United Nations Department of Economic and Social Affairs. *World Population Prospects: The 2019 Revision.* New York: United Nations; 2019.

pregnancy complications.[37] Teen parents also experience long-term adverse economic disadvantages related to lower levels of education; reduced occupational opportunities; and the costs of providing food, housing, and other necessities for their offspring.[38] The adolescent fertility rate can be reduced with interventions that increase access to sexuality education, improve access to contraception, prevent early marriage, and reduce coerced sex.[39]

11.5 Contraception

Contraception is the intentional prevention of pregnancy. Modern contraceptive methods include barriers, medications, and surgery (**Figure 11.9**).[40] A **condom** is a thin sheath that is used as a physical barrier during sexual contact. Condoms prevent sperm from coming into contact with an egg after sexual contact and reduce the risk of some types of STIs. Another example of a barrier method is a contraceptive sponge, which is placed over the cervix prior to intercourse. Sponges are often used with spermicides to increase their effectiveness at preventing sperm from entering the uterus.

Oral contraceptives are pills that prevent ovulation when taken as prescribed so no eggs are released from the ovaries and a pregnancy cannot occur.[41] In many parts of the world, oral contraceptives are called the "family planning pill" in recognition of their importance for birth spacing. Oral contraceptive pills must be taken at about the same time every day, without skipping any doses, for this method to be effective. Some women prefer a longer-term method of pregnancy prevention and choose hormonal contraceptives that are delivered through a weekly patch, monthly injections, or vials placed under the skin of the upper arm that release medication for up to five years.

An **intrauterine device (IUD)** is a small T-shaped copper or plastic object that is placed in the womb to act as a contraceptive. IUDs prevent fertilization of eggs by creating a uterine environment that is unfavorable to sperm, which must pass through the uterus to reach unfertilized eggs.[42] IUDs may also inhibit the implantation of fertilized eggs in the endometrium that lines the uterus.

Permanent **sterilization** is the use of surgical or medical procedures to intentionally make it difficult or impossible for a person to reproduce. Tubal ligation surgery for females and vasectomies for males are sterilization procedures. Because only abstinence and condoms help to prevent the spread of STIs, sexually active people who have taken steps to permanently prevent pregnancy must still use methods to prevent contracting and spreading STIs.

Sexual **abstinence** is the practice of refraining from sexual intercourse and other types of genital contact. Complete sexual abstinence is the only guaranteed way to prevent pregnancy. Some couples practice periodic abstinence and avoid intercourse during the days after ovulation since the risk of conception is highest when an egg has just been released from an ovary. However, this is an imperfect method because it can be difficult for a woman to recognize when ovulation is imminent or has just occurred.

Abortion is the termination or loss of a pregnancy. A **miscarriage** is the spontaneous loss of a pregnancy prior to the fetal age of viability. A miscarriage is also called a **spontaneous abortion**. An **induced abortion** is a chemically or surgically terminated pregnancy. Induced abortions are not a form of contraception because they terminate a pregnancy rather than prevent pregnancy. Increased access to contraception reduces the number of induced abortions by preventing unplanned pregnancies.

Type	Approach	Approximate Pregnancy Rate in First Year of Typical Use	Protection Against STIs?	Notes
Complete abstinence	Abstinence	0%	Yes	No intercourse
Male sterilization (vasectomy)	Surgery	~0%	No	Permanent
Subdermal implant contraceptives	Hormones	~0%	No	Effective for about 3–5 years after implantation
Female sterilization (tubal ligation)	Surgery	<1%	No	Permanent
Intrauterine device (IUD)	IUD	<1%–2%	No	Effective for 5 or more years after insertion
Injection contraceptives	Hormones	<1%–3%	No	One injection every 1–3 months
Oral contraceptives	Hormones	8%	No	Pill must be taken daily to be effective
Transdermal (patch) contraceptives	Hormones	8%	No	The patch must be replaced weekly
Intravaginal (ring) contraceptives	Hormones	8%	No	The vaginal ring must be replaced monthly
Male condom	Barrier	15%	Yes	Must be used during every act of intercourse
Diaphragm or cervical cap with spermicide	Barrier 1 spermicide	20%	No	Must be used during every act of intercourse
Female condom	Barrier	21%	Some	Must be used during every act of intercourse
Spermicide alone	Spermicide	29%	No	Must be used during every act of intercourse
Periodic abstinence (methods based on fertility awareness)	Behavior	12%–25%	No	Requires daily monitoring of body functions and periods of abstinence
Withdrawal method	Behavior	27%	No	Must be used during every act of intercourse
No contraceptive method used	None	85%	No	

Figure 11.9 Contraceptive methods.

Data from Black KI, Gupta S, Rassi A, Kubba A. Why do women experience untimed pregnancies? A review of contraceptive failure rates. *Best Pract Res Clin Obstet Gynaecol.* 2010;24:443–455.

Worldwide, about 45% of reproductive-aged women (ages 15–49 years) are using a modern form of contraception (male or female sterilization, IUDs, oral contraceptive pills, injectable contraceptives, hormonal implants, condoms, or female barrier methods), about 4% are using a traditional form of family planning (such as periodic abstinence or use of medicinal plants), and about 11% would like to use contraception but are not using it.[43] In total, about 23% of reproductive-aged women who would like to use modern contraception are not using any modern contraceptive method, and the rate of unmet demand is higher in low-income countries (**Figure 11.10**).[43]

The goal of family planning programs is for all adolescents and adults who want to delay or prevent pregnancy to have access to modern forms of contraception. Family planning programs do not aim to have all women use contraception but rather to ensure access to those who want it. About 40% of reproductive-aged women do not want to use contraception. Women who are married or in partnerships are more likely than unpartnered women to use contraception because they are more likely to be having sex, but many partnered women are actively seeking to become pregnant and therefore make the decision not to use contraception (**Figure 11.11**).[43]

Most countries and communities now recognize the importance of all adults and adolescents, both males and females, understanding their options for contraception and family planning. The SDGs call for monitoring progress toward ensuring that all women of reproductive age have access to modern methods of family planning (SDG 3.7.1).[1] Although millions of people who would like to use modern forms of contraception still do not have access to family planning services, there are thousands of healthcare providers, governmental agencies, UN Population Fund (UNFPA) partners, Planned Parenthood affiliates, and other organizations seeking to provide information and supplies to adolescents and adults worldwide who want to make informed reproductive decisions. In addition to domestic government and out-of-pocket spending on family planning, billions of external dollars have been invested

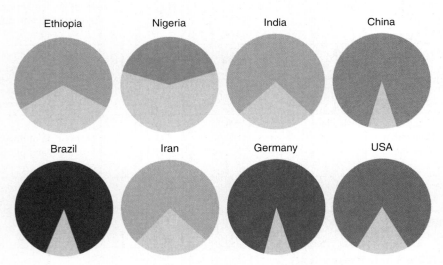

Figure 11.10 Percentage of all women aged 15–49 years who would like to limit or delay childbearing who are using modern contraception.

Data from *State of World Population 2021*. New York: United Nations Population Fund (UNFPA); 2021.

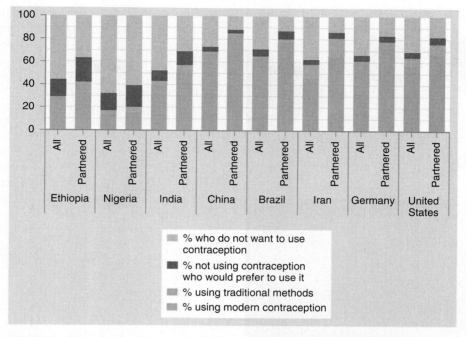

Figure 11.11 Percentage of all women and married/partnered women aged 15–49 years who are using modern contraception, traditional methods of contraception (such as periodic abstinence or use of medicinal plants), or no contraception.

Data from *State of World Population 2021*. New York: United Nations Population Fund (UNFPA); 2021.

in supporting family planning initiatives in low- and middle-income countries since 2000.[44]

11.6 Healthy Pregnancy

Safe motherhood programs promote maternal health from the months prior to conception through the postpartum period.[45] **Antenatal care** checkups, also called **prenatal care**, are routine preventive healthcare consultations during pregnancy that allow clinicians to identify and ameliorate potential health problems in a woman or fetus. These sessions are also times for clinicians to provide pregnant individuals and their partners with information about how to stay healthy, eat well, and recognize

potential pregnancy complications so they can be treated as soon as possible.[46] Women who have existing health concerns, those who have a high-risk pregnancy or have experienced complications in previous pregnancies, and those who are having twins or higher numbers of children may require additional prenatal services.

Several medical problems in the first trimester of pregnancy may require clinical treatment. **Hyperemesis gravidarum** is relentless nausea and vomiting during pregnancy that causes severe dehydration and significant weight loss.[47] An **ectopic pregnancy** occurs when a fertilized egg implants in a fallopian tube or another location outside the uterus. These nonviable pregnancies may cause severe internal bleeding, which can cause death if the affected woman does not have access to emergency surgery.[48] Miscarriages

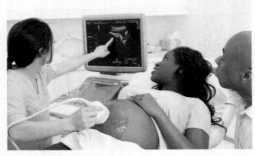

© Monkey Business Images/Shutterstock

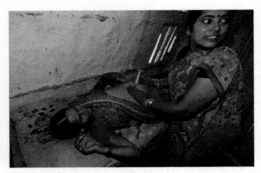

© Travel Stock/Shutterstock

may also cause hemorrhage or infection that requires surgical or medical treatment.

As a pregnancy progresses, women may require treatment for anemia, hypertension, gestational diabetes, and other conditions. Most women are able to safely continue their usual routines throughout pregnancy, but premature labor and other complications may require reduced activity levels. For example, placental issues like **placenta previa**, in which the placenta covers part or all of the cervix and causes bleeding, or **placental abruption**, in which the placenta separates from the uterine wall prior to delivery, may necessitate extended periods of bed rest or emergency delivery.

Elevated blood pressure can occur at any time during pregnancy. **Preeclampsia** is a combination of worsening hypertension in the final months of pregnancy along with the presence of protein in the urine. Pregnant women with severe preeclampsia may sustain kidney and liver damage. When the condition progresses to eclampsia, seizures occur,

and there is a risk of organ failure and death. The only cure for preeclampsia is delivery of the placenta.[49] Up to 5% of pregnant women develop preeclampsia,[50] and many of those pregnancies require preterm deliveries, which carry health risks for the babies but are necessary for the survival and health of the mother.

Childbirth occurs in three stages. The first stage is labor, when contractions dilate the cervix to about 10 centimeters in diameter. The second stage is the delivery of the neonate. The third stage is the delivery of the **placenta**, or afterbirth, which is the organ that lines the uterus during pregnancy and provides oxygen and nutrients to a fetus during fetal development. Complications can occur during any stage of labor. During the first stage, problems may arise from unsatisfactorily slow progress of labor. For example, prolonged labor may occur when the fetus is poorly positioned, such as being in a transverse or breech position rather than head down. During the second stage, fetal distress characterized by an unusually slow or fast fetal heart rate may occur, often as a result of the umbilical cord becoming compressed and cutting off the blood supply to the fetus. A birthing parent is at risk of severe tearing during delivery. During the third stage, there is a risk of excessive bleeding, which can lead to shock. Many of these complications are preventable or manageable with skilled clinical care.[51]

The need for medical care does not end with labor and delivery.[52] Postnatal care ensures that people who have given birth are recovering and their babies are healthy. Mothers and newborns should be carefully monitored in the hours after parturition and clinically examined several weeks later to check for problems.

When complications occur during or after pregnancy, it is important for women and newborns to have access to skilled care. A **skilled birth attendant** (SBA) is an obstetrician or gynecologist, another type of physician, a midwife, a nurse, or another licensed clinician who is proficient in recognizing and treating potential complications of

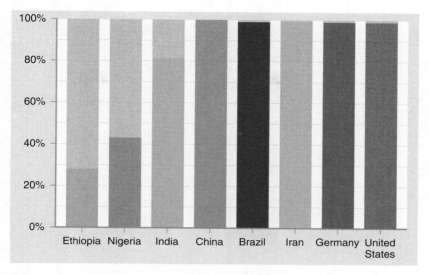

Figure 11.12 Percentage of births attended by skilled health personnel.

Data from *State of World Population 2021*. New York: United Nations Population Fund (UNFPA); 2021.

women and newborns during and after labor and delivery.[53] (In some countries, midwives train as nurses first and then complete extra training to become nurse-midwives; in other countries, midwifery is a direct-entry clinical field that requires several years of formal education and training.[54]) About 80% of births are now attended by SBAs, including nearly 100% of deliveries in higher-income countries but only about 60% of births in low-income countries (**Figure 11.12**).[43] A **traditional birth attendant** (TBA) is a lay midwife who has been trained through an apprenticeship rather than a formal educational program. A TBA may be able to handle uncomplicated births but does not have the advanced training to safely manage complications.[55]

11.7 Maternal Mortality

Maternal mortality is the death of a woman from a pregnancy-related cause during pregnancy, childbirth, or the six weeks after delivery. Most maternal deaths occur in lower-income countries (**Figure 11.13**).[56] There are significant variations in the per-pregnancy and lifetime risk of pregnancy-related mortality between countries and also within many countries, with higher-income women experiencing lower mortality rates than lower-income women.[57] The number of maternal deaths per year dropped from more than 500,000 women in 1990 to about 300,000 in 2015, but the number remained far higher than it should be given that most of those deaths were preventable.[58]

For many pregnant adolescents and adults, the hours of labor and delivery are precarious ones. Without timely access to obstetric services, pregnancy and delivery complications can cause a rapid death or lead to permanent disabilities. For example, **obstructed labor** is an obstetric complication that occurs when the unborn baby is wedged so tightly into the birth canal that blood flow to surrounding tissues is cut off and the tissues start to die. Women who do not have access to surgery may be in labor for several days. If a woman survives obstructed labor, the outcome is often the formation of an **obstetric fistula**, a hole between the rectum or bladder and the vagina that constantly leaks urine or feces. Because of the odor, most women with an obstetric fistula

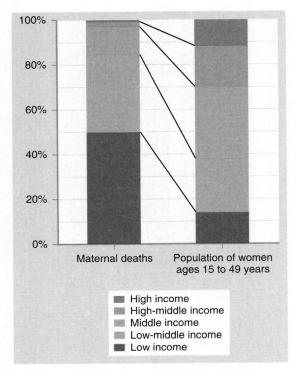

Figure 11.13 Distribution of maternal deaths, by country sociodemographic index.

Data from GBD 2019 Diseases and Injuries Collaborators. Global burden of 369 diseases and injuries in 204 countries and territories, 1990–2019: a systematic analysis for the Global Burden of Disease Study 2019. *Lancet*. 2020;396:1204–1222; GBD 2019 Demographics Collaborators. Global age-sex-specific fertility, mortality, health life expectancy (HALE), and population estimates in 204 countries and territories, 1950–2019: a comprehensive demographic analysis for the Global Burden of Disease Study 2019. *Lancet*. 2020;396:1160–1203.

are ostracized by their communities. Some women are left paralyzed because of nerve damage, and many are left infertile. In nearly all of these cases, the baby is stillborn. More than 1 million women worldwide may be living with an obstetric fistula.[59] Fistulas can be surgically corrected, but the better option is preventing obstructed labor by delaying pregnancy until females are fully grown and ensuring access to medical professionals during delivery if help is needed.

The most frequent causes of maternal mortality include hemorrhage, eclampsia and other types of maternal hypertension, and sepsis (**Figure 11.14**).[56] **Postpartum hemorrhage** is severe bleeding within several hours after giving birth, usually caused by uterine atony (failure of the uterine muscle to contract) or by retained placental tissue, trauma, or clotting problems. Eclampsia involves dangerously elevated high blood pressure. **Sepsis**, sometimes called "blood poisoning," is widespread inflammation in the body that is triggered by the chemicals released by the body's immune system in response to an infection and can lead to organ failure, shock, and death.[60]

Postpartum hemorrhage can often be prevented through the active management of the third stage of labor.[61] Active management previously consisted of three actions: (1) injecting **oxytocin**, a hormone that strengthens uterine contractions during labor and delivery and then helps control postpartum bleeding, into the mother's thigh immediately after delivery; (2) controlled cord traction until the delivery of the placenta; and

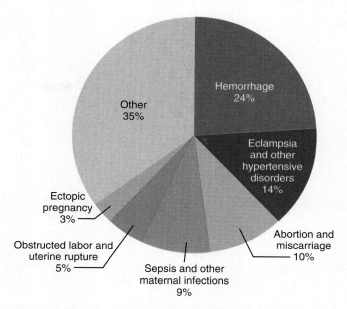

Figure 11.14 Causes of maternal mortality worldwide.

Data from GBD 2019 Diseases and Injuries Collaborators. Global burden of 369 diseases and injuries in 204 countries and territories, 1990–2019: a systematic analysis for the Global Burden of Disease Study 2019. *Lancet.* 2020;396:1204–1222.

(3) uterine massage after the delivery of the placenta to help the uterus contract. Newer protocols emphasize the importance of oxytocin or other uterotonics,[62] but suggest that controlled cord traction be performed only by skilled clinicians and that uterine massage be used only when the uterus is not contracting normally.[63]

The **perinatal period** extends from about 22 weeks of gestation through seven days after a live birth.[64] **Emergency obstetric and newborn care (EmONC)** is a core set of actions that can save the lives of women and neonates during the perinatal period. A basic EmONC (BEmONC) facility can perform seven "signal functions"[65]:

1. providing intravenous or injected antibiotics
2. providing anticonvulsants
3. providing uterotonic drugs to help the uterus contract after delivery
4. using forceps or vacuum extraction to assist with delivery
5. removing the placenta manually

6. removing retained products of conception using tools
7. performing neonatal resuscitation using a bag and mask

A comprehensive EmONC (CEmONC) facility can consistently implement all of the basic functions as well as (8) providing blood transfusions and (9) performing cesarean sections.

A **cesarean section**, often shortened to just "C-section," is the surgical delivery of a neonate through an incision in the mother's abdomen and uterus. A C-section rate of about 10%, and no more than 15%, is associated with the lowest maternal death rate.[66] The percentage of babies worldwide who are born by C-section increased from about 5% in 1990 to about 20% by 2020.[67] There is wide variation in national rates today. Only about 2% of babies in Ethiopia are delivered by C-section, while about 55% of babies in Brazil are (**Figure 11.15**).[68] The very low C-section rates in many lower-income countries raise concerns about the lack of access to advanced obstetric care leading to

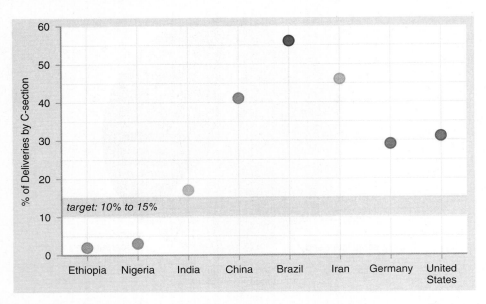

Figure 11.15 Percentage of babies delivered by cesarean section in a typical recent year. The target range is about 10%–15%.

Data from *State of the World's Children 2019*. New York: UNICEF; 2019.

the unnecessary deaths of women and babies.[69] The very high C-section rates in some middle- and high-income countries are evidence that many unnecessary surgeries are being performed.[70] Besides the short-term risks associated with surgical procedures and use of anesthesia, women who have had C-sections have an increased risk of placental problems, hemorrhage, uterine rupture, and other complications in subsequent pregnancies.[71]

The **maternal mortality ratio (MMR)** is the number of women who die of pregnancy-related causes per 100,000 live births. The **obstetric transition** is a health transition characterized by a shift from a high maternal mortality ratio to a very low ratio that typically occurs with socioeconomic development.[72] The low rate of maternal death in high-income countries is evidence that most maternal deaths in low-income countries could be prevented with currently available interventions (**Figure 11.16**). Increasing access to contraception for women who want to plan their families but do not currently have the tools to do so will help lower the MMR[73] by reducing the rate of unintended and

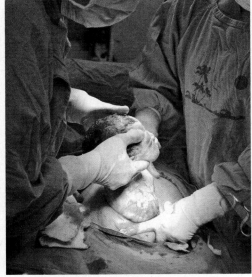

A cesarean section delivery.

© ARZTSAMUI/Shutterstock

high-risk pregnancies that might lead to unsafe abortions or serious pregnancy complications.[74] Increased access to prenatal care, assisted delivery, and postnatal care after the birth are also critical for improving maternal survival.

Level of Prevention	Primordial Prevention	Primary Prevention	Secondary Prevention	Tertiary Prevention
Goal	Prevent risk factors for maternal mortality	Mitigate risk factors during pregnancy	Detect pregnancy complications early	Manage pregnancy complications
Examples of interventions	■ Use contraceptive methods to prevent or space pregnancies ■ Eat nutritious foods	■ Treat anemia and other nutrient deficiencies ■ Manage hypertension, diabetes, and other health issues ■ Treat malaria, syphilis, and other infections ■ Vaccinate against tetanus and other infections as appropriate	■ Access routine prenatal care ■ Screen for preeclampsia ■ Have a skilled birth attendant ■ Use uterotonics after delivery to prevent postpartum hemorrhage	■ Treat complications with medications, surgery, blood transfusions, and other therapies

Figure 11.16 Examples of interventions for maternal survival.

One of the Millennium Development Goals (MDGs) was to reduce the global MMR by 75% between 1990 and 2015.[75] The MMR decreased from about 385 per 100,000 live births worldwide in 1990 to about 220 per 100,000 in 2015, but that 45% decrease fell short of the MDG target (**Figure 11.17**).[58] The SDGs aim to reduce the MMR to fewer than 70 deaths per 100,000 live births (SDG 3.1).[1] Higher-income countries already have rates that are lower than the SDG target, but most lower-income countries have rates that are above the SDG target (**Figure 11.18**).[76] The Ending Preventable Maternal Mortality initiative, led by UNFPA and the WHO, has established five milestones that if reached would indicate progress toward achieving the SDG target: (1) at least 90% of pregnant women have four or more antenatal care visits, (2) at least 90% of births are attended by skilled health personnel, (3) at least 80% of women receive routine postnatal care within two days of delivery, (4) at least 60% of people can access EmONC health facilities within two hours of travel time, and (5) at least 65% of women are able to access the information and services they need to make informed and empowered decisions about their own reproductive and sexual health.[77]

11.8 Stillbirths and Neonatal Mortality

About 140 million babies are born each year, and the vast majority of these babies are born healthy.[13] However, not all pregnancies result in

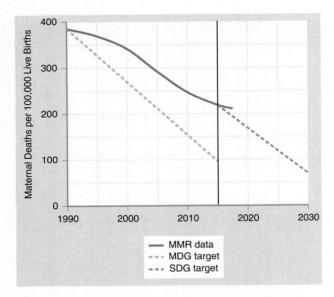

Figure 11.17 Progress toward achieving Millennium Development Goal (MDG) and Sustainable Development Goal (SDG) targets for the maternal mortality ratio (MMR) per 100,000 live births.

Data from *Trends in Maternal Mortality, 1990 to 2015: Estimates by WHO, UNICEF, UNFPA, World Bank Group and the United Nations Population Division.* Geneva: World Health Organization; 2015; *Trends in Maternal Mortality 2000 to 2017: Estimates by WHO, UNICEF, UNFPA, World Bank Group and the United Nations Population Division.* Geneva: World Health Organization; 2019.

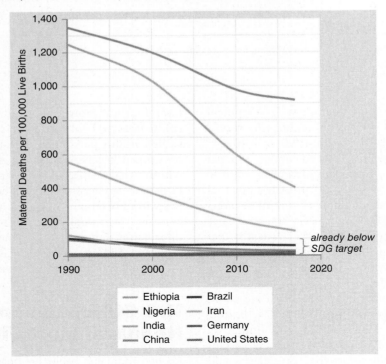

Figure 11.18 The maternal mortality ratio (MMR) per 100,000 live births in selected countries.

Data from *Trends in Maternal Mortality, 1990 to 2015: Estimates by WHO, UNICEF, UNFPA, World Bank Group and the United Nations Population Division.* Geneva: World Health Organization; 2015; *Trends In Maternal Mortality 2000 to 2017: Estimates by WHO, UNICEF, UNFPA, World Bank Group and the United Nations Population Division.* Geneva: World Health Organization; 2019.

a live birth and a healthy newborn. A **stillbirth** is the death of a fetus late in pregnancy but prior to delivery, typically defined as occurring after the 28th week of gestation and after the fetus already weighs at least 2.2 pounds (1,000 grams).[78] Maternal infections, trauma, congenital abnormalities, umbilical cord and placental problems, uterine problems, and birth trauma cause some stillbirths, but there is often no identifiable reason for the stillbirth.[79]

In 2020, there were an estimated 14 stillbirths for every 1,000 total births after the 28th week of gestation, and the national stillbirth rate (SBR) ranged from 1 per 1,000 in some high-income countries to 32 per 1,000 in some low-income countries (**Figure 11.19**).[80] The global SBR in 2019 was 35% lower than the estimated 21 per 1,000 in 2000,[80] but it was above the Every Newborn Action Plan (ENAP) target of every country achieving an SBR of no more than 12 per 1,000 by 2030.[81] The estimated number of stillbirths per year decreased from at least 2.5 million in 2000 to about 2.0 million in 2019, and the ENAP target is to have fewer than 1.2 million stillbirths annually by 2030.[80]

A **neonate** is a newborn within his or her first 28 days (four weeks) after a live birth. The major causes of neonatal mortality include preterm delivery, birth traumas such as asphyxia,

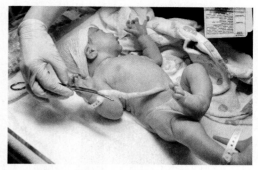
© Paul Hakimata Photography/Shutterstock

and infections.[56] Some babies are born extremely prematurely, experience severe birth trauma, or have congenital abnormalities that are incompatible with survival. These newborns may live for only a few minutes or hours after birth. About 2.5 million neonatal deaths occurred annually in recent years, and nearly 2 million of those deaths occurred within the first week after birth.[56] **Perinatal mortality** encompasses stillbirths and deaths within the first seven days (one week) after a live birth. As of 2020, about 4 million perinatal deaths—about 2 million stillbirths plus 2 million early neonatal deaths—were occurring each year.

A typical pregnancy is about 40 weeks long. **Preterm birth** is the delivery of a baby before the 37th week of pregnancy. About 10%

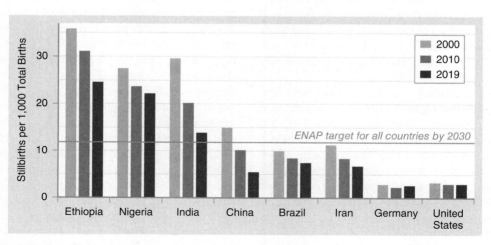

Figure 11.19 Stillbirths per 1,000 total births in selected countries.

Data from *A Neglected Tragedy: The Global Burden of Stillbirths: Report of the UN Inter-agency Group for Child Mortality Estimation, 2020.* New York: United Nations Inter-agency Group for Child Mortality Estimation; 2020.

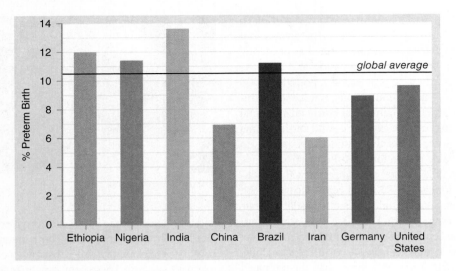

Figure 11.20 Preterm birth rate per 100 live births.

Data from Chawanpaiboon S, Vogel JP, Moller AB, et al. Global, regional, and national estimates of levels of preterm birth in 2014: a systematic analysis and modelling analysis. *Lancet Glob Health*. 2019;7:e37–e46.

of babies are born prematurely (**Figure 11.20**).[82] Each year, about 15 million preterm babies are born, and more than 1 million of those preterm babies die at a young age from complications associated with being born too soon.[83] Survivors, especially those born very or extremely prematurely, may have long-term special needs related to learning disabilities, visual impairment, and other neurodevelopmental problems.[84] Most cases of preterm birth are spontaneous, rather than being induced because of preeclampsia or other threats to the health of the mother or baby.[85] The causal factors for many of these spontaneous early deliveries remain poorly understood.[86]

Most babies who are born too early have **low birthweight** (LBW), which is defined as a birthweight of less than 5.5 pounds (2,500 grams). LBW can also occur in full-term babies, often as a result of their mothers being undernourished when they became pregnant and not taking in adequate nutrients during pregnancy.[87] The overall prevalence of LBW decreased from about 17.5% in 2000 to 14.6% in 2015, but the rate of improvement was not on track to meet the WHO/UNICEF target of reducing the prevalence to 10.5% by 2025 (**Figure 11.21**).[88] Rates

of LBW are highest in lower-income countries, especially in southern Asia.[89] Many babies with LBW develop typically, but those with very low weights at birth have an increased risk of neurodevelopmental difficulties, vulnerability to infections and other illnesses, and poor growth during infancy and childhood.[90]

Some newborns sustain injuries during the birthing process. **Birth asphyxia** is a birth complication that occurs when a newborn fails to take a first breath immediately after delivery and is therefore deprived of oxygen. Neonatal resuscitation can save the lives of some of these babies,[91] but they may have permanent brain damage because of the hypoxia. Some newborns suffer birth traumas like bruising, fractures, and nerve damage as a result of the physical pressures exerted on their bodies during delivery. For example, a brachial plexus injury to the nerves of the shoulder, arm, and hand can occur when shoulder dystocia occurs because a baby's shoulder is wedged behind the mother's pubic bone during delivery.[92] About 1 in 400 newborns has **cerebral palsy** (CP), a neuromuscular disorder that is associated with birth trauma (and with very low birthweight) and is characterized by permanent difficulties

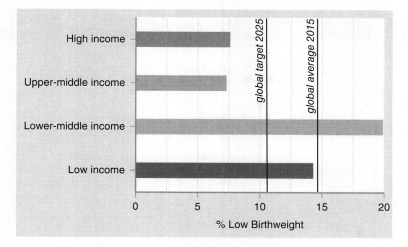

Figure 11.21 Percentage of newborns with low birthweight (less than 2,500 grams at birth) in 2015 (14.6%) and target for 2025 (10.5%).

Data from *UNICEF-WHO Low Birthweight Estimates: Levels and Trends 2000–2015*. Geneva: World Health Organization; 2019.

with movement, balance, and posture.[93] While many of the symptoms of CP are permanent, they typically do not get worse over time. Physical therapy, occupational therapy, speech therapy, and other forms of habilitation therapy can improve physical performance, mobility, and communication for children with CP.[94]

A variety of infectious diseases can be fatal for newborns, including neonatal sepsis, which can be caused by several pathogens, including group B *Streptococcus* and *Staphylococcus*,[95] as well as pneumonia, diarrhea, and neonatal tetanus.[96] The word **tetanus** means sustained muscle contraction. Neonatal tetanus occurs when a neurotoxin from the bacterium *Clostridium tetani* causes painful muscle spasms in a neonate, starting as lockjaw, which interferes with feeding, and eventually affecting the full body and posing a significant risk of death.[97] Tetanus is a risk when babies are born in unclean environments, such as homes with dirt floors, which allow the umbilical cord to come into contact with soil that might contain tetanus spores. Maternal immunization with tetanus toxoid prior to delivery protects both pregnant people and newborns.

Neonatal deaths currently account for nearly half of all under-5 child mortality,[56] so neonatal survival interventions are critical for improving overall child survival rates (**Figure 11.22**). Neonatal survival begins with universal access to prenatal care and intrapartum care provided by skilled birth attendants.[98] After birth, routine care for newborns includes keeping them warm, breastfeeding them at regular intervals starting soon after birth, and preventing infections through handwashing and hygienic cord care.[99] Babies with breathing difficulties, signs of infection, yellow skin suggesting jaundice, or other problems require clinical treatment.[100] The best outcomes for preterm births and LBW babies occur when the neonate has access to thermal care to keep the body temperature warm, assistance with consumption of breast milk, prevention of infections through careful hygiene and appropriate use of antiseptics, and safe use of supplemental oxygen.[83] Babies in high-income countries usually have access to well-equipped neonatal intensive care units in hospitals. In resource-limited settings, the survival of preterm babies is enhanced by the use of kangaroo mother care, which consists of skin-to-skin contact between a parent and newborn, frequent breastfeeding, and early discharge from the hospital to reduce the risk of infection.[101]

Level of Prevention	Primordial Prevention	Primary Prevention	Secondary Prevention	Tertiary Prevention
Goal	Prevent risk factors for neonatal mortality	Mitigate risk factors among neonates	Detect neonatal complications early	Manage neonatal complications
Examples of interventions	■ Support healthy pregnancies and maternal nutrition, including supplemental folic acid and iron ■ Maintain good hygiene and environmental cleanliness	■ Use skilled birth attendants ■ Keep neonates warm, clean, and dry ■ Initiate early breastfeeding ■ Maintain cord care and other types of hygiene	■ Monitor and assess health status often ■ Detect infections and birth injuries early	■ Manage breathing difficulties, jaundice, sepsis, trauma, and other health problems

Figure 11.22 Examples of interventions for neonatal survival.

11.9 Infertility

Infertility is the inability to achieve a pregnancy when sexually active and not using contraception or the inability to maintain a pregnancy through to a live birth. Male infertility may be caused by congenital abnormalities, injuries, infections, endocrine disorders, or genetics, but in about half of clinically treated cases there is no identifiable cause for low levels of sperm, abnormalities with sperm shape and motility, or problems with the ejection of semen.[102] Female infertility may be associated with blocked fallopian tubes (which may be the result of untreated STIs), uterine and ovarian disorders (such as fibroids or polycystic ovaries), endocrine disorders, and other conditions.[103] More than 50 million couples worldwide with a female partner of childbearing age have been unable to have a child after five years of attempting to become pregnant.[104]

Primary infertility is infertility in someone who has never achieved a live birth, and it is usually diagnosed when conception does not occur within a year of attempting to become pregnant. **Secondary infertility** is the inability to have additional offspring when attempting to conceive after giving birth. About 2% of women who are 20–44 years old have primary infertility after 5 years of attempting to conceive, and about 10.5% of women who have had a live birth have secondary infertility.[105] Infertility rates tend to be highest in the places with the highest fertility rates because many cases of secondary infertility are attributable to complications from prior pregnancies.[106]

Treatments for infertility include the use of medications to stimulate egg production, surgery to remove fibroids in the uterus and blockages in the fallopian tubes, medication and surgery to improve male reproductive function, and procedures like intrauterine insemination.[107] **Assisted reproductive technologies** (ART) are fertility treatments that handle eggs or embryos. The most often used form of ART is **in vitro fertilization**

(IVF) in which a woman's eggs are extracted from her ovaries, fertilized with sperm in a laboratory setting, and then the resulting embryos are transferred to the uterus. However, ART is costly even in high-income countries, and it is not widely available to residents of lower-income countries.

Infertility can adversely affect mental and social health. People experiencing infertility may develop depression and anxiety, be excluded from social activities with their families and communities, and face steep economic burdens associated with the costs of fertility treatments; in some communities, people with infertility, especially women, are subjected to violence, divorce, and poverty as a result of not having biological offspring.[108] Treatment for infertility is a low priority for healthcare systems in countries with high birth rates. Lack of access to infertility treatment may exacerbate the ostracism of women without children who live in communities where having numerous children is the cultural norm.[106]

11.10 Gynecological Health

Menstruation is the shedding of the lining of the uterus (the endometrium) that occurs approximately monthly for most nonpregnant females of childbearing age. **Menarche** is the first menstrual period. A century ago, the average age at menarche was about 14.5 years; today, the average age at menarche is about 12.5 years.[109] The reason for the apparent shift toward earlier menarche is not well understood.[110] **Menopause** is the cessation of menstruation. Natural menopause occurs when a formerly menstruating adult goes 12 months without having a period and the cessation of menses was not due to medical or surgical interventions (such as cancer treatments or a hysterectomy). The average age at menopause is about 51 years,[111] but healthy women experience menopause during a wide range of ages (approximately 45 to 55 years).[112] Menopause is typically preceded by several years of perimenopause, which may be accompanied by hot flashes, night sweats, and other signs of hormonal changes.[113]

Many individuals who menstruate experience abdominal cramps, back pain, headaches, bloating, mood swings, and other types of discomfort at various stages of the menstrual cycle. Premenstrual syndrome (PMS), which when severe may be termed premenstrual dysphoric disorder (PMDD), is present when the physical and emotional effects of hormonal changes during a menstrual cycle are severe enough to interfere with usual daily activities.[114] Even if PMS or PMDD is not experienced, periods can interfere with the ability to attend school, go to work, and participate in community events. For example, students who do not have access to menstrual hygiene products, sanitation facilities, privacy, and time for hygiene during the school day may miss several days of school every month or even drop out of school due to concerns about dignity, safety, and comfort.[115] The stigma associated with menstruation in most cultures means that many girls are not prepared for their first periods, many people with irregular periods and PMDD do not seek medical help for them, and many individuals experience "period poverty" because they are not able to access menstrual hygiene products because of their cost or the embarrassment or shame they feel when purchasing them.[116]

Female reproductive health is about much more than pregnancy care. Uterine fibroids, endometriosis, polycystic ovary syndrome (PCOS), and genital prolapse are frequently occurring gynecological disorders that can reduce the quality of life.[56] **Fibroids** are benign tumors (leiomyomas) in the uterus that can cause heavy bleeding and pelvic pain.[117] **Endometriosis** is a condition in which some of the tissue that lines the uterus is located on the ovaries or in other parts of the abdominal cavity. That tissue bleeds with each menstrual cycle, often causing pain and resulting in the formation of scar tissue and adhesions.[118] PCOS is a hormonal disorder (hyperandrogenism) that is characterized by irregular menstrual cycles, hirsutism (excess hair on the face), acne, and weight gain.[119] Genital prolapse occurs when the reproductive organs are displaced from their usual locations in the pelvis due to weak or damaged connective tissues, and it often causes urinary incontinence.[120] Females are also at risk of a diversity of cancers of the reproductive system, including breast cancer, cervical cancer, uterine (endometrial) cancer, and ovarian cancer as well as STIs, benign breast diseases that cause pain or discomfort, sexual dysfunction, and gender-based violence.

11.11 Men's Reproductive Health

Males may experience a variety of health issues related to reproduction and sexual function, including infertility, STIs, injuries, and cancers of the reproductive system. Testicular cancer occurs very infrequently, but the incidence rate is higher among younger men than older men.[121] For older men, prostate health often becomes a significant health concern. **Benign prostatic hyperplasia** (BPH) is an enlargement of the prostate gland that may cause difficulty with urination and sexual performance, and the prevalence of BPH is very high among older men.[122] Many men develop prostate cancer as they age, and treatments for prostate cancer may cause urinary incontinence and erectile dysfunction (ED).[123] ED may also occur as a result of neurological conditions, diabetes, hypertension, cardiovascular disease, some types of medications, trauma, and a variety of other exposures and aging-related physiological conditions.[124] Medications, lifestyle changes, stress management, and other tools may be helpful for treating ED.[125] Reproductive health clinics usually focus on women's care, and men may have more difficulty than women in accessing specialty care for their reproductive and sexual health problems.[126]

11.12 Sexual Minority Health

Members of sexual and gender minority groups often have difficulty accessing high-quality health services. One of the steps toward improving access to health services is making sure that health and social service workers understand the various aspects of sexuality and gender and use appropriate terms when working with clients.[127]

Sexual orientation is a function of an individual's sexual attraction, identity, and behavior. Sexual attraction is about the type of person an individual desires sexually, romantically, emotionally, and in other ways. Heterosexual individuals are sexually attracted to people of the opposite gender, homosexual individuals are attracted to people of the same gender, bisexual individuals are attracted to people of multiple genders, pansexual individuals are attracted to people of all genders, asexual individuals experience little sexual attraction to people of any gender, and some people use other terms to describe their sexual and romantic attractions. Sexual identity is about how people perceive their sexual and romantic attractions and how they present their sexuality to others, with some people being very private about their sexual identity and others very open.

Sexual behavior is about the sexual actions in which a person engages. Some people choose to be celibate. Some people engage in sexual activities that do not align with their sexual attraction or identity. People with opposite-gender attractions may be involved in homosexual relationships, and people with same-gender attractions may be involved in heterosexual relationships. For example, the term **MSM** is a classification that emphasizes sexual behavior rather than sexual identity by encompassing all **m**en who have **s**ex with **m**en.

Some MSM identify as homosexual, some identify as bisexual, and some identify as heterosexual and are happily married to women even though they also have sex with men.

Terms related to sexual orientation are in a different domain than terms related to **gender identity**, which is an individual's sense of maleness or femaleness. **Cisgender** describes a person whose gender identity aligns with the sex assigned to that individual at birth, and **transgender** describes a person whose gender identity does not match the sex assigned at birth. Individuals who identify as nonbinary or genderfluid do not identify exclusively with one gender. The acronym LGBT—short for lesbian, gay, bisexual, and transgender—mixes terms about sexual orientation and gender identity. So do longer acronyms such as LGBTQ+ (which adds a Q for queer and a plus to represent others) and LGBTQIA (which adds terms for questioning, intersex, and asexual).

Members of LGBTQ+ populations often experience stigma and discrimination, including in healthcare settings.[128]

Transgender individuals have a higher than typical risk of STIs, substance abuse, mental health disorders related to chronic stress, and injuries from violence.[129] Similarly elevated risks have been observed in sexual minority populations.[130] While some countries have enacted laws that protect the human rights of LGBTQ+ people and ensure equitable access to health services, other countries are moving in the opposite direction by codifying laws that discriminate against LGBTQ+ people and make it dangerous for LGBTQ+ individuals to seek medical care or be honest with their clinicians about their health needs.[131]

Achieving the SDGs will require all adolescents and adults to have equitable access to health services (SDG 3.8), including reproductive health services (SDG 3.7), as well as having social, economic, and political inclusion (SDG 10.2) and freedom from violence (SDG 16.1).[1] The SDGs cannot be achieved when sexual and gender majority and minority populations do not have equal access to health and safety.

References

1. *Transforming Our World: The 2030 Agenda for Sustainable Development.* New York: United Nations; 2015.
2. McIntosh CA, Finkle JL. The Cairo Conference on Population and development: a new paradigm? *Popul Dev Rev.* 1995;21:223–260.
3. *International Conference on Population and Development Program of Action: 20th anniversary edition.* New York: United Nations Population Fund (UNFPA); 2014.
4. *Religion, Women's Health and Rights: Points of Contention and Paths of Opportunities.* New York: United Nations Population Fund (UNFPA); 2016.
5. Cook RJ, Fathalla MF. Advancing reproductive rights beyond Cairo and Beijing. *Int Family Plann Perspect.* 1996;22:115–121.
6. *The Beijing Declaration and Platform for Action Turns 20.* New York: UN Women; 2015.
7. *Reproductive Rights Are Human Rights: A Handbook for National Human Rights Institutions.* New York: United Nations Population Fund (UNFPA); 2014.
8. Ringheim K, Gribble J, Foreman M. *Integrating Family Planning and Maternal and Child Health Care: Saving Lives, Money, and Time.* Washington DC: Population Reference Bureau; 2011.
9. *Sexual Health and Its Linkages to Reproductive Health: An Operational Approach.* Geneva: World Health Organization; 2017.
10. Starrs AM, Ezeh AC, Barker G, et al. Accelerate progress: sexual and reproductive health and rights for all: report of the Guttmacher-Lancet Commission. *Lancet.* 2018;391:2642–2692.
11. Stenberg K, Sweeny K, Axelson H, Temmerman M, Sheehan P. Returns on investment in the continuum of care for reproductive, maternal, newborn, and

child health (chapter 16). In: Black RE, Laxminarayan R, Temmerman M, Walker N, eds. *Disease Control Priorities: Reproductive, Maternal, Newborn, and Child Health*. 3rd ed. Vol. 2. Washington DC: IBRD/World Bank; 2016:299–318.

12. Kirk D. Demographic transition theory. *Popul Studies*. 1996;50:361–387.

13. United Nations Department of Economic and Social Affairs. *World Population Prospects: The 2019 Revision*. New York: United Nations; 2019.

14. Espenshade TJ, Guzman JC, Westoff CF. The surprising variation in replacement fertility. *Popul Res Pol Rev*. 2003;22:575–583.

15. Ezeh AC, Bongaarts J, Mberu B. Global population trends and policy options. *Lancet*. 2012;380: 142–148.

16. Bhatia R, Sasser JS, Ojeda D, Hendrixson A, Nadimpally S, Foley EE. A feminist exploration of 'populationism': engaging contemporary forms of population control. *Gender Place Culture*. 2020;27:333–350.

17. United Nations Department of Economic and Social Affairs. *World Population Policies 2013*. New York: United Nations; 2013.

18. Upadhyay UD, Gipson JD, Withers M, et al. Women's empowerment and fertility: a review of the literature. *Soc Sci Med*. 2014;115:111–120.

19. Canning D, Schultz TP. The economic consequences of reproductive health and family planning. *Lancet*. 2012;380:165–171.

20. Cavenaghi S, Diniz Alves JE. The everlasting outmoded contraceptive method mix in Brazil and its legacy. *Rev Bras Estud Popul*. 2019;36:1–29.

21. Khamenei SA. Ayatollah Ali Khamenei on Iran's population policy. *Popul Develop Rev*. 2014;40: 573–575.

22. Hesketh T, Zhu WX. The one child family policy: the good, the bad, and the ugly. *BMJ*. 1997;314:1685–1687.

23. Hesketh T, Lu L, Xing ZW. The effect of China's one-child family policy after 25 years. *N Engl J Med*. 2005;353:1171–1177.

24. Hvistendahl M. Has China outgrown the one-child policy? *Science*. 2010;329:1458–1461.

25. Zhu WX, Lu L, Hesketh T. China's excess males, sex selective abortion, and one child policy: analysis of data from 2005 national intercensus survey. *BMJ*. 2009;338:b1211.

26. Chao F, Gerland P, Cook AR, Alkema L. Systematic assessment of the sex ratio at birth for all countries and estimation of national imbalance and regional reference levels. *Proc Natl Acad Sci U S A*. 2019;116:9303–9311.

27. Zeng Y, Hesketh T. The effects of China's universal two-child policy. *Lancet*. 2016;388:1930–1938.

28. Abrahamson P. End of an era? China's one-child policy and its unintended consequences. *Asian Soc Work Pol Rev*. 2016;10:326–338.

29. Basten S, Jiang Q. Fertility in China: an uncertain future. *Popul Stud*. 2015;69:S97–S105.

30. Lee R, Mason A, NTA Network. Is low fertility really a problem? Population aging, dependency, and consumption. *Science*. 2014;346:229–234.

31. Luci-Greulich A, Thévenon O. The impact of family policies on fertility trends in developed countries. *Eur J Popul*. 2013;29:387–416.

32. Harper S. Economic and social implications of aging societies. *Science*. 2014;346:587–591.

33. Conde-Agudelo A, Rosas-Bermudez A, Castaño F, Norton MH. Effects of birth spacing on maternal, perinatal, infant, and child health: a systematic review of causal mechanisms. *Stud Fam Plann*. 2012;43:93–114.

34. Moore Z, Pfitzer A, Gubin R, Charurat E, Elliott L, Croft T. Missed opportunities for family planning: an analysis of pregnancy risk and contraceptive method use among postpartum women in 21 low- and middle-income countries. *Contraception*. 2015;92:31–39.

35. Ezeh A, Bankole A, Cleland J, García-Moreno C, Temmerman M, Ziraba AK. Burden of reproductive ill health (chapter 2). In: Black RE, Laxminarayan R, Temmerman M, Walker N, eds. *Disease Control Priorities: Reproductive, Maternal, Newborn, and Child Health*. 3rd ed. Vol. 2. Washington DC: IBRD/World Bank; 2016:25–50.

36. Santelli JS, Song X, Garbers S, Sharma V, Viner RM. Global trends in adolescent fertility, 1990–2012, in relation to national wealth, income inequalities, and educational expenditures. *J Adolesc Health*. 2017;60:161–168.

37. Ganchimeg T, Ota E, Morisaki N, et al. Pregnancy and childbirth outcomes among adolescent mothers: a World Health Organization multicountry study. *BJOG*. 2014;121(Suppl 1):40–48.

38. Patton GC, Olsson CA, Skirbekk V, et al. Adolescence and the next generation. *Nature*. 2018;554:458–466.

39. Chandra-Mouli V, Camacho AV, Michaud PA. WHO guidelines on preventing early pregnancy and poor reproductive outcomes among adolescents in developing countries. *J Adolesc Health*. 2013;52:517–522.

40. Black KI, Gupta S, Rassi A, Kubba A. Why do women experience untimed pregnancies? A review of contraceptive failure rates. *Best Pract Res Clin Obstet Gynaecol*. 2010;24:443–455.

41. Rivera R, Yacobson I, Grimes D. The mechanism of action of hormonal contraceptives and intrauterine contraceptive devices. *Am J Obstet Gynecol*. 1999;181:1263–1269.

42. Mishell DR Jr. Intrauterine devices: mechanisms of action, safety, and efficacy. *Contraception*. 1998;58 (3 Suppl):S45–S53.

43. *State of World Population 2021*. New York: United Nations Population Fund (UNFPA); 2021.

44. Kates J, Wexler A, Lief E. *Donor Government Funding for Family Planning in 2019*. San Francisco, CA: Kaiser Family Foundation; 2021.

45. Campbell OMR, Graham WJ, The Lancet Maternal Survival Series Steering Group. Strategies for reducing maternal mortality: getting on with what works. *Lancet.* 2006;368:1284–1299.

46. *WHO Recommendations on Antenatal Care for a Positive Pregnancy Experience*. Geneva: World Health Organization; 2016.

47. McCarthy FP, Lutomski JE, Greene RA. Hyperemesis gravidarum: current perspectives. *Int J Women's Health.* 2014;6:719–725.

48. Hajenius PJ, Mol F, Mol BWM, et al. Interventions for tubal ectopic pregnancy. *Cochrane Database Syst Rev.* 2007;2007:CD000324.

49. Young BC, Levine RJ, Karumanchi SA. Pathogenesis of preeclampsia. *Annu Rev Pathol Mech Dis.* 2010;5:173–192.

50. Abalos E, Cuesta C, Grosso AL, Chou D, Say L. Global and regional estimates of preeclampsia and eclampsia: a systematic review. *Eur J Obstet Gynecol Reprod Biol.* 2013;170:1–7.

51. *Managing Complications in Pregnancy and Childbirth: A Guide for Midwives and Doctors*. 2nd ed. Geneva: World Health Organization; 2017.

52. Miller S, Abalos E, Chamillard M, et al. Beyond too little, too late and too much, too soon: a pathway towards evidence-based, respectful maternity care worldwide. *Lancet.* 2016;388:2176–2192.

53. *Making Pregnancy Safer: The Critical Role of the Skilled Attendant: A Joint Statement by WHO, ICM and FIGO*. Geneva: World Health Organization; 2004.

54. *State of the World's Midwifery*. Geneva: World Health Organization; 2021.

55. Lassi ZS, Kumar R, Bhutta ZA. Community-based care to improve reproductive, maternal, newborn, and child health (chapter 14). In: Black RE, Laxminarayan R, Temmerman M, Walker N, eds. *Disease Control Priorities: Reproductive, Maternal, Newborn, and Child Health*. 3rd ed. Vol. 2. Washington DC: IBRD/World Bank; 2016:263–284.

56. GBD 2019 Diseases and Injuries Collaborators. Global burden of 369 diseases and injuries in 204 countries and territories, 1990–2019: a systematic analysis for the Global Burden of Disease Study 2019. *Lancet.* 2020;396:1204–1222.

57. Ronsmans C, Graham WJ, The Lancet Maternal Survival Series Steering Group. Maternal mortality: who, when, where, and why. *Lancet.* 2008;368:1189–1200.

58. *Trends in Maternal Mortality, 1990 to 2015: Estimates by WHO, UNICEF, UNFPA, World Bank Group and the United Nations Population Division*. Geneva: World Health Organization; 2015.

59. Adler AJ, Ronsmans C, Calvert C, Filippi V. Estimating the prevalence of obstetric fistula: a systematic review and meta-analysis. *BMC Pregnancy Childbirth.* 2013;13:246.

60. Cohen J, Vincent JL, Adhikari NKJ, et al. Sepsis: a roadmap for future research. *Lancet Infect Dis.* 2015;15:581–614.

61. Leduc D, Senikas V, Lalonde AB, et al. Active management of the third stage of labour: prevention and treatment of postpartum hemorrhage. *J Obstet Gynaecol Can.* 2009;31:980–993.

62. *WHO Recommendations: Uterotonics for the Prevention of Postpartum Haemorrhage*. Geneva: World Health Organization; 2018.

63. Tunçalp Ö, Souza JP, Gülmezoglu M, World Health Organization. New WHO recommendations on prevention and treatment of postpartum hemorrhage. *Int J Gynaecol Obstet.* 2013;123:254–256.

64. Nguyen RH, Wilcox AJ. Terms in reproductive and perinatal epidemiology: 2. perinatal terms. *J Epidemiol Community Health.* 2005;59:1019–1021.

65. *Monitoring Emergency Obstetric Care: A Handbook*. Geneva: WHO/UNPF/UNICEF; 2009.

66. Betran AP, Torloni MR, Zhang JJ, Gülmezoglu AM, WHO working group on Caesarean section. WHO statement on Caesarean section rates. *BJOG.* 2016;123:667–670.

67. Betran AP, Ye J, Moller AB, Souza JP, Zhang J. Trends and projections of caesarean section rates: global and regional estimates. *BMJ Glob Health.* 2021;6:e005671.

68. *State of the World's Children 2019*. New York: UNICEF; 2019.

69. Bollinger LA, Kruk ME. Innovations to expand access and improve quality of health services (chapter 15). In: Black RE, Laxminarayan R, Temmerman M, Walker N, eds. *Disease Control Priorities: Reproductive, Maternal, Newborn, and Child Health*. 3rd ed. Vol. 2. Washington DC: IBRD/World Bank; 2016:285–298.

70. Boerma T, Ronsmans C, Melesse DY, et al. Global epidemiology of use of and disparities in caesarean sections. *Lancet.* 2018;392:1341–1348.

71. Sandall J, Tribe RM, Avery L, et al. Short-term and long-term effects of caesarean section on the health of women and children. *Lancet.* 2018;392:1349–1357.

72. Souza JP, Tunçalp Ö, Vogel JP, et al. Obstetric transition: the pathway towards ending preventable maternal deaths. *BJOG.* 2014;121(Suppl 1):1–4.

73. Ahmed S, Li Q, Liu L, Tsui AO. Maternal deaths averted by contraceptive use: an analysis of 172 countries. *Lancet.* 2012;380:111–125.

74. Cleland J, Conde-Agudelo A, Peterson H, Ross J, Tsui A. Contraception and health. *Lancet.* 2012; 380:149–156.

75. *The Millennium Development Goals Report 2015*. New York: United Nations; 2015.

76. *Trends in Maternal Mortality 2000 to 2017: Estimates by WHO, UNICEF, UNFPA, World Bank Group and the United Nations Population Division*. Geneva: World Health Organization; 2019.

77. *Ending Preventable Maternal Mortality (EPMM): A Renewed Focus for Improving Maternal and Newborn Health and Wellbeing*. Geneva: WHO/UNFPA; 2021.

78. Lawn JE, Gravett MG, Nunes TM, Rubens CE, Stanton C, GAPPS Review Group. Global report on preterm birth and stillbirth: definitions, description of the burden and opportunities to improve data. *BMC Pregnancy Childbirth*. 2010;10(Suppl 1):S1.

79. Aminu M, Unkels R, Mdegela M, Utz B, Adaji S, van den Broek N. Causes of and factors associated with stillbirth in low- and middle-income countries: a systematic literature review. *BJOG*. 2014;121(Suppl 4):141–153.

80. *A Neglected Tragedy: The Global Burden of Stillbirths: Report of the UN Interagency Group for Child Mortality Estimation, 2020*. New York: United Nations Interagency Group for Child Mortality Estimation; 2020.

81. *Ending Preventable Newborn Deaths and Stillbirths by 2030: Moving Faster Towards High-Quality Universal Health Coverage in 2020–2025*. Geneva: World Health Organization; 2020.

82. Chawanpaiboon S, Vogel JP, Moller AB, et al. Global, regional, and national estimates of levels of preterm birth in 2014: a systematic analysis and modelling analysis. *Lancet Glob Health*. 2019;7:e37–e46.

83. *Born Too Soon: The Global Action Report on Preterm Birth*. Geneva: World Health Organization; 2012.

84. Saigal S, Doyle LW. An overview of mortality and sequelae of preterm birth from infancy to adulthood. *Lancet*. 2008;371:261–269.

85. Goldenberg RL, Culhand JF, Iams JD, Romero R. Epidemiology and causes of preterm birth. *Lancet*. 2008;371:75–84.

86. Romero R, Dey SK, Fisher SJ. Preterm labor: one syndrome, many causes. *Science*. 2014;345:760–765.

87. Kramer MS. Determinants of low birth weight: methodological assessment and meta-analysis. *Bull World Health Organ*. 1987;65:663–737.

88. *UNICEF-WHO Low Birthweight Estimates: Levels and Trends 2000–2015*. Geneva: World Health Organization; 2019.

89. Blencowe H, Krasevec J, de Onis M, et al. National, regional, and worldwide estimates of low birthweight in 2015, with trends from 2000: a systematic analysis. *Lancet Glob Health*. 2019;7:e849–e860.

90. Hack M, Klein NK, Taylor HG. Long-term developmental outcomes of low birth weight infants. *Future Child*. 1995;5:176–196.

91. *Guidelines on Basic Newborn Resuscitation*. Geneva: World Health Organization; 2012.

92. Ouzounian JG, Korst LM, Miller DA, Lee RH. Brachial plexus palsy and shoulder dystocia: obstetric risk factors remain elusive. *Am J Perinatol*. 2013;30:303–307.

93. Oskoui M, Coutinho F, Dykeman J, Jetté N, Pringsheim T. An update on the prevalence of cerebral palsy: a systematic review and meta-analysis. *Dev Med Child Neurol*. 2013;55:509–519.

94. *World Report on Disability 2011*. Geneva: World Health Organization; 2011.

95. Santos RP, Tristram D. A practical guide to the diagnosis, treatment, and prevention of neonatal infections. *Pediatr Clin North Am*. 2015;62:491–508.

96. Gülmezoglu AM, Althabe F, Souza JP, et al. Interventions to reduce maternal and newborn morbidity and mortality (chapter 7). In: Black RE, Laxminarayan R, Temmerman M, Walker N, eds. *Disease Control Priorities: Reproductive, Maternal, Newborn, and Child Health*. 3rd ed. Vol. 2. Washington DC: IBRD/World Bank; 2016:115–136.

97. Thwaites CL, Beeching NJ, Newton CR. Maternal and neonatal tetanus. *Lancet*. 2015;385:362–370.

98. Darmstadt GL, Bhutta ZA, Cousens S, Adam T, Walker N, Bernis L, Lancet Neonatal Survival Steering Team. Evidence-based, cost-effective interventions: how many newborn babies can we save? *Lancet*. 2005;365:977–985.

99. Gabrysch S, Civitelli G, Edmond KM, et al. New signal functions to measure the ability of health facilities to provide routine and emergency newborn care. *PLoS Med*. 2012;9:e1001340.

100. *Pregnancy, Childbirth, Postpartum and Newborn Care: A Guide for Essential Practice*. 3rd ed. Geneva: World Health Organization; 2015.

101. Conde-Agudelo A, Diaz-Rossello J, Cochrane Neonatal Group. Kangaroo mother care to reduce morbidity and mortality in low birthweight infants. *Cochrane Database Syst Rev*. 2016;2016:CD002771.

102. Dohle GR, Colpi GM, Hargreave TB, et al. EAU guidelines on male infertility. *Eur Urol*. 2005;48:703–711.

103. McLaren JF. Infertility evaluation. *Obstet Gynecol Clin North Am*. 2012;39:453–463.

104. Mascarenhas MN, Flaxman SR, Boerma T, Vanderpoel S, Stevens GA. National, regional, and global trends in infertility prevalence since 1990: a systematic analysis of 277 health surveys. *PLoS Med*. 2012;9:e1001356.

105. Mascarenhas MN, Flaxman SR, Boerma T, Vanderpoel S, Mathers CD, Stevens GA. Trends in primary and secondary infertility prevalence since 1990: a systematic analysis of demographic and reproductive health surveys. *Lancet*. 2013;381:S90.

106. Inhorn MC, Patrizio P. Infertility around the globe: new thinking on gender, reproductive technologies and global movements in the 21st century. *Hum Reprod Update*. 2015;21:411–426.

107. Lindsay TJ, Vitrikas KR. Evaluation and treatment of infertility. *Am Fam Physician*. 2015;91:308–314.

108. Rouchou B. Consequences of infertility in developing countries. *R Soc Public Health*. 2013;133:174–179.

109. Leone T, Brown LJ. Timing the determinants of age at menarche in low-income and middle-income countries. *BMJ Glob Health*. 2020;5:e003689.

110. Mishra GD, Cooper R, Tom SE, Kuh D. Early life circumstances and their impact on menarche and menopause. *Women's Health*. 2009;5:175–190.

111. Daan NMP, Fauser BCJM. Menopause prediction and potential implications. *Maturitas*. 2015;82:257–265.

112. Gold EB. The timing of the age at which natural menopause occurs. *Obstet Gynecol Clin North Am*. 2011;38:425–440.

113. Burger H, Woods NF, Dennerstein L, Alexander JL, Kotz K, Richardson G. Nomenclature and endocrinology of menopause and perimenopause. *Expert Rev Neurother*. 2007;7(11 Suppl):S35–S43.

114. Yonkers KA, O'Brien S, Eriksson E. Premenstrual syndrome. *Lancet*. 2008;371:1200–1210.

115. Sommer M, Caruso BA, Torondel B, et al. Menstrual hygiene management in schools: midway progress update on the "MHM in Ten" 2014–2024 global agenda. *Health Res Pol Syst*. 2021;19:1.

116. Normalizing menstruation, empowering girls. *Lancet Child Adolesc Health*. 2018;2:379.

117. Giuliani E, As-Sanie S, Marsh EE. Epidemiology and management of uterine fibroids. *Int J Gynecol Obstet*. 2020;149:3–9.

118. Chapron C, Marcellin L, Borghese B, Santulli P. Rethinking mechanisms, diagnosis and management of endometriosis. *Nat Rev Endocrinol*. 2019;15:666–682.

119. Escobar-Morreale HF. Polycystic ovary syndrome: definition, aetiology, diagnosis and treatment. *Nat Rev Endocrinol*. 2018;14:270–284.

120. Iglesia CB, Smithling KR. Pelvic organ prolapse. *Am Fam Physician*. 2017;96:179–185.

121. Cheng L, Albers P, Berney DM, et al. Testicular cancer. *Nat Rev Dis Primers*. 2018;4:29.

122. Lokeshwar SD, Harper BT, Webb E, et al. Epidemiology and treatment modalities for the management of benign prostatic hyperplasia. *Transl Androl Urol*. 2019;8:529–539.

123. Mirza M, Griebling TL, Kazer MW. Erectile dysfunction and urinary incontinence after prostate cancer treatment. *Sem Oncol Nurs*. 2011;27:278–289.

124. Shamloul R, Ghanem H. Erectile dysfunction. *Lancet*. 2013;381:153–165.

125. Mollaioli D, Ciocca G, Limoncin E, et al. Lifestyles and sexuality in men and women: the gender perspective in sexual medicine. *Reprod Biol Endocrinol*. 2020;18:10.

126. Hawkes S, Hart G. Men's sexual health matters: promoting reproductive health in an international context. *Trop Med Int Health*. 2000;5:A37–A44.

127. Mayer KH, Bradford JB, Makadon HJ, Stall R, Goldhammer H, Landers S. Sexual and gender minority health: what we know and what needs to be done. *Am J Public Health*. 2008;98:989–995.

128. Daniel H, Butkus R, Health and Public Policy Committee of American College of Physicians. Lesbian, gay, bisexual, and transgender health disparities: executive summary of a policy position paper from the American College of Physicians. *Ann Intern Med*. 2015;163:135–137.

129. Reisner SL, Poteat T, Keatley J, et al. Global health burden and needs of transgender populations: a review. *Lancet*. 2016;388:422–436.

130. Hatzenbuehler ML, McLaughlin KA, Keyes KM, Hasin DS. The impact of institutional discrimination on psychiatric disorders in lesbian, gay, and bisexual populations: a prospective study. *Am J Public Health*. 2010;100:452–459.

131. Beyrer C. Pushback: the current wave of anti-homosexuality laws and impacts on health. *PLoS Med*. 2014;11:e1001658.

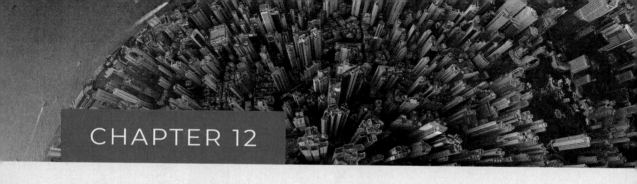

CHAPTER 12

Nutrition

In lower-income countries, hunger and micronutrient deficiencies continue to be major public health problems. In middle- and high-income countries, increasing rates of obesity are the dominant nutritional concern. Global collaborations are seeking to end child undernutrition, prevent obesity in children and adults, and ensure food security and safety as international trade in food products intensifies.

12.1 Nutrition and Global Health

Nutrition is the consumption of food that allows the body to survive, grow, heal, and be healthy and the processing of those nutrients within the body. Every person needs to eat on a regular basis to provide his or her body with energy and the materials needed to build and repair cells and tissues, fight infections, and stay warm. There is no perfect diet, but nutritionists generally recommend a diet that is mostly plant based and is minimally processed.[1] **Malnutrition** is suboptimal nutritional status that arises from deficiencies, excesses, or imbalances in the intake and processing of energy and nutrients. The types of malnutrition that are the greatest challenges at the population level vary by country income level.[2]

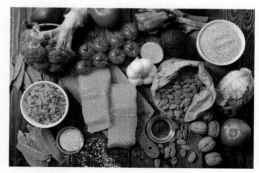

© Margouillat photo/Shutterstock

In low-income countries, the primary nutritional concern is having too little food. Many children in these areas have stunted growth because they eat too few calories and too little protein, and many infants, children, adolescents, and adults have vitamin and mineral deficiencies because the starchy staple foods that form the bulk of their diets are low in nutritional quality. Poverty is the underlying cause of nearly all cases of severe undernutrition in children, creating a cycle of malnutrition and infectious diseases that is hard to break. This reduction in child health and nutritional status can have long-term consequences. Adults who were undernourished as children tend to be shorter, less educated, less economically productive, and more likely to have low birthweight babies than adults who were not underfed in childhood.[3]

One of the driving motivations for keeping nutrition as a global health priority is the ethical imperative to protect vulnerable children no matter where they happen to have been born.[4] Children born in low-income countries have, on average, worse nutritional status than children born in high-income countries. Within every country, children born to low-income households have, on average, worse nutritional status than higher-income households.[2] Food aid has been a key part of international health initiatives for many decades.[5] The continuing challenges of undernutrition are the target of Sustainable Development Goal (SDG) 2, which aims to "end hunger, achieve food security and improved nutrition, and promote sustainable agriculture."[6]

In middle-income and high-income countries, and a growing number of communities within low-income countries, the biggest nutritional concern is obesity.[2] People who live in wealthier areas have access to a great variety of nutritious foods, but they also eat more refined and processed foods along with more fats. Obesity-related health concerns like diabetes and hypertension are becoming more prevalent in industrialized and industrializing economies as more adults and children are physically inactive and overweight.

The **nutrition transition** is a health transition characterized by a shift from having undernutrition and nutrient deficiencies as the most prevalent nutritional concerns in a population to having overweight and obesity as the dominant nutritional disorders.[7] During the process of shifting from a pre-transition profile toward a post-transition profile, countries often experience a dual burden of nutritional problems, with undernutrition continuing to be prevalent among children, especially those living in rural areas and in low-income urban communities, while adult obesity becomes more prevalent.[8] Thus, obesity is not just a problem of high-income countries but one that affects countries across the income spectrum, including low-income countries. Collaborative efforts are needed to understand the causes of obesity and identify effective interventions for obesity prevention. Global cooperation is also required to ensure food safety as international trade in food products increases.

12.2 Macronutrients

Healthy nutrition requires an appropriate amount of daily food that includes a diversity of types of nutrients. A **macronutrient** is nutrient such as a carbohydrate, protein, fat, or oil that is required to be consumed in relatively large quantities because it provides energy. Energy in food is typically measured in units of calories. A **calorie** is the amount of energy required to raise the temperature of one gram of water by one degree Celsius. Food energy measurements are reported in units of kilocalories (kcal), with one kilocalorie eqivalent to one thousand calories (with a lowercase *c*) or one Calorie (with a capital *C*). The amount of food calories needed by a person each day varies based on age, sex, body size, activity level, climate, and pregnancy and lactation status.[9] A typical toddler requires about 1,000 kcal daily. School-aged children require approximately 1,400–2,000 kcal per day. Depending on activity levels, an adolescent girl might require about 1,600–2,400 kcal daily, and an adolescent boy might require 2,000–3,200 kcal. Young adult women require about 2,200 kcal per day, and more when pregnant or breastfeeding. Young adult men require about 2,800 kcal. The number of calories needed each day then decreases with aging. Older adult women need only about 1,600 kcal daily, and older adult men require only about 2,000 kcal.

A **carbohydrate** is a chain of sugars. Carbohydrates are found in cereal grains like rice, maize, and wheat (the three most common staple foods in the world[10]), in starchy roots like potatoes and yams, and in fruits and vegetables. When the body requires a quick source of energy, the body's cells break down carbohydrates through a process called cellular respiration. **Saccharides** are the molecular units that form carbohydrates. Simple carbohydrates are made up of short chains of sugars that are easily absorbed into the bloodstream. The galactose found in milk and the glucose and fructose found in fruits and honey are monosaccharides ("one sugar"). Table sugar, or sucrose, is a disaccharide ("two sugar") composed of glucose and fructose. Lactose is a disaccharide composed of glucose and galactose.

The complex carbohydrates (often classified as starches) found in whole-grain products like whole-wheat bread and oatmeal are made up of longer chains of sugars (polysaccharides) that take longer to digest. Eating complex carbohydrates keeps a person from feeling hungry longer than eating simple sugars. **Fiber** is a nondigestible complex carbohydrate found in unprocessed plant-based foods, and it is essential for healthy digestion because it provides bulk that moves food material through the intestines. Nutritionists recommend that carbohydrates account for 45%–65% of the daily calories consumed by the typical person.[11] In low-income countries, many people eat a starchy diet that exceeds this recommended proportion, even though they consume few nutrient-rich fruits and vegetables (**Figure 12.1**).[12]

Amino acids are organic compounds that contain carbon, hydrogen, oxygen, and

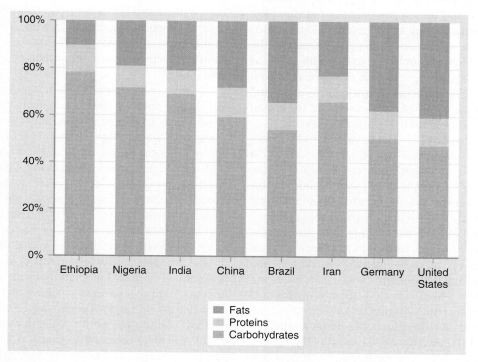

Figure 12.1 Distribution of daily calories, on average, from carbohydrates, proteins, and fats.

Data from *FAOSTAT Food Balance Sheets: New Food Balances*. Rome: Food and Agriculture Organization of the United Nations; 2020.

nitrogen. A **protein** is a chain of amino acids. Amino acids from food are broken down and reassembled in the body's cells to form new proteins. The keratin that makes up hair and nails; the hemoglobin in blood that transports oxygen; the antibodies that help the body's immune system recognize and fight infection; the actin and myosin that contract and relax muscles; and the collagen in ligaments, tendons, and skin are all types of proteins. About 20 different kinds of amino acids are recognized as critical for human biochemistry.

An **essential amino acid** is one that cannot be produced by the human body and must be acquired from food. A **complete protein** contains all nine essential amino acids. Proteins from animal-based foods are usually complete proteins. **Complementary proteins** are foods that individually lack some types of essential amino acids but provide all the essential amino acids when consumed together. Plant proteins are usually incomplete proteins, but all of the essential amino acids can be consumed in one vegetarian meal by combining complementary proteins, such as eating maize (corn) with beans or nuts with whole-wheat bread. Nutritionists recommend that 10%–35% of daily calories for the typical person come from high-quality proteins.[11]

A **lipid** is a fatty acid, which is a hydrocarbon chain with other chemical groups at the ends of the chain. Both fats and oils are types of lipids. A **fat** is a lipid of animal origin that is solid at room temperature, like butter and lard. An **oil** is a lipid of plant origin that is a liquid at room temperature, like corn oil and olive oil. Lipids contain more energy per gram than any other biological molecule and provide long-term energy storage, insulation, protective padding around internal organs, and assistance with nutrient absorption. Lipids are needed for the processing of some vitamins (A, D, E, and K) and are used by the body to make other compounds, such as steroid hormones. Nutritionists recommend that about

20%–35% of calories consumed in a day come from healthy fats and oils.[11] People who live in high-income countries often exceed the recommended amount, while people who live in low-income countries often consume too few fats and oils.[12]

Not all fatty acids are equally healthy. The relative healthiness of lipids is related to the amount of hydrogen they contain. An **unsaturated fatty acid** contains at least one double bond in the carbon chain. Both monounsaturated fats like those found in olive oil, avocados, and nuts and the polyunsaturated fats in cold-water fish like salmon (which contain omega-3 fatty acids) seem to be protective against heart disease.[13] A **saturated fatty acid** has only single bonds between its carbon atoms. No more hydrogen can be added to the molecule because it is already "saturated" with hydrogen. Saturated fatty acids are found in meat, butter, and other animal products. A **trans fat** is a liquid oil that has been transformed into a semisolid fat through hydrogenation. Trans fats, which are found in margarine and other processed foods, are associated with adverse cardiovascular disease outcomes.[14]

Water is not a nutrient, but it is an essential part of the diet. Every cell in the body needs a way to take in oxygen and nutrients along with a way to get rid of carbon dioxide and waste. Blood is about 92% water, and it is the medium for transporting gases, nutrients, and wastes throughout the body. Blood volume is a function of the amount of water in the body. When a human does not have an adequate volume of blood, the blood pressure decreases, and it is difficult for the body's cells to function. A person who loses a lot of blood due to an injury or a lot of water due to excessive vomiting or diarrhea can go into hypovolemic shock, which is shock caused by too little blood volume. Water also helps the body regulate its temperature by sweating and helps the body get rid of waste through urination and defecation.

An adult loses about 2–3 quarts of water a day by urinating, sweating, and exhaling humidified air.[15] More may be lost in hot climates, during intense physical activity, or when a person has diarrhea. This lost water must be replaced to avoid dehydration. Severe dehydration can cause an acid–base imbalance in the blood and lead to organ failure (especially of the kidneys) and death.

12.3 Breastfeeding and Infant Nutrition

Breast milk contains all of the nutrients and water babies need, and it also includes digestive enzymes as well as antibodies and other immune factors that protect against harmful infections and promote health.[16] New mothers are encouraged to breastfeed their babies so that nutrients and disease-fighting antibodies will be delivered to them. **Colostrum**, the breast milk produced in the first days after giving birth, is especially beneficial because it contains large quantities of proteins and antibodies that stimulate the newborn's immune system development.[17] **Early breastfeeding** means initiating breastfeeding within the first hour after giving birth. Early breastfeeding increases the neonatal survival rate,[18] but less than half of newborns worldwide receive breast milk within one hour after birth.[19]

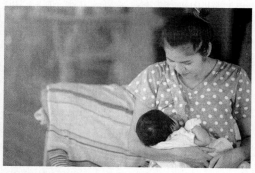

© Warongdech Digital/Shutterstock

Exclusive breastfeeding means that breast milk is the only substance a baby consumes and that no supplemental water, juice, cow or goat milk, porridge, rice water, or any other foods are fed to the baby. UNICEF and the WHO recommend that infants should be exclusively breastfed for the first six months of life.[20] Only about two in five infants younger than six months old are exclusively breastfed,[19] and this low percentage contributes to infant illnesses and deaths from undernutrition and diarrhea.[21]

Complementary foods are soft, semisolid, or solid foods introduced into an infant's diet while continuing to breastfeed the child until the baby's second birthday or later (**Figure 12.2**).[20] "Complementary" means that the foods accompany breast milk and do not immediately replace it.[22] About two in three children aged 12–23 months receive at least some breast milk daily.[19] UNICEF recommends that the minimum acceptable daily diet for children aged 6–23 months include foods from at least several different food groups (such as grains, legumes, dairy, meat, eggs, fruits, and vegetables) consumed at appropriate frequencies (at least two or three meal or snack times daily for breastfed children and four times for nonbreastfed children).[23] Only about 20% of children in this age group meet the criteria for at least a minimally acceptable diet (**Figure 12.3**).[19]

Not all mothers are able to exclusively breastfeed. Some mothers do not produce adequate milk for their babies and must supplement

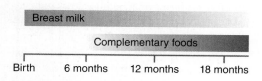

Figure 12.2 Global nutrition standards recommend exclusive breastfeeding for six months followed by the introduction of complementary foods with continued breastfeeding.

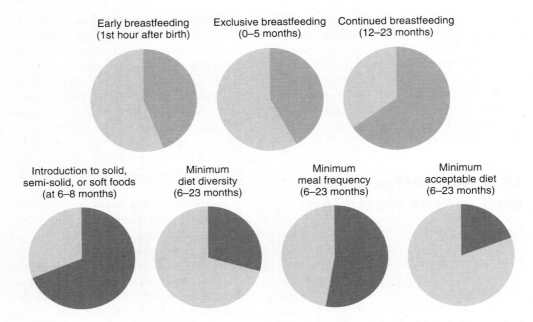

Figure 12.3 Percentage of neonates, infants, and young children being breastfed and receiving recommended nutrition.

Data from *State of the World's Children 2019.* New York: UNICEF; 2019.

with formula at an early age. Some have HIV infection and do not want to risk passing the virus to their babies through breast milk. Some have work schedules that do not allow them to feed their babies every few hours.[24] Newborns whose mothers have died in childbirth are also not able to be breastfed by their biological mothers. When breast milk is not available at all or in sufficient quantities, alternative nutritional options are necessary.

Breast-milk substitutes for infants must provide hydration plus all of the essential nutrients. Commercial infant formula is usually the best substitute for breast milk because cow's milk, tea, rice water, and other substitutes do not provide all the nutrients of breast milk or infant formula. However, using infant formula can be a challenge for parents and caregivers who lack access to clean water, have difficulties reading and following the mixing instructions, or have limited incomes to pay for commercial products.

Additional concerns about the use of formula in lower-income countries stem from the marketing strategies used by Nestlé and

other infant formula companies in the 1970s.[25] Hospital maternity wards in some developing countries were sponsored by formula companies, and new mothers were sent home with formula samples and no lactation education. New mothers who do not breastfeed will quickly lose the ability to produce milk and must then rely on breast-milk substitutes, so providing a limited amount of free formula may create a dependency on the product. Worse, some companies hired "milk nurses" to go into communities in nursing uniforms and advertise formula, implying that formula was better than breast milk. In 1981, the World Health Assembly adopted an **International Code of Marketing of Breast-milk Substitutes** that bans problematic marketing of infant formula. The code stresses that breast milk is the best option for feeding babies, and it requires new mothers who are given information about the use of infant formula to be informed about the financial and health costs of formula adoption. The code stipulates that marketing personnel should not directly contact pregnant women or new mothers, even if those salespeople are healthcare professionals; that health facilities should not promote formula use; and that samples of formula should not be distributed at hospitals or by retailers. Many of the major international formula producers have adopted the code and no longer directly market to pregnant women or new parents, but few countries have enacted laws that enforce the entire code.[26]

Parents need to be provided with the information to make informed decisions about whether and how long to breastfeed. Attitudes toward breastfeeding also need to be changed in settings that discourage breastfeeding. Employers rarely have a private room available for mothers who would like to use a breast pump. Mothers are not always free to breastfeed in public areas, even the "public" areas of their own homes. New grandmothers who bottle fed their own babies may discourage their daughters from choosing breastfeeding. The advice that "breast is best" needs to be accompanied by conditions that support breastfeeding, especially in places where breastfeeding is not the cultural norm.[27]

12.4 Child Growth

Anthropometry is the measurement of the human body. Height, weight, waist circumference, body fat percentage, and other measurements can be useful indicators of a person's nutritional status. For children, height-for-age, weight-for-height, and weight-for-age are frequently used measures of healthy growth. **Stunting** is a condition in which a child has low height-for-age. **Wasting** is a condition in which a child has low weight-for-height (also called weight-for-length). A **mid-upper arm circumference (MUAC)** that shows a low arm-circumference-for-age is another sign of wasting in a child. **Underweight** is a condition in which a child has a low weight-for-age. Stunting and wasting are often used by global child nutrition initiatives as metrics for tracking progress toward achieving goals related to macronutrient undernutrition. Stunting is a sign of chronic undernutrition. Wasting is a sign of acute undernutrition characterized by rapidly

decreasing nutritional health status. Children can experience stunting and wasting separately or at the same time.

Global growth standards for children from birth through age 60 months are provided by the World Health Organization (WHO).[28] The WHO growth charts display the average measurements for healthy children of a particular age along with the range of normal measurements that fall above and below that mean. The WHO growth charts can be used worldwide because scientific evidence shows that infants and children from geographically diverse regions experience very similar growth patterns when their health and nutritional needs are met.[29] (One limitation of many growth standards for children is that they require caregivers to know the birth date of the child, and some children who were born at home or orphaned do not have a record of this date. When this information is not available, it can be difficult to determine if a child is growing well.)

Since the distribution of anthropometric measurements follows a bell-shaped curve, child growth measurements can be translated to z-scores and percentiles. A standard deviation is a statistical indicator for the width of a distribution, and a **z-score** is an indicator of how many standard deviations away from the population mean an individual's measure is. A height-for-age z-score of $z = 1$ indicates

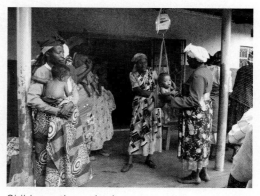

Child growth monitoring.

CDC Connects/CAPT, USPHS, Pamela Ching, MS, ScD, RD/LD, Health Scientist, Center for Global Health. Reference to specific commercial products, manufacturers, companies, or trademarks does not constitute its endorsement or recommendation by the U.S. Government, Department of Health and Human Services, or Centers for Disease Control and Prevention.

a child whose measurements fall one standard deviation above the mean. A z-score of 1 is equivalent to the child's height-for-age being at the 84th percentile, which means that the child is taller than 84% of healthy children of the same age and shorter than 16% of healthy same-age children. A height-for-age z-score of z = –2 indicates a child whose height-for-age falls two standard deviations below the mean, which is equivalent to being at the 2nd percentile of height-for-age for healthy children. This child would be referred for medical evaluation based on being shorter than 98% of healthy children of the same age.

Figure 12.4 shows a sample weight-for-age chart for girls.[30] The graph plots age in months on the x-axis and weight on the y-axis. The graph allows a parent or healthcare worker to easily determine if a child of a particular age is underweight (below the 15th percentile) or severely underweight (under the 3rd percentile) for his or her age. The sample curve for Child 1 shows a child of healthy weight. The sample curve for Child 2 shows an underweight child. Both children lost weight just after their first birthdays, most likely because of an episode of diarrheal disease or another infectious illness. For Child 1, this was a minor event that had almost no effect on her growth trajectory. For Child 2, this bout of diarrhea pushed her into severe malnutrition and could easily have caused her death. Children should be weighed often, especially when they are very young, so that growth trends can emerge. A child like Child 2 who loses weight or fails to gain weight needs medical attention.

Significant progress toward reducing child hunger worldwide has been made over the past 20 years.[31] The percentage of children

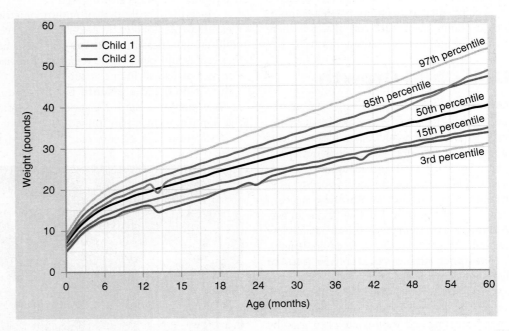

Figure 12.4 A sample child growth chart showing weight-for-age curves for girls from birth to the fifth birthday.

Percentile curve data from WHO Multicentre Growth Reference Study Group. *WHO Child Growth Standards: Length/Height-for-Age, Weight-for-Age, Weight-for-Length, Weight-for-Height and Body Mass Index-for-Age: Methods and Development.* Geneva: World Health Organization; 2006.

less than five years old who have stunting decreased from 32.5% in 2000 to about 22% in 2020, but that meant that about 150 million under-5 children still had moderately or severely stunted growth. About 7% of under-5 children had moderate or severe wasting in 2020, which meant that at least 50 million young children were too thin. Cases of childhood malnutrition are not evenly distributed (**Figure 12.5**).[31] About 30% of under-5 children in South Asia and sub-Saharan Africa have stunting, and about 15% of children in South Asia and 7% in sub-Saharan Africa have wasting.[31]

In 2012, the World Health Assembly approved six Global Nutrition Targets, which aim to improve the nutritional status of the global maternal, infant, and young child populations by 2025 by doing the following:

1. Reducing the number of under-5 children who have stunting by 40% so that fewer than 100 million young children in 2025 will have stunting
2. Reducing anemia in women of reproductive age by 50% so that the prevalence is less than 15%

3. Reducing the percentage of newborns with low birthweight (less than 2,500 grams) by 30%
4. Preventing a rise in the proportion of children who are overweight
5. Increasing the rate of exclusive breastfeeding in the first six months of life to at least 50%
6. Reducing the prevalence of childhood wasting to less than 5%, which will require a reduction of nearly 40%[32]

By 2020, modest progress had been made on reducing low birthweight (target #3) and increasing exclusive breastfeeding rates (#5) at the overall worldwide level, but the world was not on track to achieve the goals related to stunting (#1), anemia (#2), overweight (#4), or wasting (#6) (**Figure 12.6**).[2] Most low- and middle-income countries were not expected to achieve the Global Nutrition Targets for child growth by 2025.[33]

The SDGs aim to "end hunger and ensure access by all people, in particular the poor and people in vulnerable situations, including infants, to safe, nutritious, and sufficient food all year round" (SDG 2.1) and "end all forms of malnutrition" by achieving growth

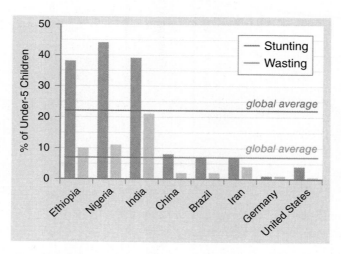

Figure 12.5 Percentage of under-5 children (ages 0–59 months) in selected countries who are more than two standard deviations below the median of the WHO Child Growth Standards.

Data from *State of the World's Children 2019.* New York: UNICEF; 2019.

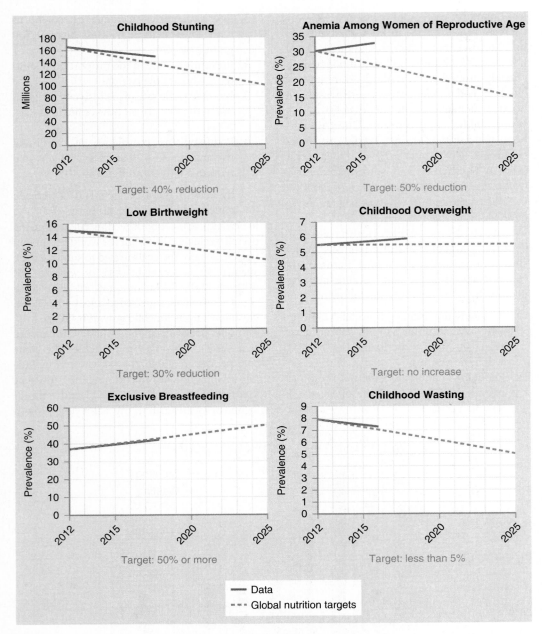

Figure 12.6 Progress toward the Global Nutrition Targets for 2012–2025.

Data from *2020 Global Nutrition Report: Action on Equity to End Malnutrition*. Bristol UK: Development Initiatives; 2020.

targets in children under five years of age and satisfying "the nutritional needs of adolescent girls, pregnant and lactating women, and older persons" (SDG 2.2).[6] Improving access

to nutrition is a foundational requirement for achieving the other health goals spelled out in the SDGs. The lack of progress toward achieving the WHO Global Nutrition Targets for 2025 means that the world is also not on track to achieve the SDG goal of having zero malnutrition by 2030.

12.5 Severe Acute Malnutrition

Undernutrition is malnutrition resulting from deficiencies in the amount of food or types of nutrients eaten or from poor absorption of the nutrients that have been consumed. There are two main categories of undernutrition related to inadequate diets: deficiencies of macronutrients and deficiencies of vitamins and minerals. These forms of undernutrition often occur concurrently. For example, too little fat in the diet means that fat-soluble vitamins cannot be processed.

Nearly half of all under-5 child deaths have undernutrition as a contributing factor.[34]

Even mild and moderate undernutrition can significantly increase a child's risk of illness and death due to infectious diseases such as diarrhea, pneumonia, and measles.[35] The Global Hunger Index is a metric that combines the percentage of the total population that consumes too few calories with statistics about wasting, stunting, and mortality among children who are less than five years old. Severe hunger is rare in most high- and upper-middle-income countries, but many low- and lower-middle-income countries continue to experience significant child undernutrition (**Figure 12.7**).[36] Poor nutritional status in childhood can have long-term adverse impacts on growth and health. Young children who survive severe undernutrition often experience lifelong complications that reduce school performance and then impair work productivity in adulthood.[37]

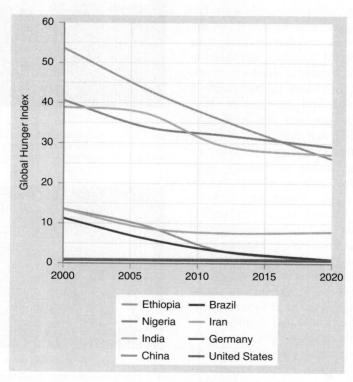

Figure 12.7 Global Hunger Index (0 = best situation [no hunger] and 100 = worst situation).

Data from *2020 Global Hunger Index: One Decade to Zero Hunger.* Bonn/Dublin: Welthungerhilfe and Concern Worldwide; 2020.

Long-term insufficiencies in the intake of protein and calories can lead to a life-threatening state of protein energy malnutrition that requires urgent (acute) medical care.[38] **Severe acute malnutrition** (SAM) is a state of extreme undernutrition that is present when a child has a weight-for-height z-score below $z = -3$. Moderate acute malnutrition (MAM) is defined as a weight-for-height z-score between -2 and -3. Alternatively, children with a MUAC of less than 11.5 centimeters are considered to have SAM, and those with measurements between 11.5 and 12.4 centimeters are classified as having MAM.[39]

SAM presents in two ways, as kwashiorkor and as marasmus.[40] **Kwashiorkor** is caused by chronic dietary protein deficiency, and it is characterized by very low weight-for-height accompanied by pitting edema. **Edema** is fluid retention in extracellular spaces that causes swelling of the tissues in the arms, legs, and face. Pitting means that when a swollen body part is pressed, a depression forms and remains for at least several seconds after the pressure is removed. Children with kwashiorkor may have somewhat adequate calorie intake but lack the dietary protein necessary for healthy growth and development. Most children with kwashiorkor also have weak muscles and pale hair and skin, and they may have a distended abdomen because their nutrient-deficient bodies are retaining water and the abdominal walls are so weak that the internal organs sag out. Kwashiorkor is associated with early weaning, which often happens when an infant's mother becomes pregnant again soon after giving birth. **Marasmus** is caused by prolonged calorie deprivation, and it is characterized by very low weight-for-height without edema. Children with marasmus are emaciated, weak, and lethargic. They look skeletal, have loose and wrinkled skin, and have too little energy to move or cry. Eventually, their body systems begin to fail. Both marasmus and kwashiorkor increase susceptibility to infection and put children at risk of permanent disability and death.

SAM requires urgent medical care.[41] Infants with SAM require inpatient care so they can be fed specially formulated therapeutic

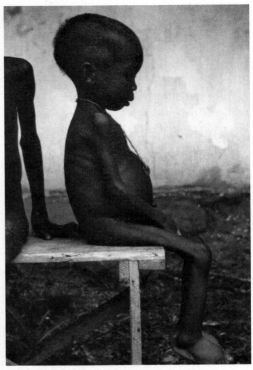

Kwashiorkor.

CDC/Dr. Lyle Conrad. Reference to specific commercial products, manufacturers, companies, or trademarks does not constitute its endorsement or recommendation by the U.S. Government, Department of Health and Human Services, or Centers for Disease Control and Prevention.

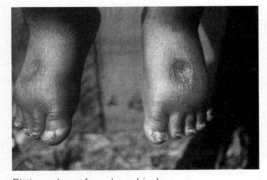

Pitting edema from kwashiorkor.

CDC/Dr. Lyle Conrad. Reference to specific commercial products, manufacturers, companies, or trademarks does not constitute its endorsement or recommendation by the U.S. Government, Department of Health and Human Services, or Centers for Disease Control and Prevention.

milks and receive other medical treatments. Children with SAM who are more than one year old, have no appetite, and are suffering from medical complications also usually require inpatient hospital care so they can receive therapeutic nutrition; fluid and electrolyte management; and treatment for diarrhea, malaria, intestinal parasites, and other infections. These undernourished children are typically fed **ready-to-use therapeutic foods** (RUTF), which are premade food products that are high in energy and protein and are often made from a peanut base.[42] Children with SAM who have an appetite and do not have other serious medical conditions can often be treated in community-based programs that offer RUTF and basic medical care. Community-based management of acute malnutrition (CMAM) programs also provide care for children who have gained enough weight to be discharged from inpatient nutritional care but require continued monitoring.[43]

Effective community-based strategies for improving child and family nutrition include promoting breastfeeding, educating about complementary feeding, providing food supplements or conditional cash transfers to vulnerable households, and using WHO recommended case management strategies for clinically treating children with SAM.[44] Access to safe drinking water and sanitation, sustainable agricultural practices, and other aspects of environmental health are foundations for good community nutritional status.[45] Since the underlying cause of nearly all SAM in children is poverty, population-level improvements in education, employment, gender equality, and other socioeconomic factors are also associated with improvements in child nutrition.[46]

12.6 Food Security and Food Systems

Food security exists when all members of a household or community reliably have access to enough food to be healthy, active, and productive.[47] Food security is dependent on food being physically available, economically affordable, and nutritionally valuable. The available food must also be safe to consume, culturally acceptable, and fairly allocated to individuals within households (such as ensuring that children receive adequate nutrition even when they eat from a shared dish more slowly than adults).[48] At the household level, access to food means being able to produce, purchase, or otherwise acquire an adequate quantity, quality, and variety of food during the entire year.[49]

Households and communities may experience seasonal food insecurity as food stocks dwindle prior to a new harvest. Transitory food insecurity at the household level may also occur at unpredictable times due to unemployment or illness or at the community or national level due to economic shocks or natural disasters. Members of food insecure households may report feeling hungry but not eating, worrying that their food will run out, running out of food and not having enough money to buy more, eating only a limited variety of low-cost foods, cutting the size of meals, skipping meals, and not eating for a whole day.[50] Some households experience chronic food insecurity. Chronically undernourished people often lack the strength and stamina to be productive, and that reduction in productivity often exacerbates the poverty that is the underlying cause of food insecurity.[51]

Food insecurity affects households in countries across the income spectrum. Some lower-income countries struggle to produce or import enough food to meet the daily requirements of their residents. A large proportion of households that can afford enough calories may not be able to afford sufficiently nutritious foods (**Figure 12.8**).[52] In higher-income countries, the number of calories available per person each day far exceeds the required number of calories (**Figure 12.9**),[12] but low-income households may still be unable to afford diets with sufficient food diversity.

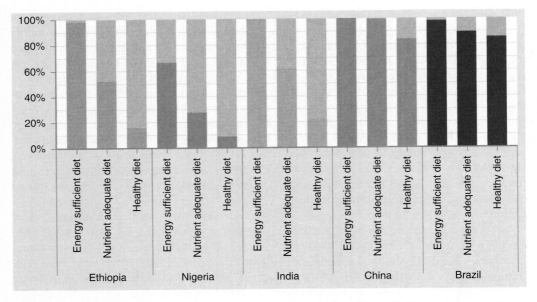

Figure 12.8 Percentage of households that can afford an energy sufficient diet that meets short-term needs for subsistence, a nutrient adequate diet that meets required levels for all essential nutrients, or a healthy diet that includes food group diversity.

Data from *The State of Food Security and Nutrition in the World 2020.* Rome: Food and Agriculture Organization of the United Nations; 2020.

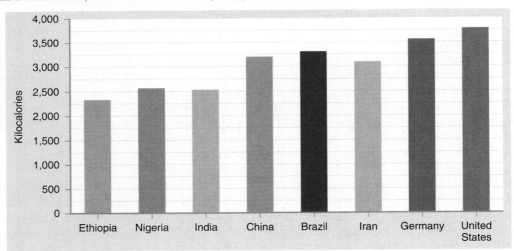

Figure 12.9 Food supply (kilocalories per capita per day).

Data from *FAOSTAT Food Balance Sheets: New Food Balances.* Rome: Food and Agriculture Organization of the United Nations; 2020.

Chronic population food insecurity may spiral into humanitarian catastrophes. **Famine** occurs when a large proportion of a population has very low food security. Famines are partially attributable to demographics (such as population growth) and environmental factors (such as drought), but they are largely the result of economic and political dysfunction. Food shortages may occur because of reduced food production, but they also happen because of increased food prices and interruptions in the supply chain that transports food from producers to consumers. In the words of Amartya Sen, a Nobel Prize–winning economist from India, "starvation is a matter of some people not *having* enough food to eat, and not a matter of there *being* not enough food to eat."[53]

Food security is about the distribution and affordability of food as much as it is about food production. The **food system** encompasses the entire process of growing or producing food, processing and packaging food, distributing and selling food (which may require transportation and storage), and preparing and consuming food. SDG 2 emphasizes that the ability of people to have food security is dependent on healthy food systems. The overall goal is to "end hunger, achieve food security and improved nutrition, and promote sustainable agriculture," and the pathways toward ending hunger (SDG 2.1) and undernutrition (SDG 2.2) include increasing the agricultural productivity of small-scale food producers (SDG 2.3) and ensuring that food production systems are sustainable and preserve ecosystem health (SDG 2.4).[6] A disruption in any part of the food system may cause food insecurity.

As the world population increases and available croplands shrink, crop yields will have to increase to meet the growing demand for food. The best way to ensure that everyone is food secure is to increase food production while also increasing environmental protection.[54] This means developing new agricultural techniques or choosing to use time-tested techniques such as crop rotation that cause as little damage to the environment as possible and also increase yields.[55] Food supplies can be further maximized when as little food as possible is wasted, eaten by animals, or allowed to spoil during transportation and storage. Food distribution systems need to be strengthened so that those who are unable to produce enough food for their families have access to the surplus food produced by others. Additionally, trade policies that make it attractive for growers to produce crops for local consumption rather than export may help alleviate hunger.[56]

12.7 Micronutrients

A **micronutrient** is a nutrient that the body requires in small amounts. Micronutrients include both minerals and vitamins. A **mineral** is an inorganic chemical element. Macrominerals (also called major minerals) are needed in relatively large quantities. Trace minerals (also called microminerals) are required in very small amounts. As with any nutrient, either a deficiency or an excess of minerals (such as an overdose of supplemental minerals) can be harmful.

A **vitamin** is an organic compound that typically cannot be synthesized by the body. A **water-soluble vitamin** is easily dissolved in the body but is not able to be stored in body tissues. Water-soluble vitamins must be consumed daily for maximum health, and any excess amounts ingested in a day are excreted in the urine. The B vitamins and vitamin C are water-soluble vitamins that are necessary for regulation of energy use and critical cellular functions. A **fat-soluble vitamin** is able to be stored in body tissues. The fat-soluble vitamins (vitamins A, D, E, and K) contribute to bone health, vision, and other important body functions. People with too little fat in their diets and

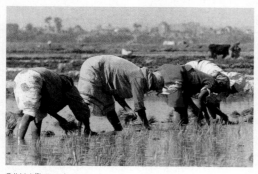
© Hajakely/Shutterstock

those who have disorders that limit fat absorption from the intestines may have deficiencies of fat-soluble vitamins. People who consume too many fat-soluble vitamins, usually by overdosing on supplements, may accumulate elevated levels of these vitamins in their bodies.

About 30 vitamins and minerals have been identified as essential components of the human diet (**Figure 12.10**). Micronutrient deficiencies are a frequent form of undernutrition in both children and adults. Vitamin and mineral deficiencies are sometimes called "hidden hunger" because they may not cause obvious symptoms but they do contribute to diminished health status.[36] A large proportion of the world's population remains at risk of deficiencies of iron, iodine, vitamin A, zinc, and other micronutrients.[57] Most people with severe micronutrient deficiencies live in lower-income countries, but there are also pockets of micronutrient deficiencies in some high-income populations because of dietary habits.

The best way to consume micronutrients is through food. When a person's diet does not provide enough nutrients or the body is not absorbing enough nutrients from food, nonfood sources may be helpful.[58] **Supplementation** is the process of delivering micronutrients through a pill, tablet, capsule, or other nonfood substance. For example, prenatal vitamins for women who may become pregnant, vitamin D and iron for infants, and vitamin D and calcium for older adults all have demonstrated health benefits.[59]

Another option is to add extra micronutrients to foods. **Enrichment** is the process of adding nutrients lost during handling, processing, or storage back to food products. **Fortification** is the process of adding micronutrients not naturally present in a food's ingredients to a food product. Examples of enriched and fortified foods include vitamin A fortified sugar, vitamin D fortified milk, folic acid and iron enriched flours, and iodized salt.[60] However, not all supplements and enriched and fortified foods provide vitamins and minerals in a form that has a high bioavailability. **Bioavailability** is the proportion of a consumed nutrient that is able to be absorbed and used by the body. Absorption can be increased by taking supplements with food.[61] For example, fat-soluble vitamins work best when taken with fat or oil, and iron absorption is boosted by vitamin C.

12.8 Iron Deficiency Anemia

Iron is a mineral that the body uses to make red blood cells (RBCs, also called erythrocytes), which carry oxygen from the lungs to the rest of the cells in the body. **Hemoglobin** is a molecule made from iron that holds the oxygen inside the RBCs. A person with too

Vitamins		Minerals	
Water-Soluble Vitamins	**Fat-Soluble Vitamins**	**Macrominerals**	**Trace Minerals**
■ Thiamine (vitamin B_1) ■ Riboflavin (vitamin B_2) ■ Niacin (vitamin B_3) ■ Pantothenic acid (vitamin B_5) ■ Pyridoxine (vitamin B_6) ■ Biotin (vitamin B_7) ■ Folate (vitamin B_9) ■ Cobalamin (vitamin B_{12}) ■ Vitamin C (ascorbic acid)	■ Vitamin A (retinol, beta-carotene) ■ Vitamin D (cholecalciferol) ■ Vitamin E (tocopherol) ■ Vitamin K	■ Calcium ■ Chloride ■ Magnesium ■ Phosphorus ■ Potassium ■ Sodium ■ Sulfur	■ Chromium ■ Copper ■ Fluoride ■ Iodine ■ Iron ■ Manganese ■ Molybdenum ■ Selenium ■ Zinc

Figure 12.10 Essential vitamins and minerals.

little iron is not able to make enough RBCs to efficiently transport oxygen. **Anemia** is a deficiency of RBCs or hemoglobin. Symptoms of anemia include pale skin, fatigue, weakness, shortness of breath, headaches, an increased heart rate, and a limited ability to concentrate at work or school. Children, pregnant women, and menstruating adolescents and adults are at high risk of anemia.[62] Children need extra iron as their body grows and their blood volume increases. Pregnant women need extra iron as their blood volume expands and to reduce the risk of dying during childbirth. People who menstruate or have recently given birth may have depleted RBCs and iron from blood loss.

Several processes can cause anemia, including inadequate production of healthy RBCs (which may occur due to a genetic disorder such as sickle cell disease or thalassemia), infections like malaria that destroy RBCs, blood loss (including blood loss associated with menstruation and childbirth), and micronutrient deficiencies (such as deficiencies of folate, vitamin B_{12}, vitamin A, or vitamin C).

Iron deficiency anemia (IDA) occurs when the body produces too few RBCs due to inadequate iron intake.[63] IDA is the most frequent cause of anemia worldwide.[64]

The prevalence of mild, moderate, and severe anemia has decreased in recent decades,[65] dropping from an overall prevalence of about 40% in 1990 to about 33% in 2010 and less than 25% in 2020.[64] However, population growth means that the number of people with anemia has not changed much. In 2020, there were still about 1.7 billion people with at least mild anemia, including at least 1 billion people with anemia due to dietary iron deficiencies.[64] More than 40% of under-5 children, about 40% of pregnant women, and nearly 33% of all reproductive-age females are anemic.[66] The Global Nutrition Targets aim to reduce the prevalence of anemia among women ages 15–49 years by 50% between 2012 and 2025, achieving a rate of less than 15% (**Figure 12.11**).[2] Over the first five years of this period, the prevalence increased from 30% to 33% rather than decreasing.[67]

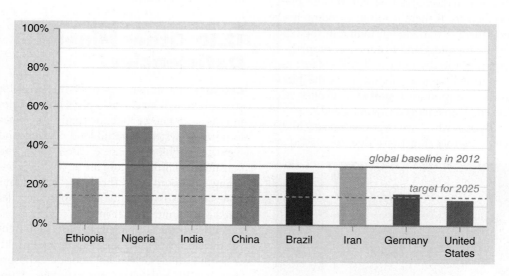

Figure 12.11 Percentage of women ages 15–49 years with mild, moderate, or severe anemia (a hemoglobin concentration less than 120 g/L for nonpregnant women and lactating women or less than 110 g/L for pregnant women) in 2016. The Global Nutrition Targets aim to reduce the anemia prevalence rate in each country and worldwide by 50% between 2012 and 2025.

Data from *2020 Global Nutrition Report: Action on Equity to End Malnutrition.* Bristol, UK: Development Initiatives; 2020.

IDA can be prevented and treated by increasing iron intake. Iron is present in both animal- and plant-based food sources. Heme iron is naturally found in blood and meat from animals, birds, and fish, and about 15%–35% of consumed heme iron is absorbed by the body; nonheme iron is found in plants, eggs, and milk, but less than 10% is absorbed.[68] Iron can also be consumed via supplements or added to fortified foods like pastas and flours. Treating infections that cause internal bleeding (like hookworm and schistosomiasis) and destroy RBCs (like malaria) is also important for preventing and alleviating the burden from anemia.[69]

12.9 Iodine Deficiency Disorders

Metabolism is the rate at which a person's body uses energy. **Iodine** is an element that is critical for regulating metabolism. The thyroid gland, located in the neck, uses iodine to create thyroid hormones, which are the chemical messengers that control the body's metabolism. If there is too little iodine in the diet, there is not enough iodine in the blood for the thyroid gland to function properly. In response, the thyroid gland will enlarge as it tries to collect more iodine from the blood, and it will produce a **goiter**, a swollen neck caused by an enlarged thyroid gland.

People who have hypothyroidism (underactive thyroid function) due to inadequate iodine intake or other causes cannot produce enough thyroid hormones, and they often have slow metabolisms and feel cold, fatigued, and constipated. Babies born to mothers who have hypothyroidism may be stillborn or born with congenital hypothyroidism (previously called cretinism), which describes the brain damage and stunted growth that occurs when fetal development is impaired due to inadequate maternal iodine levels. Even relatively minor iodine deficiencies may cause impaired mental function in children and adults.[70]

Iodine deficiency disorders (IDD) encompass the thyroid disorders and intellectual disabilities caused by a lack of dietary iodine. Iodized salt is a cost-efficient way to reduce the population-level burden from IDD, and a growing proportion of commercial table salt is iodized. As the prevalence of households using iodized salt increased from 20% in 1990 to nearly 90% by 2020, the worldwide prevalence of goiters decreased from about 13% to about 3%.[71] However, IDD remains among the most frequent causes of impaired cognitive function in the world.[72]

12.10 Other Mineral Deficiencies

Calcium is a mineral used by the body for strengthening bones. It also plays critical roles in muscle and nerve functions and contributes to immune system health, blood clotting, and regulation of blood pressure. Adolescents who consume too little calcium are at risk of developing osteoporosis as they age, and porous bones can lead to hip fractures and other life-threatening injuries later in life.

Fluoride is a mineral that is essential for the development of strong teeth. Dental health is optimized by a level of fluoride exposure that is neither deficient nor excessive. Fluoride is often added to commercial toothpaste and sometimes added to drinking water at low concentrations.[73] High concentrations of fluoride are avoided because excess fluoride (fluorosis) can cause the teeth to stain and become

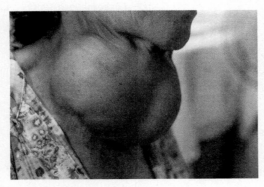

A woman with a goiter.
© Karan Bunjean/Shutterstock

pitted and weak when fluoride replaces some of the calcium in the teeth.

Zinc is a mineral that is important for immune function and wound healing. Even mild zinc deficiency is associated with increased susceptibility to infection; slow wound healing; and a higher risk of death from diarrhea, malaria, and pneumonia.[74] Zinc is found primarily in animal sources, so people who consume a mostly plant-based diet often benefit from taking zinc supplements or eating food fortified with zinc.[75]

Deficiencies in other minerals can also impair growth, health, and healing.[76] Magnesium is used for protein formation, muscle contraction, immune function, and nerve signal transmission, and a deficiency can cause constipation. Phosphorus is necessary for energy production within cells and contributes to skeletal health, acid–base balance, and regulation of other functions. Chloride, potassium, and sodium are important for maintaining fluid balance within the body, and deficiencies can lead to fatigue, weakness, and serious complications related to electrolyte imbalances. Sulfur plays a role in stabilizing proteins. Chromium contributes to glucose tolerance. Copper is necessary for RBC production, so copper deficiency causes anemia.[77] Manganese, molybdenum, and selenium contribute to cell functioning.

12.11 Vitamin A Deficiency

Vitamin A is a fat-soluble vitamin that is critical for vision. Vitamin A from animal sources occurs in the form of retinol, and plant-based vitamin A occurs in the form of beta-carotene. **Vitamin A deficiency** (VAD) causes visual impairment. The first symptom of advanced VAD is night blindness, which is poor vision at night or in low light conditions. Continued VAD causes **xerophthalmia**, a severe dryness of the eye that occurs as keratin builds up in the conjunctiva (the whites of the eyes). Untreated VAD can progress from the formation of Bitot's spots (dry patches on the conjunctiva) to corneal xerosis and then the ulceration and scarring of the cornea (keratomalacia). For children, VAD also increases the risk of death from infectious diseases, especially measles and diarrhea.

Young children and pregnant women experience the greatest adverse health outcomes from VAD. The prevalence of mild, moderate, or severe VAD among children less than five years old who live in low- and middle-income countries decreased from about 40% in 1990 to less than 30% by 2015.[78] Even though there has been continued progress toward reducing the prevalence of VAD, about 100 million under-5 children currently have serum retinol concentrations of <0.70 μmol/L, a level of deficiency that is associated with a heightened risk of VAD-related infectious disease complications.[64] More than 1 million children have night blindness, most of whom live in sub-Saharan Africa or south Asia.[79] Many pregnant women in low-income countries are also vitamin A deficient, and about half of pregnant women with VAD have night blindness.[79]

Yellow, orange, and dark green vegetables are the best dietary sources of vitamin A, in addition to some animal sources, such as liver. Because vitamin A is fat soluble and will only be absorbed by the body if it is eaten with fats or oils, dietary prevention of VAD requires a consistent source of both vegetables and oil. In some countries, milk, sugar, or other commercial products are fortified with vitamin A, but fortified foods are not available to all households that need them. Some genetically modified food products that are high in vitamin A are in development, but they are not yet widely available.[80] Oil-filled vitamin A capsule supplements are relatively inexpensive and are effective at lowering under-5 child morbidity and mortality from diarrhea, measles, and other causes in places where VAD is a public health problem.[81] However, distribution can be a challenge, and frequent redistribution must occur because the benefits of the capsules last for only a few months.[82]

12.12 Other Vitamin Deficiencies

A severe deficiency of any vitamin or mineral can cause significant impairment of a person's health status. For example, the B vitamins are critical for metabolism, and people with B vitamin deficiencies tend to lack energy. Each B vitamin plays a unique role in body function. For example, **thiamine** is a B vitamin (vitamin B$_1$) that is necessary for nerve, muscle, and heart function, and **niacin** is a B vitamin (vitamin B$_3$) that is necessary for skin health and digestive and nervous system function. Thiamine deficiency is called **beriberi**. Infants with beriberi may experience heart failure, and older children and adults with thiamine deficiency may experience leg weakness and confusion.[83] Niacin deficiency is called **pellagra**. The three key symptoms of pellagra are dermatitis, dementia, and chronic diarrhea.[84] The skin of people with pellagra becomes scaly, darkens, and sloughs off the body.

Folate is a B vitamin (vitamin B$_9$) that is critical for fetal development as well as growth and RBC production. Women of childbearing age need to make sure that they have an adequate daily intake of folate because deficiency during the first weeks of pregnancy is associated with neural tube defects in developing fetuses.[85] The most frequently occurring neural tube defects are anencephaly, a fatal condition in which the brain fails to develop, and spina bifida, in which the spinal cord does not develop properly. These defects occur very early in the pregnancy, usually before a woman knows she is pregnant, so all adolescents and adults who might become pregnant are advised to take a daily multivitamin. Folate is naturally found in foods like liver and spinach. **Folic acid** is a synthetic form of folate that can be added to foods or supplements.

Antioxidants reduce the free radicals in cells that may damage cell membranes. **Vitamin C** is an antioxidant that is essential for collagen formation and iron absorption and is also involved in immune system function. People with vitamin C deficiency develop **scurvy**, which is characterized by bleeding gums, loose teeth, weakness, anemia, and leg pain.[86]

Vitamin D is necessary for bone health because it assists the body with calcium absorption.[87] Vitamin D deficiency (VDD) in children, whose bones are still growing, is called **rickets** or, informally, "knock knees." VDD in adults, whose bones have stopped growing, is called **osteomalacia**. Rickets and osteomalacia can cause the bones to become soft and prone to breaking. Vitamin D, known as the "sun vitamin," can be made by the body when skin is exposed to sunlight for about 15 minutes daily, but adequate sun exposure is not always possible.[88] Low levels of vitamin D in the blood are frequently found among students, workers, and older adults who often remain indoors all day; people who consistently wear skin-covering clothes when outdoors; people who live far from the equator and experience several months of outdoor darkness each year; and individuals with dark skin pigmentation.[89]

Deficiencies of riboflavin, pantothenic acid, pyridoxine, biotin, cobalamin, vitamin E (which is an antioxidant), and vitamin K (which is critical for blood clotting) can also cause health problems.

12.13 Overweight and Obesity

Overnutrition is a form of malnutrition caused by excessive intake of calories and nutrients. Overnutrition is usually classified based on the **body mass index (BMI)**, a measure of body composition calculated by taking weight in kilograms and dividing it by the square of the person's height in meters:

$$BMI = \frac{\text{weight (kg)}}{\text{height (m)} \times \text{height (m)}}$$
$$= 703 \times \frac{\text{weight (lb)}}{\text{height (in)} \times \text{height (in)}}.$$

For adults, international classifications generally suggest that a BMI of less than 18.5 indicates underweight, a BMI of 25 to 29.9 indicates **overweight**, and a BMI of 30 or greater indicates **obesity**.[90] For children and adolescents, BMI percentiles by age group are typically used to identify overweight and obesity.[91] Additional anthropometric measures can complement the BMI by providing further information about health risks. For example, having a waist circumference greater than 35 inches for a woman or 40 inches for a man is associated with an increased risk of diabetes and heart disease.[92]

The BMI and other anthropometric measurements have limitations as measures of health status.[93] The BMI does not adjust for the body fat percentage, so people who are trim but have a lot of muscle mass may incorrectly be classified as overweight. The BMI also does not measure physical fitness levels. People with any BMI who have poor cardiovascular endurance are at risk of a diversity of adverse health outcomes. However, scientific studies consistently find that obesity is associated with an increased risk of many diseases, including type 2 diabetes, hypertension (high blood pressure), heart disease, strokes, gallstones and other digestive disorders, back pain, arthritis of the back and hip, and several types of cancer.[94] Treatment of health problems attributed to high BMIs currently costs health systems nearly $1 trillion per year, with those expenditures accounting for about $1 of every $8 spent on health services.[95]

Over the past several decades, most countries have experienced steady increases in their average adult BMIs (**Figure 12.12**).[96] The global adult prevalence of overweight and obesity combined (BMI ≥25) increased from less than 30% in 1980 to nearly 40%

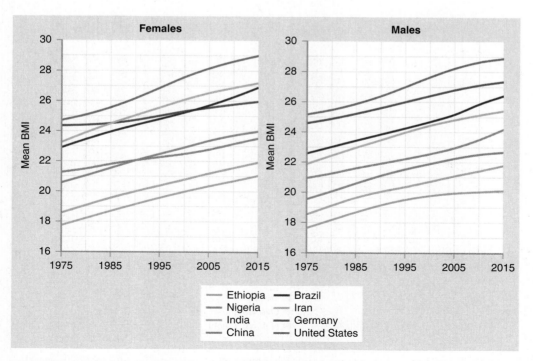

Figure 12.12 Mean adult BMI (ages 20+ years), 1975–2015.

Data from NCD Risk Factor Collaboration (NCD-RisC). Worldwide trends in body-mass index, underweight, overweight, and obesity from 1975 to 2016: a pooled analysis of 2416 population-based measurement studies in 128.9 million children, adolescents, and adults. *Lancet.* 2017;390:2627–2642.

in 2015,[97] and more than 10% of the world's adults now have obesity (BMI ≥30).[98] In many high-income countries and a growing number of middle-income countries, more than half of adults are now overweight or obese (**Figure 12.13**).[96] Overweight and obesity are also becoming more prevalent in pediatric populations. The percentage of school-aged children and adolescents (ages 5–19 years) who are overweight or obese worldwide is now nearly double the percentage who are underweight (**Figure 12.14**).[99]

The **obesity transition** describes the typical progression of which demographic groups develop obesity as the nutrition transition occurs.[100] The prevalence of obesity typically increases first among adult women, especially urban women with higher socioeconomic status. In low-income countries today, women tend to have a significantly higher prevalence of obesity than men.[96] Next, the prevalence of obesity among adults increases across all income groups and locations, and the differences in obesity rates by sex narrow. During this phase, a growing proportion of children and adolescents also become overweight or obese. These changes have been observed in many middle-income countries, especially upper-middle-income ones.[98] In the third phase of the obesity transition, the prevalence of obesity among individuals with lower socioeconomic status rises above the rate for people with higher socioeconomic status.[101] This is the current pattern in most high-income countries today, where rural residents tend to have lower incomes and slightly higher rates of obesity than urban residents (**Figure 12.15**).[102] A hypothesized fourth stage would be characterized by the rates of obesity decreasing in the highest-income populations, but this has not yet been observed anywhere.[100]

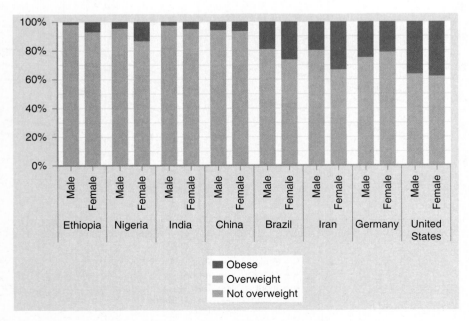

Figure 12.13 Prevalence of obesity and overweight among adult males and females (ages 20+ years).

Data from NCD Risk Factor Collaboration (NCD-RisC). Worldwide trends in body-mass index, underweight, overweight, and obesity from 1975 to 2016: a pooled analysis of 2416 population-based measurement studies in 128.9 million children, adolescents, and adults. *Lancet.* 2017;390:2627–2642.

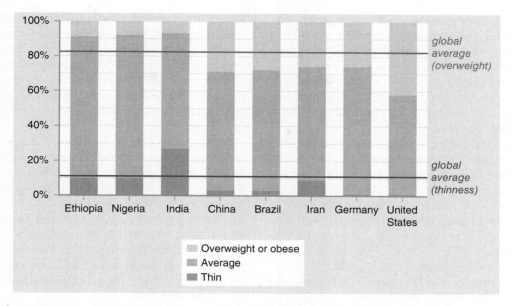

Figure 12.14 Percentage of school-aged children (ages 5–19 years) who are thin (<–2 standard deviations from the median for body mass index of the WHO growth reference for school-age children and adolescents) or overweight (>1 standard deviation from the median for BMI).

Data from *State of the World's Children 2019*. New York: UNICEF; 2019.

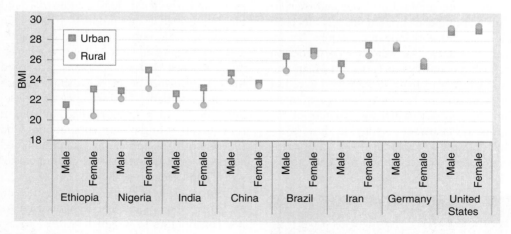

Figure 12.15 Mean body mass index (BMI) among adults (ages 20+ years), by sex and country of residence.

Data from NCD Risk Factor Collaboration (NCD-RisC). Rising rural body-mass index is the main driver of the global obesity epidemic in adults. *Nature*. 2019;569:260–264.

12.14 Obesity Interventions

The transition toward overnutrition as the dominant global nutrition concern is primarily a function of the dietary changes associated with economic development.[103] These new practices often include increased portion sizes, more snacking, more meals eaten outside the home, replacing water with sweetened beverages, eating more animal protein, cooking with more oil, adding more sweeteners to the diet, and shifting from consuming whole grains to refined grains.[7] Genetic changes do not explain why obesity has become so much more prevalent in recent decades. Genes influence metabolic rate, body shape (where a person carries excess weight), and the efficiency of the body at storing extra calories, but it takes generations for genetic adaptations to occur. By contrast, it takes only a short time to change dietary and exercise habits. A person who consistently takes in more calories than the body uses will gain weight, become overweight, and then develop obesity.

Dietary behaviors are guided by sociocultural eating practices and by attitudes about acceptable and preferred weights, body shapes, and definitions of physical beauty.[104] In industrialized societies today, being underweight is often an indication of wealth because richer households have the time and money to prepare healthy foods and exercise while working-class households rely on cheap fast foods and work long hours at jobs that are often sedentary. The women who model on the fashion runways in Paris and Milan and those who are Hollywood stars tend to reflect this standard for beauty by being extremely thin. By contrast, when the painters of the European Renaissance wanted to show beautiful, powerful femininity, they portrayed women with rolls of fat and rounded curves.

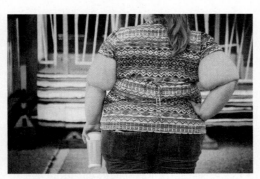

© Suzanne Tucker/Shutterstock

In some cultures today, larger women are still seen as having ideal body shapes and greater weight is perceived to indicate fertility. When resources are scarce, having greater weight is often a sign of wealth because it shows that the household has more than enough calories and does not need to expend so many of them in physical labor.

Observations about how obesity clusters within social networks have led some researchers to consider obesity to be a "contagious" condition.[105] One person's weight gain may increase the likelihood that friends and family members will also gain weight.[106] In places where the typical person is obese, people who have obesity may not consider themselves or others in their social networks to be overweight because body size is evaluated relative to community norms.[107]

An individual's body perceptions and dietary choices are also influenced by a variety of globalization processes, including global media, urbanization, intensified international trade, and new technologies. Industrial food processing often creates products that are high in salt, trans fat, saturated fats, added sugars, and total calories and low in fruits, vegetables, nuts, legumes, and whole grains. Processed food products may be the only dietary options that are affordable to lower-income households or the only items readily available in some urban settings. Since communities tend to have similar socioeconomic status and food access, poor nutritional status tends to cluster socially and geographically.

Although reducing caloric intake and exercising longer and more vigorously are key contributors to weight loss, the process of losing weight and maintaining that weight loss is not as simple as "calories in, calories out."[108] Adults with obesity who lose a lot of weight may permanently lower their resting metabolic rates, and it can be difficult to prevent weight regain when their bodies expend fewer calories at rest and during exercise after losing weight.[109] Individuals with similar ages, body weights, and activity levels often have different metabolic rates and energy expenditures,[110] so some individuals have to restrict more calories from their diets and exercise longer than others to make similar progress toward achieving weight goals. The biological, psychological, social, economic, environmental, and other factors that contribute to weight gain also often make weight loss difficult.

Because increasing rates of obesity are related to sociocultural factors, economics, national and international policies, industrialized food systems, environmental changes, and a host of other contributors,[111] initiatives to reverse this trend will require an equally complex set of interventions. Individuals seeking to prevent weight gain, lose weight, or maintain weight loss must adopt and sustain healthy diets and physically active lifestyles. Those individual efforts can be supported through community nutrition programs. Community initiatives can be supported by state and national nutrition policy interventions, such as ones that fund nutrition education, regulate the nutrition information provided on food packages, limit the marketing of unhealthy foods to children, tax unhealthy foods to increase their prices and decrease consumption, and subsidize healthy foods to lower their prices.[112]

At the broader policy level, the World Obesity Federation calls for a variety of new approaches for responding to obesity as a global public health issue, including greater recognition that obesity has serious implications for individuals, societies, and economies; more research to elucidate the causes of obesity and identify strategies for preventing and treating it; the development, testing, and implementation of obesity prevention strategies across the life span; the use of evidence-based, person-centered, nonstigmatizing, dignified, multimodal treatments for obesity; and the use of systems-based approaches to strengthen health systems and mitigate the underlying social, commercial, and environmental roots of obesity.[95]

12.15 Food Safety

The globalization of food systems is evident in changing eating habits, the increasing variety of foods on grocery store shelves, the growing number of international restaurant chains, and the global marketing of food products. International food markets have grown significantly in recent decades. For example, the proportion of food consumed in the United States that is imported increased from 12% in 1990 to nearly 20% by 2015 (**Figure 12.16**).[113] This increased cross-border trade in foods has created a new set of concerns about food safety.[114] Because these threats can be mitigated only through international agreements, food safety has become a global health issue.

More than 2 billion cases of foodborne diseases and intoxications occur every year, and foodborne infectious diseases cause more than 1 million deaths each year.[115] A wide variety of foods have been implicated in outbreaks, including fruits and vegetables, meats and poultry, eggs, seafood, dairy products, bakery items, nuts, and unpasteurized fruit juices.[116] The major causes of foodborne illness and death include norovirus, *E. coli*, *Salmonella*, *Campylobacter*, *Shigella*, and hepatitis A virus.[117] Other foodborne infectious diseases include brucellosis; cholera; listeriosis; *Mycobacterium bovis*; paratyphoid; typhoid[118]; and parasitic infections like cryptosporidiosis, cyclosporiasis (*Cyclospora cayetanensis*), giardiasis, and toxoplasmosis

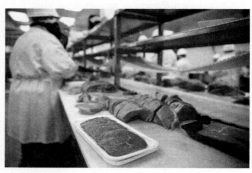

© El Nariz/Shutterstock

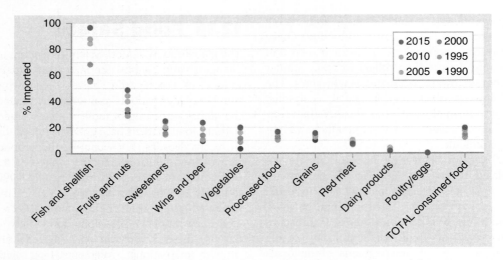

Figure 12.16 Percentage of foods consumed in the United States that are imported, by year.

Data from *U.S. Food and Agricultural Imports: Safeguards and Selected Issues (R46440).* Washington DC: Congressional Research Service; 2020.

(*Toxoplasma gondii*).[119] In addition to microbial contamination, chemical contaminants are increasing threats to health.[120] Concerns have been raised about heavy metal poisoning from mercury in fish, pesticide residues, chemical additives and preservatives, and other substances.[121] Most outbreaks of foodborne diseases are caused by locally grown and processed foods because most foods consumed around the world are still ones that were produced in the home countries of the people eating them, but an increasing number of foodborne outbreaks are traced back to imported foods.[122]

Food producers, processors, distributors, and consumers all have a role to play in ensuring that foods remain safe along the supply chain. The **Codex Alimentarius** international food standards, developed by scientific panels hosted by the United Nations, are a compilation of specific guidelines for keeping food products safe.[123] For example, **pasteurization**, a process of heating foods to kill the bacteria that might be present in milk, dairy and egg products, beer, fruit juices, and

other products, is recommended for some food items. However, the *Codex* is not binding on countries or food producers, and the standards can be difficult to enforce. Additionally, labeling requirements are not standardized across markets, and countries have different expectations about the use of additives and preservatives, fortification and enrichment with vitamins and minerals, and the use and labeling of genetically modified organisms.

The hazard analysis and critical control point (HACCP) system is an approach to food safety that has been widely adopted by commercial food processors and distributors.[124] Several simple food safety practices can help protect consumers at home and in restaurants, including careful cleaning, separation of uncooked and ready-to-eat foods, and keeping foods at appropriate temperatures.[125] However, food preparers have limited ability to combat some types of food contamination. As the food industry becomes increasingly global, it may become more difficult for governments and consumers to have confidence that their food supply is safe.

References

1. Katz DL, Meller S. Can we say what diet is best for health? *Ann Rev Public Health.* 2014;35:83–103.

2. *2020 Global Nutrition Report: Action on Equity to End Malnutrition.* Bristol UK: Development Initiatives; 2020.

3. Victora CG, Adair L, Fall C, et al. Maternal and child undernutrition: consequences for adult health and human capital. *Lancet.* 2008;371:340–357.

4. Jonsson U. Nutrition and the convention on the rights of the child. *Food Policy.* 1996;21:41–55.

5. Barrett BD, Maxwell DG. *Food Aid after Fifty Years: Recasting Its Role.* New York: Routledge; 2005.

6. *Transforming Our World: The 2030 Agenda for Sustainable Development.* New York: United Nations; 2015.

7. Popkin BM. Global nutrition dynamics: the world is shifting rapidly toward a diet linked with noncommunicable diseases. *Am J Clin Nutr.* 2006;84:289–298.

8. Popkin BM, Adair LS, Ng SW. The global nutrition transition: the pandemic of obesity in developing countries. *Nutr Rev.* 2012;70:3–21.

9. *Dietary Guidelines for Americans, 2020–2025.* 9th ed. Washington DC: U.S. Department of Agriculture; 2020.

10. *FAO Statistical Pocketbook: World Food and Agriculture 2020.* Rome: Food and Agriculture Organization of the United Nations; 2020.

11. *Dietary Reference Intakes for Energy, Carbohydrate, Fiber, Fat, Fatty Acids, Cholesterol, Protein, and Amino Acids.* Washington DC: National Academies Press; 2005.

12. *FAOSTAT Food Balance Sheets: New Food Balances.* Rome: Food and Agriculture Organization of the United Nations; 2020.

13. Sacks FM, Lichtenstein AH, Wu JHY, et al. Dietary fats and cardiovascular disease: a presidential advisory from the American Heart Association. *Circulation.* 2017;136:e1–e23.

14. de Souza RJ, Mente A, Maroleanu A, et al. Intake of saturated and trans unsaturated fatty acids and risk of all cause mortality, cardiovascular disease, and type 2 diabetes: systematic review and meta-analysis of observational studies. *BMJ.* 2015;351:h3978.

15. Popkin BM, D'Anci KE, Rosenberg IH. Water, hydration and health. *Nutr Rev.* 2010;68:439–458.

16. Gura T. Nature's first functional food. *Science.* 2014;345:747–749.

17. Jones KDJ, Berkley JA, Warner JO. Perinatal nutrition and immunity to infection. *Pediatr Allergy Immunol.* 2010;21(4 Pt 1):564–576.

18. Debes AK, Kohli A, Walker N, Edmond K, Mullany LC. Time to initiation of breastfeeding and neonatal mortality and morbidity: a systematic review. *BMC Public Health.* 2013;13(Suppl 3):S19.

19. *The State of the World's Children 2019.* New York: UNICEF; 2019.

20. *Breastfeeding: A Mother's Gift, for Every Child.* New York: UNICEF/World Health Organization; 2018.

21. Victora CG, Bahl R, Barros AJD, et al. Breastfeeding in the 21st century: epidemiology, mechanisms, and lifelong effect. *Lancet.* 2016;387:475–490.

22. *From the First Hour of Life: Making the Case for Improved Infant and Young Child Feeding Everywhere.* New York: UNICEF; 2016.

23. *Indicators for Assessing Infant and Young Child Feeding Practices.* Geneva: World Health Organization; 2010.

24. Rollins NC, Bhandari N, Hajeebhoy N, et al. Why invest, and what will it take to improve breastfeeding practices? *Lancet.* 2016;387:491–504.

25. Brady JP. Marketing breast milk substitutes: problems and perils throughout the world. *Arch Dis Child.* 2012;97:529–532.

26. *Marketing of Breast-Milk Substitutes: National Implementation of the International Code, Status Report 2020.* Geneva: World Health Organization; 2020.

27. Meedya S, Fahy K, Kable A. Factors that positively influence breastfeeding duration to 6 months: a literature review. *Women Birth.* 2010;23:135–145.

28. WHO Child Growth Standards. *Length/Height-for-Age, Weight-for-Age, Weight-for-Length, Weight-for-Height and Body Mass Index-for-Age: Methods and Development.* Geneva: World Health Organization; 2006.

29. Onyango AW, de Onis M, Caroli M, et al. Field-testing the WHO Child Growth Standards in four countries. *J Nutr.* 2007;137:149–152.

30. WHO Multicentre Growth Reference Study Group. *WHO Child Growth Standards: Length/Height-for-Age, Weight-for-Age, Weight-for-Length, Weight-for-Height and Body Mass Index-for-Age: Methods and Development.* Geneva: World Health Organization; 2006.

31. *Levels and Trends in Child Malnutrition: UNICEF/WHO/World Bank Group Joint Child Malnutrition Estimates.* New York: UNICEF; 2019.

32. *Global Nutrition Targets 2025: Policy Brief Series.* Geneva: World Health Organization; 2014.

33. Local Burden of Disease Child Growth Failure Collaborators. Mapping child growth failure across low- and middle-income countries. *Nature.* 2020; 577:231–234.

34. Black RE, Victora CG, Walker SP, et al. Maternal and child undernutrition and overweight in low-income and middle-income countries. *Lancet.* 2013;382:427–451.

35. Caulfield LE, de Onis M, Blössner M, Black RE. Undernutrition as an underlying cause of child deaths

associated with diarrhea, pneumonia, malaria, and measles. *Am J Clin Nutr.* 2004;80:193–198.

36. *2020 Global Hunger Index: One Decade to Zero Hunger.* Bonn/Dublin: Welthungerhilfe/Concern Worldwide; 2020.

37. Smith LC, Haddad L. Reducing child undernutrition: past drivers and priorities for the post-MDG era. *World Dev.* 2015;68:180–204.

38. Grover Z, Ee LC. Protein energy malnutrition. *Pediatr Clin North Am.* 2009;56:1055–1068.

39. *WHO Child Growth Standards and the Identification of Severe Acute Malnutrition in Infants and Children: A Joint Statement by the World Health Organization and the United Nations Children's Fund.* Geneva/New York: World Health Organization/UNICEF; 2009.

40. Bhutta ZA, Berkley JA, Bandsma RHJ, Kerac M, Trehan I, Briend A. Severe childhood malnutrition. *Nat Rev Dis Primers.* 2017;3:17067.

41. *Guideline: Updates on the Management of Severe Acute Malnutrition in Infants and Children.* Geneva: World Health Organization; 2013.

42. Brown KH, Nyirandutiye DH, Jungjohann S. Management of children with acute malnutrition in resource-poor settings. *Nat Rev Endocrinol.* 2009;5:597–603.

43. Bhutta ZA, Wazny K, Lenters L. Management of severe and moderate acute malnutrition in children (chapter 11). In: Black RE, Laxminarayan R, Temmerman M, Walker N, eds. *Disease Control Priorities: Reproductive, Maternal, Newborn, and Child Health.* 3rd ed. Vol. 2. Washington DC: IBRD/World Bank; 2016:205–224.

44. Bhutta ZA, Das JK, Rizvi A, et al. Evidence-based interventions for improvement of maternal and child nutrition: what can be done and at what cost? *Lancet.* 2013;382:452–477.

45. Gillespie S, Haddad L, Mannar V, et al. The politics of reducing malnutrition: building commitment and accelerating progress. *Lancet.* 2013;382:552–569.

46. Ruel MT, Alderman H, Maternal and Child Nutrition Study Group. Nutrition-sensitive interventions and programmes: how can they help to accelerate progress in improving maternal and child nutrition? *Lancet.* 2013;382:536–551.

47. *Trade Reforms and Food Security: Conceptualizing the Linkages.* Rome: Food and Agriculture Organization of the United Nations; 2003.

48. Jones AD, Ngure FM, Pelto G, Young SL. What are we assessing when we measure food security? A compendium and review of current metrics. *Adv Nutr.* 2013;4:481–505.

49. Barrett CB. Measuring food insecurity. *Science.* 2010;327:825–828.

50. Bickel G, Nord M, Price C, Hamilton W, Cook J. *Guide to Measuring Household Food Security.* Alexandria VA: U.S. Department of Agriculture; 2000.

51. *An Introduction to the Basic Concepts of Food Security.* Rome: Food and Agriculture Organization of the United Nations; 2008.

52. *The State of Food Security and Nutrition in the World 2020.* Rome: Food and Agriculture Organization of the United Nations; 2020.

53. Sen A. Ingredients of famine analysis: availability and entitlements. *Q J Econ.* 1981;96:433–464.

54. Godfray HCJ, Beddington JR, Crute IR, et al. Food security: the challenge of feeding 9 billion people. *Science.* 2010;327:812–818.

55. Godfray HC, Crute IR, Haddad L, et al. The future of the global food system. *Philos Trans R Soc Lond B Biol Sci.* 2010;365:2769–2777.

56. Maxwell S, Slater R. Food policy old and new. *Dev Policy Rev.* 2003;21:531–553.

57. Bailey RL, West KP Jr, Black RE. The epidemiology of global micronutrient deficiencies. *Ann Nutr Metab.* 2015;66(Suppl 2):22–33.

58. Rautiainen S, Manson JE, Liechtenstein AH, Sesso HD. Dietary supplements and disease prevention: a global overview. *Nat Rev Endocrinol.* 2016;12:407–420.

59. Manson JE, Bassuk SS. Vitamin and mineral supplements: what clinicians need to know. *JAMA.* 2018;319:859–860.

60. Allan L, de Benoist B, Dary O, Hurrell R. *Guidelines on Food Fortification with Micronutrients.* Geneva: World Health Organization/Food and Agriculture Organization of the United Nations; 2006.

61. Yetley EA. Multivitamin and multimineral dietary supplements: definitions, characterization, bio-availability, and drug interactions. *Am J Clin Nutr.* 2007;85:S269–S276.

62. Camaschella C. Iron-deficiency anemia. *N Engl J Med.* 2015;372:1832–1843.

63. Lopez A, Cacoub P, Macdougall IC, Peyrin-Biroulet L. Iron deficiency anaemia. *Lancet.* 2016;387:907–916.

64. GBD 2019 Diseases and Injuries Collaborators. Global burden of 369 diseases and injuries in 204 countries and territories, 1990–2019: a systematic analysis for the Global Burden of Disease Study 2019. *Lancet.* 2020;396:1204–1222.

65. Kassebaum NJ, Jasrasaria R, Naghavi M, et al. A systematic analysis of global anemia burden from 1990 to 2010. *Blood.* 2014;123:615–624.

66. Stevens GA, Finucane MM, De-Regil LM, et al. Global, regional, and national trends in haemoglobin concentration and prevalence of total and severe anaemia in children and pregnant and non-pregnant women for 1995–2011: a systematic analysis of population-representative data. *Lancet Glob Health.* 2013;1:e16–e25.

67. *Global Anaemia Reduction Efforts among Women of Reproductive Age: Impact, Achievement of Targets and the Way Forward for Optimizing Efforts.* Geneva: World Health Organization; 2020.

68. Zimmermann MB, Hurrell RF. Nutritional iron deficiency. *Lancet.* 2007;370:511–520.

69. *Nutritional Anaemias: Tools for Effective Prevention and Control.* Geneva: World Health Organization; 2017.

70. Li M, Eastman CJ. The changing epidemiology of iodine deficiency. *Nat Rev Endocrinol.* 2012;8:434–440.

71. Gorstein JL, Bagriansky J, Pearce EN, Kupka R, Zimmerman MB. Estimating the health and economic benefits of universal salt iodization programs to correct iodine deficiency disorders. *Thyroid.* 2020;30:1802–1809.

72. Zimmermann MB, Boelaert K. Iodine deficiency and thyroid disorders. *Lancet Diabetes Endocrinol.* 2015;3:286–295.

73. *Inadequate or Excess Fluoride: A Major Public Health Concern.* Geneva: World Health Organization; 2019.

74. Yakoob MY, Theodoratou E, Jabeen A, et al. Preventive zinc supplementation in developing countries: impact on mortality and morbidity due to diarrhea, pneumonia and more. *BMC Public Health.* 2011;11:S23.

75. Gupta S, Brazier AKM, Lowe NM. Zinc deficiency in low- and middle-income countries: prevalence and approaches for mitigation. *J Hum Nutr Dev.* 2020;33:624–643.

76. Gharibzahedi SMT, Jafari SM. The importance of minerals in human nutrition: bioavailability, food fortification, processing effects and nanoencapsulation. *Trends Food Sci Tech.* 2017;62:119–132.

77. Myint ZW, Oo TH, Thein KZ, Tun AM, Saeed H. Copper deficiency anemia: review article. *Ann Hematol.* 2018;97:1527–1534.

78. Stevens GA, Bennett JE, Hennocq Q, et al. Trends and mortality effects of vitamin A deficiency in children in 138 low-income and middle-income countries between 1991 and 2013: a pooled analysis of population-based surveys. *Lancet Glob Health.* 2015;3:e528–e536.

79. *Global Prevalence of Vitamin A Deficiency in Populations at Risk 1995–2005: WHO Global Database on Vitamin A Deficiency.* Geneva: World Health Organization; 2009.

80. Moghissi AA, Pei S, Liu Y. Golden rice: scientific, regulatory and public information processes of a genetically modified organism. *Crit Rev Biotechnol.* 2016;36:535–541.

81. Irmad A, Mayo-Wilson E, Herzer K, Bhutta ZA. Vitamin A supplementation for preventing morbidity and mortality in children from six months to five years of age. *Cochrane Database Syst Rev.* 2017;3:CD008524.

82. Mason J, Greiner J, Shrimpton R, Sanders D, Yukich J. Vitamin A policies need rethinking. *Int J Epidemiol.* 2015;44;283–292.

83. Whitfield KC, Bourassa MW, Adamolekun B, et al. Thiamine deficiency disorders: diagnosis, prevalence, and a roadmap for global control programs. *Ann N Y Acad Sci.* 2018;1430:3–43.

84. Hegyi J, Schwartz RA, Hegyi V. Pellagra: dermatitis, dementia, and diarrhea. *Int J Dermatol.* 2004;43:1–5.

85. Ami N, Bernstein M, Boucher F, Rieder M, Parker L. Folate and neural tube defects: the role of supplements and food fortification. *Pediatr Child Health.* 2016;21:145–154.

86. Byard RW, Maxwell-Stewart H. Scurvy: characteristic features and forensic issues. *Am J Forensic Med Pathol.* 2019;40:43–46.

87. Roth DE, Abrams SA, Aloia J, et al. Global prevalence and disease burden of vitamin D deficiency: a roadmap for action in low- and middle-income countries. *Ann N Y Acad Sci.* 2018;1430:44–79.

88. Wacker M, Holick MF. Sunlight and vitamin D: a global perspective for health. *Dermatoendocrinol.* 2013;5:51–108.

89. Van Schoor NM, Lips P. Worldwide vitamin D status. *Best Pract Res Clin Endocrinol Metab.* 2011;25:671–680.

90. *Obesity: Preventing and Managing the Global Epidemic.* Geneva: World Health Organization; 2000.

91. Cole TJ, Lobstein T. Extended international (IOTF) body mass index cut-offs for thinness, overweight and obesity. *Pediatr Obes.* 2012;7:284–294.

92. Klein S, Allison DB, Heymsfield SB, et al. Waist circumference and cardiometabolic risk: a consensus statement from Shaping America's Health: Association for Weight Management and Obesity Prevention; NAASO, The Obesity Society; the American Society for Nutrition; and the American Diabetes Association. *Am J Clin Nutr.* 2007;85:1197–1202.

93. Prentice AM, Jebb SA. Beyond body mass index. *Obes Rev.* 2001;2:141–147.

94. Field AE, Coakley EH, Must A, et al. Impact of overweight on the risk of developing common chronic diseases during a 10-year period. *Arch Intern Med.* 2001;161:1581–1586.

95. *Obesity: Missing the 2025 Global Targets: Trends, Costs and Country Reports.* London: World Obesity Federation; 2020.

96. NCD Risk Factor Collaboration (NCD-RisC). Worldwide trends in body-mass index, underweight, overweight, and obesity from 1975 to 2016: a pooled analysis of 2416 population-based measurement studies in 128.9 million children, adolescents, and adults. *Lancet.* 2017;390:2627–2642.

97. Ng M, Fleming T, Robinson M, et al. Global, regional and national prevalence of overweight and obesity in children and adults 1980–2013: a systematic analysis. *Lancet.* 2014;384:766–781.

98. GBD 2015 Obesity Collaborators. Health effects of overweight and obesity in 195 countries over 25 years. *N Engl J Med.* 2017;377:13–27.

99. *State of the World's Children 2019.* New York: UNICEF; 2019.

100. Jacks LM, Vandevijvere S, Pan A, et al. The obesity transition: stages of the global epidemic. *Lancet Diabetes Endocrinol.* 2019;7:231–240.

101. Ameye H, Swinnen J. Obesity, income and gender: the changing global relationship. *Global Food Security.* 2019;23:267–281.

102. NCD Risk Factor Collaboration (NCD-RisC). Rising rural body-mass index is the main driver of the global obesity epidemic in adults. *Nature.* 2019;569:260–264.

103. Malik VS, Willett WC, Hu FB. Global obesity: trends, risk factors and policy implication. *Nat Rev Endocrinol.* 2013;9:13–27.

104. Swami V, Frederick DA, Aavik T, et al. The attractive female body weight and female body dissatisfaction in 26 countries across 10 world regions: results of the International Body Project I. *Pers Soc Psychol Bull.* 2010;36:309–325.

105. Powell K, Wilcox J, Clonan A, et al. The role of social networks in the development of overweight and obesity among adults: a scoping review. *BMC Public Health.* 2015;15:996.

106. Christakis NA, Fowler JH. The spread of obesity in a large social network over 32 years. *N Engl J Med.* 2007;357:370–379.

107. Robinson E. Overweight but unseen: a review of the underestimation of weight status and a visual normalization theory. *Obes Rev.* 2017;18:1200–1209.

108. Ludwig DS, Ebbeling CB. The carbohydrate–insulin model of obesity: beyond 'calories in, calories out.' *JAMA Intern Med.* 2018;178:1098–1103.

109. Fothergill E, Guo J, Howard L, et al. Persistent metabolic adaptation 6 years after "The Biggest Loser" competition. *Obesity.* 2016;24:1612–1619.

110. Piaggi P. Metabolic determinants of weight gain in humans. *Obesity.* 2019;27:691–699.

111. Swinburn BA, Kraak VI, Allender S, et al. The global syndemic of obesity, undernutrition, and climate change: The Lancet Commission report. *Lancet.* 2019;393:791–846.

112. Cecchini M, Sassi F, Lauer JA, Lee YY, Guajardo-Barron V, Chisholm D. Tackling of unhealthy diets, physical inactivity, and obesity: health effects and cost-effectiveness. *Lancet.* 2010;376:1775–1784.

113. *U.S. Food and Agricultural Imports: Safeguards and Selected Issues (R46440).* Washington DC: Congressional Research Service; 2020.

114. Käferstein FK, Motarjemi Y, Bettcher DW. Foodborne disease control: a transnational challenge. *Emerg Infect Dis.* 1997;3:503–510.

115. Kirk MD, Pires SM, Black RE, et al. World Health Organization estimates of the global and regional disease burden of 22 foodborne bacterial, protozoal, and viral diseases, 2010: a data synthesis. *PLoS Med.* 2015;12:e1001921.

116. Hoffman S, Devleesschauwer B, Aspinall W, et al. Attribution of global foodborne disease to specific foods: findings from a World Health Organization structured expert elicitation. *PLoS One.* 2017;12:e0183641.

117. Havelaar AH, Kirk MD, Torgerson PR, et al. World Health Organization global estimates and regional comparisons of the burden of foodborne diseases in 2010. *PLoS Med.* 2015;12:e1001923.

118. Kirk MD, Pires SM, Black RE, et al. Global and regional disease burden of 22 foodborne bacterial, protozoal, and viral diseases, 2010: a data synthesis. *PLoS Negl Trop Dis.* 2015;12:e1001921.

119. Torgerson PR, Devleesschauwer B, Praet N, et al. World Health Organization estimates of the global and regional disease burden of 11 foodborne parasitic diseases, 2010: a data synthesis. *PLoS Negl Trop Dis.* 2015;12:e1001920.

120. *Bad Bug Book: Foodborne Pathogenic Microorganisms and Natural Toxins Handbook.* 2nd ed., updated. Silver Spring MD: FDA Center for Food Safety and Applied Nutrition; 2017.

121. Fung F, Wang HS, Menon S. Food safety in the 21st century. *Biomed J.* 2018;41:88–95.

122. Gould LH, Kline J, Monahan C, Vierk K. Outbreaks of disease associated with food imported into the United States, 1996–2014. *Emerg Infect Dis.* 2017;23:525–528.

123. *Codex Alimentarius: Understanding Codex.* 5th ed. Rome: Food and Agriculture Organization of the United Nations/World Health Organization; 2018.

124. *Food Quality and Safety Systems: A Training Manual on Food Hygiene and the Hazard Analysis and Critical Control Point (HACCP) System.* Rome: Food and Agriculture Organization of the United Nations; 1998.

125. *Five Keys to Safer Food Manual.* Geneva: World Health Organization; 2006.

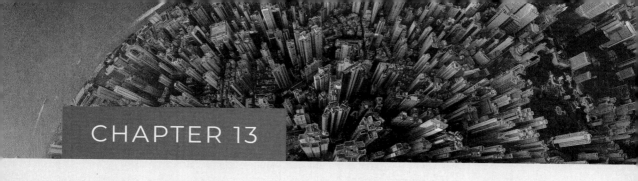

CHAPTER 13

Cardiovascular Diseases

Heart attacks, strokes, and other cardiovascular diseases are the leading cause of death among men and women in every world region. Much of the disability and premature mortality from CVDs could be prevented with behavior change, increased access to medications that control hypertension and reduce cholesterol levels, and other low-cost interventions.

13.1 Cardiovascular Disease and Global Health

A **cardiovascular disease (CVD)** is a disorder of the heart or blood vessels. The heart is the organ responsible for pumping blood throughout the body. Deoxygenated blood is returned through the vena cava to the right atrium of the heart; passes through the right ventricle; and is pumped to the lungs, where gas exchange occurs. After carbon dioxide and other wastes have been removed from the blood and oxygen has been added to the blood, the oxygenated blood is returned through the pulmonary veins to the left atrium of the heart, passes through the left ventricle, and is delivered to the rest of the body via the aorta. Arteries carry blood away from the heart, and veins carry blood back to the heart. Any problem with the structure or function of the heart or the major blood vessels can have detrimental effects on the whole body.

CVD is a concern shared by every country in the world. This is first and foremost because CVD is the most frequent cause of death for both men and women in nearly every country. One in three deaths worldwide—about 18.5 million deaths each year—is attributable to CVDs (**Figure 13.1**).[1] However, most people with CVD do not live symptom-free and then,

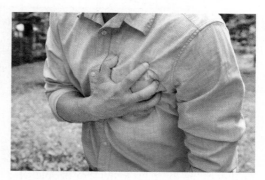

© Africa Studio/Shutterstock

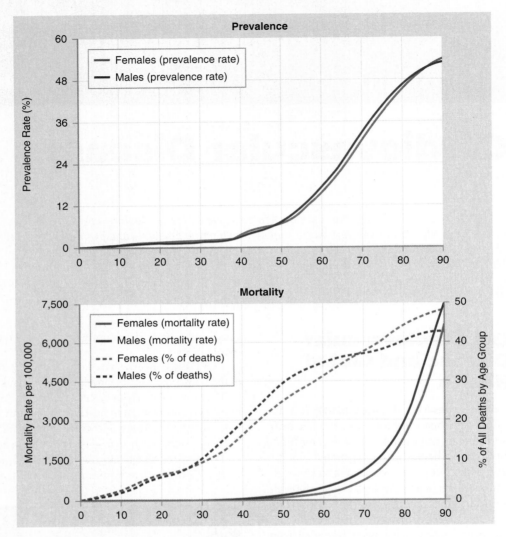

Figure 13.1 Prevalence rate per 100,000 people, mortality rate per 100,000 people, and percentage of deaths from cardiovascular diseases, by sex and age.

Data from GBD 2019 Diseases and Injuries Collaborators. Global burden of 369 diseases and injuries in 204 countries and territories, 1990–2019: a systematic analysis for the Global Burden of Disease Study 2019. *Lancet.* 2020;396:1204–1222.

with no warning, drop dead from a heart attack or stroke. Many people with chronic CVD experience reduced productivity and quality of life for many years. For people who suffer acute CVD crises, nonfatal events may cause long-term impairment. Heart attack survivors may require months of rehabilitation and never regain the stamina they had

before the infarction. Stroke victims may be permanently bedridden and unable to speak.

The disability caused by CVD is very expensive for families and nations, including patients who incur healthcare expenses and cannot work, family members who physically and financially care for relatives with CVD-related disability, and communities and nations that provide social services and health care for people with long-term CVD.[2] Each year, CVD already costs the world more than $900 billion, including more than $400 billion in direct healthcare costs and about $500 billion in lost productivity, and the annual costs of CVD will exceed $1 trillion by 2030.[3] Much of the burden from CVD is preventable. Global health interventions are seeking to decrease premature mortality, prevent disability, and reduce the burden CVD places on affected individuals, families, and societies.

13.2 The Epidemiologic Transition

Everyone will eventually die of something, so the goal of public health is not to prevent death. The goal of public health is to prevent premature death—death before late adulthood—while promoting health across the life span. Today, there are staggering differences in the distribution of deaths by age in countries with different income levels (**Figure 13.2**).[4] About 37% of the people who died in low-income countries in a typical recent year were infants and children who were less than 15 years old, while less than 1% of the people who died in high-income countries were children (and most of those deaths occurred among newborns with complicated health issues). By contrast, almost 20% of the people who died in high-income countries in a typical recent year were adults who were at least 90 years old, while in low-income countries only about 1% of deaths occurred among very old adults.

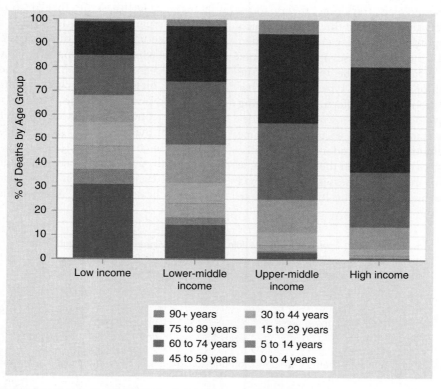

Figure 13.2 Percentage of deaths by age and country income level.

Data from United Nations Department of Economic and Social Affairs. *World Population Prospects: The 2019 Revision.* New York: United Nations; 2019.

The **epidemiologic transition** (also called the epidemiological transition) is a health transition characterized by a shift from infectious diseases to chronic noncommunicable diseases (NCDs) being the primary cause of deaths and disability in a population. In pre-transition populations, infections cause a large proportion of deaths, and the child mortality rate is high. In post-transition populations, most people live into older adulthood, and NCDs are responsible for most of the disease burden. The epidemiologic transition often follows the demographic transition as the economic status of a population improves, the fertility rate decreases, the infant and child survival rates improve, and the population ages.[5] Shifting the burden of illness, disability, and death from children and young adults to older adults is considered to be a good population-level health outcome.

Epidemiologic transition theory does not specify the economic threshold at which the proportional increase in the burden from NCDs begins to rise. It also does not provide details about the timeline for the transition or the specific types of NCDs that become prominent at different stages during the transition process. However, the epidemiologic transition does accurately describe the general trends observed in burden of disease metrics over time.[6] In the lowest-income countries, infectious diseases of childhood remain a higher public health priority than NCDs in older adults; in high-income countries, the vast majority of deaths are attributable to NCDs (**Figure 13.3**).[1] A transition toward a higher burden from NCDs has occurred in nearly all middle-income countries and most low-income countries over the past 25 years (**Figure 13.4**).[1] During these years of transition, many countries are experiencing a dual burden of disease (sometimes called a double burden) because children in some low-income communities within transitioning countries continue to have a significant burden from infectious diseases while many adults experience a significant burden from NCDs.

Health transitions theory highlights the powerful influence that socioeconomic conditions have on the diseases experienced by individuals and populations. The epidemiologic transition describes the significant differences in health status that are observed when comparing populations with different income levels. These differences can be observed when comparing two countries with divergent economic profiles, and they are also often evident when comparing richer and poorer states or provinces within the same country or comparing the health profiles of the richest and poorest residents within one country.[7]

Health transitions theory also emphasizes that every population at every income level has health concerns. Every country in

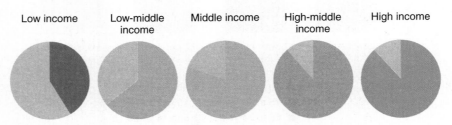

Figure 13.3 Percentage of deaths from noncommunicable diseases, by country sociodemographic group.

Data from GBD 2019 Diseases and Injuries Collaborators. Global burden of 369 diseases and injuries in 204 countries and territories, 1990–2019: a systematic analysis for the Global Burden of Disease Study 2019. *Lancet.* 2020;396:1204–1222.

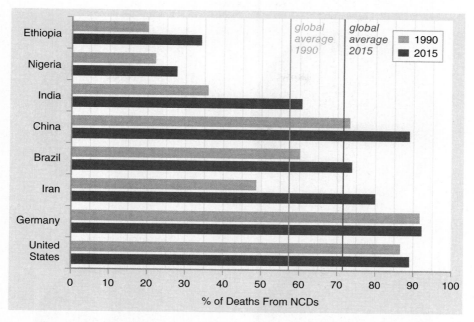

Figure 13.4 The percentage of deaths from NCDs increased in many low- and middle-income countries between 1990 and 2015.

Data from GBD 2019 Diseases and Injuries Collaborators. Global burden of 369 diseases and injuries in 204 countries and territories, 1990–2019: a systematic analysis for the Global Burden of Disease Study 2019. *Lancet.* 2020;396:1204–1222.

the world experiences a mix of deaths from infections, NCDs, injuries, and other causes, even though the relative proportion of these causes of morbidity and mortality differs according to the country's income level. Reducing deaths from infections, childbirth, and undernutrition is an excellent public health achievement because these conditions tend to kill children and young adults, but those averted deaths will be replaced with other causes of death because everyone eventually dies. The majority of people who survive to their fifth birthdays will die as adults from an NCD. As more people survive to old age, the population health profile will shift toward a greater burden from CVD, cancers, and other NCDs. The epidemiologic transition transfers disease burden to an older population with a different set of illnesses and disabilities, but it does not necessarily reduce the costs of healthcare.

13.3 CVD Epidemiology

CVD is the most frequent cause of mortality worldwide for both women and men, and there is a heavy burden from CVD-related disability in both high-income and low-income regions of the world.[1] The prevalence of CVD and the likelihood of dying from it increases with age. Because high-income countries have the greatest proportion of older adults in their populations, the overall (all-ages) CVD mortality rates per 100,000 residents are higher in high-income countries than in low-income countries. However, when age-specific rates are compared, the opposite pattern is observed: high-income countries have much lower age-specific rates of CVD death than low-income countries (**Figure 13.5**).[1] A 60-year-old woman is much more likely to die from CVD if she lives in a low-income country than in a high-income country. A 75-year-old

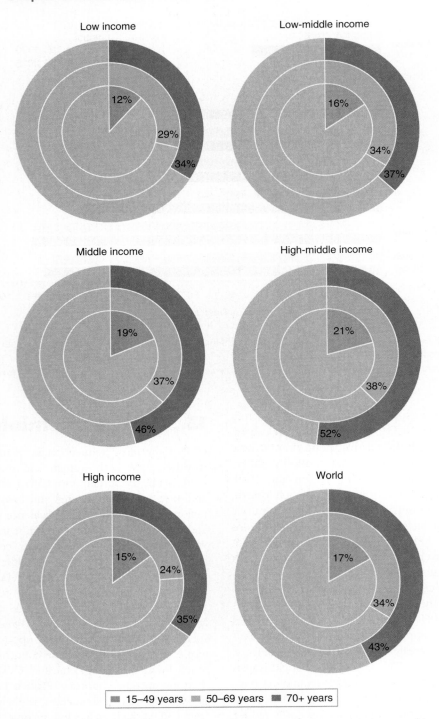

Figure 13.5 Percentage of deaths that are due to CVD, by age and country sociodemographic group.

Data from GBD 2019 Diseases and Injuries Collaborators. Global burden of 369 diseases and injuries in 204 countries and territories, 1990–2019: a systematic analysis for the Global Burden of Disease Study 2019. *Lancet.* 2020;396:1204–1222.

man is much more likely to die from CVD if he lives in a low-income country instead of a high-income country. This trend applies to all gender and age groups.

Age-standardized statistics allow the burden of disease in two or more populations to be compared after removing the differences that are caused by some populations being younger than average and others being older than average. Age-standardized rates are calculated by applying the age-group-specific rates from each country to the age distribution of the global population to generate a new age-standardized summary statistic. This new metric answers the question "If the distribution of people by age in this country (or another population) were the same as the distribution of the global population by age, what would the mortality rate be?" (The all-ages and age-standardized rates are identical for the global population when the global population is used as the standard population for age standardization.) When age-standardized mortality rates for CVD are compared, the rates for males and females are higher in low- and middle-income countries than in high-income countries (**Figure 13.6**).[1]

The global CVD mortality rate decreased slightly between 1990 and 2015 (after using age-standardization methods to adjust for the world population getting older during that 25-year period), but the number of deaths from CVD continued to increase because the total number of adults worldwide increased.[8] If most of the people dying from CVD were very old, the rise in the number of CVD deaths might not be considered problematic. Many adults report that their preference is to die in their sleep, without pain or suffering.[9] By this standard, dying quickly from a heart attack or stroke would be considered preferable to a slow death from cancer, chronic respiratory disease, or diabetes (or death after a long period of disability resulting from a CVD). Increasing the percentage of deaths that are

attributable to CVD rather than to less preferred causes of death could be considered a public health improvement if CVD fatalities always occurred among very old adults, but that is not what is observed.

Only 65% of CVD deaths occur among people who are 70 years old or older. About 2% of people who die from CVD are in their 30s, about 4% are in their 40s, about 10% are in their 50s, and about 18% are in their 60s (**Figure 13.7**).[1] About one-third of the people who died from CVD in a typical recent year were young and middle-aged adults. A 30-year-old man has a greater than 10% chance of dying from CVD before his 70th birthday, and a 30-year-old woman has about a 6.7% likelihood of dying from CVD before her 70th birthday.[10] Those fatalities will be considered to be premature, and preventing premature deaths is a global health priority. Specifically, the Sustainable Development Goals (SDGs) aim to "reduce by one-third premature mortality from noncommunicable diseases through prevention and treatment" by 2030 (SDG 3.4).[11] Achieving this goal will require improvements in preventing, postponing, and managing CVD. While the SDG target focuses on mortality, CVD is also a cause of disability (**Figure 13.8**).[1] The interventions that reduce the burden from premature death due to CVD also reduce the burden from CVD-related disability.

13.4 CVD Prevention

Many modifiable risk factors for CVD have been identified, including uncontrolled hypertension (high blood pressure), hypercholesterolemia (high blood cholesterol levels), and diabetes (high blood glucose levels); tobacco use; a high body mass index (overweight and obesity); and health behaviors such as physical inactivity and a diet high in salt, alcohol, processed meat, and trans fats and low in fruits, vegetables, fiber,

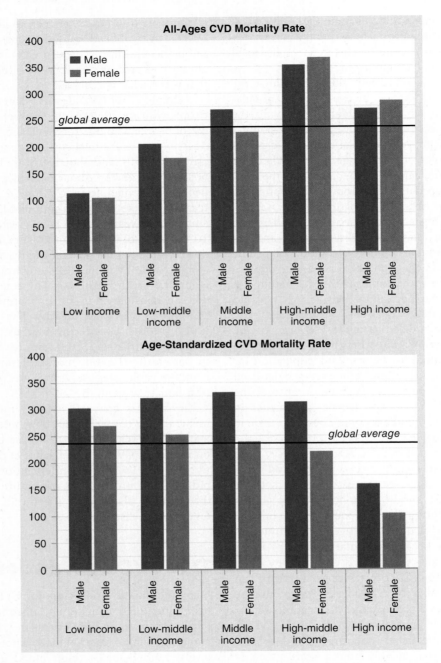

Figure 13.6 For people of the same age, the CVD mortality rate is usually higher in low- and middle-income countries than in high-income countries.

Data from GBD 2019 Diseases and Injuries Collaborators. Global burden of 369 diseases and injuries in 204 countries and territories, 1990–2019: a systematic analysis for the Global Burden of Disease Study 2019. *Lancet.* 2020;396:1204–1222.

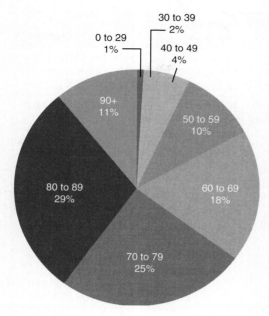

Figure 13.7 Percentage of global deaths from cardiovascular disease by age group.

Data from GBD 2019 Diseases and Injuries Collaborators. Global burden of 369 diseases and injuries in 204 countries and territories, 1990–2019: a systematic analysis for the Global Burden of Disease Study 2019. *Lancet.* 2020;396:1204–1222.

and whole grains.[12] Additional risk factors relate to the health systems structures and policies that enable or inhibit access to CVD prevention, diagnosis, and management.[13] Understanding the major risk factors for a disease enables primary, secondary, and tertiary prevention strategies to be developed and implemented (**Figure 13.9**).

At the population level, about half of all CVD deaths are thought to be attributable to modifiable risk factors.[14] That means that nearly 10 million deaths each year could be prevented, including millions of premature deaths. The remainder of annual CVD deaths are attributed to nonmodifiable risk factors like age or to events that are not preventable or treatable with current science and technologies. The best option for population health is for every individual to practice a healthy lifestyle and access recommended primary care for cardiovascular health.[15] If a large proportion of individuals in a population implement and sustain healthy behaviors,

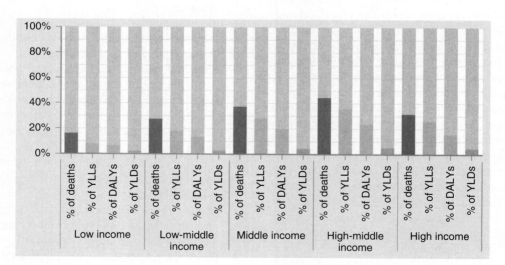

Figure 13.8 Burden of disease from cardiovascular disease by country sociodemographic group.

Data from GBD 2019 Diseases and Injuries Collaborators. Global burden of 369 diseases and injuries in 204 countries and territories, 1990–2019: a systematic analysis for the Global Burden of Disease Study 2019. *Lancet.* 2020;396:1204–1222.

Level of Prevention	Primordial Prevention	Primary Prevention	Secondary Prevention	Tertiary Prevention
Goal	Prevent risk factors in people without CVD	Mitigate risk factors in people without CVD	Detect CVD before it becomes symptomatic	Manage CVD after it becomes symptomatic
Examples of interventions	■ Exercise often ■ Eat a nutritious diet ■ Maintain a healthy weight ■ Avoid tobacco ■ Avoid harmful use of alcohol	■ Use medication to control blood pressure, cholesterol levels, and blood glucose levels in people without known CVD ■ Quit smoking	■ Screen for atherosclerosis, hypertension, aortic aneurysms, and other types of CVD	■ Use medication to reduce the severity of heart failure and other types of CVD ■ Use surgery to open or bypass blocked coronary arteries or to implant a pacemaker device ■ Receive rehabilitation therapy after surviving a heart attack or stroke

Figure 13.9 Examples of interventions for cardiovascular disease.

the number of premature deaths from CVD in the population will decrease.

At the individual level, it is rarely possible to have certainty about the causal pathways that lead to CVD events.[16] Healthy behaviors do not guarantee long-term health and survival for any individual. Even young adults who adhere to all the recommendations for nutrition and fitness and never smoke can develop and die from CVD, cancer, and other health issues. However, the existence of many nonmodifiable risk factors for CVD, including age and genetics, is not a reason not to adopt and maintain a healthy, active lifestyle. "Heart-healthy" habits may reduce the likelihood of developing a variety of NCDs, postpone the age at onset of NCDs, and facilitate management of existing NCDs so that they do not decrease quality of life.

The World Health Organization (WHO) promotes a six-component package of interventions for reducing the burden of CVD that is summarized by the acronym HEARTS[17]:

- Promoting **h**ealthy lifestyles through counseling about nutrition, exercise, and tobacco cessation
- Encouraging the implementation of **e**vidence-based treatment protocols that improve the quality of health care
- Ensuring **a**ccess to health technologies (like stethoscopes and devices for measuring blood pressure) and essential medicines (like aspirin, cholesterol-lowering statins, and antihypertensive medications)
- Using a **r**isk-based management strategy that refers high-risk individuals for advanced care
- Implementing **t**eam care and task sharing in which community health workers support advanced medical professionals
- Developing **s**ystems for monitoring patient outcomes

The *H* in the WHO's HEARTS technical package focuses on individual health behavior changes, while most of the other elements aim to improve health systems responses. Achieving the SDG target of reducing the burden from NCDs will require substantial investments in preventing and treating hypertension and CVD-related medical conditions, reducing tobacco use, and attending to other health and behavioral contributors to CVD.[18]

13.5 Health Behavior Change

A **health behavior** is an individual's intentional or unintentional action that either enhances or impairs health.[19] **Behavior change** is the process of an individual intentionally adopting and maintaining healthier behaviors. There are many types of behavior changes that are effective in reducing the risk of NCDs. The "healthy-lifestyle counseling" component of the WHO's HEARTS technical package focuses on individual health behavior changes related to unhealthy diets, insufficient physical activity, tobacco use, and harmful use of alcohol.[17] Examples of behavior changes related to these domains include deciding to lose weight and then adopting a nutritious lower-calorie diet, shedding pounds, and maintaining the new, lower weight for many years; deciding to start an exercise program, following through with increasing fitness levels through daily exercise, and maintaining that new routine for many years; and deciding to stop using tobacco products, following through with a smoking cessation plan, and remaining tobacco free for many years after the initial decision. Behavior change is difficult because it requires a long-term commitment to a healthy lifestyle.

A variety of health behavior theories provide insight about the stages of behavior change.[20] The **rational model**, or KAP model, considers behavior change to be a function of knowledge, attitudes (or beliefs or perceptions), and practices (or behaviors).[21] The KAP model emphasizes the importance of health education for enabling behavior change. Once individuals know why a behavior is healthy and believe that it is worth the effort to make a change, it is easier for them to choose to engage in healthier behaviors. The **activated health education model** describes a three-step process: an experiential phase of engaging individuals in personal health assessments, an awareness phase of promoting desirable health behaviors, and a responsibility phase of supporting implementation of healthier behaviors.[22] These stages align with the components of the rational model, with the experiential phase building knowledge, the awareness phase shaping attitudes, and the responsibility phase supporting new health practices.

Self-efficacy is an individual's confidence in his or her ability to successfully achieve a performance goal. The **health belief model** states that individual behavior change is a function of personal perceptions of the severity of the disease, susceptibility to the disease, the likely benefits from adopting healthier behaviors, the barriers to action, cues to action, and the self-efficacy to enact change.[23] People will not adopt new health behaviors if they do not perceive themselves to be at risk of an adverse health condition like CVD or if they do not think the health condition is a serious one. A **cue to action** is an internal or external stimulus that prompts an individual to implement a recommended health behavior. A cue to action could be the hospitalization of a friend for heart disease; a personal health scare like chest pain; a package warning label; a magazine column written by a trusted health expert; or any other encounter that shapes perceptions of severity, susceptibility, benefits, and barriers. Cues to action like reminder notices about health checkups and referrals from clinicians are important for triggering behavior change because they support self-efficacy by stating the action that should be taken.

The **stages of change model**, also called the **transtheoretical model**, describes individual behavior change as a multistage process of moving from pre-contemplation to contemplation, preparation for action, action, and maintenance.[24] The **theory of reasoned action** says that follow-through on implementing plans for a healthier lifestyle is dependent on the individual's belief that the outcome of the change will be worth the effort and his or her confidence that others will support the change.[25] The **theory of planned behavior** builds on the theory of reasoned action by adding the importance of an individual's perceived self-efficacy and control over the change.[26]

Health behavior models provide frameworks for creating risk- or disease-specific interventions that are tailored to specific populations. For example, the "5 As and 5 Rs" model of health behavior change, which builds on the health belief model, was developed to support tobacco cessation interventions and was then adopted to support other CVD-related behavior changes (**Figure 13.10**).[27]

The ability of an individual to implement behavior change is not solely a function of knowledge or willpower. It is also dependent on access to the tools for health. The **social ecological model** is a theoretical framework that considers individual health and health behaviors to be a function of the social environment, which includes intrapersonal (individual), interpersonal, institutional (organizational), community, and public policy dimensions. **Social cognitive theory** acknowledges that behavior change is about both inner motivation and environmental realities because behavior is a function of personal factors, behaviors, and environmental conditions.[28]

The **diffusion of innovations model** describes a process of behavior change in communities that unfolds as new ideas and actions are adopted by community members.[29] Innovators demonstrate the benefits of the change,

5 As		5 Rs	
Ask	Ask about the health behavior	**Relevance** (perceived susceptibility)	Identify how the current behavior adversely affects the individual
Advise	Advise about the preferred health behavior	**Risks** (perceived severity)	Identify the negative consequences of not changing the behavior
Assess	Assess the individual's readiness to adopt new health behaviors and perceived self-efficacy to make the change	**Rewards** (perceived benefits)	Identify the benefits of adopting the new health behavior
Assist	Assist in development of a plan of action	**Roadblocks** (perceived barriers to action)	Identify barriers to adopting the new health behavior
Arrange	Arrange follow-up support	**Repetition**	Repeat the 5 As to assess readiness to change the health behavior

Figure 13.10 5 As and 5 Rs of health behavior change.

Data from Fiore MC, Jaén CR, Baker TB, et al. *Treating Tobacco Use and Dependence: 2008 Update: Clinical Practice Guideline.* Rockville MD: U.S. Public Health Service, Department of Health and Human Services; 2008.

then early adopters generate enthusiasm for it. More and more residents decide to participate in the change. Eventually, only a small number of residents remain who have not adopted it. Clinical care providers; governments; community organizations; and others involved in health education, health promotion, and health communication can all play a role in increasing knowledge about the risk of disease and the benefits of healthier behaviors, creating policies that facilitate healthier behaviors, improving access to health resources, and communicating with clients and constituents.

13.6 Physical Inactivity and Sedentariness

Regular aerobic exercise is associated with reduced body weight, lower blood pressure, more favorable blood cholesterol profiles, increased insulin sensitivity, improved oxygen consumption, and other benefits for cardiovascular health.[30] The WHO recommends that children aged 5–17 years engage in at least 60 minutes of moderate or vigorous physical activity daily; that adults average at least 30 minutes of moderate or 15 minutes of vigorous physical activity daily along with doing strength-building exercises at least two days each week; and that older adults add balance training to their routines and maintain their physical activity levels for as long as they are able to do so.[31]

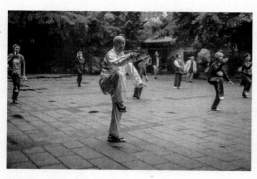

© WHYFRAME/Shutterstock

Physical inactivity is the failure to regularly engage in exercise of moderate or vigorous intensity. Physical inactivity is associated with an increased risk of morbidity and mortality from numerous NCDs.[32] At least one in four adults (ages 18+ years) worldwide does not meet the WHO standard of being physically active for at least 150 minutes of moderately intense activity or 75 minutes of vigorous activity each week (**Figure 13.11**).[33] The rates of inactivity are especially high among women and in high-income countries. About 80% of adolescents (ages 11–17 years) do not meet the WHO standard of being physically active for at least one hour daily (**Figure 13.12**).[34]

A related but distinct concept is **sedentariness**, which is characterized by sitting for long durations each day. Sedentariness is associated with an increased risk of NCDs, an increased likelihood of having other risk factors for NCDs, and a higher mortality rate.[35] Sedentariness is often linked to screen time (the hours spent watching television or another electronic device), but sedentarism is also built into many work and school environments. It is possible for a person to exercise enough to be classified as physically active and, at the same time, sit enough to be considered to have a sedentary lifestyle.[36] For example, people who spend eight hours a day at a desk job might be classified as sedentary even if they run five miles every day after work.

Although nearly everyone who is physically inactive or sedentary would benefit from adopting a more active lifestyle, there are many barriers to behavior change.[37] There may be perceived time barriers. Sleep, leisure, occupation, transportation, and home-based activities (a framework known as the SLOTH model) may be higher priorities than exercise.[38] There may be cultural barriers. For example, in places where women and older adults traditionally have not been physically active, they may feel uncomfortable doing something outside of cultural norms. There may be environmental

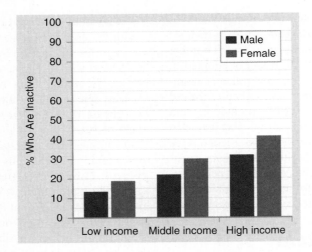

Figure 13.11 Age-standardized percentage of adults (ages 18+ years) who are physically inactive, by sex and country income level.

Data from Guthold R, Stevens GA, Riley LA, Bull FC. Worldwide trends in insufficient physical inactivity from 2001 to 2016: a pooled analysis of 358 population-based surveys with 1.9 million participants. *Lancet Glob Health.* 2018;6:e1077–e1086.

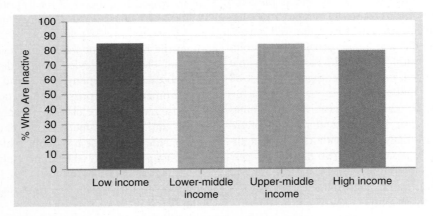

Figure 13.12 Age-standardized percentage of adolescents (ages 11–17 years) who are physically inactive, by sex and country income level.

Data from Guthold R, Stevens GA, Riley LA, Bull FC. Worldwide trends in insufficient physical inactivity among adolescents: a pooled analysis of 298 population-based surveys with 1.6 million participants. *Lancet Glob Health.* 2020;4:e23–e35.

barriers, especially in urban environments where homes are crowded; there are no sidewalks; and few parks, schoolyards, and sports facilities are available. Exercising more often is about more than just learning that exercise is valuable, having the fortitude to establish a new exercise routine, and being physically able to do aerobic exercise.[39] It is also dependent on having social support to make time for exercise and reduce periods of sedentariness, living in a community that considers exercise to be culturally acceptable, and having access to a safe and convenient environment in which to exercise.[40] Effective physical activity promotion campaigns combine community-, school-, and work-based health education and exercise programs with environmental and policy strategies that enable healthy practices to continue.[41]

13.7 Ischemic Heart Disease

Half of all CVD deaths are due to ischemic heart disease (**Figure 13.13**).[1] Just like every other organ in the body, the tissues that make up the heart require a constant supply of oxygenated blood. **Ischemia** means reduced blood supply. Ischemia may occur as a result of **atherosclerosis**, which is the thickening and hardening of the walls of the arteries that carry oxygen-rich blood from the heart to the rest of the body, including to the heart muscle itself. As atherosclerotic plaque narrows the diameter of those blood vessels, the blood supply to the tissues fed by those arteries becomes limited. People with **peripheral artery disease** have narrowed blood vessels in their extremities that impair blood circulation and can cause severe leg pain and cramping when walking (a symptom called claudication). **Ischemic heart disease** (IHD), also called **coronary artery disease** or coronary heart disease, occurs when atherosclerosis in the arteries that provide blood to the heart reduces blood flow to the heart muscle.

The initial symptom of IHD might be **angina**, which is chest pain or tightness caused by the heart muscle not getting an adequate supply of oxygen. A **myocardial infarction**, or heart attack, is the death or damage of a portion of the heart muscle due to lack of oxygen. Heart attacks occur when a coronary blood vessel becomes mostly or fully occluded (blocked), either due to atherosclerosis or to blood clots (thromboses) forming

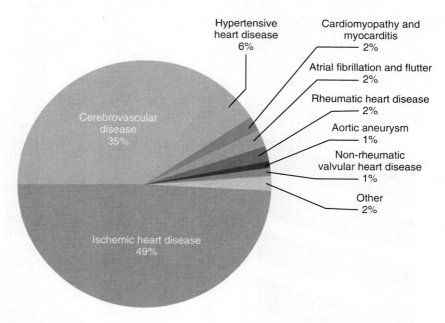

Figure 13.13 Distribution of causes of death from cardiovascular diseases.

Data from GBD 2019 Diseases and Injuries Collaborators. Global burden of 369 diseases and injuries in 204 countries and territories, 1990–2019: a systematic analysis for the Global Burden of Disease Study 2019. *Lancet.* 2020;396:1204–1222.

CIRCULATION OF BLOOD THROUGH THE HEART

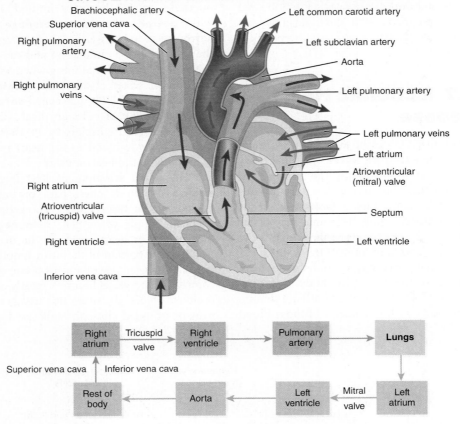

Brachiocephalic artery
Superior vena cava
Right pulmonary artery
Right pulmonary veins
Right atrium
Atrioventricular (tricuspid) valve
Right ventricle
Inferior vena cava

Left common carotid artery
Left subclavian artery
Aorta
Left pulmonary artery
Left pulmonary veins
Left atrium
Atrioventricular (mitral) valve
Septum
Left ventricle

Right atrium	Tricuspid valve	Right ventricle		Pulmonary artery		**Lungs**

Superior vena cava   Inferior vena cava

Rest of body		Aorta		Left ventricle	Mitral valve	Left atrium

© Ducu59us/Shutterstock

STAGES OF ATHEROSCLEROSIS

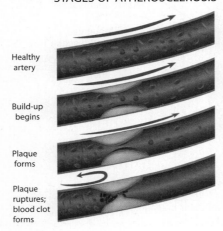

Healthy artery

Build-up begins

Plaque forms

Plaque ruptures; blood clot forms

© Alila Medical Media/Shutterstock

on the plaque surface in an atherosclerotic vessel.[42] People experiencing an acute myocardial infarction typically have chest pain or chest pressure and tightness, and they may also experience pain in one or both arms, the back, neck, or jaw along with nausea, shortness of breath, and other forms of discomfort. Women may experience fatigue, sleep disturbances, and shortness of breath rather than the typical chest discomfort.[43] Heart attacks can cause irregular heartbeats that lead to cardiac arrest and death.

The best way to reduce the costs of IHD for individuals and for health systems is to invest in prevention. The major risk factors for IHD are the same behavioral and metabolic factors that apply to CVD as a whole:

inactive lifestyles and unmanaged comorbidities like hypertension, elevated blood glucose levels, and hypercholesterolemia.[12] Medications can control high blood pressure, stabilize blood sugar levels in people with type 2 diabetes, and reduce blood levels of cholesterol.

Cholesterol is a waxy lipid (fat) that is a major component of the plaque that causes atherosclerosis. Cholesterol is a necessary substance because it is used by the body to insulate nerves, make cell membranes, and produce some types of hormones. Two types of lipoproteins transport cholesterol between cells in the body: low-density lipoprotein (LDL), which is associated with the formation of atherosclerosis, and high-density lipoprotein (HDL), which is associated with reduced CVD risk.[44] Triglycerides are a different type of body fat that is often measured at the same time as cholesterol levels because high triglyceride levels combined with high LDL or low HDL are associated with inflammation and atherosclerosis.[45]

Anatomy of a heart attack

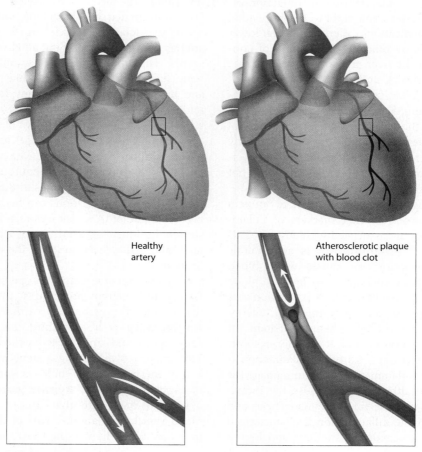

Healthy artery

Atherosclerotic plaque with blood clot

LDL, HDL, and triglycerides are part of the standard lipid profile that is used to evaluate cardiovascular risk.

Most of the cholesterol that is detected in a blood test is produced by the liver. Additional cholesterol is acquired by eating animal products such as meat, eggs, shrimp, and dairy products, but dietary cholesterol accounts for only about 10%–15% of the LDL in blood.[46] People with high cholesterol levels are often advised to eat a nutritious diet that limits consumption of foods that are high in cholesterol and fats,[47] but dietary changes typically have at most a modest impact on cholesterol levels and their associated CVD risk.[48] Weight loss and exercise are also associated with a more favorable cholesterol profile, but they are often not sufficient to lower cholesterol to recommended levels.[49] Medications called statins that lower LDL levels by blocking production of cholesterol in the liver are very effective, cause few side effects, and are safe for most individuals.[50] Widespread use of statins in high-income countries has decreased cholesterol levels in those populations, while rates of hypercholesterolemia have remained mostly stable over the past several decades in lower-income countries where medications are not as widely used.[51]

Statins also lower C-reactive protein (CRP) levels and other markers of inflammation that are associated with adverse CVD outcomes.[52] **Inflammation** is an immune system response that causes white blood cells to release chemicals that increase blood flow to local tissues. Acute inflammation may be triggered by an injury, infection, allergy, autoimmune disorder, chemical irritant, or another exposure, and it usually resolves within a few days. Chronic inflammation is persistent inflammation that can damage the DNA of healthy cells and cause the formation of scar tissue through angiogenesis and fibrosis. Acute inflammation is characterized by pain, heat, redness, swelling, and loss of function, while chronic inflammation generates nonspecific symptoms such as fatigue, chronic pain, and digestive issues. Low-grade, systemic chronic inflammation is associated with a variety of noncommunicable diseases, including CVD, cancer, asthma, diabetes, rheumatoid arthritis, inflammatory bowel disease, and periodontitis.[53] It is also associated with atherosclerosis and may increase cholesterol levels.[54]

Nearly 200 million people worldwide have IHD, more than 100 million people worldwide are living with peripheral artery disease, and about 9 million people die each year from IHD; the rate of deaths is decreasing over time with improved medical care, but the number of deaths is increasing due to population aging.[8] The medications deemed essential for cardiovascular health include antianginal agents that relax the muscles in the walls of arteries to increase blood flow, antiarrhythmic agents, antihypertensive agents, antithrombotic agents (blood thinners) like aspirin, and lipid-lowering agents.[55] Many low- and middle-income countries do not yet have reliable stocks of all of these types of medications,[56] but most of these countries are working with global partners to increase access to quality medications.[57] Health education provided to individuals and groups through community health organizations can help people become aware of their risk factors, adopt and sustain healthier behaviors, and access the medications they need to lower the risk of a heart attack.[58]

In high-income countries, people with IHD can undergo procedures that help restore blood flow to the cardiac tissue. **Angioplasty** is a procedure that physically opens and unclogs a blocked artery. This may involve placing a stent, which is a tiny mesh tube that holds a previously blocked vessel open. **Bypass surgery** is a surgical procedure that uses a healthy blood vessel from another part of the body to restore blood flow to the heart muscle by bypassing the damaged vessel. These surgical therapies are rarely available in lower-income countries and are cost prohibitive in many middle-income countries.[59] The heart muscle of a heart attack survivor can heal by forming scar tissue,[60] but the heart may no longer be strong enough to pump blood efficiently. Cardiac rehabilitation after surviving a heart attack is beneficial but is underused, especially in low- and middle-income countries.[61]

13.8 Stroke

Cerebrovascular disease is characterized by reduced blood flow to the brain. A **stroke** occurs when cells in the brain die due to lack of oxygen.[62] The typical symptoms of a stroke include weakness on one or both sides of the face and body, confusion, trouble speaking (expressive aphasia) or understanding language (receptive aphasia), vision disturbances, a loss of balance, and a severe headache.

There are two major pathological processes that cause strokes: ischemia and hemorrhage. An **ischemic stroke** occurs when a blocked blood vessel cuts off blood flow to a portion of the brain. This is a similar process to the pathology of heart attacks. Many ischemic strokes are due to blood clots in the vessels that supply oxygenated blood to the brain. A **transient ischemic attack** (TIA), sometimes called a mini stroke or warning stroke, occurs when a temporary blockage of an artery causes stroke-like symptoms that quickly resolve. TIA episodes are signs that an individual is at imminent risk of a severe ischemic stroke. Individuals who are experiencing TIAs are often prescribed blood-thinning medications, and in higher-income countries they may be referred for surgery or angioplasty to remove atherosclerotic plaque from the carotid arteries, which carry blood from the heart to the brain. Once a stroke occurs, urgent medical care is required to prevent death and disability. The symptoms of an ischemic stroke are often permanent when the affected individual does not receive clot-busting intravenous thrombolytic medications within just a few hours of the onset of stroke symptoms.

A **hemorrhagic stroke** occurs when a blood vessel ruptures and causes bleeding in the brain. There are two main types of hemorrhagic strokes: intracerebral and subarachnoid. Intracerebral hemorrhages cause bleeding within the brain, and strokes of this type are associated with uncontrolled high blood pressure. Subarachnoid hemorrhages cause blood to fill the space between the skull and the brain, and strokes of this type are typically caused by a ruptured aneurysm. An **aneurysm** is a bulge in a blood vessel that can cause the vessel to rupture. The main symptom of a subarachnoid hemorrhagic stroke is a sudden severe headache. Hemorrhagic strokes can sometimes be treated with medications to slow the bleeding or surgery to stop the bleeding and relieve pressure on the brain, but there is a higher case fatality rate for hemorrhagic strokes than for ischemic strokes.[63] In low- and middle-income countries where computed tomography (CT) scans are not routinely available, clinicians have limited ability to distinguish between ischemic and hemorrhagic strokes. This makes it difficult to decide whether to administer blood thinners, which are essential for ischemic strokes but dangerous for hemorrhagic strokes.[64]

About 12 million people had a stroke each year in typical recent years, including about 7.5 million ischemic strokes and about 4.5 million hemorrhagic strokes; about 6.5 million of those individuals died from their strokes, and the remainder joined the more than 100 million living stroke survivors.[8] There are significant differences by country in the relative distribution of ischemic and hemorrhagic strokes, the case fatality rates

Brain Stroke

Ischemic Stroke

Hemorrhagic Stroke

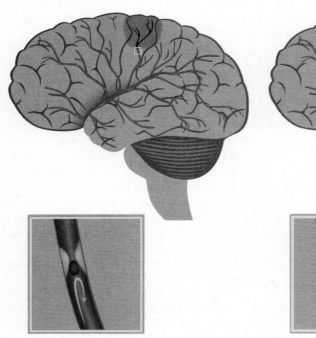

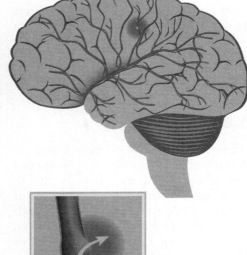

Blockage of blood vessels; lack of blood flow to affected area

Rupture of blood vessels; leakage of blood

© Alila Medical Media/Shutterstock

for strokes, and the comparative burden of ischemic heart disease and strokes. Countries that have a higher proportion of hemorrhagic strokes tend to have higher death rates from stroke. In most high-income countries, strokes are a much less frequent cause of death than IHD, but that pattern is not observed in all lower- and middle-income countries (**Figure 13.14**).[1]

A large proportion of the global burden from stroke is attributed to modifiable risk factors, including health behaviors, metabolic conditions, and environmental exposures like air pollution.[65] One of the most well-established risk factors for stroke is uncontrolled high blood pressure.[66] Antihypertensive medications are a key component of primary prevention of stroke, along with the other elements of CVD prevention plans.[67] For people who have already had strokes, access to emergency medical care and long-term rehabilitation is important for allowing the greatest chances for regaining function.[68] Rehabilitative care is scarce in most low- and middle-income countries,[69] and it is costly in most high-income countries.[70] More than half of stroke survivors have persistent physical and/or cognitive impairment.[68]

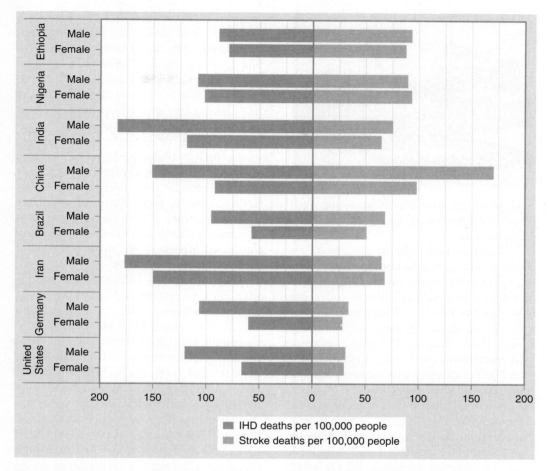

Figure 13.14 Comparison of age-standardized mortality rates per 100,000 people from ischemic heart disease (left) and cerebrovascular disease (right).

Data from GBD 2019 Diseases and Injuries Collaborators. Global burden of 369 diseases and injuries in 204 countries and territories, 1990–2019: a systematic analysis for the Global Burden of Disease Study 2019. *Lancet.* 2020;396:1204–1222.

13.9 Hypertension

Blood pressure is typically reported as a ratio of two numbers, like 110/70 or 135/85. The top number is the **systolic blood pressure** (SBP), the pressure in the blood vessels when the heart beats. The bottom number is the **diastolic blood pressure** (DBP), the pressure in the blood vessels when the heart is at rest between beats. The units are "millimeters

of mercury" (mm Hg), a measurement of pressure. **Hypertension** is high blood pressure, and it is typically defined as having an SBP of 140 mm Hg or higher and/or a DBP of 90 mm Hg or higher.[71] Hypertension usually causes no symptoms that are apparent to the individual with high blood pressure, but uncontrolled hypertension significantly increases the risk of having heart failure, strokes, and coronary heart disease.[72] Over time, uncontrolled

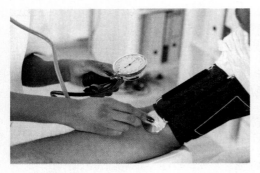

© Andrey_Popov/Shutterstock

high blood pressure also increases the likelihood of kidney failure, vision loss, and other complications.[73]

Blood pressure checks are one of the many health screening tests for which there is no obvious cutoff point to distinguish between a person with disease and a person without disease. Using an SBP cutoff of 130 mm Hg, or an even lower number, would result in a much higher prevalence of hypertension than using a cutoff of 140 mm Hg. For diseases with no treatment and diseases with treatments that are expensive and potentially harmful, it is better to avoid false-positive diagnoses by having a high threshold for declaring that a person has the condition. For conditions like hypertension that can often be managed and for which early intervention can prevent serious complications, it may be beneficial to set a low threshold for classifying an individual with a borderline test result as having the disease. In the past, the recommended cutoff for classifying a person as having hypertension was an SBP of 160 mm Hg or above. Some scientific studies suggest that it is healthiest to have an SBP below 115 mm Hg, which is significantly below the current 140 mm Hg threshold for a hypertension diagnosis.[74] Based on this research, the threshold for a hypertension diagnosis may be reduced to below 140 mm Hg in the future.[75]

Blood pressure can be lowered with medications such as angiotensin-converting enzyme (ACE) inhibitors, like captopril, enalapril, and ramipril, and angiotensin receptor blockers (ARBs), which relax blood vessels; beta blockers like atenolol and metoprolol, which cause the heart to beat more slowly; calcium-channel blockers like amlodipine, which help the heart beat less forcefully; and diuretics like hydrochlorothiazide, which reduce fluid volume in the body.[76] Blood pressure medications are not effective at controlling hypertension in everyone who takes them,[77,78] but having access to more classes of affordable medications that reduce blood pressure is associated with a greater likelihood of achieving blood pressures below the threshold for hypertension.[76]

More than 1.4 billion people worldwide have hypertension, including about 34% of men and 32% of women who are 30–79 years old.[79] More than 55% of people with high blood pressure who live in high-income countries take antihypertensive medication, but only about 30% of people with hypertension who live in low- and middle-income countries receive medications to reduce their blood pressure.[80] Because so many people with hypertension do not know they have high blood pressure, are not taking medications for it, and are not successfully controlling their blood pressure with prescribed medications (**Figure 13.15**), about 28% of men and 25% of women worldwide have uncontrolled hypertension.[79]

In most higher-income countries, the increased use of antihypertensive medications has led to a decrease in the prevalence of uncontrolled hypertension over the past several decades; in lower-income countries where these medications are not widely used, the prevalence of hypertension is not decreasing (**Figure 13.16**).[81] Blood pressure levels typically increase with age (**Figure 13.17**).[82] As life expectancies increase in low- and middle-income countries, the

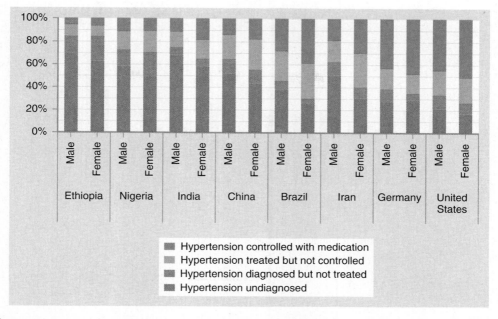

Figure 13.15 Age-standardized percentage of adults (ages 30–79 years) with hypertension that is controlled, treated but not controlled, diagnosed but not treated, and undiagnosed.

Data from NCD Risk Factor Collaboration (NCD-RisC). Worldwide trends in hypertension prevalence and progress in treatment and control from 1990 to 2019: a pooled analysis of 1201 population-representative studies with 104 million participants. *Lancet.* 2021;398:957–980.

prevalence of hypertension will increase. The number of adults with hypertension worldwide doubled between 1990 and 2020,[79] and that number is expected to continue to increase as the global population grows and ages. The current need for antihypertensive medications in low- and middle-income countries is not being met, and demand for these medications will rise considerably in the coming years.[83]

The sodium in salt (sodium chloride) is associated with higher blood pressures among people with hypertension, so hypertensive individuals are often encouraged to reduce their salt consumption.[84] Much of the sodium that people consume comes from processed foods rather than from the table salt that is added to food at mealtimes. Without being able to check food labels, people may not be aware of how much sodium

they are ingesting. The Global Nutrition Targets aim for a population mean intake of 2 grams of salt per day, and the typical adult currently consumes at least twice that amount (**Figure 13.18**).[85] The SHAKE package of policies recommended by the WHO promotes lower salt intake through[86]:

- **S**urveillance of salt use
- **H**arnessing industry to reduce salt in processed and prepared foods
- **A**dopting standards for labeling and marketing
- Improving **K**nowledge about the value of low salt intakes
- Developing a supportive **E**nvironment for healthy eating

Other behavioral strategies for controlling blood pressure include maintaining a healthy weight, exercising, avoiding tobacco

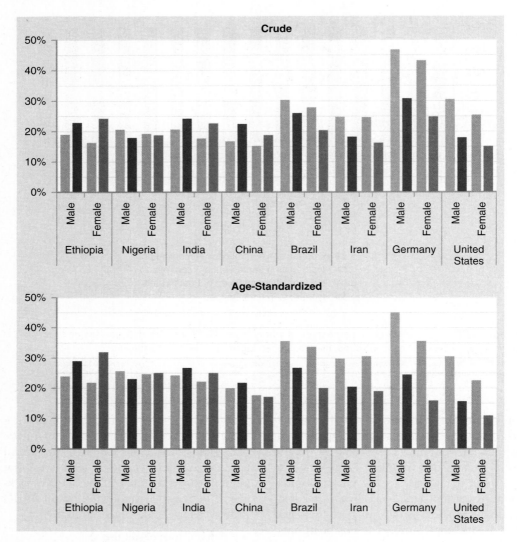

Figure 13.16 Age-standardized percentage of adults (aged 18+ years) with hypertension (a systolic blood pressure of ≥140 mm Hg and/or a diastolic blood pressure of ≥90 mm Hg, with or without medication to control it) in 1975 and 2015.

Data from NCD Risk Factor Collaboration (NCD-RisC). Worldwide trends in blood pressure from 1975 to 2015: a pooled analysis of 1479 population-based measurement studies with 19.1 million participants. *Lancet.* 2017;389:37–55.

and excess intake of alcohol, consuming adequate dietary potassium,[87] getting sufficient amounts of sleep, and managing stress.[88] Combinations of medications and behavioral change are likely to yield the best outcomes for individuals with high blood pressure.

13.10 Other Cardiovascular Diseases

Numerous other types of CVDs also contribute to disability and death worldwide. Some

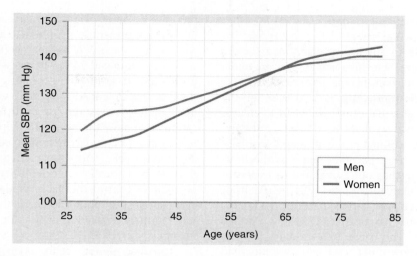

Figure 13.17 The mean systolic blood pressure increases with age.

Data from Forouzanfar MH, Liu P, Roth GA, et al. Global burden of hypertension and systolic blood pressure of at least 110 to 115 mm Hg, 1990–2015. *JAMA*. 2017;317:165–182.

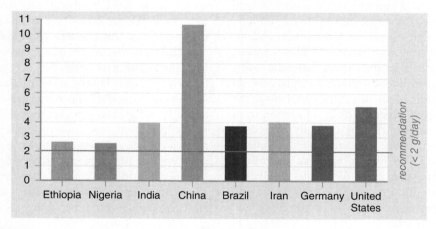

Figure 13.18 Mean population intake of salt (grams/day) among adults (aged 25+ years).

Data from *2020 Global Nutrition Report: Action on Equity to End Malnutrition*. Bristol UK: Development Initiatives; 2020.

CVDs are anatomical. Some babies are born with congenital heart anomalies, and some children and adults develop scarring of the valves within the heart. For example, **rheumatic heart disease** is an inflammatory condition that causes irreversible damage to the heart and heart valves as a result of an untreated infection with group A *Streptococcus*, like strep throat or scarlet fever.[89] Most new cases of rheumatic fever occur in children and adolescents.[90] About 40 million people worldwide are living with heart or valve damage from rheumatic heart disease.[8] Valves can also calcify or degenerate with aging. In higher-income countries, valves can be surgically replaced; in low- and middle-income countries, this type of surgery is rarely available.[91] People may also develop an **aortic aneurysm**, a bulge in the aorta that can rupture and cause rapid death from internal bleeding.

When tobacco users and members of other risk groups are screened for aneurysms,[92] it is possible to surgically repair them before they rupture. Screening and surgery are rarely available in lower-income countries.

Cardiomyopathy is a disease of the heart muscles that causes the heart to enlarge and become weaker. In dilated cardiomyopathy, the volume of the atria and ventricles inside the heart becomes larger as the heart muscle stretches out and thins. In hypertrophic cardiomyopathy, the cells in the heart muscle get bigger, and the resulting thickening of the tissue may restrict blood flow through the heart. The cause of cardiomyopathy is often unknown, but some cases are inherited and others are due to harmful use of alcohol.[93]

The walls of the heart are composed of three layers of muscle: the endocardium on the inside, the myocardium in the middle, and the epicardium on the outside. Inflammation of the heart muscle is called carditis. Some types of carditis affect particular layers of the heart. Endocarditis is an inflammation of the inside of the heart that can damage the heart valves. Myocarditis is inflammation of the myocardium that is typically caused by a viral infection. Pericarditis is an inflammation of the fibrous sac that surrounds the heart. Many cases of carditis resolve on their own, but they can become chronic and cause problems such as cardiomyopathy and arrhythmias.[94]

An **arrhythmia** is an abnormal heartbeat that is too fast (tachycardia), too slow (bradycardia), or irregularly paced. **Atrial fibrillation** occurs when the atria (the upper chambers of the heart) quiver fast and irregularly rather than contracting and relaxing at a regular pace.[95] People with atrial fibrillation may form blood clots in the heart because the blood stagnates in the atria instead of quickly being moved out of those chambers. If these clots enter the bloodstream and block a vessel in the brain, the blockage can cause a stroke. While some arrhythmias occur because of the presence of other cardiovascular conditions, many cases present in people who are otherwise healthy. Nearly 60 million people worldwide are estimated to be living with atrial fibrillation.[8] Use of blood-thinning medications is recommended for people with atrial fibrillation to reduce the risk of stroke. Medications that slow the heart can help regulate heart rates, and antiarrhythmic medications, ablation surgery, and implanted pacemaker devices and cardioverter-defibrillators can be used to control the heart rhythm. However, surgical solutions for arrhythmias are not routinely available in low- and middle-income countries.[96]

Cardiac arrest occurs when the heart abruptly stops beating. Heart attacks and other forms of CVD can lead to cardiac arrest, but cardiac arrest is an "electrical" problem while ischemic CVDs are considered to be "plumbing" problems. **Ventricular tachycardia** is an arrhythmia that occurs when the ventricles (the lower chambers of the heart) begin contracting extremely rapidly, and this can quickly lead to cardiac arrest. The automated external defibrillators (AEDs) available in many public places in high-income countries are intended to save the lives of people who collapse due to an episode of ventricular tachycardia. Both "electrical" and "plumbing" problems are major contributors to disease burden in countries across the income spectrum.

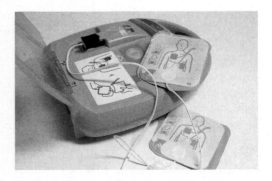

Automated external defibrillator.

© Sakunrat Panyapor/Shutterstock

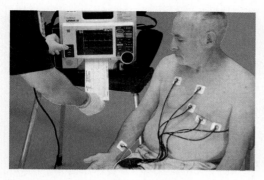

© Jones and Bartlett Learning. Courtesy of MIEMSS.

Heart failure is a chronic condition in which the heart is not able to pump enough blood to meet the body's need for oxygen. Cardiac arrest occurs quickly; heart failure is a slow process. Congestive heart failure occurs when blood and fluid back up into the lungs and tissues (often causing edema of the legs and ankles) because the heart is not pumping enough blood volume with each beat. Almost any type of CVD can lead to chronic heart failure.[97] People with heart failure may have symptoms like fatigue and shortness of breath that reduce their quality of life for many years. Diuretics and other medications can assist with management of symptoms.

While the prevention and treatment strategies for various CVDs must be tailored to the particular issue of concern, there are some general interventions that promote cardiovascular health, including health behavior modifications, such as increased physical activity; use of medications to reduce blood pressure, cholesterol levels, and blood clot formation; management of comorbidities such as diabetes; and access to affordable primary and advanced healthcare services for CVD and related conditions.[98]

References

1. GBD 2019 Diseases and Injuries Collaborators. Global burden of 369 diseases and injuries in 204 countries and territories, 1990–2019: a systematic analysis for the Global Burden of Disease Study 2019. *Lancet.* 2020;396:1204–1222.
2. Abejunde DO, Mathers CD, Adam T, Ortegon M, Strong K. The burden and costs of chronic diseases in low-income and middle-income countries. *Lancet.* 2007;370:1929–1938.
3. Reddy S, Riahi F, Dorling G, Callahan R, Patel H. *Innovative Approaches to Prevention: Tackling the Global Burden of Cardiovascular Disease.* Doha: World Innovation Summit for Health; 2016.
4. United Nations Department of Economic and Social Affairs. *World Population Prospects: The 2019 Revision.* New York: United Nations; 2019.
5. Omran AR. The epidemiologic transition: a theory of the epidemiology of population change. *Milbank Mem Fund Q.* 1971;29:509–538.
6. Caldwell JC. Population health in transition. *Bull World Health Organ.* 2001;79:159–170.
7. Braveman P, Tarimo E. Social inequalities in health within countries: not only an issue for affluent nations. *Soc Sci Med.* 2002;54:1621–1635.
8. Roth GA, Mensah G, Johnson CO, et al. Global burden of cardiovascular diseases and risk factors, 1990–2019: update from the GBD 2019 Study. *J Am Coll Cardiol.* 2020;76:2982–3021.
9. Meier EA, Gallegos JV, Thomas LP, Depp CA, Irwin SA, Jeste DV. Defining a good death (successful dying): literature review and a call for research and public dialogue. *Am J Geriatr Psychiatry.* 2016;24:261–271.
10. Roth GA, Huffman MD, Moran AE, et al. Global and regional patterns in cardiovascular mortality from 1990 to 2013. *Circulation.* 2015;132:1667–1678.
11. *Transforming Our World: The 2030 Agenda for Sustainable Development.* New York: United Nations; 2015.
12. Tzoulaki I, Elliott P, Kontis V, Ezzati M. Worldwide exposures to cardiovascular risk factors and associated health effects: current knowledge and data gaps. *Circulation.* 2016;133:2314–2333.
13. Joseph P, Leong D, McKee M, et al. Reducing the global burden of cardiovascular disease, part 1: the epidemiology and risk factors. *Circ Res.* 2017;121:677–694.
14. *Global Atlas on Cardiovascular Disease Prevention and Control.* Geneva: World Health Organization, World Heart Federation, and World Stroke Organization; 2011.

15. Schwalm JD, McKee M, Huffman MD, Yusuf S. Resource effective strategies to prevent and treat cardiovascular disease. *Circulation.* 2016;133:742–755.

16. WHO CVD Risk Chart Working Group. World Health Organization cardiovascular disease risk charts: revised models to estimate risk in 21 global regions. *Lancet Glob Health.* 2019;7:e1332–e1345.

17. *HEARTS Technical Package for Cardiovascular Disease Management in Primary Health Care.* Geneva: World Health Organization; 2016.

18. Roth GA, Nguyen G, Forouzanfar MH, Mokdad AH, Naghavi M, Murray CJL. Estimates of the global and regional premature cardiovascular mortality in 2025. *Circulation.* 2015;132:1270–1282.

19. Short SE, Mollborn S. Social determinants and health behaviors: conceptual frames and empirical advances. *Curr Opin Psychol.* 2015;5:78–84.

20. *Health Education:Theoretical Concepts, Effective Strategies and Core Competencies: A Foundation Document to Guide Capacity Development of Health Educators.* Cairo: World Health Organization Regional Office for the Eastern Mediterranean; 2012.

21. Valente TW, Paredes P, Poppe PR. Matching the message to the process: the relative ordering of knowledge, attitudes, and practices in behavior change research. *Hum Commun Res.* 1998;24:366–385.

22. Dennison D, Golaszewski T. The activated health education model: refinement and implications for school health education. *J School Health.* 2002;72:23–26.

23. Rosenstock IM, Stretcher VJ, Becker MH. Social learning theory and the health belief model. *Health Educ Q.* 1988;15:175–183.

24. Prochaska JO, DiClemente CC. Transtheoretical therapy: toward a more integrative model of change. *Psychother Theory Res Pract.* 1982;19:276–288.

25. Fishbein M. A theory of reasoned action: some applications and implications. *Nebr Symp Motiv.* 1980;27:65–116.

26. Ajzen I. The theory of planned behavior. *Organ Behav Human Decision Processes.* 1991;50:179–211.

27. Fiore MC, Jaén CR, Baker TB, et al. *Treating Tobacco Use and Dependence: 2008 Update: Clinical Practice Guideline.* Rockville MD: U.S. Public Health Service, Department of Health and Human Services; 2008.

28. Bandura A. Health promotion from the perspective of social cognitive theory. *Psychol Health.* 1998;13:623–649.

29. Haider M, Kreps GL. Forty years of diffusion of innovations: utility and value in public health. *J Health Commun.* 2004;9(Suppl 1):3–11.

30. Myers J. Exercise and cardiovascular health. *Circulation.* 2003;107:e2–e5.

31. *WHO Guidelines on Physical Activity and Sedentary Behaviour.* Geneva: World Health Organization; 2020.

32. Lee IM, Shiroma EJ, Lobelo F, Puska P, Blair SN, Katzmarzyk PT. Effect of physical inactivity on major non-communicable diseases worldwide: an analysis of burden of disease and life expectancy. *Lancet.* 2012;380:219–229.

33. Guthold R, Stevens GA, Riley LA, Bull FC. Worldwide trends in insufficient physical inactivity from 2001 to 2016: a pooled analysis of 358 population-based surveys with 1.9 million participants. *Lancet Glob Health.* 2018;6:e1077–e1086.

34. Guthold R, Stevens GA, Riley LA, Bull FC. Worldwide trends in insufficient physical inactivity among adolescents: a pooled analysis of 298 population-based surveys with 1.6 million participants. *Lancet Glob Health.* 2020;4:e23–e35.

35. Katzmarzyk PT. Physical activity, sedentary behavior, and health: paradigm paralysis or paradigm shift? *Diabetes.* 2010;59:2717–2725.

36. Ekelund U, Steene-Johannessen J, Brown WJ, et al. Does physical activity attenuate, or even eliminate, the detrimental association of sitting time with mortality? A harmonized meta-analysis of data from more than 1 million men and women. *Lancet.* 2016;388:1302–1310.

37. Kohl HW 3rd, Craig CL, Lambert EL, et al. The pandemic of physical inactivity: global action for public health. *Lancet.* 2012;380:294–305.

38. Pratt M, Macera CA, Sallis JF, O'Donnell M, Frank LD. Economic interventions to promote physical activity: application of the SLOTH model. *Am J Prev Med.* 2004;27(Suppl 3):136–145.

39. Reis RS, Salvo D, Ogilvie D, et al. Scaling up physical activity interventions worldwide: stepping up to larger and smarter approaches to get people moving. *Lancet.* 2012;388:1337–1348.

40. Bauman AE, Reis RS, Sallis JF, Wells JC, Loos RJF, Martin BW. Correlates of physical activity: why are some people physically active and others not? *Lancet.* 2012;380:258–271.

41. Heath GW, Parra DC, Sarmiento OL, et al. Evidence-based intervention in physical activity: lessons from around the world. *Lancet.* 2012;380:272–281.

42. Reed GW, Rossi JE, Cannon CP. Acute myocardial infarction. *Lancet.* 2017;389:197–210.

43. McSweeney JC, Cody M, O'Sullivan P, Elberson K, Moser DK, Garvin BJ. Women's early warning signs of acute myocardial infarction. *Circulation.* 2003;108:2619–2623.

44. Soliman GA. Dietary cholesterol and the lack of evidence in cardiovascular disease. *Nutrients.* 2018;10:780.

45. Miller M, Stone NJ, Ballantyne C, et al. Triglycerides and cardiovascular disease: a scientific statement from the American Heart Association. *Circulation.* 2011;123:2292–2333.

46. Schaefer EJ, Brousseau ME. Diet, lipoproteins, and coronary heart disease. *Endocrinol Metab Clin North Am.* 1998;27:711–732.

47. Carson JAS, Lichtenstein AH, Anderson CAM, et al. Dietary cholesterol and cardiovascular risk: a science advisory from the American Heart Association. *Circulation.* 2020;141:e39–e53.

48. Berger S, Raman G, Vishwanathan R, Jacques PF, Johnson EJ. Dietary cholesterol and cardiovascular disease: a systematic review and meta-analysis. *Am J Clin Nutr.* 2015;102:276–294.

49. Clifton PM. Diet, exercise and weight loss and dyslipidaemia. *Pathology.* 2019;51:222–226.

50. Adhyaru BB, Jacobson TA. Safety and efficacy of statin therapy. *Nat Rev Cardiol.* 2018;15:757–769.

51. NCD Risk Factor Collaboration (NCD-RisC). Repositioning of the global epicentre of non-optimal cholesterol. *Nature.* 2020;582:73–77.

52. Biasucci LM, Biasillo G, Stefanelli A. Inflammatory markers, cholesterol and statins: pathophysiological role and clinical importance. *Clin Chem Lab Med.* 2010;48:1685–1691.

53. Egger G, Dixon J. Beyond obesity and lifestyle: a review of 21st century chronic disease determinants. *Biomed Res Int.* 2014;2014:731685.

54. Tsoupras A, Lordan R, Zaetakis I. Inflammation, not cholesterol, is a cause of chronic disease. *Nutrients.* 2018;10:604.

55. *World Health Organization Model List of Essential Medicines, 22nd List.* Geneva: World Health Organization; 2021.

56. Khatib R, McKee M, Shannon H, et al. Availability and affordability of cardiovascular disease medicines and their effect on use in high-income, middle-income, and low-income countries: an analysis of the PURE study data. *Lancet.* 2016;387:61–69.

57. Wirtz VJ, Kaplan WA, Kwan GF, Laing RO. Access to medications for cardiovascular diseases in low- and middle-income countries. *Circulation.* 2016;133:2076–2085.

58. Dugani SB, Moran AE, Bonow RO, Gaziano TA. Ischemic heart disease: cost-effective acute management and secondary prevention (chapter 8). In: Prabhakaran D, Anand S, Gaziano TA, Mbanya J-C, Wu Y, Nugent R, eds. *Disease Control Priorities: Cardiovascular, Respiratory, and Related Diseases.* 3rd ed. Vol. 5. Washington DC: IBRD/World Bank; 2017:135–156.

59. Brouwer ED, Watkins D, Olson Z, Goett J, Nugent R, Levin C. Provider costs for prevention and treatment of cardiovascular and related conditions in low- and middle-income countries: a systematic review. *BMC Public Health.* 2015;15:1183.

60. Sun Y, Weber KT. Infarct scar: a dynamic tissue. *Cardiovasc Res.* 2000;46:250–256.

61. Turk-Adawi KI, Grace SL. Narrative review comparing the benefits of and participation in cardiac rehabilitation in high-, middle- and low-income countries. *Heart Lung Circ.* 2015;24:510–520.

62. Prabhakaran S, Ruff I, Bernstein RA. Acute stroke intervention: a systematic review. *JAMA.* 2015;313:1451–1462.

63. Andersen KK, Skyhøj Olsen T, Dehlendorff C, Kammersgaard LP. Hemorrhagic and ischemic strokes compared: stroke severity, mortality, and risk factors. *Stroke.* 2009;40:2068–2072.

64. Berkowitz AL. Managing acute stroke in low-resource settings. *Bull World Health Organ.* 2016;94:554–556.

65. Yan L, Li C, Chen J, et al. Stroke (chapter 9). In: Prabhakaran D, Anand S, Gaziano TA, Mbanya J-C, Wu Y, Nugent R, eds. *Disease Control Priorities: Cardiovascular, Respiratory, and Related Diseases.* 3rd ed. Vol. 5. Washington DC: IBRD/World Bank; 2017:157–172.

66. Lawes CMM, Bennett DA, Feigin VL, Rodgers A. Blood pressure and stroke: an overview of published reviews. *Stroke.* 2004;35:776–785.

67. Strong K, Mathers C, Bonita R. Preventing stroke: saving lives around the world. *Lancet Neurol.* 2007;6:182–187.

68. Teasell R, Hussein N, Foley N, Cotoi A. *Evidence-Based Review of Stroke Rehabilitation.* London ON: Canadian Partnership for Stroke Recovery; 2015.

69. Bernhardt J, Urimubenshi G, Gandhi DBC, Eng JJ. Stroke rehabilitation in low-income and middle-income countries: a call to action. *Lancet.* 2020;396:1452–1462.

70. Di Carlo A. Human and economic burden of stroke. *Age Ageing.* 2009;38:4–5.

71. Poulter NR, Prabhakaran D, Caulfield M. Hypertension. *Lancet.* 2015;386:801–812.

72. Ettehad D, Emdin CA, Kiran A, et al. Blood pressure lowering for prevention of cardiovascular disease and death: a systematic review and meta-analysis. *Lancet.* 2016;387:957–967.

73. Unger T, Borghi C, Charchar F, et al. 2020 International Society of Hypertension global hypertension practice guidelines. *J Hypertens.* 2020;38:982–1004.

74. Rapsomaniki E, Timmis A, George J, et al. Blood pressure and incidence of twelve cardiovascular diseases: lifetime risks, healthy life-years lost, and age-specific associations in 1.25 million people. *Lancet.* 2014;383:1899–1911.

75. Egan BM, Kjeldsen SE, Grassi G, Esler M, Mancia G. The global burden of hypertension exceeds 1.4 billion people: should a systolic blood pressure target below 130 become the universal standard? *J Hypertens.* 2019;37:1148–1153.

76. Attaei MW, Khatib R, McKee M, et al. Availability and affordability of blood pressure-lowering medicines

and the effect on blood pressure control in high-income, middle-income, and low-income countries: an analysis of the PURE study data. *Lancet Public Health.* 2017;2:e411–e419.

77. NCD Risk Factor Collaboration (NCD-RisC). Long-term and recent trends in hypertension awareness, treatment, and control in 12 high-income countries: an analysis of 123 nationally representative surveys. *Lancet.* 2019;394:639–651.

78. Geldsetzer P, Manne-Goehler J, Marcus ME, et al. The state of hypertension care in 44 low-income and middle-income countries: a cross-sectional study of nationally representative individual-level data from 1.1 million adults. *Lancet.* 2019;394:652–662.

79. NCD Risk Factor Collaboration (NCD-RisC). Worldwide trends in hypertension prevalence and progress in treatment and control from 1990 to 2019: a pooled analysis of 1201 population-representative studies with 104 million participants. *Lancet.* 2021;398:957–980.

80. Mills KT, Bundy JD, Kelly TN, et al. Global disparities of hypertension prevalence and control: a systematic analysis of population-based studies from 90 countries. *Circulation.* 2016;134:441–450.

81. NCD Risk Factor Collaboration (NCD-RisC). Worldwide trends in blood pressure from 1975 to 2015: a pooled analysis of 1479 population-based measurement studies with 19.1 million participants. *Lancet.* 2017;389:37–55.

82. Forouzanfar MH, Liu P, Roth GA, et al. Global burden of hypertension and systolic blood pressure of at least 110 to 115 mm Hg, 1990–2015. *JAMA.* 2017;317:165–182.

83. Olsen MH, Angell SY, Asma S, et al. A call to action and a lifecourse strategy to address the global burden of raised blood pressure on current and future generations: the Lancet Commission on hypertension. *Lancet.* 2016;388:2665–2712.

84. Sacks FM, Svetkey LP, Vollmer WM, et al. Effects on blood pressure of reduced dietary sodium and the Dietary Approaches to Stop Hypertension (DASH) diet. *N Engl J Med.* 2001;344:3–10.

85. *2020 Global Nutrition Report: Action on Equity to End Malnutrition.* Bristol UK: Development Initiatives; 2020.

86. *The SHAKE Technical Package for Salt Reduction.* Geneva: World Health Organization; 2016.

87. Mills KT, Stefanescu A, He J. The global epidemiology of hypertension. *Nature Rev Nephrol.* 2020;16:223–237.

88. Valenzuela PL, Carrera-Bastos P, Gálvz BG, et al. Lifestyle interventions for the prevention and treatment of hypertension. *Nat Rev Cardiol.* 2021;18:251–275.

89. Marijon E, Mirabel M, Celermajer DS, Jouven X. Rheumatic heart disease. *Lancet.* 2012;379:953–964.

90. Zühlke L, Karthikeyan G, Engel ME, et al. Clinical outcomes in 3343 children and adults with rheumatic heart disease from 14 low- and middle-income countries: two-year follow-up of the Global Rheumatic Heart Disease Registry (the REMEDY Study). *Circulation.* 2016;134:1456–1466.

91. Zilla P, Bolman RM III, Boateng P, Sliwa K. A glimpse of hope: cardiac surgery in low- and middle-income countries (LMICs). *Cardiovasc Diagn Ther.* 2020;10:336–349.

92. Aune D, Schlesinger S, Norat T, Riboli E. Tobacco smoking and the risk of abdominal aortic aneurysm: a systematic review and meta-analysis of prospective studies. *Sci Rep.* 2018;8:14786.

93. Brieler J, Breeden MA, Tucker J. Cardiomyopathy: an overview. *Am Fam Physician.* 2017;96:640–646.

94. Oakley CM. Myocarditis, pericarditis and other pericardial diseases. *Heart.* 2000;84:449–454.

95. Lip GYH, Tse HF, Lane DA. Atrial fibrillation. *Lancet.* 2012;379:648–661.

96. Bestawros M. Electrophysiology in the developing world: challenges and opportunities. *Cardiol Clin.* 2017;31:49–58.

97. Metra M, Teerlink JR. Heart failure. *Lancet.* 2017;390:1981–1995.

98. Leong DP, Joseph PG, McKee M, et al. Reducing the global burden of cardiovascular disease, part 2: prevention and treatment of cardiovascular disease. *Circ Res.* 2017;121:695–710.

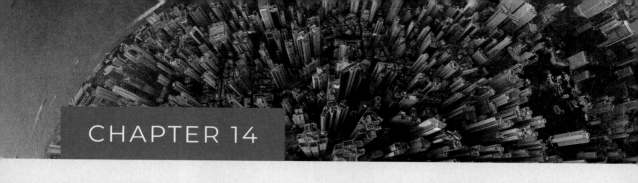

Cancer

Cancers are among the most frequent causes of adult death in every country, and many types of cancer cannot be prevented with current knowledge and technologies. Reducing the global burden from cancer will require improving access to affordable and effective prevention, screening, early diagnosis, and treatment interventions.

14.1 Cancer and Global Health

Cancer is a major cause of illness, disability, and death among adults in every country. High-income countries have higher cancer incidence rates than low-income countries. This is partly because average life expectancies are higher in high-income countries, so more people live long enough to develop cancer. However, even after adjusting for differences in the age structures of populations and accounting for differential access to screening and diagnostic tests, people who live in high-income countries are more likely to develop cancer than people who live in low-income countries. The percentage of cancers that occur in countries with very high human development levels is disproportionately high compared to the percentage of the world's people who live in these areas (**Figure 14.1**).[1]

Although the cancer incidence rate is currently highest in high-income countries, the number of new cases of cancer each year in lower-income countries will increase significantly over the next several decades (**Figure 14.2**).[2] Many residents of lower-income countries do not have access to screening and diagnostic tests that are able to detect early-stage cancers, so cancers are often at an advanced stage when they are diagnosed. After diagnosis, many people with cancer who live in lower-income countries do not have access to surgery, chemotherapy, radiation, and other types of cancer treatment. Because of the many financial, geographic, and other barriers to cancer diagnosis and treatment, the cancer survival rates are much lower in lower-income countries than in high-income countries.[3]

There is significant diversity in which types of cancer cause the greatest economic and epidemiological burdens by country income level and geographic region, but all countries will benefit from discoveries that enable primary prevention of various types of cancer and innovations that improve cancer detection and treatment. Global collaborations are the most efficient way to accelerate the

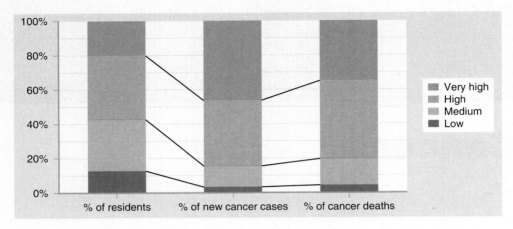

Figure 14.1 Distribution of new cancer cases, cancer deaths, and the total population, by country human development index level.

Data from Sun H, Ferlay J, Siegel RL, et al. Global cancer statistics 2020: GLOBOCAN estimates of incidence and mortality worldwide for 36 cancers in 185 countries. *CA Cancer J Clin.* 2021;71:209–249.

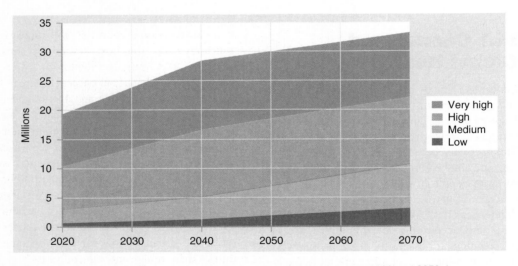

Figure 14.2 Projected number of new cases of cancer per year between 2020 and 2070, by country human development index level.

Data from Ferlay J, Laversanne M, Ervik M, et al. *Global Cancer Observatory: Cancer Tomorrow.* Lyon France: International Agency for Research on Cancer; 2020; Soerjomataram I, Bray F. Planning for tomorrow: global cancer incidence and the role of prevention 2020–2070. *Nat Rev Clin Oncol.* 2021;18:663–672.

process of making scientific breakthroughs, translating those findings into improved medical care, and increasing access to affordable and effective tools for cancer prevention, screening, diagnosis, and treatment.

14.2 Cancer Biology

Cancer is a disease that occurs when abnormal cells in the body begin to reproduce uncontrollably, often invading nearby tissues and then spreading to other parts of the body. Normal cells are genetically stable, and if mutations or other types of damage cannot be repaired, the cell will undergo **apoptosis**, a process of programmed cell death. Cancer cells, in contrast, are genetically unstable and undergo unlimited reproductive cycles.

A **tumor** is an abnormal growth of a body tissue. Tumors are sometimes called **neoplasms**, a term derived from root words meaning "new formation." A **benign tumor** is a noncancerous growth that will not spread to another part of the body. Benign does not mean that the tumor is not harmful. A benign tumor might cause pain, hormone disfunction, or other health issues. Some types of benign tumors may change over time into cancerous tumors if they are not surgically removed or otherwise treated. An **in situ tumor** is a noninvasive precancerous group of abnormal cells. A **malignant tumor** is a cancerous growth that can spread to other parts of the body.

A **metastasis** is a secondary cancerous tumor that is located at a different site in the body than the primary tumor. Cells from a primary malignant tumor that invade the walls of blood vessels or lymph vessels can travel to other parts of the body, proliferate (multiply) there, and form new tumors at that distant site. The cells in that secondary tumor will be the same as the cells at the primary cancer site. For example, a breast cancer metastasis in a lung will be composed of breast cells and not lung cells. Cancer cells can stimulate **angiogenesis**, the formation of new blood vessels that nourish a new cancerous tumor.

Cancers are named for the part of the body where they originate and for the specific type of cell that has become cancerous. A **carcinoma** is a cancer that formed in epithelial tissues, which usually line the inside or outside of the body. A **sarcoma** is a cancer that arose from connective tissues like bones or muscles. Leukemias and myelomas are cancers that formed in the blood or in the bone marrow where blood is produced by the body. Cancers are also classified based on whether the cancer cells remain noninvasive and local, if they have spread to regional lymph nodes, or if they have spread to distant parts of the body. There are several staging systems. One assigns a stage based on the TNM classification system, which categorizes the size of the original tumor, the number of lymph nodes near the primary tumor that have cancer cells in them, and whether metastasis has occurred. Another classifies cancers using a four-stage scale. Precancerous lesions like carcinoma *in situ* are classified as Stage 0 cancers. Stage I cancers are localized. Stage II and III cancers have spread regionally. Stage IV cancers have spread to distant sites.

There are several hundred types of cancer, and each has a unique set of causes, characteristics, and treatment approaches. The signs and symptoms of cancer are specific to the site and stage of the cancer, but the general warning signs of malignancy are often summarized using the acronym CAUTION: a change in bowel or bladder habits, a skin or mouth sore that does not heal, unusual bleeding or discharge, a thickening or lump, indigestion or difficulty swallowing, obvious changes to skin blemishes, or a nagging cough or hoarseness. People with cancer may also experience fatigue, weight loss, pain, fevers, sensory disturbances, and other discomforts.

The treatment approach recommended at the time of diagnosis is based on the type and stage of the cancer. A **relative survival rate** compares the likelihood of survival to selected time points after diagnosis of an adverse health condition with survival rates for people of the same age who do not have the condition. In the United States, the all-stages five-year relative survival rate for all cancers combined is currently about 67%, which means that people with cancer are about 33% more likely to die during a five-year observation period than people who are the same age but do not have

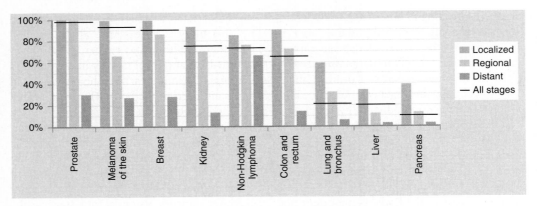

Figure 14.3 Five-year relative survival rates by cancer site in the United States, by stage at diagnosis.
Data from Siegel RL, Miller KD, Fuchs HE, Jemal A. Cancer statistics, 2021. *CA Cancer J Clin.* 2021;71:7–33.

cancer.[4] Five- and 10-year relative survival rates after diagnosis are higher when cancers are diagnosed at early stages (**Figure 14.3**).[4]

14.3 Cancer Epidemiology

About one in six deaths worldwide each year is now due to some type of cancer (**Figure 14.4**).[5] The percentage of deaths from cancer is increasing as more children live into adulthood and more adults live to older ages.[6] The number of people diagnosed with cancer each year is expected to rise from about 19 million in 2020 to 30 million in 2040 due to population growth and aging, and the number of cancer deaths per year is expected to increase from about 10 million to 16 million over those 20 years.[7]

The cancer incidence rate is higher in high-income countries than in low-income countries (**Figure 14.5**).[5] Even after adjusting for differences in population age structures, a person who lives in a high-income country is several times more likely to receive a cancer diagnosis as a person of the same age who lives in a low-income country.[5] This is partly due to people who live in high-income countries having greater access to cancer screening and diagnostic tests. In

high-income countries where access to testing enables most cancers to be diagnosed, the incidence rate and the detection rate are similar. In low-income countries, where only the most advanced cancers are clinically diagnosed, the incidence rate might be much higher than the reported rate of detected cancers. However, people who live in high-income countries also have higher levels of exposure to many of the known risk factors for cancer.[8] After accounting for differences in age structures and case detection rates, cancer incidence rates remain much higher in high-income countries than in low-income countries.

Although the age-standardized cancer incidence rates are significantly higher in higher-income countries than in lower-income countries, age-standardized cancer mortality rates are similar across country income groups.[5] The similarity in mortality rates despite the differences in incidence is due to the cancer survival rate in lower-income countries being much lower than the survival rate in higher-income countries. Cancer survival rates have increased in high-income countries as diagnosis and treatment options have improved.[9] Cancer survival rates in lower-income countries have also improved, but they continue to lag behind the rates in higher-income countries.[9]

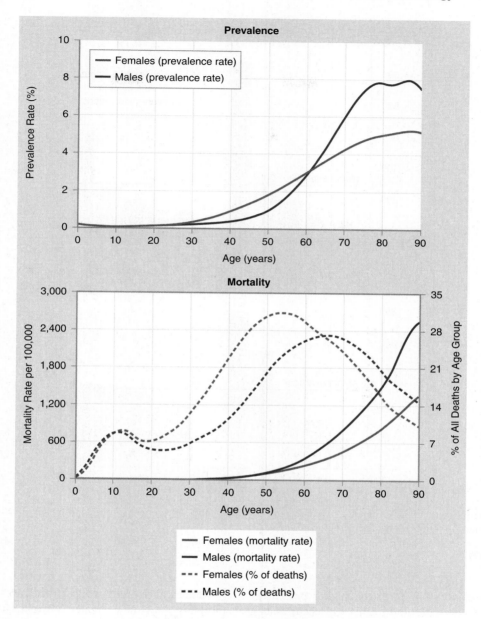

Figure 14.4 Prevalence rate per 100,000 people, mortality rate per 100,000 people, and percentage of deaths from cancer, by sex and age.

Data from GBD 2019 Diseases and Injuries Collaborators. Global burden of 369 diseases and injuries in 204 countries and territories, 1990–2019: a systematic analysis for the Global Burden of Disease Study 2019. *Lancet.* 2020;396:1204–1222.

Older adults have a much higher rate of cancer incidence and death than younger people (**Figure 14.6**).[7] More than 60% of

cancer diagnoses and more than 70% of cancer deaths worldwide occur in people who are at least 60 years old (**Figure 14.7**).[7] As the world

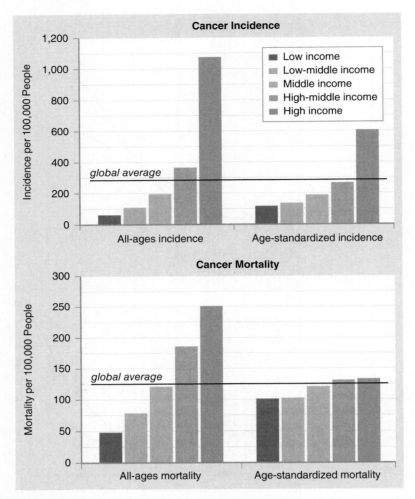

Figure 14.5 All-ages and age-standardized cancer incidence and cancer mortality rates per 100,000 people, by country sociodemographic group.

Data from GBD 2019 Diseases and Injuries Collaborators. Global burden of 369 diseases and injuries in 204 countries and territories, 1990–2019: a systematic analysis for the Global Burden of Disease Study 2019. *Lancet.* 2020;396:1204–1222.

population ages, an even higher percentage of cancer cases and deaths will occur among older adults. However, cancers can and do occur at every age. If progress on preventing and treating cancer does not accelerate, about 7% of today's 30-year-olds will die from cancer before their 70th birthdays.[6]

Males have higher cancer incidence and mortality rates than females (**Figure 14.8**).[5] Globally, the most frequently occurring cancers by site among males are lung cancer, prostate cancer, colorectal cancer, nonmelanoma skin cancer, and stomach cancer, and the most frequent causes of cancer death

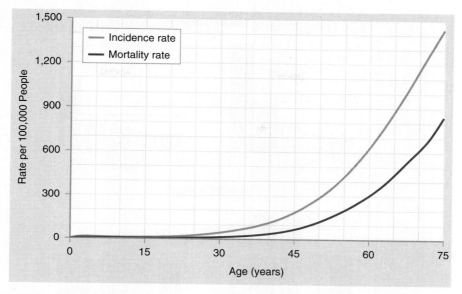

Figure 14.6 Worldwide cancer incidence and mortality rates per 100,000 people by age.

Data from Sung H, Ferlay J, Siegel RL, et al. Global cancer statistics 2020: GLOBOCAN estimates of incidence and mortality worldwide for 36 cancers in 185 countries. *CA Cancer J Clin.* 2021;71:209–249; Ferlay J, Laversanne M, Ervik M, et al. *GLOBOCAN 2020 Database Version 2.0.* Lyon: International Agency for Research on Cancer; 2020.

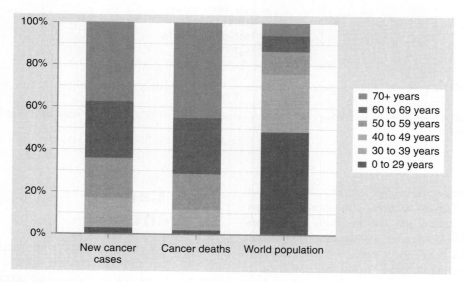

Figure 14.7 Proportion of worldwide cancer cases and deaths by age group.

Data from Ferlay J, Laversanne M, Ervik M, et al. *GLOBOCAN 2020 Database Version 2.0.* Lyon: International Agency for Research on Cancer; 2020; United Nations Department of Economic and Social Affairs. *World Population Prospects: The 2019 Revision.* New York: United Nations; 2019.

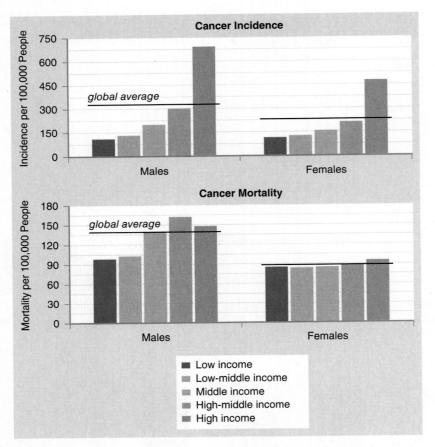

Figure 14.8 Age-standardized cancer incidence and cancer mortality rates per 100,000 people, by sex and country sociodemographic group.

Data from GBD 2019 Diseases and Injuries Collaborators. Global burden of 369 diseases and injuries in 204 countries and territories, 1990–2019: a systematic analysis for the Global Burden of Disease Study 2019. *Lancet.* 2020;396:1204–1222.

are lung cancer, liver cancer, colorectal cancer, stomach cancer, and prostate cancer; for females, the cancers with the highest incidence rates are breast cancer, colorectal cancer, lung cancer, cervical cancer, and non-melanoma skin cancer, and the most frequent causes of cancer death are breast cancer, lung cancer, colorectal cancer, cervical cancer, and stomach cancer.[1] The types of cancers that occur most often and cause the greatest number of deaths vary considerably by country and world region (**Figure 14.9**).[1]

14.4 Cancer Prevention

Cancer is a genetic disease, but it usually results from mutations rather than inheritance.[10] About 5% of the genetic mutations that lead to cancer are inherited; about 30% are associated with health behaviors, environmental exposures, and other modifiable risk factors; and about two-thirds are random mutations without a currently known cause.[11]

	World	Ethiopia	Nigeria	India	China	Brazil	Iran	Germany	USA
Cancer Incidence among Males	Lung Prostate CRC	CRC Prostate Leukemia	Prostate CRC NHL	LOC Lung Stomach	Lung Stomach CRC	Prostate CRC Lung	Stomach Prostate Lung	Prostate Lung CRC	Prostate Lung CRC
Cancer Deaths among Males	Lung Liver CRC	CRC Leukemia Prostate	Prostate Liver CRC	LOC Lung Esophagus	Lung Liver Stomach	Lung Prostate CRC	Stomach Lung Prostate	Lung Prostate CRC	Lung Prostate CRC
Cancer Incidence among Females	Breast CRC Lung	Breast Cervix CRC	Breast Cervix NHL	Breast Uterus Ovary	Breast Lung CRC	Breast CRC Thyroid	Breast CRC Stomach	Breast CRC Lung	Breast Lung CRC
Cancer Deaths among Females	Breast Lung CRC	Breast Cervix CRC	Breast Cervix Ovary	Breast Cervix Ovary	Lung CRC Stomach	Breast Lung CRC	Breast Stomach Lung	Breast Lung CRC	Lung Breast CRC

CRC: colorectal cancer; LOC: lip and oral cavity cancer; NHL: non-Hodgkin lymphoma

Figure 14.9 Top three most frequent incident cancers (excluding nonmelanoma skin cancers) and causes of cancer death for males and females in selected countries. The shade of the box represents the most frequent cancer type for each category.

Data from Sun H, Ferlay J, Siegel RL, et al. Global cancer statistics 2020: GLOBOCAN estimates of incidence and mortality worldwide for 36 cancers in 185 countries. *CA Cancer J Clin.* 2021;71:209–249.

Cancers are often the result of several mutations being present together, and a variety of different sets of exposures may lead to the development of the same type of cancer. Age is the dominant risk factor for many types of cancer, and because aging is not modifiable, the burden from cancers associated with aging will increase as life expectancies increase.[12]

The genetic mutations that lead to cancer can occur via numerous pathways.[13] Chemicals in tobacco can damage cells in the lungs, mouth, pharynx, larynx, esophagus, pancreas, urinary bladder, and kidneys.[14] Occupational carcinogens can also damage cells. For example, benzene increases the risk of leukemia; asbestos has been linked to a kind of lung cancer called mesothelioma; and arsenic, cadmium, chromium, and other chemicals increase the risk of cancers of the lungs, bronchi, and trachea.[15] Environmental hazards such as air pollution, residential radon, and arsenic in drinking water can induce cellular damage.[16] An unhealthy diet, obesity, and physical inactivity may also impair cellular function.[10]

Additionally, chronic infections may cause inflammation that damages body tissues.[17] Chronic infections are estimated to cause more than 2 million new cases of cancer worldwide each year (**Figure 14.10**),[18] contributing to more than 1 in 4 cancers in lower-income areas and about 1 in 14 cancers in in higher-income areas.[19] The **cancer transition** describes a shift from many cancers being associated with chronic infections (such as cervical cancer linked to HPV, stomach cancer associated with *Helicobacter pylori* infection, and liver cancer linked to hepatitis B and C) to few cancers being caused by untreated chronic infections.[20]

Infection	Associated Cancer(s)
Clonorchis sinensis	Bile duct cancer
Epstein–Barr virus (EBV)	Nasopharyngeal carcinoma, Hodgkin lymphoma, Burkitt lymphoma
Helicobacter pylori	Stomach cancer
Hepatitis B virus (HBV)	Liver cancer
Hepatitis C virus (HCV)	Liver cancer
Human herpes virus type 8 (HHV-8)	Kaposi sarcoma
Human papillomavirus (HPV)	Cervical cancer, oropharyngeal cancers, anogenital cancers
Human T-cell lymphotropic virus (HTLV)	Adult T-cell leukemia and lymphoma
Opisthorchis viverrini	Bile duct cancer
Schistosoma haematobium	Bladder cancer

Figure 14.10 Examples of cancers associated with chronic infections.

Data from de Martel C, Georges D, Bray F, Ferlay J, Clifford GM. Global burden of cancer attributable to infections in 2018: a worldwide incidence analysis. *Lancet Glob Health*. 2020;8:e180–e190.

At the global population level, about one-third of cancer deaths are attributed to nine modifiable lifestyle and environmental factors: smoking, alcohol use, low fruit and vegetable intake, overweight and obesity, physical inactivity, unsafe sex (which is associated with HPV and other chronic infections), urban air pollution, indoor smoke from household use of solid fuels, and contaminated injections in healthcare settings (which can transmit HIV and other pathogens that increase susceptibility to cancer).[21] At the individual level, however, it is rarely possible to know with certainty which factors led to the development of cancer.

The **ecological fallacy** is the incorrect assumption that individuals follow the trends observed in population-level data. For example, while the link between tobacco use and lung cancer is well established, there are many individuals whose experience does not align with that general association. Many people who develop lung cancer have never smoked,[22] many people who smoke for decades never develop lung cancer, and some people who smoke develop lung cancer as a result of a mutation that is unrelated to tobacco exposure. Everyone is encouraged to follow the guidelines for cancer prevention, but even people who adhere to all the scientific recommendations for good health must remain vigilant about screening and seeking medical care for symptoms that might indicate the presence of cancer.

Only about half of cancers occurring globally today are ones that could be prevented with current scientific knowledge and technologies,[23] but advances in prevention science are reducing the burden from some types of cancer. For example, surgery to remove intestinal polyps before they become cancerous prevents colon cancer, and the HPV vaccine is associated with a significant reduction in cervical cancer risk.[24] One of the key steps toward reducing the global burden from cancer will be identifying additional modifiable risk factors and developing interventions that will prevent new cancers from developing. The multicausal origins of most cancers means that there are many possible pathways for improving cancer prevention.[25]

14.5 Cancer Screening

When cancer cannot be prevented, the next best option is to detect cancer at an early stage through screening. **Screening** is a type of secondary prevention in which all members of a well-defined group of people are encouraged to be tested for a disease based on evidence that members of the population are at risk for the disease and early intervention improves health outcomes. The goal of cancer screening programs is to identify precancerous lesions or early-stage, localized cancers in people who have no symptoms of cancer (**Figure 14.11**). When diagnostic tests are conducted in people who already have signs and symptoms of cancer in order to confirm the presence of cancerous cells, those tests are diagnostic tests rather than screening tests.

Population-based screening initiatives target large demographic groups, such as all women aged 40–79 years. **High-risk screening** recommendations apply to people who are known to have an elevated risk of a particular disease. Individuals may have a higher than typical risk of cancer due to family history (genetics), occupational exposures, tobacco use, or other risk factors. Inherited mutations are responsible for relatively few cases of cancer, and most people diagnosed with cancer do not have a family history of that type of cancer. However, people with a family history may benefit from being screened more often than is recommended for the general population and may be advised to start screening at a younger age than is typically recommended.

An excellent screening test will have values near 100% for five statistics that measure various aspects of test performance. The **diagnostic accuracy** is the proportion of people who receive a test whose results are true positives or true negatives. A good screening test will have a high diagnostic accuracy, with nearly 100% of test results being true positives or true negatives and almost no results being false positives or false negatives. A good screening test will also have nearly 100% sensitivity and specificity. The **sensitivity** of a test is the proportion of people who truly have the disease who test positive for the disease. The **specificity** of a test is the proportion of people who

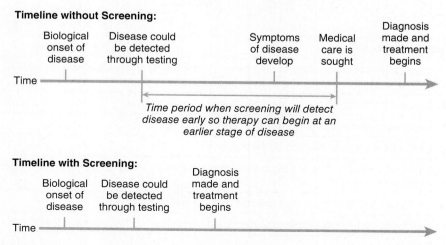

Figure 14.11 Timeline for the natural history of disease.

are truly free of the disease who test negative for it. Additionally, a good screening test will have positive and negative predictive values near 100%. The **positive predictive value** (PPV) is the proportion of people who test positive for the disease who truly have the disease. The **negative predictive value** (NPV) is the proportion of people who test negative for the disease who truly do not have the disease. The PPV and NPV are based, in part, on the percentage of people in the population being tested who have the disease. A test will have a higher PPV in a population with a high prevalence of disease than in one with a low prevalence.

Diseases that are targeted by screening programs are usually severe, treatable, and have a relatively high prevalence rate (**Figure 14.12**). More screening is not necessarily better. **Overdiagnosis** describes the detection of cancers (or other conditions) that would have gone away on their own or caused no symptoms during the diagnosed individual's lifetime. Overdiagnosis often leads to **overtreatment**, the unnecessary provision of therapy for cancer (or other diseases) when the cancer is unlikely to cause health problems during the diagnosed individual's lifetime and the therapy has harmful side effects. Decisions about when to

implement a screening program and which population subgroups to target are made by health professionals, policymakers, and communities after considering the most important local health conditions.

High-income countries often recommend population-based screening for several types of cancer (**Figure 14.13**).[26] Fewer screening tests are available in lower-income countries.[27] In lower-income countries, the most cost-effective cancer screening tests include clinical breast exams and cervical cancer visualization.[28] A more extensive set of screening tests that involve more expensive procedures are cost effective in higher-income countries that have higher cancer incidence rates and spend more money on cancer treatment.[29]

14.6 Cancer Treatment

The three most frequently used cancer treatments are surgery, chemotherapy, and radiation therapy. **Surgery** is an operation to confirm whether a disease is present or to remove a tumor or repair a part of the body. Cancer surgery typically involves sedating a patient with anesthesia, making an incision

The disease is life threatening.
There is an early asymptomatic stage of the disease in which early diagnosis is possible with an available test.
Early diagnosis significantly improves survival rates or other outcomes.
The screening test has high sensitivity and high specificity.
The screening test is acceptable to the target population.
The target population has access to additional testing and treatment if a screening test indicates the likely presence of disease.
The disease has a relatively high prevalence rate in the target population.
Economic analyses have demonstrated that the screening program is likely to be cost effective.

Figure 14.12 Characteristics of good screening programs.

Type of Cancer	Examples of Screening Tests
Breast cancer	■ Breast self-examination ■ Clinical breast examination ■ Mammography
Cervical cancer	■ Papanicolaou test (Pap smear, cervical cytology) ■ Visual inspection with acetic acid (VIA)
Colorectal cancer	■ Fecal occult blood test (FOBT) ■ Flexible sigmoidoscopy ■ Colonoscopy
Esophageal cancer	■ Endoscopy
Oral cancers	■ Physical examination of the mouth
Prostate cancer	■ Digital rectal examination ■ Prostate-specific antigen (PSA) test
Skin cancers	■ Physical examination of the skin

Figure 14.13 Examples of cancer screening tests.

Data from Sankaranarayanan R. Screening for cancer in low- and middle-income countries. *Ann Global Health.* 2014;80:412–417; Ebell MH, Thai TN, Royalty KJ. Cancer screening recommendations: an international comparison of high income countries. *Public Health Rev.* 2018;39:7.

through the skin with a scalpel in a sterile environment, excising cancerous tissues, and then closing the wound with sutures or staples. Some cancer surgeries are diagnostic. A **biopsy** is the examination of tissue removed from a living body in order to test for the presence or absence of disease. Small samples of cells or tissues collected through an incision or with a needle can be examined for the presence or absence of cancer. After a diagnosis is confirmed, a surgical procedure may be used to stage the cancer. The areas around the primary tumor, including nearby lymph nodes, may be examined. When cancers are localized, surgery can entirely remove a cancerous lesion or tumor. Some surgical procedures reduce the mass of a tumor prior to or after initiating other forms of therapy. Surgery can also be used to manage the complications of advanced cancer, such as intestinal obstructions, and to reduce discomfort and pain. Additionally, reconstructive surgery can restore function and appearance after successful cancer treatment.

Chemotherapy is the treatment of disease using chemical substances. More than 100 different types of chemotherapeutic agents are available to kill cancerous cells, slow the growth of cancerous masses, and keep cancer from spreading to other parts of the body. Chemotherapeutic medications can be delivered orally, intravenously, by injection, or via other mechanisms. They typically must be administered according to strict protocols for dosage and timing, often using several cycles of treatment and rest periods. Chemotherapy can be used alone for some types of cancers. For others, it may be used as neoadjuvant therapy to shrink tumors before surgery or radiation or as adjuvant therapy to kill any cancer cells remaining after other types of treatments. Chemotherapy often causes fatigue and may cause other side effects, such as nausea, skin and mouth sores, and hair loss.

Radiation therapy uses high-energy ionizing radiation to damage the DNA of actively dividing cells, which causes the cells to stop dividing or die. Because cancer cells

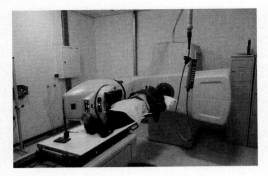

usually divide quickly, they are more likely than healthy cells to be affected by radiation. Even so, healthy cells near the tumor may also be damaged. External beam radiation therapy uses photon beams (or other types of radiation, such as proton therapy) from a machine outside the body to deliver targeted radiation to selected sites. Internal radiation therapy, also called brachytherapy, implants a radioactive isotope in or near the tumor. Systemic radiation therapy injects radioisotopes so they can circulate throughout the body. Radiation may be used alone or in conjunction with other therapies. Fatigue and skin damage are common side

effects, and there is a small risk of a secondary cancer being caused by the exposure to radiation.

A comprehensive cancer care plan includes access to prevention, screening, diagnosis, various types of treatment, and psychosocial support for people with cancer and their caregivers.[30] **Palliative care** includes clinical interventions that improve the quality of life of people with serious chronic illnesses by managing pain, reducing emotional distress, and providing other types of support to patients and their families.[31] Palliative care is typically provided concurrently with curative care interventions. When a patient with a chronic disease is not expected to survive for longer than a few more months, that individual may opt to stop receiving invasive interventions and transition into supportive end-of-life care. **Hospice care** services provide end-of-life comfort care for people with end-stage illnesses and support for their families.[32]

There are significant disparities in access to cancer care by country income level (**Figure 14.14**).[33] Rural residents often have fewer options for cancer treatment than urban residents. Surgery is widely available

Resource Environment	Basic	Limited	Enhanced	Maximal
Location	Low-income countries	Rural areas of middle-income countries	Urban areas of middle-income countries	High-income countries
Screening and treatment of precancerous conditions	Very limited availability	Limited availability	Available	Widely available
Surgery	Limited availability	Limited availability	Widely available	Widely available
Chemotherapy	Not available	Limited availability	Available	Widely available
Radiation therapy	Not available	Very limited availability	Widely available	Widely available

Figure 14.14 Typical resources for cancer care by country income level and location.

Data from Horton S, Gauvreau CL. Cancer in low- and middle-income countries: an economic overview (chapter 16). In: Gelband H, Jha P, Sankaranarayanan R, Horton S, eds. *Disease Control Priorities: Cancer*. 3rd ed. Vol. 3. Washington DC: IBRD/World Bank; 2015:263–280.

in high-income countries, but it may be inaccessible in rural areas of middle-income countries and almost completely unavailable in low-income countries.[34] Chemotherapy may be so expensive in low- and middle-income countries that it is not available to most cancer patients. Radiation therapy remains nonexistent in most low-income countries (**Figure 14.15**).[35] Advanced treatment options, such as immunotherapies (like the use of monoclonal antibodies) and stem cell transplants, are also not widely available outside of high-income countries. Improved access to advanced therapies would enable many more people to survive for many years after being diagnosed with cancer.

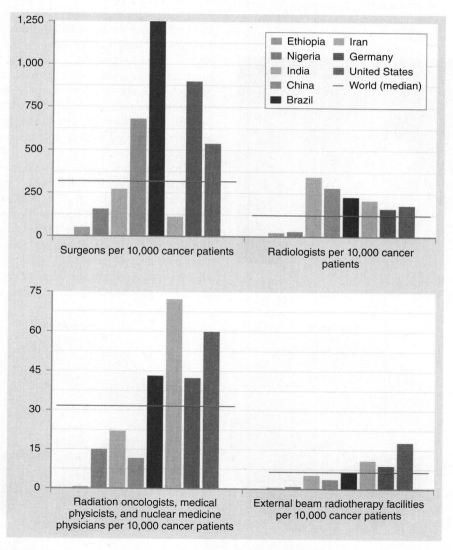

Figure 14.15 Health system capacity and workforce per 10,000 cancer patients in selected countries.

Data from *WHO Cancer Country Profiles 2020*. Geneva: World Health Organization; 2020.

14.7 Lung Cancer

Lung cancer is the most frequent cause of cancer death worldwide, accounting for nearly one in five cancer deaths. In a typical recent year, about 2.2 million adults were diagnosed with lung cancer worldwide and nearly 1.8 million deaths were attributed to lung cancer.[1] Lung cancer is the most frequent cause of cancer deaths among males, accounting for about 22% of male cancer deaths, and lung cancer is the second most frequent cause of cancer

deaths among females after breast cancer, accounting for about 14% of female cancer deaths (**Figure 14.16**).[1]

About 65% of lung cancer deaths are attributable to tobacco smoking.[36] There is wide variation in the lung cancer incidence and mortality rates by country and region, with the highest lung cancer rates occurring in Eastern Europe and Eastern Asia and the lowest rates in sub-Saharan Africa.[5] This geographic pattern closely mirrors the prevalence of tobacco smoking.[37] Differences in lung cancer rates by sex also mirror tobacco use rates. About 65% of lung cancer cases and deaths occur among males,[1] and about 85% of daily tobacco smokers are male.[37] Indoor and outdoor air pollution and some occupational hazards are also associated with an increased risk of lung cancer.[38]

The five-year relative survival rate after a diagnosis of cancer of the lung, bronchus, or trachea remains below 20% even in many high-income countries.[39] Because the treatment options for lung cancer are limited, the most effective lung cancer interventions focus on primary prevention (**Figure 14.17**). The most cost-effective interventions for reducing lung cancer incidence and mortality are tobacco control

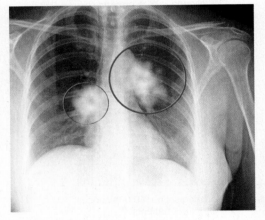

Lung cancer.
© Muratart/Shutterstock

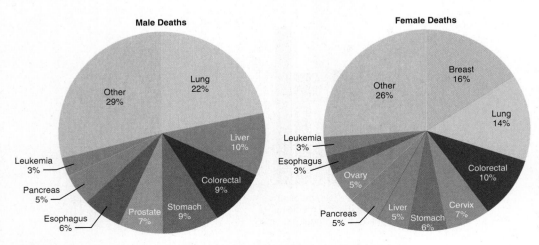

Figure 14.16 Distribution of cancer deaths by site among males and females.

Data from Sun H, Ferlay J, Siegel RL, et al. Global cancer statistics 2020: GLOBOCAN estimates of incidence and mortality worldwide for 36 cancers in 185 countries. *CA Cancer J Clin.* 2021;71:209–249.

Level of Prevention	Primordial Prevention	Primary Prevention	Secondary Prevention	Tertiary Prevention
Goal	Prevent risk factors in people without cancer	Mitigate risk factors in people without cancer	Detect cancer before it becomes symptomatic	Manage cancer after it becomes symptomatic
Examples of interventions	■ Avoid tobacco products ■ Exercise often ■ Eat a nutritious diet	■ Quit smoking ■ Reduce exposure to radon gas, asbestos, and other carcinogens	■ X-rays or low-dose CT scans	■ Surgery ■ Chemotherapy ■ Radiation therapy ■ Palliative care

Figure 14.17 Examples of interventions for lung cancer.

initiatives like warning labels and taxation.[40] Tobacco control initiatives also help reduce the incidence of lip, mouth, and other oral cancers.[41]

14.8 Breast Cancer

Breast cancer is the most frequently diagnosed cancer among women, with more than 2.2 million new cases occurring worldwide each year (**Figure 14.18**).[1] Breast cancer is responsible for about 25% of cancer diagnoses and 16% of cancer deaths among women.[1] The age-standardized breast cancer incidence rate is higher in higher-income countries than it is in lower-income countries, but the mortality rate from breast cancer among women (that is, the rate of death from breast cancer among all women, including those with and

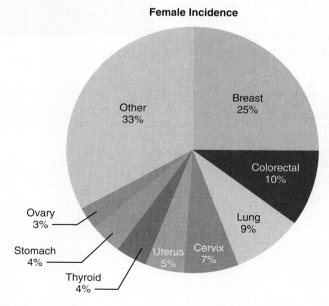

Figure 14.18 Distribution of cancer incidence by site among females (after excluding nonmelanoma skin cancers).

Data from Sun H, Ferlay J, Siegel RL, et al. Global cancer statistics 2020: GLOBOCAN estimates of incidence and mortality worldwide for 36 cancers in 185 countries. *CA Cancer J Clin.* 2021;71:209–249.

without cancer) is higher in lower-income countries than in higher-income countries.[1] Lower-income countries also have a higher breast cancer case fatality rate (that is, a higher proportion of women with breast cancer who die from the disease) and a lower relative survival rate among people diagnosed with breast cancer than is observed in higher-income countries. While the five-year relative breast cancer survival rate exceeds 85% in most high-income countries, the rates are below 70% in some lower-income countries.[39]

The less favorable relative survival rate in lower-income countries is a result of limited access to screening, early diagnosis, and treatment (**Figure 14.19**). Early detection of breast cancer is associated with better outcomes.[42] A mammogram is an X-ray of a breast that is generated using low-dose radiation. In most middle- and high-income areas, routine mammography is available; in low-income countries, the options for early detection are typically limited to clinical breast exams.[43] Women diagnosed with breast cancer in higher-income areas usually have early-stage breast cancers (Stage 0, I, or II), while women diagnosed with breast cancer in lower-income areas often have advanced stage breast cancers (Stage III or IV).[44]

The available treatment options also differ by country income level. For women with breast cancer who live in low-income countries, a mastectomy followed by use of the drug tamoxifen is likely to be the best

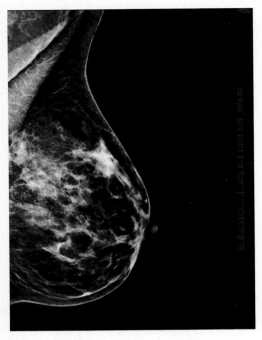

Mammogram.
© Serdar Tibet/Shutterstock

Level of Prevention	Primordial Prevention	Primary Prevention	Secondary Prevention	Tertiary Prevention
Goal	Prevent risk factors in people without cancer	Mitigate risk factors in people without cancer	Detect cancer before it becomes symptomatic	Manage cancer after it becomes symptomatic
Examples of interventions	▪ Maintain a healthy weight ▪ Avoid harmful use of alcohol ▪ Exercise often	▪ Chemoprevention and/or preventive surgery for women with a strong family history of breast cancer	▪ Clinical breast exams ▪ Mammography (X-ray) and other types of imaging (such as ultrasound and MRI)	▪ Surgery (such as lumpectomy or mastectomy) ▪ Hormone therapy (such as tamoxifen) ▪ Radiation therapy ▪ Chemotherapy ▪ Palliative care

Figure 14.19 Examples of interventions for breast cancer.

available option. In high-income countries, breast-conserving surgery followed by reconstruction is often offered, and a diversity of chemotherapy, radiation, endocrine therapies, and biological therapies provide additional pathways to long-term survival.[43]

14.9 Cervical Cancer

Cancers of the female reproductive system are significant contributors to the burden of disease in some populations. In recent years, about 600,000 women were diagnosed with cervical cancer annually.[1] The uterine cervix is the lowest part of the uterus, located immediately above the vagina. During pregnancy, the cervix helps protect the developing fetus; during delivery, the cervix relaxes to allow the baby to pass through the birth canal. The development of abnormal cervical cells, a condition called cervical dysplasia, is not uncommon among women of reproductive age. **Human papillomavirus (HPV)** is a virus associated with the majority of cases of cervical dysplasia.[45] In most women, the viral infection will clear on its own. In some women, the infection becomes chronic and causes additional damage to the cervical cells,

eventually leading to cervical cancer.[46] As the malignant cells multiply, invasive cervical cancer may spread to nearby tissues and then metastasize to other organs.

HPV vaccination is a primary prevention intervention that protects against cervical cancer (**Figure 14.20**). Early detection of cervical dysplasia so that precancerous lesions can be treated is another way to prevent cervical cancer from developing. Pap smears in which cervical cells are collected and histologically examined in a cytology laboratory are the traditional form of cervical cancer screening, but this requires access to laboratory facilities. **VIA**, **v**isual **i**nspection with **a**cetic acid, is an inexpensive method for detecting signs of cervical cancer. In VIA, a diluted vinegar solution applied to the cervix with a cotton swab causes areas that are inflamed or have cellular damage to turn white.[47] Lesions that are observed during VIA screening can be treated with cryotherapy, a procedure that does not require surgery or general anesthesia.[48]

HPV vaccination is not yet available in most lower-income countries, but it is now included in the national vaccination schedules of most higher-income countries.[49] In

Level of Prevention	Primordial Prevention	Primary Prevention	Secondary Prevention	Tertiary Prevention
Goal	Prevent risk factors in people without cancer	Mitigate risk factors in people without cancer	Detect cancer before it becomes symptomatic	Manage cancer after it becomes symptomatic
Examples of interventions	■ Practice safer sex to reduce the risk of sexually transmitted infections that increase the risk of contracting HPV ■ Avoid tobacco products	■ HPV vaccination ■ Use cryotherapy to remove precancerous lesions	■ Visual inspection with acetic acid (VIA) ■ Cytology and HPV DNA tests	■ Surgery (such as trachelectomy or hysterectomy) ■ Chemotherapy ■ Radiation therapy ■ Palliative care

Figure 14.20 Examples of interventions for cervical cancer.

lower-income countries, where HPV vaccines and cervical screening are rarely accessible, cervical cancer continues to be a significant cause of death among women.[50] In higher-income countries, where screening for cervical dysplasia is routinely available, the incidence of cervical cancer has decreased significantly in recent decades.[51] (Since women who have been vaccinated against some strains of HPV are still at risk of cervical cancer from other causes, screening for cervical dysplasia is recommended for most women regardless of their HPV vaccination status.) The disparities between the cervical cancer incidence and mortality rates by country income level are evidence that most of the deaths from cervical cancer worldwide could have been prevented.[52]

Less frequently occurring cancers of the female reproductive system include ovarian cancer and uterine cancer. Ovarian cancer is difficult to diagnose at an early stage, and

the five-year relative survival rate is less than 50% in most countries.[53] Endometrial cancer (cancer of the lining of the uterus) and other uterine cancers usually occur in postmenopausal women. Women who are able to receive surgery for uterine cancer while the cancer is at an early stage typically have favorable outcomes.[54]

14.10 Prostate Cancer

The two most frequently diagnosed cancers among men are lung cancer and prostate cancer, each responsible for about one in seven new cancers (**Figure 14.21**).[1] Most older men develop benign prostatic hyperplasia (BPH), a noncancerous enlargement of the prostate gland that may make urination difficult. At least one in four men experiences moderate to severe symptoms of BPH during his lifetime.[55] Increased age is the dominant risk factor for

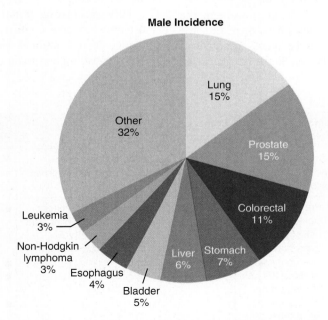

Male Incidence

Lung 15%

Prostate 15%

Other 32%

Colorectal 11%

Leukemia 3%

Non-Hodgkin lymphoma 3%

Esophagus 4%

Bladder 5%

Liver 6%

Stomach 7%

Figure 14.21 Distribution of cancer incidence by site among males (after excluding nonmelanoma skin cancers).

Data from Sun H, Ferlay J, Siegel RL, et al. Global cancer statistics 2020: GLOBOCAN estimates of incidence and mortality worldwide for 36 cancers in 185 countries. *CA Cancer J Clin.* 2021;71:209–249.

prostate cancer, and cancerous cells are often found in the prostate tissues of older men with BPH.[56] About one-third of 70-year-old men, half of 80-year-old men, and nearly 100% of 100-year-old men have cancerous cells in their prostates.[57] Over time, cancers that begin in the prostate may metastasize to lymph nodes, bones, and other parts of the body.

Prostate cancer is the most frequently diagnosed cancer (other than nonmelanoma skin cancers) among men in the Americas, Western Europe, Australia, New Zealand, Japan, and many African countries.[1] The incidence rate is increasing in most world regions due to population aging. Detection rates are also rising as a result of increased access to screening and diagnostic tests like digital rectal examination and prostate-specific antigen (PSA).[58]

The relative survival rate for early-stage prostate cancer is very high in most countries. Many older men die with prostate cancer but not because of it. However, there are so many diagnoses of prostate cancer worldwide each year that the cumulative number of deaths is substantial. Also, because relative survival rates adjust for life expectancy, cancers that primarily occur in older adults tend to have relative survival rates that appear more favorable than some other types of mortality statistics. For example, the United States reports a 98% relative five-year survival rate for prostate cancer, yet more than 30,000 American men die of prostate cancer each year.[59] The typical 50-year-old man has a very high likelihood of surviving to his 55th birthday, so an advanced prostate cancer diagnosis at age 50 may significantly reduce his relative likelihood of survival to age 55 compared to men the same age who do not have any type of cancer. By contrast, a 90-year-old man is unlikely to survive to his 95th birthday even if he is very healthy on his 90th birthday. A 90-year-old who dies of prostate cancer will be included in a count of prostate cancer deaths in his country, but because there are so many other health issues that might cause death prior to the 95th birthday, a prostate cancer diagnosis might not significantly change the survival expectation.

Most interventions for prostate cancer emphasize early detection and symptom management (**Figure 14.22**). Surgery and radiation therapy can be effective treatments for prostate cancer, but both can cause adverse side effects related to urinary, bowel, and sexual function.[60] Improvements in the effectiveness of prostate cancer treatments have led to a decrease in the case fatality rate from prostate cancer in many countries, but access to therapies remains limited in most low-income countries.[61]

Level of Prevention	Primordial Prevention	Primary Prevention	Secondary Prevention	Tertiary Prevention
Goal	Prevent risk factors in people without cancer	Mitigate risk factors in people without cancer	Detect cancer before it becomes symptomatic	Manage cancer after it becomes symptomatic
Examples of interventions	■ Eat a nutritious diet ■ Maintain a healthy weight	—	■ Digital rectal exam ■ Prostate-specific antigen (PSA) test	■ Surgery (prostatectomy) ■ Radiation therapy ■ Hormone therapy ■ Chemotherapy ■ Palliative care

Figure 14.22 Examples of interventions for prostate cancer.

14.11 Liver Cancer

Many cases of liver cancer are attributed to chronic viral hepatitis infections (**Figure 14.23**).[5] Chronic hepatitis B virus (HBV) infection, often acquired in infancy, can trigger a pathologic process that damages liver cells and leads to hepatocellular carcinoma (HCC), the most prevalent type of liver cancer.[62] Most cases of liver cancer currently occur in the places within East Asia, South Asia, and sub-Saharan Africa that had high rates of infant HBV infection before hepatitis B vaccines became available.[63] Besides HBV, other major risk factors for liver cancer include hepatitis C virus (HCV), alcohol use, tobacco smoking, obesity, and exposure to aflatoxins, which are toxic molds found in some foods.[64] Alcohol is a direct risk factor for liver cancer and also

accelerates the progression of the liver damage caused by HBV and HCV.[65] Because males consume significantly more alcohol than females, males have a significantly higher incidence of liver cancer than females.

The best currently available option for preventing future cases of liver cancer is hepatitis B vaccine (**Figure 14.24**).[66] To prevent mother-to-child transmission of the virus, the first dose of the vaccine is typically given to neonates shortly after birth.[67] The vaccine prevents new HBV infections, but it does not stop cancer from developing in adults whose livers have already been scarred by chronic infection. The five-year relative survival rate for liver cancer currently is less than 20%, even in many of the countries with the most favorable outcomes,[39] so liver cancer will continue to be a major cause of cancer death among adults

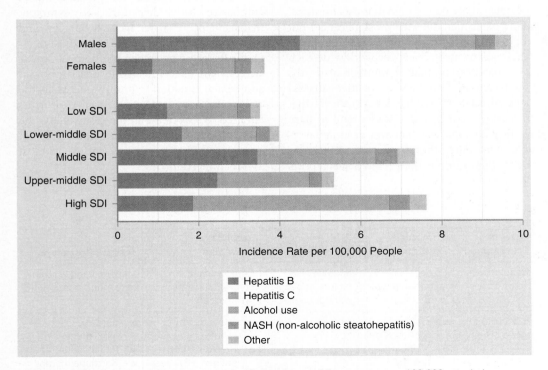

Figure 14.23 Age-standardized, cause-specific incidence of liver cancer per 100,000 people by sex and country sociodemographic index (SDI) group.

Data from GBD 2019 Diseases and Injuries Collaborators. Global burden of 369 diseases and injuries in 204 countries and territories, 1990–2019: a systematic analysis for the Global Burden of Disease Study 2019. *Lancet.* 2020;396:1204–1222.

Level of Prevention	Primordial Prevention	Primary Prevention	Secondary Prevention	Tertiary Prevention
Goal	Prevent risk factors in people without cancer	Mitigate risk factors in people without cancer	Detect cancer before it becomes symptomatic	Manage cancer after it becomes symptomatic
Examples of interventions	■ Avoid harmful use of alcohol ■ Maintain a healthy weight ■ Practice food safety to avoid fluke infections ■ Reduce exposures to aflatoxins produced by *Aspergillus* fungi (which grow on some agricultural crops)	■ Hepatitis B vaccination ■ Prevent and treat hepatitis B virus (HBV), hepatitis C virus (HCV), liver flukes, and other chronic infections	—	■ Surgery ■ Radiation therapy ■ Palliative care

Figure 14.24 Examples of interventions for liver cancer.

who already have liver damage. However, the incidence of HCC is expected to decrease significantly in future decades because today's infant vaccination programs are preventing many chronic HBV infections.

14.12 Esophageal, Stomach, and Colorectal Cancers

The incidence rates for cancers of the digestive tract—esophageal cancers, stomach cancers, and colon and rectal cancers—vary significantly by country and world region.[5] Esophageal cancer incidence rates are highest in Central and Eastern Asia and in eastern and southern Africa. Most esophageal cancers are squamous cell carcinomas, and some are esophageal adenocarcinomas.[68] The risk factors for squamous cell carcinomas include tobacco use, alcohol use, and some nutritional exposures as well as heritable genes.[69] The major risk factors for esophageal adenocarcinomas are obesity and gastroesophageal reflux

disease (GERD), which increases the risk of a precancerous condition called Barrett's esophagus.[70] Early detection and treatment of chronic acid reflux and Barrett's esophagus can help prevent the development of adenocarcinomas. The five-year relative survival rate for esophageal cancer in most countries is currently about 10% to 30%.[9]

Stomach cancer rates are highest in Central and Eastern Asia, Eastern Europe, and South America.[5] Stomach cancers are classified as cardia gastric cancers if they are located near the esophagus and as noncardia gastric cancers if they are not. For cardia gastric cancers, age, tobacco smoking, and obesity are associated with increased incidence; for noncardia stomach cancers, age and *Helicobacter pylori* infection are confirmed risk factors, and dietary habits (such as low consumption of fruits, vegetables, and fiber and high intake of salty and smoked foods) may also influence the risk.[71] Because early-stage stomach cancer causes few symptoms, most stomach cancers are diagnosed at an advanced stage when the five-year relative survival rate is about 20% to 40%.[9]

Colorectal cancer incidence rates are highest in high-income countries. Obesity, physical inactivity, and diets that are high in fat and processed meat are associated with increased risk of the disease.[72] Although most cases of colorectal cancer occur in older adults, the rate of colorectal cancer in younger adults is increasing in some places.[73] Many colon and rectal cancers could be prevented through screening for polyps and surgical removal of any observed precancerous lesions (**Figure 14.25**), but these procedures are expensive.[74] Colorectal cancer rates are decreasing in high-income countries, where colonoscopies and other screening tools are widely available, but incidence rates are increasing in some middle-income areas.[75]

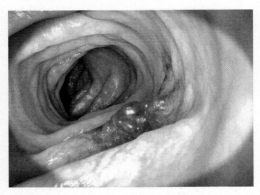

Colorectal cancer.

© Juan Gaertner/Shutterstock

14.13 Other Cancers

Cancer can occur in any part of the body, and a diversity of cancers contribute to the global burden from cancer, including cancers of the brain and nervous system, kidneys, thyroid, and other organs. For example, pancreatic cancer has a relatively low incidence rate, but it has a five-year relative survival rate of only 5% to 15% in most countries.[9] Because of the high case fatality rate, pancreatic cancer is responsible for nearly 5% of cancer deaths, even though it is not among the 10 most frequently occurring cancers.[1] Tobacco use might account for about 20% of pancreatic cancer cases worldwide and obesity for about 10% of cases, but about two-thirds of cases are not associated with currently known modifiable risk factors.[76]

Leukemia is a blood cancer that begins in the bone marrow, which produces the body's blood. There are several types of leukemia, and the risk of each type varies by age. Acute myelogenous leukemia (AML) and various types of chronic leukemias mostly affect older adults.[77] Acute lymphoblastic leukemia (ALL) is the most frequently occurring childhood cancer, responsible for about one-third of all cancers in children.[78]

Lymphoma is an immune system cancer that affects white blood cells and lymph nodes. Lymphomas are divided into two main groups,

Level of Prevention	Primordial Prevention	Primary Prevention	Secondary Prevention	Tertiary Prevention
Goal	Prevent risk factors in people without cancer	Mitigate risk factors in people without cancer	Detect cancer before it becomes symptomatic	Manage cancer after it becomes symptomatic
Examples of interventions	■ Eat a nutritious diet ■ Maintain a healthy weight ■ Avoid tobacco products	■ Surgically remove precancerous intestinal polyps	■ Fecal occult blood test ■ Colonoscopy	■ Surgery ■ Chemotherapy ■ Radiation therapy ■ Pain management/palliative care

Figure 14.25 Examples of interventions for colorectal cancer.

Hodgkin lymphoma and non-Hodgkin lymphoma (NHL), with Hodgkin lymphoma diagnosed based on the presence of Reed-Sternberg cells. NHL is further divided into subtypes, such as diffuse large B-cell lymphomas, follicular lymphomas, and Burkitt lymphoma. Hodgkin lymphoma accounts for about 10% of lymphomas, typically affects young adults, and is usually treatable; NHL typically affects older adults.[79] The distribution of particular subtypes of NHL varies significantly between and within world regions.[80] NHL is associated with some types of chronic infections,[81] but it is not currently possible to prevent most lymphomas from occurring.

About 80% of bladder cancer cases are considered to be preventable.[82] Because the toxins from smoke that are filtered out of the bloodstream by the kidneys are stored in the bladder prior to urination and may damage the cells lining the bladder, more than half of bladder cancer cases are linked to tobacco use.[83] The higher rate of tobacco use by men is a large contributor to men having higher bladder cancer rates than women. Some urinary bladder cancers are associated with exposure to arsenic in drinking water or to occupational exposure to aromatic amines and other harmful chemicals.[84] Additionally, some bladder cancers that occur in Africa and Asia are linked to chronic infection with the parasitic worms that cause schistosomiasis.[85]

Most skin cancers have a very low mortality rate (such as basal cell carcinomas and squamous cell carcinomas), but malignant **melanoma**, a cancer that originates in melanin-producing skin cells, can be deadly. Most cases of malignant melanoma occur in people with pale skin who have a history of sunburns in childhood,[86] but melanoma can occur in people with any skin tone. The characteristics of skin cancers are often described using the acronym ABCDE: **a**symmetrical rather than round shapes, irregular **b**orders, uneven **c**olors, large **d**iameters, and **e**volution in appearance or size over time. Removal of precancerous and early-stage cancerous lesions improves outcomes (**Figure 14.26**).

Although only about 1% of all new cancers occur among children younger than 15 years old, more than 200,000 children each year develop cancer.[87] The most frequently diagnosed cancers in children are leukemias, central nervous system tumors (such as neuroblastoma, a type of brain cancer), and lymphomas.[78] The proportion of child deaths that are attributable to cancer is increasing as deaths from infectious diseases decrease.[5] One of the ways to reduce the future burden of cancer on today's children and adolescents is to use primary prevention interventions now to reduce their risks as they age into

Level of Prevention	Primordial Prevention	Primary Prevention	Secondary Prevention	Tertiary Prevention
Goal	Prevent risk factors in people without cancer	Mitigate risk factors in people without cancer	Detect cancer before it becomes symptomatic	Manage cancer after it becomes symptomatic
Examples of interventions	—	■ Limit sun exposure by wearing protective clothing and using sunscreen ■ Avoid tanning lamps and beds ■ Surgically remove precancerous skin lesions	■ Check moles that are asymmetrical, have an irregular border, or are changing in color or diameter	■ Surgery ■ Chemotherapy ■ Radiation therapy ■ Pain management/palliative care

Figure 14.26 Examples of interventions for melanoma skin cancer.

adulthood and then older adulthood. Interventions that discourage uptake of tobacco use, prevent and treat chronic infections, promote healthy and active lifestyles, and minimize the risks associated with occupational and environmental carcinogens may help reduce future cancer incidence and mortality rates.[13]

References

1. Sun H, Ferlay J, Siegel RL, et al. Global cancer statistics 2020: GLOBOCAN estimates of incidence and mortality worldwide for 36 cancers in 185 countries. *CA Cancer J Clin.* 2021;71:209–249.

2. Soerjomataram I, Bray F. Planning for tomorrow: global cancer incidence and the role of prevention 2020–2070. *Nat Rev Clin Oncol.* 2021;18:663–672.

3. Ilbawi AM, Anderson BO. Cancer in global health: how do prevention and early detection strategies relate? *Sci Trans Med.* 2015;7:278.

4. Siegel RL, Miller KD, Fuchs HE, Jemal A. Cancer statistics, 2021. *CA Cancer J Clin.* 2021;71:7–33.

5. GBD 2019 Diseases and Injuries Collaborators. Global burden of 369 diseases and injuries in 204 countries and territories, 1990–2019: a systematic analysis for the Global Burden of Disease Study 2019. *Lancet.* 2020;396:1204–1222.

6. *WHO Report on Cancer: Setting Priorities, Investing Wisely and Providing Care for All.* Geneva: World Health Organization; 2020.

7. Ferlay J, Laversanne M, Ervik M, et al. *Global Cancer Observatory: Cancer Tomorrow.* Lyon France: International Agency for Research on Cancer; 2020.

8. Wu S, Zhu W, Thompson P, Hannun YA. Evaluating intrinsic and non-intrinsic cancer risk factors. *Nat Commun.* 2018;9:3490.

9. Allemani C, Matsuda T, Di Carlo V, et al. Global surveillance of trends in cancer survival 2000–14 (CONCORD-3): analysis of individual records for 37,513,025 patients diagnosed with one of 18 cancers from 322 population-based registries in 71 countries. *Lancet.* 2018;391:1023–1075.

10. *Food, Nutrition, Physical Activity, and the Prevention of Cancer: A Global Perspective.* Washington DC: American Institute for Cancer Research/World Cancer Research Fund International; 2007.

11. Tomasetti C, Li L, Vogelstein B. Stem cell divisions, somatic mutations, cancer etiology, and cancer prevention. *Science.* 2017;355:1330–1334.

12. Pilleron S, Soto-Perez-de-Celis E, Vignat J, et al. Estimated global cancer incidence in the oldest adults in 2018 and projections to 2050. *Int J Cancer.* 2021;148:601–608.

13. Vineis P, Wild CP. Global cancer patterns: causes and prevention. *Lancet.* 2014;383:549–557.

14. Sasco AJ, Secretan MB, Straif K. Tobacco smoking and cancer: a brief review of recent epidemiological evidence. *Lung Cancer.* 2004;45(Suppl 2):S3–S9.

15. Charbotel B, Fervers B, Droz JP. Occupational exposures in rare cancers: a critical review of the literature. *Crit Rev Oncol Hematol.* 2014;90:99–134.

16. Boffetta P, Nyberg F. Contribution of environmental factors to cancer risk. *Br Med Bull.* 2003;68:71–94.

17. Rakoff-Nahoum S. Why cancer and inflammation? *Yale J Biol Med.* 2006;79:123–130.

18. de Martel C, Georges D, Bray F, Ferlay J, Clifford GM. Global burden of cancer attributable to infections in 2018: a worldwide incidence analysis. *Lancet Glob Health.* 2020;8:e180–e190.

19. Oh JK, Weiderpass E. Infection and cancer: global distribution and burden of diseases. *Ann Glob Health.* 2014;80:384–392.

20. Gersten O, Barbieri M. Evaluation of the cancer transition theory in the US, select European nations, and Japan by investigating mortality of infectious- and noninfectious-related cancers, 1950–2018. *JAMA Netw Open.* 2021;4:e215322.

21. Danaei G, Vander Hoorn S, Lopez AD, Murray CJ, Ezzati M, Comparative Risk Assessment Collaborating Group (cancers). Causes of cancer in the world: comparative risk assessment of nine behavioural and environmental risk factors. *Lancet.* 2005;366:1784–1793.

22. Islami F, Torre LA, Jemal A. Global trends of lung cancer mortality and smoking prevalence. *Transl Lung Cancer Res.* 2015;4:327–338.

23. *AACR Cancer Progress Report 2016.* Philadelphia PA: American Association for Cancer Research; 2016.

24. St Laurent J, Luckett R, Feldman S. HPV vaccination and the effects on rates of HPV-related cancers. *Curr Probl Cancer.* 2018;42:493–506.

25. Thun MJ, DeLancey JO, Center MM, Jemal A, Ward EM. The global burden of cancer: priorities for prevention. *Carcinogenesis.* 2010;31:100–110.

26. Ebell MH, Thai TN, Royalty KJ. Cancer screening recommendations: an international comparison of high income countries. *Public Health Rev.* 2018;39:7.

27. Sankaranarayanan R. Screening for cancer in low- and middle-income countries. *Ann Global Health*. 2014; 80:412–417.

28. Sullivan T, Sullivan R, Ginsburg OM. Screening for cancer: considerations for low- and middle-income countries (chapter 12). In: Gelband H, Jha P, Sankaranarayanan R, Horton S, eds. *Disease Control Priorities: Cancer*. 3rd ed. Vol. 3. Washington DC: IBRD/World Bank; 2015:211–222.

29. Smith RA, Andrew KS, Brooks D, et al. Cancer screening in the United States, 2019: a review of current American Cancer Society guidelines and current issues in cancer screening. *CA Cancer J Clin*. 2019;69:184–210.

30. Gospodarowicz M, Trypuc J, Cruz AD, et al. Cancer services and the comprehensive cancer center (chapter 11). In: Gelband H, Jha P, Sankaranarayanan R, Horton S, eds. *Disease Control Priorities: Cancer*. 3rd ed. Vol. 3. Washington DC: IBRD/World Bank; 2015:195–210.

31. Knaul FM, Farmer PE, Krakauer EL, et al. Alleviating the access abyss in palliative care and pain relief—and imperative of universal health coverage: the Lancet Commission report. *Lancet*. 2018;391:1391–1454.

32. Hui D, De La Cruz M, Mori M, et al. Concepts and definitions for "supportive care," "best supportive care," "palliative care," and "hospice care" in the published literature, dictionaries, and textbooks. *Support Care Cancer*. 2013;21:659–685.

33. Horton S, Gauvreau CL. Cancer in low- and middle-income countries: an economic overview (chapter 16). In: Gelband H, Jha P, Sankaranarayanan R, Horton S, eds. *Disease Control Priorities: Cancer*. 3rd ed. Vol. 3. Washington DC: IBRD/World Bank; 2015:263–280.

34. Sullivan R, Alatise OI, Anderson BO, et al. Global cancer surgery: delivering safe, affordable, and timely cancer surgery. *Lancet Oncol*. 2015;16:1193–1224.

35. Jaffray DA, Gospodarowicz MK. Radiation therapy for cancer (chapter 14). In: Gelband H, Jha P, Sankaranarayanan R, Horton S, eds. *Disease Control Priorities: Cancer*. 3rd ed. Vol. 3. Washington DC: IBRD/World Bank; 2015:239–248.

36. Yang X, Man J, Chen H, et al. Temporal trends of the lung cancer mortality attributable to smoking from 1990 to 2017: a global, regional, and national analysis. *Lung Cancer*. 2021;152:49–57.

37. Drope J, Hamill S, eds. *The Tobacco Atlas*. 7th ed. Chicago IL: Vital Strategies; 2022.

38. Corrales L, Rosell R, Cardona AF, Martín C, Zatarain-Barrón ZL, Arrieta O. Lung cancer in never smokers: the roles of different risk factors other than tobacco smoking. *Crit Rev Oncol Hematol*. 2020;148:102895.

39. Allemani C, Weir HK, Carreira H, et al. Global surveillance of cancer survival 1995–2009: analysis of individual data for 25,676,887 patients from 279 population-based registries in 67 countries (CONCORD-2). *Lancet*. 2015;385:977–1010.

40. Jha P, MacLennan M, Yurekli A, et al. Global hazards of tobacco and the benefits of smoking cessation and tobacco tax (chapter 10). In: Gelband H, Jha P, Sankaranarayanan R, Horton S, eds. *Disease Control Priorities: Cancer*. 3rd ed. Vol. 3. Washington DC: IBRD/World Bank; 2015:175–194.

41. Sankaranarayanan R, Ramadas K, Amarasinghe H, Subramanian S, Johnson N. Oral cancer: prevention, early detection, and treatment (chapter 5). In: Gelband H, Jha P, Sankaranarayanan R, Horton S, eds. *Disease Control Priorities: Cancer*. 3rd ed. Vol. 3. Washington DC: IBRD/World Bank; 2015:85–100.

42. Ginsburg O, Yip CH, Brooks A, et al. Breast cancer early detection: a phased approach to implementation. *Cancer*. 2020;126:2379–2393.

43. Anderson BO, Lipscomb J, Murillo RH, Thomas DB. Breast cancer (chapter 3). In: Gelband H, Jha P, Sankaranarayanan R, Horton S, eds. *Disease Control Priorities: Cancer*. 3rd ed. Vol. 3. Washington DC: IBRD/World Bank; 2015:45–68.

44. *Global Cancer Facts & Figures*. 4th ed. Atlanta GA: American Cancer Society; 2018.

45. Ho GY, Burk RD, Klein S, et al. Persistent genital human papillomavirus infection as a risk factor for persistent cervical dysplasia. *J Natl Cancer Inst*. 1995;87:1365–1371.

46. Bulkmans NWJ, Berkhof J, Bulk S, et al. High-risk HPV type-specific clearance rates in cervical screening. *Br J Cancer*. 2007;96:1417–1424.

47. *Comprehensive Cervical Cancer Control: A Guide to Essential Practice*. 2nd ed. Geneva: World Health Organization; 2014.

48. Denny L, Herrero R, Levin C, Kim JJ. Cervical cancer (chapter 4). In: Gelband H, Jha P, Sankaranarayanan R, Horton S, eds. *Disease Control Priorities: Cancer*. 3rd ed. Vol. 3. Washington DC: IBRD/World Bank; 2015:69–84.

49. Gallagher KE, LaMontagne DS, Watson-Jones D. Status of HPV vaccine introduction and barriers to country uptake. *Vaccine*. 2018;36:4761–4667.

50. Brisson M, Kim JJ, Canfell K, et al. Impact of HPV vaccination and cervical screening on cervical cancer elimination: a comparative modelling analysis in 78 low-income and lower-middle-income countries. *Lancet*. 2020;395:22–28.

51. Simms KT, Steinberg J, Caruana M, et al. Impact of scaled up human papillomavirus vaccination and cervical screening and the potential for global elimination of cervical cancer in 181 countries, 2020–99: a modelling study. *Lancet Oncol*. 2019;20:394–407.

52. Arbyn M, Weiderpass E, Bruni L, et al. Estimates of incidence and mortality of cervical cancer in 2018: a worldwide analysis. *Lancet Glob Health*. 2020;8:e191–e203.

53. Matz M, Coleman MP, Carreira H, et al. Worldwide comparison of ovarian cancer survival: histological

group and stage at diagnosis (CONCORD-2). *Gynecol Oncol.* 2017;144:396–404.

54. Morice P, Leary A, Creutzberg C, Abu-Rustum N, Darai E. Endometrial cancer. *Lancet.* 2016;387:1094–1108.

55. Lee SWH, Chan EMC, Lai YK. The global burden of lower urinary tract symptoms suggestive of benign prostatic hyperplasia: a systematic review and meta-analysis. *Sci Rep.* 2017;7:7984.

56. Alcaraz A, Hammerer P, Tubaro A, Schröder FH, Castro R. Is there evidence of a relationship between benign prostatic hyperplasia and prostate cancer? Findings of a literature review. *Eur Urol.* 2008;55:864–873.

57. Haas GP, Delongchamps N, Brawley OW, Yang CY, de la Roza G. The worldwide epidemiology of prostate cancer: perspectives from autopsy studies. *Can J Urol.* 2008;15:3866–3871.

58. Pernar CH, Ebot EM, Wilson KM, Mucci LA. The epidemiology of prostate cancer. *Cold Spring Harb Perspect Med.* 2018;8:a030361.

59. *Cancer Facts and Figures 2021.* Atlanta GA: American Cancer Society; 2021.

60. Ávila M, Patel L, López S, et al. Patient-reported outcomes after treatment for clinically localized prostate cancer: a systematic review and meta-analysis. *Cancer Treat Rev.* 2018;66:23–44.

61. Culp MB, Soerjomataram I, Efstathiou JA, Bray F, Jemal A. Recent global patterns in prostate cancer incidence and mortality rates. *Eur Urol.* 2020;77:38–52.

62. El-Serag HB. Epidemiology of viral hepatitis and hepatocellular carcinoma. *Gastroenterology.* 2012;142:1264–1273.

63. Maucort-Boulch D, de Martel C, Franceschi S, Plummer M. Fraction and incidence of liver cancer attributable to hepatitis B and C viruses worldwide. *Int J Cancer.* 2018;142:4271–4277.

64. Bosetti C, Turati F, La Vecchia C. Hepatocellular carcinoma epidemiology. *Best Pract Res Clin Gastroenterol.* 2014;28:753–770.

65. Matsushita H, Takaki A. Alcohol and hepatocellular carcinoma. *BMJ Open Gastroenterol.* 2019;6:e000260.

66. Chang MH. Prevention of hepatitis A virus infection and liver cancer. *Recent Results Cancer Res.* 2014;193:75–95.

67. Hepatitis B vaccines: WHO position paper – July 2017. *Wkly Epidemiol Rec.* 2017;92:369–392.

68. Uhlenhopp DJ, Then EO, Sunkara T, Gaduputi V. Epidemiology of esophageal cancer: update in global trends, etiology and risk factors. *Clin J Gastroenterol.* 2020;13:1010–1021.

69. Huang FL, Yu SJ. Esophageal cancer: risk factors, genetic association, and treatment. *Asian J Surg.* 2018;41:210–215.

70. Rustgi AK, El-Serag HB. Esophageal carcinoma. *New Engl J Med.* 2014;371:2499–2509.

71. Karimi P, Islami F, Anandasabapathy S, Freedman ND, Kamangar F. Gastric cancer: descriptive epidemiology, risk factors, screening, and prevention. *Cancer Epidemiol Biomarkers Prev.* 2014;23:700–713.

72. Keum N, Giovannucci E. Global burden of colorectal cancer: emerging trends, risk factors and prevention strategies. *Nat Rev Gastroenterol Hepatol.* 2019;16:713–732.

73. El Din KS, Loree JM, Sayre EC, et al. Trends in the epidemiology of young-onset colorectal cancer: a worldwide systematic review. *BMC Cancer.* 2020;20:288.

74. Rabeneck L, Horton S, Zauber AG, Earle C. Colorectal cancer (chapter 6). In: Gelband H, Jha P, Sankaranarayanan R, Horton S, eds. *Disease Control Priorities: Cancer.* 3rd ed. Vol. 3. Washington DC: IBRD/World Bank; 2015:101–120.

75. Arnold M, Sierra MS, Laversanne M, Soerjomataram I, Jemal A, Bray F. Global patterns and trends in colorectal cancer incidence and mortality. *Gut.* 2017;66:683–691.

76. Maisonneuve P, Lowenfels AB. Risk factors for pancreatic cancer: a summary review of meta-analytic studies. *Int J Epidemiol.* 2015;44:186–198.

77. Baeker Bispo JA, Pinheiro PS, Kobetz EK. Epidemiology and etiology of leukemia and lymphoma. *Cold Spring Harb Perspect Med.* 2020;10:a034819.

78. Bhakta N, Force LM, Allemani C, et al. Childhood cancer burden: a review of global estimates. *Lancet Oncol.* 2019;20:e42–e53.

79. Armitage JO, Gascoyne RD, Lunning MA, Cavalli F. Non-Hodgkin lymphoma. *Lancet.* 2017;390:298–310.

80. Müller AM, Ihorst G, Mertelsmann R, Engelhardt M. Epidemiology of non-Hodgkin's lymphoma (NHL): trends, geographic distribution, and etiology. *Ann Hematol.* 2005;84:1–12.

81. Engels EA. Infectious agents as causes of non-Hodgkin lymphoma. *Cancer Epidemiol Biomarkers Prev.* 2007;16:401–404.

82. Al-Zalabani AH, Stewart KFJ, Wesselius A, Schols AMWJ, Zeegers MP. Modifiable risk factors for the prevention of bladder cancer: a systematic review of meta-analyses. *Eur J Epidemiol.* 2016;31:811–851.

83. Boffetta P. Tobacco smoking and risk of bladder cancer. *Scand J Urol Nephrol Suppl.* 2008;42(218):45–54.

84. Letašiová S, Medved'ová A, Šovčíková A, et al. Bladder cancer, a review of the environmental risk factors. *Environ Health.* 2012;11:S11.

85. Parkin DM. The global burden of urinary bladder cancer. *Scand J Urol Nephrol Suppl.* 2008;42(218):12–20.

86. Erdmann F, Lortet-Tieulent J, Schüz J, et al. International trends in the incidence of malignant melanoma 1953–2008: are recent generations at higher or lower risk? *Int J Cancer.* 2013;132:385–400.

87. Ward ZJ, Yeh JM, Bhakta N, Frazier AL, Atun R. Estimating the total incidence of global childhood cancer: a simulation-based analysis. *Lancet Oncol.* 2019;20:483–493.

CHAPTER 15

Diabetes, Chronic Respiratory Diseases, and Other Noncommunicable Diseases

Cardiovascular diseases, cancer, diabetes, chronic respiratory diseases, and other noncommunicable diseases (NCDs) cause many early deaths in countries of all income levels, and nonfatal NCDs cause significant reductions in quality of life. Behavior change, medications, tobacco control, and other interventions can facilitate healthy aging and reduce the disability associated with NCDs.

15.1 Noncommunicable Diseases and Global Health

A **noncommunicable disease (NCD)** is an adverse health condition that is not contagious. Cardiovascular diseases, cancers, chronic respiratory diseases, diabetes, other endocrine and metabolic disorders, kidney diseases, liver diseases, digestive diseases, musculoskeletal diseases, skin diseases, and neurological disorders are all classified as NCDs. Most NCDs are chronic diseases that develop gradually and last for a long time.

The need for strategies to reduce the burden from disability and premature death caused by NCDs in adult populations applies to countries across the income spectrum.[1] The percentage of deaths from NCDs is highest in high-income countries because relatively few people who live in high-income countries die from infectious diseases and injuries in a typical year, but the age-specific death rates from NCDs per 100,000 people are highest in lower-income countries (**Figure 15.1**).[2] After age standardizing population health statistics to adjust for the differences in age distributions that make the high-income countries with the oldest populations look like the highest-burden

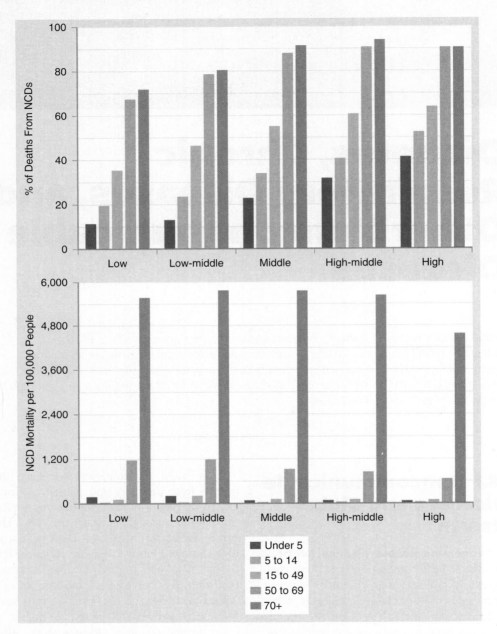

Figure 15.1 Percentage of deaths from noncommunicable diseases (NCDs) and rate of deaths from NCDs per 100,000 people in a typical (nonpandemic) year, by age and country sociodemographic group. (These percentages exclude deaths from communicable diseases, maternal and neonatal disorders, nutritional deficiencies, and injuries.)

Data from GBD 2019 Diseases and Injuries Collaborators. Global burden of 369 diseases and injuries in 204 countries and territories, 1990–2019: a systematic analysis for the Global Burden of Disease Study 2019. *Lancet*. 2020;396:1204–1222.

areas, the rates of disability from NCDs are similar across country income levels, and the rates of early death from NCDs are much higher in lower-income countries than in higher-income countries (**Figure 15.2**).[2]

Modifiable behavioral and metabolic risk factors are thought to be responsible for about two-thirds of all deaths from NCDs.[3] NCDs that can be prevented through behavior change are sometimes called **lifestyle diseases** because

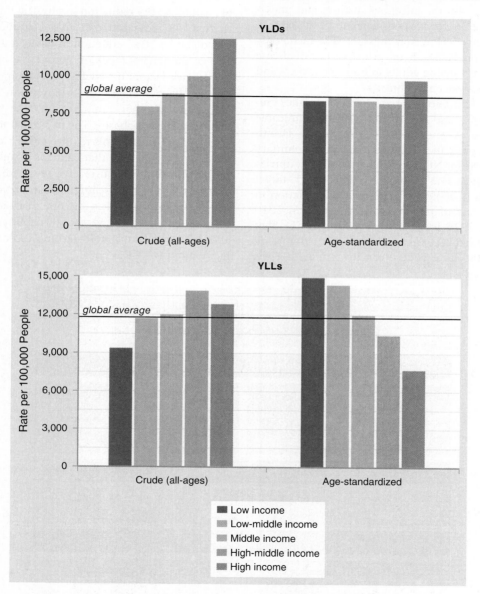

Figure 15.2 All-ages and age-standardized years of life lived with disability (YLDs) and years lost to early death (YLLs) per 100,000 people, by country sociodemographic group.

Data from GBD 2019 Diseases and Injuries Collaborators. Global burden of 369 diseases and injuries in 204 countries and territories, 1990–2019: a systematic analysis for the Global Burden of Disease Study 2019. *Lancet.* 2020;396:1204–1222.

they are associated with health-related behaviors such as unhealthy diets, sedentariness, tobacco use, and heavy alcohol consumption.[4] These NCDs have also been called "diseases of affluence," a way of contrasting these conditions with the infectious diseases and undernutrition that are considered to be "diseases of poverty."[5] However, this is a false dichotomy because NCDs are the primary cause of disease burden among adults in both the lowest- and highest-income countries.[6]

The Global Action Plan for the Prevention and Control of Noncommunicable Diseases endorsed by the World Health Assembly in 2013 spells out nine voluntary targets for NCD control in member countries (**Figure 15.3**).[7] The overall "25 × 25" target aims to achieve a 25% relative reduction in the rate of premature death between 2010 and 2025 for four high-priority NCDs that together account for about 80% of premature deaths from NCDs: cardiovascular diseases (CVDs), cancers, diabetes, and chronic respiratory diseases (CRDs) (**Figure 15.4**).[2] Four of the other eight targets focus on health behaviors linked to a diversity of NCDs, aiming for a 10% reduction in harmful use of alcohol, a 10% reduction in physical inactivity, a 30% reduction in mean salt (sodium) intake, and a 30% reduction in tobacco use. Two of the targets focus on modifiable biological risk factors for NCDs: one aiming to reduce the prevalence of hypertension by 25% and the other aiming to halt the rising prevalence of obesity. The two remaining targets focus on the tools required to achieve the 25 × 25 goal: one that calls for a higher proportion of adults to receive the medications and health counseling that can prevent heart attacks and strokes and one that seeks to substantially increase the availability of affordable health technologies and essential medicines for NCDs.

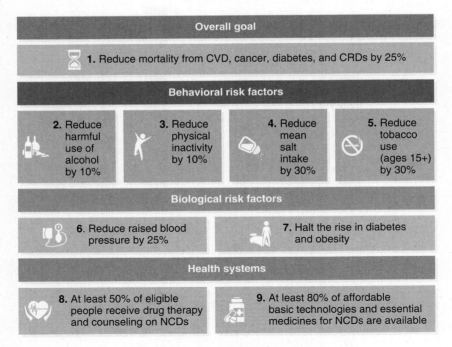

Figure 15.3 Nine voluntary global targets for NCDs for 2010–2025.

Data from *Global Action Plan for the Prevention and Control of Noncommunicable Diseases 2013–2020*. Geneva: World Health Organization; 2013.

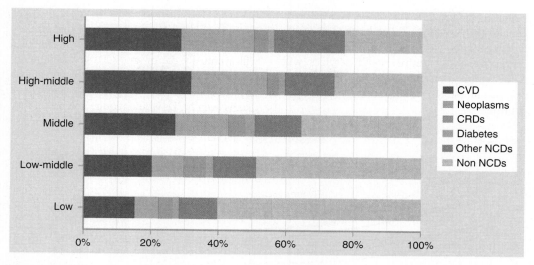

Figure 15.4 Age-standardized years of life lost to early death (YLLs) per 100,000 people, by causes and country sociodemographic group.

Data from GBD 2019 Diseases and Injuries Collaborators. Global burden of 369 diseases and injuries in 204 countries and territories, 1990–2019: a systematic analysis for the Global Burden of Disease Study 2019. *Lancet.* 2020;396:1204–1222.

The focus on the four featured behavioral risk factors associated with the four high-priority NCDs is referred to as the "4 × 4 framework." This model has been criticized for excluding environmental and occupational risk factors for NCDs and for omitting other NCDs with high prevalence rates, such as musculoskeletal disorders, kidney diseases, and mental health disorders.[8] There is also some concern about how population-level observations about health behaviors are inappropriately used to blame individuals for developing NCDs and to shame people for having some types of chronic health issues. The onset and progression of NCDs is a function of age, genetics, environmental exposures, health behaviors, and many other factors. "Healthy" lifestyles do not guarantee health, and "unhealthy" lifestyles do not guarantee ill health. Many people who are very active and avoid risky activities develop NCDs at young ages, and some people who engage in all four of the unhealthy behaviors featured in the 4 × 4 framework remain healthy into older

adulthood. At the population level, increasing the proportion of people who practice healthy behaviors is critical for reversing the growing burden from NCDs.[9] At the individual level, there are many reasons why people might not adopt and sustain the actions recommended for NCD prevention and management. No matter what combination of factors contributed to an individual's health status, all people deserve compassion and respect.

The Sustainable Development Goals (SDGs) aim to "reduce by one-third premature mortality from noncommunicable diseases through prevention and treatment" between 2015 and 2030 (SDG 3.4).[10] A key metric for evaluating progress toward this goal during the SDG era is the percentage of 30-year-olds who are predicted to die from cardiovascular diseases, cancers, chronic respiratory diseases, or diabetes before their 70th birthdays if current age-specific mortality rates from these diseases remain unchanged (SDG 3.4.1). Based on current mortality rates, about 18% of today's 30-year-olds will die from one of these NCDs before their 70th birthdays (**Figure 15.5**), including about 21% of males and 14% of females (**Figure 15.6**).[11] The hope is that new health technologies and expanded access to preventive and curative health services will reduce those percentages to much closer to 0% before today's young adults reach older adulthood.

The SDGs do not to seek to reduce the total number of deaths from NCDs or the proportion of deaths attributable to NCDs. Most adults will eventually die of an NCD, so the number of deaths from NCDs will increase as the global population ages. Lowering the percentage of deaths from NCDs would require an undesirable

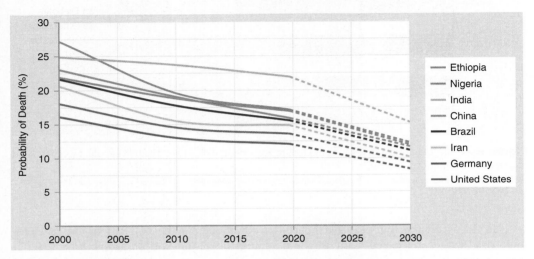

Figure 15.5 Probability (%) that a 30-year-old in selected countries will die from CVD, cancer, chronic respiratory disease, or diabetes before age 70, from 2000 through the targets for 2030.

Data from *World Health Statistics 2021*. Geneva: World Health Organization; 2021.

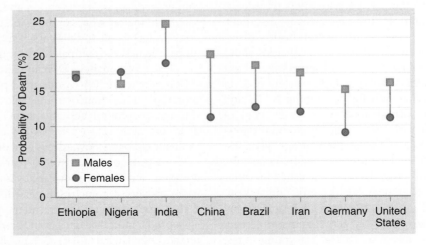

Figure 15.6 Probability (%) that a 30-year-old in selected countries will die from CVD, cancer, chronic respiratory disease, or diabetes before age 70, by sex (2019).

Data from *Global Health Estimates 2021*. Geneva: World Health Organization; 2021.

increase in deaths from infections and injuries. Instead, the SDGs aim for adults to enjoy as many healthy years of life as possible before developing and dying from an NCD in very old age.

Many inexpensive interventions can help reduce tobacco use, harmful use of alcohol, unhealthy diets, and physical inactivity; manage cardiovascular diseases and diabetes; and prevent and detect cancer. A package of "NCD best buys" costing about $1 per person per year in low- and middle-income countries could prevent millions of premature deaths and generate about $7 in economic gains over the next decade for each $1 invested in NCD interventions.[12] However, this return on investment will be generated only if several billion additional dollars per year are invested in NCD interventions. Achieving the health and socioeconomic goals spelled out in the SDGs will require increased funding for both preventing NCDs via risk factor reduction and improving case management for people with one or more NCDs.[13]

15.2 Diabetes

Insulin is a hormone produced by the pancreas that helps the body maintain a relatively constant level of glucose (sugar) in the bloodstream so cells have a relatively consistent supply of energy. **Diabetes** is a metabolic disorder characterized by an impairment in the production of or response to insulin. There are two major types of diabetes. **Type 1 diabetes** (previously called juvenile-onset diabetes or insulin-dependent diabetes) is a form of diabetes that occurs when the body does not produce enough insulin.[14] Type 1 diabetes typically has a sudden onset in childhood. Type 1 diabetes is not related to weight, and there are currently no methods for preventing or curing the disease. People with type 1 diabetes require frequent insulin injections to maintain safe blood sugar levels. Waiting too long between injections allows a blood chemistry imbalance called diabetic ketoacidosis to develop as blood sugar levels increase and dehydration occurs. Untreated

ketoacidosis can lead to seizures, coma, and death. More than 1.1 million children and adolescents and millions of adults have type 1 diabetes.[15] Most of these individuals live in higher-income countries where people with diabetes have access to the insulin they need to survive.[16] In low-income places where insulin is not routinely available, type 1 diabetes is often a fatal condition.

Type 2 diabetes (formerly known as adult-onset diabetes or non-insulin-dependent diabetes) is a form of diabetes in which the body develops insulin resistance and stops responding appropriately to insulin even when the hormone is still being produced by the body.[17] Type 2 diabetes typically has a gradual onset in adulthood. Approximately 5% of people in their 30s, 10% of people in their 40s, 15% of people in their 50s, and 20% of people in their 60s and older have diabetes (**Figure 15.7**).[15] Almost all of these cases of diabetes are type 2 diabetes. (Both type 1 and type 2 diabetes are sometimes called diabetes mellitus to distinguish them from diabetes insipidus, a rare condition that is caused by fluid imbalances due to overproduction of urine. Type 1 diabetes accounts for only a tiny percentage of all people with diabetes mellitus.) Type 2 diabetes is considered to be a preventable disease because the major risk factors include obesity and related lifestyle characteristics, such as physical inactivity and an unhealthy diet. The connection between obesity and type 2

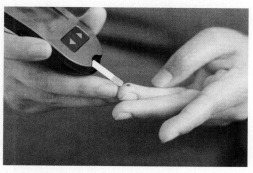

© Kwangmoozaa/Shutterstock

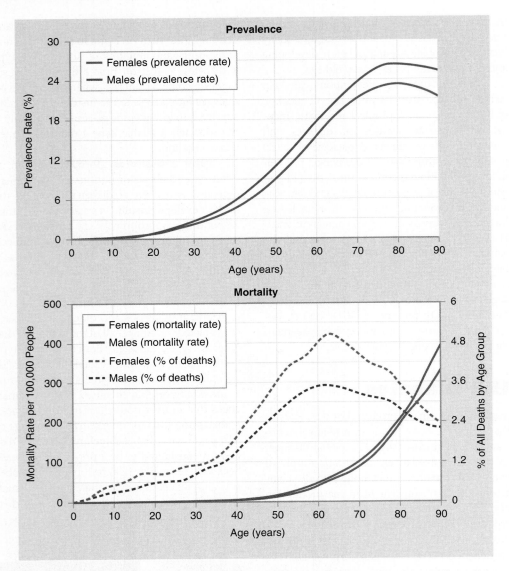

Figure 15.7 Prevalence (%), mortality rate per 100,000 people, and percentage of deaths from diabetes mellitus, by sex and age.

Data from GBD 2019 Diseases and Injuries Collaborators. Global burden of 369 diseases and injuries in 204 countries and territories, 1990–2019: a systematic analysis for the Global Burden of Disease Study 2019. *Lancet.* 2020;396:1204–1222.

diabetes is so strong that some researchers refer to type 2 diabetes as "diabesity."[18] The percentage of adults with type 2 diabetes worldwide increased over the past few decades in parallel with rising average body weights and increasing rates of obesity (**Figure 15.8**).[19]

Signs of the initial onset of diabetes may include excessive thirst, frequent urination, unexplained weight loss, and fatigue. Diagnosis is based on blood sugar tests.[20] Fasting plasma glucose levels of ≥126 mg/dL (7.0 mmol/L) at two points in time indicate diabetes. A random

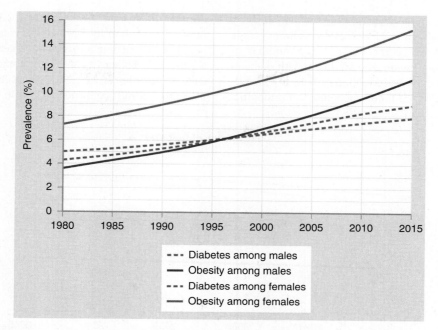

Figure 15.8 Age-standardized prevalence of diabetes and obesity among adults (ages 18+ years) worldwide, 1980–2015.

Data from NCD Risk Factor Collaboration (NCD-RisC). Worldwide trends in diabetes since 1980: a pooled analysis of 751 population-based studies with 4.4 million participants. *Lancet.* 2016;387:1513–1530; NCD Risk Factor Collaboration (NCD-RisC). Worldwide trends in body-mass index, underweight, overweight, and obesity from 1975 to 2016: a pooled analysis of 2416 population-based measurement studies in 128.9 million children, adolescents, and adults. *Lancet.* 2017;390:2627–2642.

(nonfasting) plasma glucose level of ≥200 mg/dL (11.1 mmol/L) suggests diabetes but must be confirmed with other tests, such as a two-hour oral glucose tolerance test. Levels of glycated hemoglobin (HbA1c), a measure of the average plasma glucose over the 8–12 weeks prior to the test, are not diagnostic tests but provide insight about diabetes management.[21]

Prediabetes describes elevated blood glucose levels that are below the threshold for a type 2 diabetes diagnosis. Impaired glucose tolerance and impaired fasting glucose (sometimes called nondiabetic hyperglycemia or intermediate hyperglycemia because the blood sugar levels are somewhere between normal and diabetic levels) are associated with a high risk for developing type 2 diabetes in the future and experiencing cardiovascular and other complications.[22] In 2020, about 460 million (9.3%) of the 5 billion 20- to 79-year-olds

worldwide had diabetes, and about 370 million (7.5%) were classified as having prediabetes.[15] Weight loss and other lifestyle modifications can reduce the likelihood of prediabetes advancing to type 2 diabetes.

Gestational diabetes is elevated blood sugar that is first diagnosed during pregnancy and typically resolves after delivery. In 2020, about 16% of pregnant women experienced hyperglycemia, which means that more than 20 million women had gestational diabetes.[15] Women who have had gestational diabetes have an increased likelihood of subsequently developing type 2 diabetes.[23]

Between 1980 and 2015, the global diabetes prevalence rate nearly doubled from 4.7% to 8.5%, after standardizing the 1980 rates to the age distribution in 2015 to remove the effects of an aging global population.[19] The prevalence is expected to continue to climb in the coming decades, to more than 10% by 2030 and nearly 11% by 2045, as more people worldwide become obese.[15] The number of adults worldwide who are living with diabetes increased from 110 million in 1980 to 420 million in 2015.[19] If current trends continue, that number will rise to 580 million by 2030 and nearly 700 million by 2045.[15] Diabetes affects people of all income levels. The percentage of adults with diabetes in middle-income countries is now almost as high as the percentage in high-income countries (**Figure 15.9**).[15]

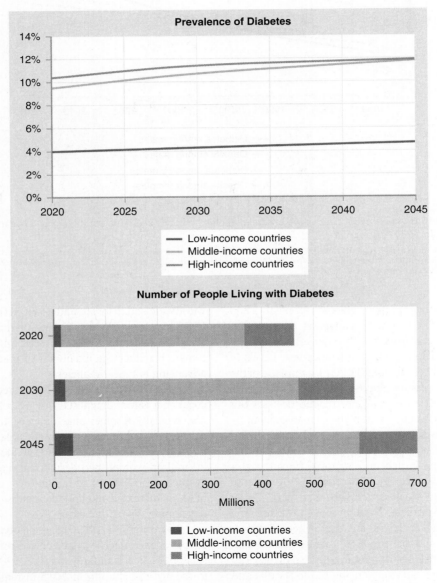

Figure 15.9 Projected diabetes prevalence (%) and total number of cases among adults (ages 20–79 years) by country income level, 2020–2045.

Data from *IDF Diabetes Atlas*. 9th ed. Brussels: International Diabetes Federation; 2019.

About 75% of the world's people live in middle-income countries, and about 75% of individuals with diabetes live in middle-income countries.[24]

Diabetes prevalence estimates are projected from population-based serosurveys that test the blood of randomly sampled people who represent the demographics of the total population. The percentage of participants in serological studies who have elevated blood sugar is usually much higher than the percentage of survey participants who report that they have ever been diagnosed as having diabetes. Recent serosurveys suggest that about half of adults with type 2 diabetes do not know that they have the condition (**Figure 15.10**).[15] In low-income countries, only about one in three adults with diabetes has received a diagnosis. People with diabetes who have not been clinically diagnosed are not receiving treatment for the condition, and they may develop complications that could have been prevented if their blood sugar levels had been better managed.

Diabetes and its complications have become major causes of disability and premature death in middle- and high-income countries.[25] Diabetes is also an expensive health issue, already costing more than $760 billion each year in health expenditures.[26] The goal of diabetes management is to keep blood sugar levels from becoming too high (hyperglycemia) or too low (hypoglycemia). When blood sugar levels are not carefully maintained, complications like blindness (from diabetic retinopathy), heart disease, kidney failure, nerve damage (diabetic neuropathy), and foot ulcers leading to amputation may develop over time.[27] For people with type 2 diabetes, the disease often can be controlled with weight loss, a careful diet, and sometimes also oral medications such as metformin, which reduces glucose production by the liver and improves the insulin sensitivity of body tissues.[28] Management of diabetes requires access to health and nutrition education, medication for diabetes and cardiovascular comorbidities, routine clinical examinations (including eye exams and foot checks), and referrals to advanced care when complications arise (**Figure 15.11**).

15.3 Chronic Respiratory Diseases

Chronic respiratory diseases (CRDs) are long-term NCDs of the airway, bronchi, and lungs, such as asthma, chronic obstructive pulmonary disease, lung diseases associated with occupational exposures, sleep apnea, pulmonary hypertension (increased pressure in the pulmonary artery, which typically occurs secondary to other health issues), bronchiectasis, and interstitial lung diseases like sarcoidosis.[29] (Lung cancers and long-lasting infectious diseases like tuberculosis are typically not

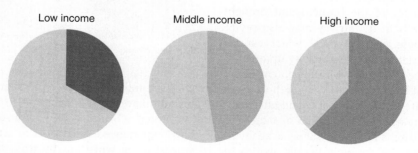

Figure 15.10 Percentage of adults (ages 20–79 years) with diabetes who have received a diagnosis, by country income level.

Data from *IDF Diabetes Atlas*. 9th ed. Brussels: International Diabetes Federation; 2019.

Level of Prevention	Primordial Prevention	Primary Prevention	Secondary Prevention	Tertiary Prevention
Goal	Prevent risk factors in people without diabetes	Mitigate risk factors in people without diabetes	Detect diabetes before it becomes symptomatic	Manage diabetes after it becomes symptomatic
Examples of interventions	<ul><li>Maintain a healthy weight</li><li>Eat a nutritious diet</li><li>Exercise often</li></ul>	<ul><li>Reduce body weight if overweight or obese</li><li>Take metformin if prescribed after diagnosis of impaired glucose tolerance</li></ul>	<ul><li>Screen for and treat prediabetes</li></ul>	<ul><li>Monitor blood sugar levels</li><li>Use dietary changes and medication to control blood sugar</li><li>Manage comorbidities such as cardiovascular disease and kidney disease</li><li>Manage complications such as nerve damage (neuropathy), foot ulcers, and vision problems (retinopathy)</li></ul>

Figure 15.11 Examples of interventions for type 2 diabetes.

included in statistics about CRDs, even when those diseases persist for many years.)

Asthma is a chronic but reversible inflammation of the airways that causes episodes of wheezing (especially when exhaling), coughing, chest tightness, and shortness of breath due to thickening of the airway wall and bronchospasms that narrow the diameter of the bronchi and bronchioles.[30] Cells in the airway may also secrete more mucus than is typical, which can further restrict airflow. Asthma symptoms can usually be managed with inhaled corticosteroids and bronchodilators when those medications are locally accessible and affordable, but severe asthma attacks can be fatal when medical care is not immediately available.[31]

About 340 million people worldwide have asthma, and the condition affects all age groups.[32] About 12% of 6- to 7-year-old

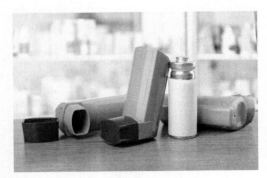
© Africa Studio/Shutterstock

children and 14% of 13- to 14-year-old adolescents have current symptoms of asthma, and about 9% of 18- to 45-year-old adults have experienced symptoms of asthma like wheezing or whistling breaths within the past year.[32] Older adults often have symptoms of asthma in combination with other

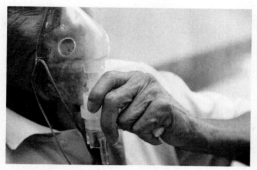

© Janthiwa Sutthiboriban/Shutterstock

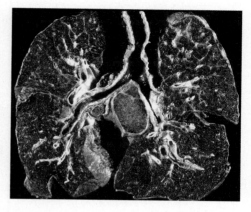

Coal worker's pneumoconiosis (anthracosilicosis).

Yale Rosen, https://flic.kr/p/8Ur4Ao. Licensed under CC BY-SA 2.0

NCDs, including other CRDs.[33] Asthma increases absenteeism from school and work and decreases learning, productivity, and quality of life.[34] In addition to appropriate use of prescription medications that keep airways open, the severity of the disease may be mitigated by reducing exposure to air pollution, cold air, and other potential environmental triggers of asthma attacks.

Chronic obstructive pulmonary disease (COPD) is a chronic, progressive respiratory disease that limits airflow and causes shortness of breath and productive coughing.[35] Two of the common presentations of COPD are chronic bronchitis and emphysema. **Bronchitis** is inflammation of the bronchi that is characterized by a productive cough, narrowing of the airways, and excess mucus production. The chronic bronchitis associated with COPD causes a persistent cough as airways progressively narrow and mucus clogs breathing passages. **Emphysema** occurs when the alveoli (the tiny air sacs in the lungs) lose elasticity and become distended or destroyed. This irreversible process reduces the surface area available for intake of oxygen and release of carbon dioxide.

The number of adults worldwide living with COPD increased from about 145 million in 2000 to more than 210 million by 2020.[2] The prevalence of COPD increases with age. COPD is the primary cause of death for more than 3 million people annually, accounting for nearly 6% of all deaths and nearly 9% of deaths of adults aged 70 years and older (**Figure 15.12**).[2] The most prominent risk factor for COPD is tobacco smoking.[36] Although COPD is not curable, many cases could be prevented by reducing exposure to tobacco smoke, indoor and outdoor air pollution, and industrial chemicals.[37] Treatment can help manage some of the symptoms of COPD,[38] but the damage to the airways and lungs is not fully reversible with current therapies. Symptoms often worsen over time.

Pneumoconiosis is a restrictive lung disease caused by exposure to various types of occupational hazards. Obstructive lung diseases like asthma and COPD make it difficult for a person to exhale all the air in the lungs. By contrast, restrictive lung diseases like pneumoconiosis make it difficult for people to fully fill their lungs with air when they inhale. Both obstructive and restrictive lung diseases cause shortness of breath, especially with exertion. The most prevalent form of pneumoconiosis is silicosis, which affects miners who inhale silica dust.[39] Other forms of pneumoconiosis include asbestosis, which is caused by prolonged periods of inhalation of asbestos fibers, and coal worker's pneumoconiosis (also called black lung disease). While pneumoconiosis

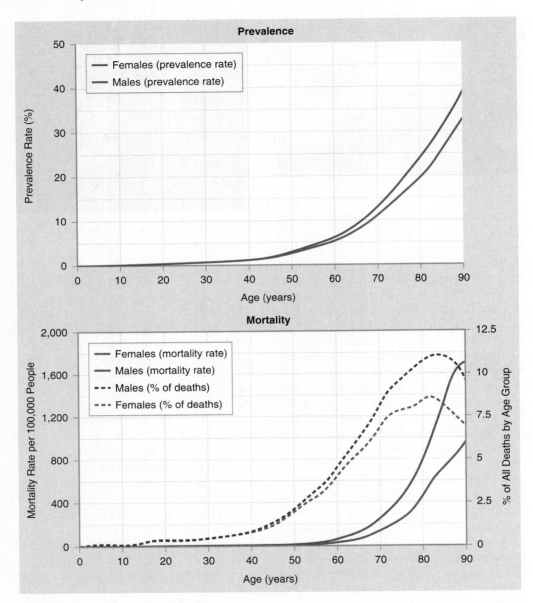

Figure 15.12 Prevalence (%), mortality rate per 100,000 people, and percentage of deaths from chronic obstructive pulmonary disease (COPD), by sex and age.

Data from GBD 2019 Diseases and Injuries Collaborators. Global burden of 369 diseases and injuries in 204 countries and territories, 1990–2019: a systematic analysis for the Global Burden of Disease Study 2019. *Lancet.* 2020;396:1204–1222.

is not a major cause of global mortality, it is important because most cases could be prevented with improved attention to worker safety, such as provision of face masks and hygiene facilities for washing dust off exposed skin.[40]

15.4 Tobacco Control

Tobacco smoke contains more than 5,300 compounds, including dozens of toxins and carcinogens.[41] The nicotine in tobacco is highly addictive.[42] It is easy for new tobacco smokers and users of electronic nicotine delivery systems, such as vaping and e-cigarettes, to become dependent on nicotine, and that addiction makes it difficult to quit using the products.[43] Smoking tobacco damages cells, stresses the cardiovascular system, alters blood chemistry, destroys the cilia that help clear mucus out of the respiratory tract, and interferes with respiration.[44] There is a dose–response relationship between tobacco and health problems, with heavier consumption of tobacco associated with steadily worsening health outcomes.[41] Over time, tobacco smokers and people frequently exposed to secondhand smoke sustain damage to nearly every body system,[45] increasing their susceptibility to a variety of diseases of the

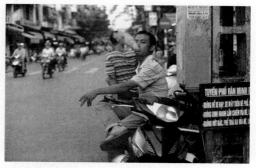

© Oxana Mamlina/Shutterstock

respiratory tract and other organs and systems. Tobacco use is the underlying cause of about one in eight deaths worldwide each year, including an estimated 67% of deaths from lung cancer, 63% from cancer of the larynx, 53% from COPD, 47% from lip and oral cavity cancer, 43% from esophageal cancer, 35% from aortic aneurysms, 34% from bladder cancer, 22% from ischemic heart disease, and 17% from strokes (**Figure 15.13**).[3]

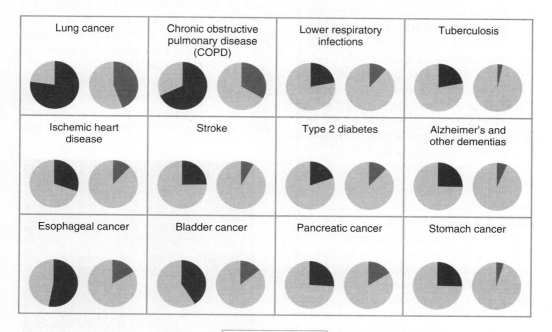

Figure 15.13 Percentage of deaths from various causes that are attributable to tobacco use, by sex.

Data from GBD 2019 Risk Factors Collaborators. Global burden of 87 risk factors in 204 countries and territories, 1990–2019: a systematic analysis for the Global Burden of Disease Study 2019. *Lancet.* 2020;396:1223–1249.

Shared global concerns about the public health burden from tobacco use led to the adoption of the **Framework Convention on Tobacco Control (FCTC)**,[46] the first global health treaty negotiated under the auspices of the World Health Organization (WHO),[47] which aims to significantly reduce the global prevalence of tobacco use.[48] The call for a treaty was approved by the World Health Assembly (WHA) in 1995. After many rounds of negotiation, the FCTC was approved by the WHA in 2003 and put into force in 2005.[49] Almost all United Nations member states have signed and ratified the FCTC. The FCTC has also been incorporated into the SDGs through a target that aims to "strengthen the implementation of the World Health Organization Framework Convention on Tobacco Control in all countries" (SDG 3.a).[10]

The FCTC strategies are operationalized with six sets of actions summarized by the acronym MPOWER:

- **M**onitor tobacco use and prevention policies
- **P**rotect people from tobacco smoke by mandating smoke-free environments
- **O**ffer help to quit tobacco use
- **W**arn about the dangers of tobacco through warnings on cigarette packages, mass media anti-tobacco campaigns, and other actions
- **E**nforce bans on tobacco advertising, promotion, and sponsorship
- **R**aise taxes on tobacco

The MPOWER measures include both demand-side interventions that reduce the desire of people to use tobacco products and supply-side interventions that reduce the availability of tobacco products.[50] The key demand-reduction measures include increasing taxes on tobacco products (Article 6 of the FCTC); banning smoking in government buildings, healthcare facilities, schools, public transportation, and other settings (Article 8); regulating the content of tobacco products (Articles 9 and 10); requiring bold health warning labels that cover a large portion of tobacco packaging (Article 11); providing education about tobacco control to health workers, educators, social workers,

and other community leaders (Article 12); banning tobacco advertising (Article 13); and providing tobacco users with support for smoking cessation, such as offering nicotine replacement therapy and counseling (Article 14). The key supply-reduction measures include eliminating illegal tobacco sales (Article 15), banning sales to minors (Article 16), and supporting alternative income-generating activities for people who currently depend on the tobacco industry for their livelihoods (Article 17).

The percentage of people who use tobacco products has decreased in most countries since the FCTC went into force in 2005.[51] In 2000, about 49% of adult males and 16% of adult females used tobacco products (including cigarettes and other smoked and smokeless tobacco products); by 2020, these rates had dropped to about 37% and 8%, respectively.[52] Men continue to have a much higher rate of tobacco use than women (**Figure 15.14**).[50] The proportion of men who use tobacco is highest in middle-income countries; for women, the tobacco prevalence rates are highest in high-income countries (**Figure 15.15**).[52]

Population growth has enabled the total number of tobacco users to remain nearly unchanged even as the percentage of people who use tobacco has decreased. There were

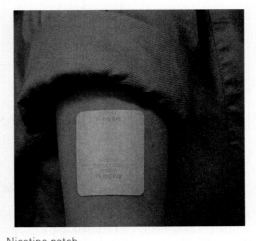

Nicotine patch.

about 1.4 billion tobacco users worldwide in 2000, and in 2020 there were still about 1.3 billion tobacco users (**Figure 15.16**).[52] The 1.1 billion people worldwide who were tobacco smokers in 2020 consumed the equivalent of more than 7 trillion cigarettes during just that one year.[51] Global efforts to reduce the morbidity and premature mortality from NCDs will not be successful without significant reductions in the number of people who use tobacco and the amount of tobacco the typical user consumes.[53]

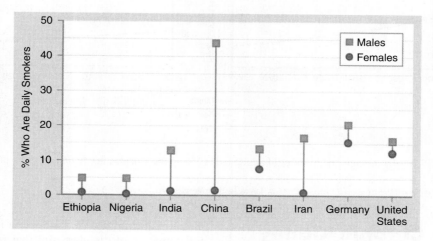

Figure 15.14 Age-standardized prevalence of daily tobacco smoking among adults (ages 15+ years) among males and females in selected countries.

Data from *WHO Report on the Global Tobacco Epidemic, 2021.* Geneva: World Health Organization; 2021.

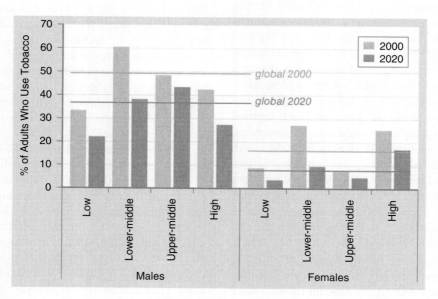

Figure 15.15 Prevalence of tobacco use among adults (ages 15+ years), by sex and country income level.

Data from *WHO Global Report on Trends in Prevalence of Tobacco Use 2000–2025.* 4th ed. Geneva: World Health Organization; 2021.

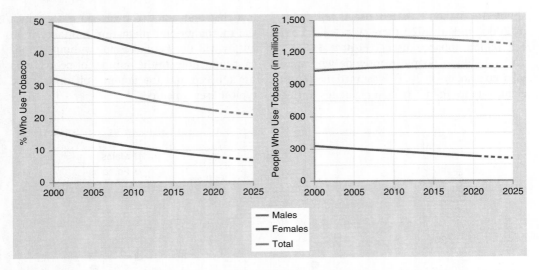

Figure 15.16 Percentage and number of adults (ages 15+ years) worldwide who use tobacco products, by sex.

Data from *WHO Global Report on Trends in Prevalence of Tobacco Use 2000–2025*. 4th ed. Geneva: World Health Organization; 2021.

15.5 Chronic Kidney Disease

The kidneys are responsible for several important functions in the body, including filtering the blood, maintaining fluid and electrolyte levels, helping control blood pressure (by producing a hormone called renin), stimulating the production of red blood cells (by producing a hormone called erythropoietin), and supporting bone health. Each kidney is composed of about one million nephrons, and each nephron contains a tiny filtering unit called a glomerulus. Healthy nephrons filter wastes out of the blood, reabsorb necessary substances, and secret excess fluid and wastes as urine. When the nephrons in a kidney are damaged, their ability to filter blood is impaired. **Kidney failure** is an acute or chronic condition that is present when kidneys are not functioning well enough for health. Untreated kidney failure can cause death.

Some kidney diseases are acute problems that start suddenly. Pyelonephritis is an acute inflammation of the kidneys caused by a bacterial infection, and it usually resolves after antibiotic therapy.[54] Glomerulonephritis is an inflammation of the glomeruli that is associated with some immune system disorders and infections.[55] An acute kidney injury, formerly called acute renal failure, is the sudden loss of kidney function due to physical trauma, poisoning (including overdoses of medications like nonsteroidal anti-inflammatory drugs), or other events.[56] Acute kidney injuries occur most often among older adults who are hospitalized for chronic diseases, and in that population acute kidney injury is a life-threatening condition.[57] However, most kidney diseases have a gradual onset.

Chronic kidney disease (CKD) is a progressive loss of kidney function characterized by a reduced glomerular filtration rate (GFR) and increased urinary albumin levels. Kidneys that are functioning well filter most creatinine (a waste product produced by muscles) out of the blood but reabsorb most proteins rather than letting them leave the body in urine. A low GFR is a sign that the kidneys are not filtering creatinine out of the blood as rapidly as they should be. An elevated amount of the protein albumin in the urine (a condition called albuminuria or proteinuria) is a sign that the kidneys are damaged.

The early stages of CKD are usually asymptomatic.[58] As the kidney damage worsens, individuals with CKD may experience fatigue, itchiness, constipation, loss of appetite, pain, difficulty sleeping, anxiety, and other symptoms.[59] CKD is also associated with a variety of adverse cardiovascular outcomes and other complications.[60] Some people with CKD progress to end-stage renal disease (ESRD) in which they require a kidney transplant or dialysis therapy to survive. **Dialysis** is the process of using a machine to filter the blood, either through hemodialysis (filtering the blood outside the body) or peritoneal dialysis (filtering the blood inside the body by adding clean fluid to the abdomen and then draining it out after it has absorbed toxins). When dialysis is used as renal replacement therapy, the hours-long process must be completed several times each week.

About 10% of the world's people—about 700 million adults—have CKD, and more than 1 million adults die from CKD each year.[61] The prevalence of CKD increases with age, rising from about 10% of 40-year-olds to more than 50% of people who are more than 80 years old (**Figure 15.17**).[2] Some forms of polycystic kidney disease are heritable, but most CKD does not result from a genetic disorder. Diabetes and hypertension are among the most prevalent causes of CKD worldwide.[62] Infections, environmental toxins, and counterfeit medications and harmful herbs used medicinally are also contributors to CKD, especially in low-income regions.[63]

There is no cure for CKD, but a variety of interventions can help reduce the burden from it (**Figure 15.18**). Medications such as angiotensin-converting enzyme (ACE) inhibitors and angiotensin II receptor blockers (ARBs), smoking cessation, low-sodium diets, management of comorbidities like hypertension and diabetes, and health technologies

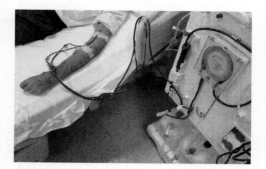

Hemodialysis.
© Trismile/iStock/Getty Images.

like dialysis can slow the progression of the disease.[58] In high-income countries, renal replacement therapy may be expensive but is routinely available to people with advanced CKD; in low-income countries, dialysis and kidney transplants are rarely available for individuals with ESRD.[64] This differential access to advanced care means that although the age-standardized CKD prevalence rates are similar across country income levels, the CKD mortality rates are significantly higher in low-income countries than in high-income countries (**Figure 15.19**).[2] Lack of access to renal replacement therapy causes hundreds of thousands of people with CKD to die prematurely each year.[65]

15.6 Liver Diseases

The liver has numerous important functions, including creating proteins that allow blood to clot, filtering some types of toxins out of the blood, and storing and releasing glucose and lipids into the bloodstream. **Cirrhosis** is irreversible scarring of the liver that impedes the flow of blood through the liver and prevents the liver from functioning well. Early stages of cirrhosis cause few symptoms, but the affected individual may feel fatigued and develop jaundice.[66] As the liver becomes more scarred, fluid may build up in the legs (edema), and then the abdomen may swell with excess fluid, a condition called ascites. Severe bleeding may

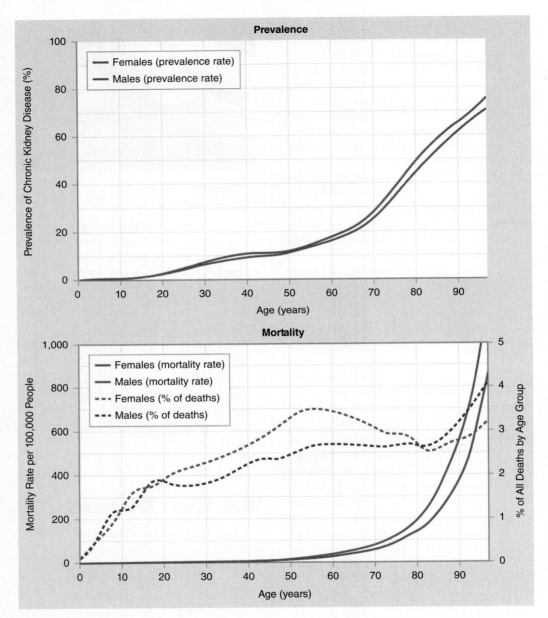

Figure 15.17 Prevalence rate (%), mortality rate per 100,000 people, and percentage of deaths from chronic kidney disease (excluding kidney cancer), by sex and age.

Data from GBD 2019 Diseases and Injuries Collaborators. Global burden of 369 diseases and injuries in 204 countries and territories, 1990–2019: a systematic analysis for the Global Burden of Disease Study 2019. *Lancet.* 2020;396:1204–1222.

Level of Prevention	Primordial Prevention	Primary Prevention	Secondary Prevention	Tertiary Prevention
Goal	Prevent risk factors in people without CKD	Mitigate risk factors in people without CKD	Detect CKD before it becomes symptomatic	Manage CKD after it becomes symptomatic
Examples of interventions	■ Exercise often ■ Eat a nutritious diet ■ Avoid tobacco products ■ Limit alcohol consumption	■ Manage hypertension ■ Manage diabetes ■ Reduce body weight if overweight or obese	■ Screen for and treat early signs of kidney damage	■ Manage comorbidities such as hypertension and diabetes ■ Use medications and dietary modifications to manage symptoms such as swelling due to fluid imbalances ■ Use a renal replacement therapy (dialysis or a kidney transplant) for end-stage renal disease (ESRD)

Figure 15.18 Examples of interventions for chronic kidney disease.

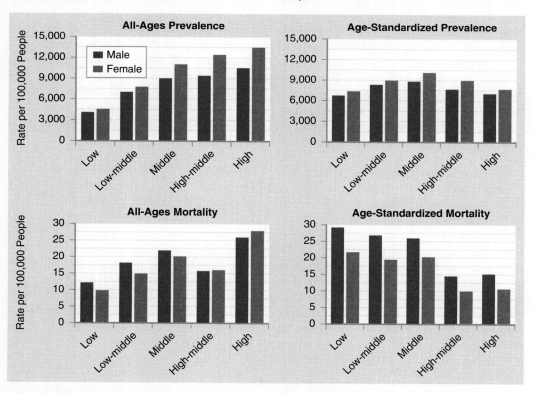

Figure 15.19 Age-standardized prevalence and mortality rates from chronic kidney disease per 100,000 people, by sex and country sociodemographic group.

Data from GBD 2019 Diseases and Injuries Collaborators. Global burden of 369 diseases and injuries in 204 countries and territories, 1990–2019: a systematic analysis for the Global Burden of Disease Study 2019. *Lancet.* 2020;396:1204–1222.

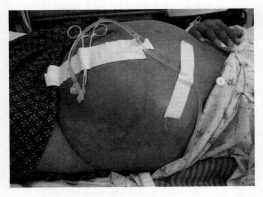

Draining ascites caused by cirrhosis of the liver.

John Campbell

occur when increased pressure in the portal vein (portal hypertension) causes the veins in the esophagus to expand (becoming esophageal varices) and possibly rupture. Cirrhosis may also cause damage to the kidneys, spleen, lungs, and other organs, and it significantly increases the risk of liver cancer.

The major causes of severe liver disease globally include alcohol abuse, hepatitis B virus, and hepatitis C virus, but many people with liver disease do not have any of these risk factors.[2] Hepatic **steatosis**, or fatty liver disease, is caused by the accumulation of lipids in the liver. Nonalcoholic fatty liver disease (NAFLD), which can progress to nonalcoholic steatohepatitis (NASH) and then to cirrhosis and liver failure, is physiologically similar to the pathology of liver disease observed in heavy drinkers.[67] At least one in five adults worldwide has steatosis, NASH, cirrhosis, or other types of liver damage.[67] More than twice as many men as women die from chronic liver diseases, and the disparity is largely attributable to higher rates of alcohol abuse by males (**Figure 15.20**).[2] A liver transplant is the only currently available cure for cirrhosis, but that option is not widely available.[68] Chronic liver diseases cause about 2 million deaths each year, including more than 1 million deaths from cirrhosis and about 500,000 from liver cancer.[68]

15.7 Digestive Diseases

Numerous digestive diseases contribute to the global burden of disease. Peptic ulcer disease is a painful wound in the lining of the stomach that may perforate and cause a fatal hemorrhage. Gastritis and duodenitis are painful inflammations of the stomach and small intestine, respectively. Pancreatitis is a severely painful inflammation of the pancreas that can cause multiple organ failure, shock, and death. Inflammatory bowel diseases, such as Crohn's disease and ulcerative colitis, cause chronic diarrhea and can significantly reduce quality of life.

Several frequently occurring digestive conditions—appendicitis, paralytic ileus and intestinal obstruction, intestinal hernias, and gallbladder and biliary diseases—often require surgical repairs. Appendicitis is an inflammation of the appendix that can perforate (rupture) and cause peritonitis, sepsis, and death. Intestinal obstructions prevent waste from passing through the intestines and out of the body, and they may cause bowel perforation, sepsis, and death. An abdominal hernia occurs when part of the intestine passes through the wall of the abdominal muscles, causing pain and possibly cutting off the blood supply to that part of the intestine. Lifting heavy objects and engaging in other forms of exertion may increase the pain, so hernias may prevent affected individuals from doing manual labor. The gallbladder stores bile and releases it into the small intestine to facilitate the digestion of lipids (fats). A gallstone (cholelithiasis) that blocks the bile duct will cause severe pain and jaundice. All of these digestive conditions can be fatal when people who experience them do not have access to emergency surgery.[69]

About 5 billion people do not have access to timely, safe, and affordable surgical services, including about 99% of people who live in low-income countries, 95% of people who

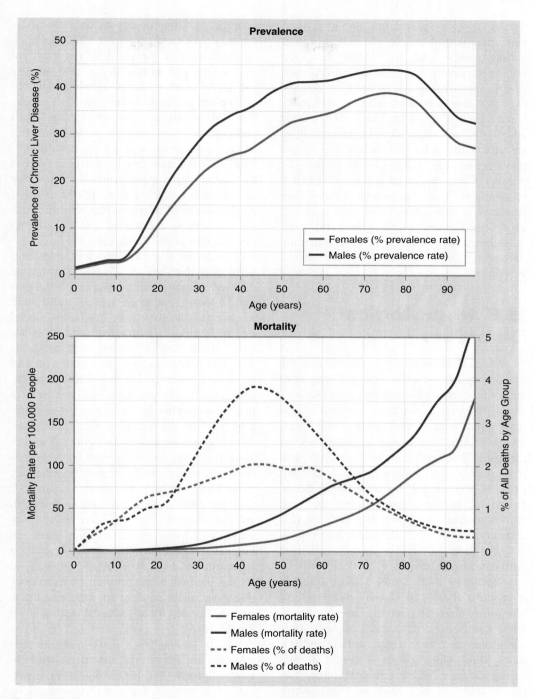

Figure 15.20 Prevalence (%), mortality rate per 100,000 people, and percentage of deaths from cirrhosis and other chronic liver diseases (excluding liver cancer), by sex and age.

Data from GBD 2019 Diseases and Injuries Collaborators. Global burden of 369 diseases and injuries in 204 countries and territories, 1990–2019: a systematic analysis for the Global Burden of Disease Study 2019. *Lancet.* 2020;396:1204–1222.

live in lower-middle-income countries, and more than half of people who live in upper-middle-income countries.[70] More than 300 million surgical procedures are needed each year for injuries, cancers, obstetric conditions, digestive disorders, and other health problems.[71] Each year, about 150 million people who live in low- and middle-income countries are unable to receive the surgical procedures they need to prevent disability or death.[72] The number of surgical procedures performed each year will only be able to increase if many more surgeons, anesthesiologists, obstetricians, and support staff (such as scrub nurses and surgical technicians) are able to receive the training they need to become members of the surgical workforce.[73]

15.8 Neurological Disorders

Neurological disorders are dysfunctions of the nervous system, such as epilepsy, migraines and other headache disorders, multiple sclerosis, Parkinson's disease, dementia, traumatic brain injuries, and amyotrophic lateral sclerosis (ALS, also known as motor neuron disease). These conditions may cause physical impairments (such as paralysis, weakness, and mobility limitations), cognitive impairments, behavioral problems, and difficulties with communication and activities of daily living.[74] Together, neurological disorders are responsible for about 7.5% of the world's years lived with disability (YLDs).[2]

Epilepsy is a chronic seizure disorder characterized by episodes of excessive and abnormal electrical activity in the brain. Epileptic seizures may cause few observable symptoms, but some trigger muscle stiffness and jerking (tonic-clonic seizures) or loss of muscle tone (atonic seizures). More than 50 million people worldwide have active epilepsy.[75] The condition affects people of all ages. Some cases of epilepsy are attributable to head trauma or other forms of brain damage, but the etiology of the disorder is unknown for most people who have epilepsy. Medications can prevent seizures in about 70% of people with epilepsy, and surgery can be curative in some people for whom anti-epileptic medications are not effective.[76] However, the majority of people with epilepsy in lower-income countries are not receiving any treatment for the condition.[77] Untreated epilepsy can be disabling and is associated with a significantly increased risk of premature death due to falls and other consequences of seizures. Many people with epilepsy encounter stigma and discrimination because of their condition.[78]

Headache disorders are very prevalent, with more than half of adults reporting that they have experienced a headache in the past year.[79] Most headaches are relatively mild tension-type headaches or headaches related to acute infections or traumas, and these last only a short time. However, some headache disorders cause moderate or severe pain and occur so frequently that they cause a significant reduction in productivity and quality of life.[80] A **migraine** is a recurrent severe headache that is often accompanied by nausea, vomiting, and sensitivity to light and sound. More than 10% of adults worldwide experience migraines, with women significantly more likely to have migraines than men.[81] Over-the-counter analgesics such as aspirin and ibuprofen are usually effective at reducing the pain from tension-type headaches. For migraines, specialized medications, such as ergotamine and sumatriptan, are necessary to control the pain. Most people who experience migraines and other disabling headache disorders do not receive any clinical treatment for the disorder.[82]

Both Parkinson's disease and multiple sclerosis are movement disorders. **Parkinson's disease** (PD) is a chronic, progressive, neurodegenerative disorder characterized by motor symptoms such as slowed movement (bradykinesia), rigidity or stiffness in an arm or leg or other body part, and tremors when a limb is resting. In addition to problems with gait, balance, and other aspects of postural stability and movement, many people with PD eventually experience nonmotor symptoms like depression and dementia.[83] PD is associated with the formation of Lewy bodies (clusters of alpha-synuclein proteins) in the brain and the loss of dopamine-producing neurons in a part of the midbrain called the substantia nigra.[84] A chemical precursor of the neurotransmitter dopamine (called L-DOPA or levodopa) helps manage the symptoms of PD, but long-term use can cause side effects such as impairment of the ability to control voluntary movements (dyskinesia).[85] An estimated 7 million people currently have PD, and this number may double by 2040 as the world's population ages.[86]

Most nerve cells are coated in myelin, an insulating material that helps speed up the transmission of signals between nerves. **Multiple sclerosis** (MS) is a chronic, progressive disease that causes inflammatory demyelination of the sheaths of nerve cells in the central nervous system. The symptoms may include vision disturbances, bladder or bowel control problems, pain, fatigue, walking difficulties, hand coordination problems, and memory issues and confusion. Most people with MS have a relapsing–remitting form of the disease characterized by periods of symptoms followed by periods of partially or fully recovered function.[87] Medications can help reduce the frequency and severity of relapses.[88] Later on, many years after the initial episode, a progressive form of the disease typically develops. In this advanced stage, the symptoms usually persist and worsen over time.[89] Nearly 3 million people worldwide have MS, about two-thirds of whom are female.[90] The first symptoms of MS typically appear at about 30 years of age, which makes MS an important contributor to the global burden of neurological diseases among younger adults.[87] Scientists have not yet identified the primary causes of or risk factors for many neurological disorders, so they have not been able to develop effective

prevention methods. Instead, current interventions focus on increasing access to treatment, supporting patients and their families, and helping to reduce the stigma associated with neurological disorders.

15.9 Genetic Blood Disorders

Genetics is the study of genes, genetic variation, and heredity, which is the passing of genes from parents to their biological offspring. Genes are sequences of nucleic acids that are part of the chromosomes found in the nucleus of every cell in the human body. This genetic material directs every function of the body, including cell replication, which is important for healing as well as for growth and development. Each cell contains identical DNA (deoxyribonucleic acid), although only some parts of the code are active in certain cells, which is why cells of a heart form different kinds of tissue than the cells lining the intestines. **Epigenetics** is the differential expression of genetic code through activation or inactivation of genes.[91]

Several types of genetic disorders can cause health problems. Some people are born with chromosomal disorders or other genetic differences. Some people inherit a disease-causing gene from one or both parents. Some diseases are caused by a genetic **mutation**, a permanent change in the sequence of bases that make up DNA that occurs after birth in response to exposure to radiation, chemicals, pollutants, or other substances. Multifactorial inheritance disorders (including many types of cancer and other NCDs) arise from a combination of inherited genes and genetic mutations.

A chromosomal disorder is caused by the presence of an extra chromosome or by missing part of a chromosome. Most people have 23 pairs of chromosomes. People with Down syndrome (trisomy 21) have an extra 21st chromosome, so they have 47 total chromosomes rather than the typical total of 46.[92]

People with Turner syndrome have only one of the two sex chromosomes, so they have only 45 total chromosomes.[93]

A **monogenic disorder** is one that can occur when a child inherits a single disease-causing gene from one or both parents. An **allele** is a version of a gene. Most genes have two alleles. A **genotype** is the set of alleles a person inherits for a particular gene. An individual has a homozygous genotype if the same allele is inherited from both parents. An individual has a heterozygous genotype if two different alleles for a gene are inherited. A **phenotype** is the way a particular set of alleles is expressed in physical appearance, the way a person develops or functions physiologically, or disease status. A **dominant gene** is an allele that will be phenotypically expressed if it is inherited from one or both parents. Huntington's disease, which causes a progressive degeneration of brain cells, is an example of a dominant monogenic disorder.[94] A **recessive gene** is an allele that must be inherited from both parents in order to be phenotypically expressed. Cystic fibrosis, which causes excess production of mucus in the lungs and digestive tract, is an example of a recessive monogenic disorder.[95]

Both thalassemia and sickle cell disease are recessive blood disorders that cause hemolytic anemia due to the breakdown of red blood cells. More than 5% of the global population carries a gene for a hemoglobinopathy.[96] The rate of disease is lower than this percentage because the symptoms of these hemoglobin disorders typically occur only when a person inherits the gene for the disorder from both parents. People who receive an allele for a gene that causes a hemoglobin disorder from just one parent are said to have the trait for the disorder (such as thalassemia trait or sickle cell trait), and they are usually asymptomatic carriers. People who receive alleles for the gene from both parents have blood disorders that cause anemia, jaundice, and an increased risk of heart failure and gallstones.

The various types of **thalassemia** are characterized by impaired production of hemoglobin, the molecules in red blood cells that carry oxygen. Individuals who inherit thalassemia alleles from both parents and survive to birth often have a serious blood disease (such as alpha thalassemia intermedia or beta thalassemia major) that requires frequent transfusions of blood.[97] In some places, recipients of blood products may be exposed to bloodborne infectious diseases. Repeated transfusions also carry a risk of iron overload that can damage the body's organs and cause cardiac complications if chelation therapy is not used to remove excess iron from the body. Bone marrow transplants can cure thalassemia, but they are not routinely available in most countries. As many as 400 million people worldwide might have thalassemia trait, and 1 million may have a form of thalassemia.[2] The prevalence of thalassemia is highest in the Mediterranean region, Africa, and Asia.[96]

Sickle cell disease is a genetic disorder that causes some red blood cells (erythrocytes) to become misshapen in a way that can cause painful blockages in small blood vessels. People who inherit the sickle cell allele from both parents form erythrocytes that look like crescents rather than having rounder donut-like shapes. Clumps of sickled cells can block blood flow within capillaries and other small blood vessels, and the resulting ischemia can cause severe pain as well as organ damage.[98] More than 400 million people worldwide have sickle cell trait, and about 5 million are estimated to have a sickle cell disorder.[2] The sickle cell gene is most prevalent among people who live in Africa, people of African heritage, and people who live in some parts of the Middle East and South Asia.[99]

Other examples of genetic blood disorders include hemophilia and glucose-6-phosphate dehydrogenase (G6PD) deficiency. The various types of hemophilia are recessive genetic blood clotting disorders, and most occur more often in males.[100] An **autosomal gene** is a gene that is not located on the sex chromosome and is therefore not sex linked. Most inherited genetic disorders are autosomal, but

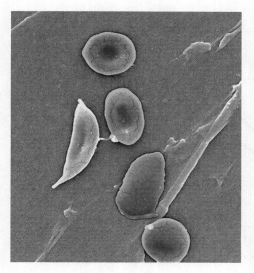

Sickle cell anemia.

hemophilia is often allosomal (sex-linked). G6PD deficiency can cause impaired metabolism of red blood cells in some carriers.[101]

15.10 Musculoskeletal Disorders

Musculoskeletal disorders include problems of the muscles, bones, tendons, ligaments, and joints. These conditions are experienced by about 20% of people each year and account for about 17% of YLDs worldwide (**Figure 15.21**).[2] Back and neck pain are responsible for more than half of the YLDs from musculoskeletal disorders, and they affect about 800 million people over the course of a year.[2] People with severe lower back pain may be completely bedridden, and the pain may cause sleep disturbances, anxiety, and other aggravations.[102] Even "short-term" back pain usually persists for more than a month, and cases frequently become chronic. For recent-onset back pain, the recommended course of treatment is remaining as active as possible, and there is little evidence that surgery is helpful; for chronic pain, physical therapy and anti-inflammatory medications may be useful, and surgical care may be appropriate for herniated discs and spinal stenosis.[103]

Arthritis is joint inflammation that causes swelling and pain, and the condition is responsible for about 2.5% of the world's YLDs.[2] The two most prevalent kinds of arthritis are osteoarthritis and rheumatoid arthritis. **Osteoarthritis** (OA) is a degenerative disease that slowly causes loss of cartilage in the joints, causing pain and stiffness. The main joints affected include the hips, knees, hands, feet, and spine. More than 500 million people worldwide have OA.[2] The most prominent risk factors for OA are age, obesity, and a history of traumatic joint injuries.[104] Some cases can be managed with pain medication, but replacement of a hip, knee, or other joint may be the only option for restoring mobility in severe cases.[105] Joint replacements are rarely available in lower-income countries.

Rheumatoid arthritis (RA) is an autoimmune disorder characterized by chronic inflammation that damages the cartilage and bones in many joints.[106] The immune system helps the body recognize and attack invaders like infectious agents and allergens. An **allergy** is an immune dysfunction in which the body is hypersensitive to foreign substances that are usually not harmful. An **autoimmune disorder** is a condition that occurs when the body has difficulty distinguishing between "self"

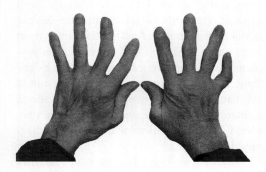

Rheumatoid arthritis.

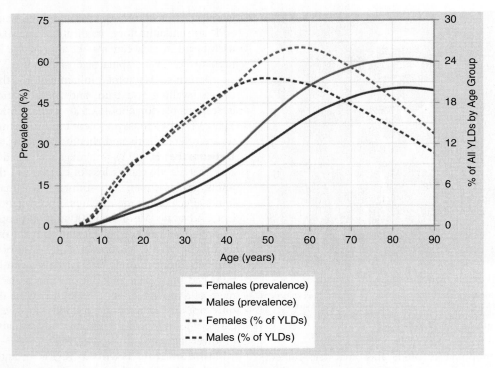

Figure 15.21 Prevalence (%) and percentage of years lived with disability (YLDs) from musculoskeletal disorders, by sex and age.

Data from GBD 2019 Diseases and Injuries Collaborators. Global burden of 369 diseases and injuries in 204 countries and territories, 1990–2019: a systematic analysis for the Global Burden of Disease Study 2019. *Lancet.* 2020;396:1204–1222.

and "nonself" and begins to attack its own cells. Autoimmune disorders are more prevalent among women than men.[107] For example, about 13 million women and 5 million men worldwide have RA.[2] When treatment for RA is accessed early after the onset of symptoms, many cases of RA can be managed with medications; without treatment, the disease is often disabling.[108] Another example of an autoimmune disorder is systemic lupus erythematosus. **Lupus** is often recognized by the "butterfly rash" it causes on the face, but it also causes swollen joints and adversely affects numerous other body systems.[109] Women are several times more likely than men to be diagnosed with lupus.[110]

The musculoskeletal disorder category also includes osteoporosis, gout, and numerous other rheumatological conditions.

Osteoporosis is a loss of bone density that significantly increases the risk of fractures of the hip, vertebrae, and other bones in older adults. Osteoporosis occurs most often among older women.[111] **Gout** is a painful swelling of a joint, usually the joint at the base of the big toe, due to elevated levels of uric acid in the blood. Gout occurs most often among older men.[112]

15.11 Vision Impairment

Adults and children with untreated or untreatable visual impairments may experience reduced quality of life, mobility, and independence.[113] Near vision impairments make it difficult or impossible to read or focus on other objects close to the eye. Distance vision impairment is present when visual acuity is less than 20/40 in the best eye,[114] which means that an individual would need to be 20 feet away from an object to see it as clearly as the typical person could see the object from 40 feet away. **Low vision** is moderate to severe vision impairment that occurs when an individual is not able to see better than 20/60 in the best eye even with corrective lenses. **Blindness** is defined as having no light perception, having vision that even with corrective lenses is no better than 20/400 in the best eye, or having a visual field of less than 10° around central fixation.

More than 2 billion people have a vision impairment; about half of those individuals can see adequately thanks to eyeglasses or other corrections, but more than 1.1 billion people—about one in seven individuals (14% of the world population)—currently have a vision impairment that could have been prevented or has yet to be corrected.[115] In total, more than 500 million people worldwide have uncorrected age-related near vision impairment (presbyopia), 250 million have mild vision impairment, 300 million have low vision, and more than 40 million are blind.[116] The prevalence of moderate or severe vision impairment or blindness increases with age, rising from about 1% of 5-year-olds to 2% of 30-year-olds, 14% of 50-year-olds, 33% of 65-year-olds, and 45% of 80-year-olds.[2]

Refractive errors are the most frequent cause of vision impairment.[115] A refractive error occurs when the length or shape of the eyeball prevents light from focusing directly on the retina, a tissue at the back of the eyeball that receives visual images that are then sent to the brain via the optic nerve. Nearsightedness (myopia), due to an eyeball that is too long, impairs distance vision. Farsightedness (hyperopia), due to an eyeball that is too short, impairs near vision. Astigmatism is an abnormal curvature of the cornea that causes vision to be distorted or fuzzy. Refractive errors can often be remediated with eyeglasses, contact lenses, or laser surgery.

Hundreds of millions of people live with poor visual acuity because they do not have access to the corrective lenses that would remediate their vision to acceptable levels.

The most frequent causes of adult vision loss leading to blindness are cataracts, glaucoma, age-related macular degeneration, diabetic retinopathy, and infections like trachoma (**Figure 15.22**).[117] A **cataract** is a clouding of the lens of an eye that makes vision fuzzy. Cataracts can be corrected with a simple surgical procedure that replaces the individual's cloudy lens with a clear artificial lens.[118] **Glaucoma** is elevated pressure within the eyeball that causes loss of peripheral vision. Eyedrops, laser therapy, and surgical procedures that reduce ocular pressure can slow disease progression.[119] **Macular degeneration** occurs when a portion of the retina deteriorates and causes loss of central vision. Medication can slow the progression of macular degeneration but cannot reverse existing damage.[120]

Population growth and aging are causing the number of people who are blind and the number who have low vision to increase rapidly even though the age-standardized prevalence of blindness has decreased over the past 30 years and the age-standardized prevalence of low vision has remained steady across those years.[116] Medical care accessed before vision has been severely impaired can prevent many types of blindness, and cost-effective interventions for uncorrected refractive errors, cataracts, and other frequent causes of vision impairment could eliminate the majority of the existing cases of vision impairment globally.[121] Some of this care can be provided at the primary health level, but there is a need to increase the number of vision care specialists, including ophthalmologists (physicians with advanced training in eye medicine and surgery), optometrists (vision testing specialists with advanced training), and opticians (technicians trained to fit corrective lenses). Many countries have severe shortages of vision health professionals.[122]

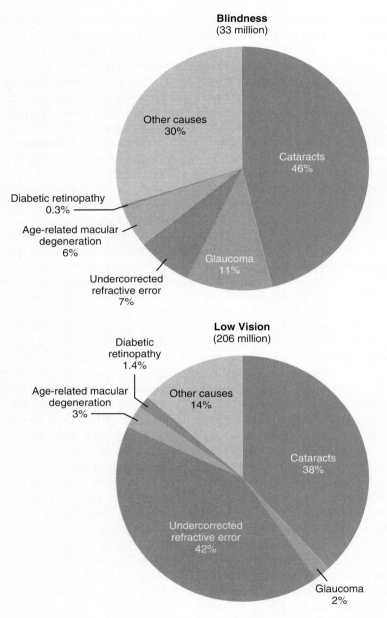

Figure 15.22 Causes of blindness and low vision (moderate or severe vision impairment) among adults ages 50 years and older.

Data from GBD 2019 Blindness and Vision Impairment Collaborators. Causes of blindness and vision impairment in 2020 and trends over 30 years, and prevalence of avoidable blindness in relation to VISION 2020: the Right to Sight: an analysis for the Global Burden of Disease Study. *Lancet Glob Health.* 2021;9:e144–e160.

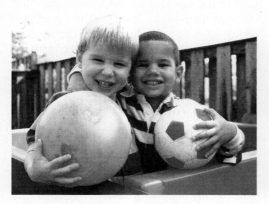

Normal vision.

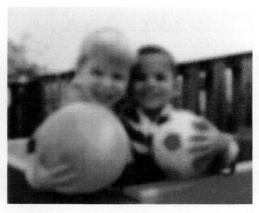

Cataracts.

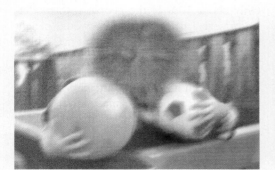

Macular degeneration.

National Eye Institute, National Institutes of Health

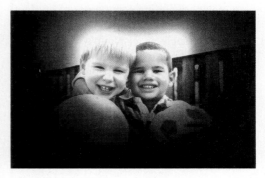

Glaucoma.

15.12 Hearing Loss

Sounds are measured in units of decibels (dB). The quietest sound the typical person with good hearing can perceive is 0 dB. A whisper might have a volume of about 20 or 30 dB, a vacuum cleaner 70 or 75 dB, and a chain saw about 110 dB. Decibels are measured using a logarithmic scale, so doubling the volume of a sound increases the loudness by 10 dB. Hearing is classified as normal if sounds less than 20 dB can be heard in a quiet environment.[123] Moderate hearing loss (the inability to hear sounds below 35 dB) makes it difficult to hear conversational speech even at close

distances. Severe hearing loss (the inability to hear sounds below 65 dB) may make it difficult to participate in conversations even when using powerful hearing aids. Individuals with profound hearing loss (the inability to hear sounds below 80 dB) or deafness (the inability to hear sounds below 95 dB) may be able to perceive sound vibrations but not hear speech or environmental noises.

More than 1.5 billion people—20% of the world population—have at least mild hearing loss (a 20 dB threshold), and more than 400 million people worldwide have at least moderate hearing loss (a permanent reduction of hearing in the better ear of 35 dB or more).[124] The prevalence of moderate or more severe hearing loss increases with age, rising from about 2% of 10-year-olds to 7% of 25-year-olds, 17% of 40-year-olds, 46% of 60-year-olds, and 77% of 80-year-olds (**Figure 15.23**).[2] Some hearing loss is conductive, which means that it originates in the ear canal or middle ear, and some is sensorineural, which means that it originates in the cochlea, auditory nerve, or other parts of the inner ear.

About half of cases of hearing loss could be prevented.[123] For children and adolescents, measles, meningitis, and chronic ear infections may cause permanent hearing damage. Additionally, some lifesaving medications may be ototoxic, including some types of antibiotics (like aminoglycosides) and some cancer treatments (such as cisplatin).[125] Preventing infections and using potentially ototoxic medications judiciously can help protect the hearing of young people. Hearing loss in adults is often noise induced. High-intensity sounds damage the special surfaces (stereocilia) of

cells in the ears that receive noise signals and transmit them to the brain.[126] The use of protective devices to reduce noise exposure in environmental, recreational, and occupational settings from childhood through adulthood helps prevent noise-induced hearing loss and the age-related hearing loss (presbycusis) that often makes it difficult for older adults to hear high frequencies.

For individuals with hearing loss, hearing technologies, sign language interpretation and other hearing assistive services (such as captioning of videos), and hearing and speech therapy may assist with communication, educational access, and social participation.[123] Only about 10% of the people with moderate or severe hearing loss who would benefit from hearing aids are using them.[127] Cochlear implants can restore some sound perception for people with severe sensorineural hearing loss for whom hearing aids are ineffective, but they are not available in most lower-income countries and are used by less than 1% of the

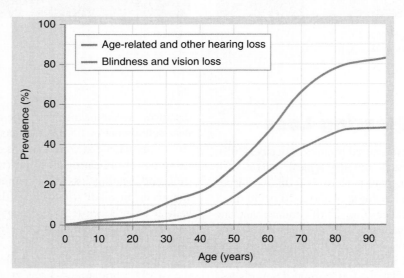

Figure 15.23 Prevalence (%) of age-related and other hearing loss (a permanent reduction of hearing in the better ear of 35 dB or more) and of blindness and vision loss (the inability to see better than 20/60 in the best eye even with corrective lenses), by age.

Data from GBD 2019 Diseases and Injuries Collaborators. Global burden of 369 diseases and injuries in 204 countries and territories, 1990–2019: a systematic analysis for the Global Burden of Disease Study 2019. *Lancet.* 2020;396:1204–1222.

people worldwide who might benefit from them.[128] Most countries do not have sufficient numbers of audiologists, otolaryngologists, speech–language therapists, teachers of the deaf, sign language interpreters, and other hearing care professionals.[129] Without access to hearing services, people with hearing loss may have difficulty accessing healthcare services, education, and social services and being fully included in economic, social, cultural, and other aspects of community life.

15.13 Skin Diseases

The skin is the largest organ of the body. Skin protects the body from the environment, provides insulation, regulates body temperature, takes in sensory information, and conducts

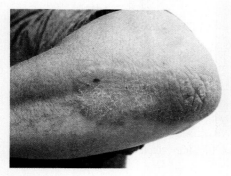

Psoriasis.
© JodiJacobson/E+/Getty Images

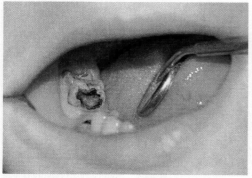

Tooth decay of lower molar.
© TRIG/Shutterstock

other important functions. While skin and subcutaneous diseases are a rare cause of death, they cause about 5% of YLDs each year.[2] Many people experience minor inconveniences from skin complaints like cuts, abrasions, blisters, dandruff, rashes, and other skin lesions, but some skin conditions can be disabling.

Various types of dermatitis, including eczema, may cause urticaria (an itchy red rash or hives) and pruritis (itchiness).[130] Psoriasis is a chronic inflammatory condition characterized by patches of discolored skin plaques.[131] Acne vulgaris is a chronic skin disease caused by blockages in the hair follicles.[132] Skin problems can also be caused by infections with bacteria, viruses, and fungi. Cellulitis is a potentially dangerous condition that occurs when bacteria like *Staphylococcus* or *Streptococcus* spread from the skin into the bloodstream.[133] Nonmelanoma skin cancers (like basal cell and squamous cell carcinomas), pyoderma (diseases that produce pus, such as impetigo), alopecia areata (hair loss due to autoimmune dysfunction), decubitus ulcers (bedsores), and other skin conditions may also cause reduced quality of life.

15.14 Dental and Oral Health

Oral health is an important part of overall health for both children and adults.[134] Dental health problems are often assessed as a function of the number of decayed, missing, or filled teeth (DMFT). Dental **caries**, colloquially called cavities, are holes in teeth created by demineralization and decay. Tooth decay is the most prevalent disease globally; about 2.5 billion people globally have untreated dental caries.[2] The typical 12-year-old has at least one DMFT, and the number of damaged teeth increases with age.[135]

Gingivitis is an inflammation of the gums associated with poor oral hygiene and the presence of bacterial plaques. **Periodontitis**

is chronic inflammation of the gums due to infection. Untreated periodontal disease can cause the teeth to become loose and fall out. More than 10% of adults worldwide have severe periodontitis.[136] **Edentulism** is the loss of most or all of one's teeth. About 7% of adults worldwide have edentulism, including nearly 20% of people ages 55 years and older and about 35% of people ages 75 years and older.[2]

The major risk factors for poor oral health include poor oral hygiene; exposure to dietary sugars that feed the bacteria that cause caries; use of tobacco products that damage tissues in the mouth and throat; lack of exposure to fluoride, an element often added to toothpaste or drinking water because it strengthens teeth; and lack of access to dental care that can prevent minor dental problems from becoming severe.[135] There are far too few dentists per capita in low-income countries to meet the demand for dental care (**Figure 15.24**),[137] especially in rural areas, so oral health problems in those regions often remain untreated.[138]

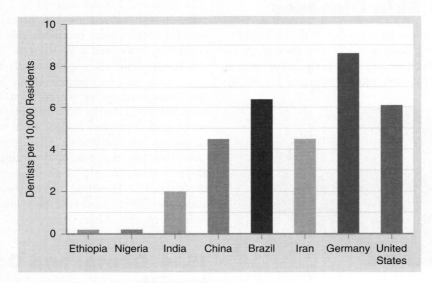

Figure 15.24 Dentists per 10,000 people in selected countries.
Data from *World Health Statistics 2021*. Geneva: World Health Organization; 2021.

References

1. Yach D, Hawkes C, Gould CL, Hofman KJ. The global burden of chronic diseases: overcoming impediments to prevention and control. *JAMA*. 2014;291:2616–2622.
2. GBD 2019 Diseases and Injuries Collaborators. Global burden of 369 diseases and injuries in 204 countries and territories, 1990–2019: a systematic analysis for the Global Burden of Disease Study 2019. *Lancet*. 2020;396:1204–1222.
3. GBD 2019 Risk Factors Collaborators. Global burden of 87 risk factors in 204 countries and territories, 1990–2019: a systematic analysis for the Global Burden of Disease Study 2019. *Lancet*. 2020;396:1223–1249.
4. *World Health Report 1997: Conquering Suffering, Enriching Humanity*. Geneva: World Health Organization; 1997.
5. Narayan KMV, Ali MK, Koplan JP. Global noncommunicable diseases: where worlds meet. *N Engl J Med*. 2010;363:1196–1198.
6. Bukhman G, Mocumbi AO, Atun R, et al. The Lancet NCDI Poverty Commission: bridging a gap in universal health coverage for the poorest billion. *Lancet*. 2020;396:991–1044.

7. *Global Action Plan for the Prevention and Control of Noncommunicable Diseases 2013–2020*. Geneva: World Health Organization; 2013.

8. Schwartz LN, Shaffer JD, Bukhman G. The origins of the 4 × 4 framework for noncommunicable disease at the World Health Organization. *SSM Popul Health*. 2021;13:100731.

9. NCD Countdown 2030 Collaborators. NCD Countdown 2030: pathways to achieving Sustainable Development Goal target 3.4. *Lancet*. 2020;396:918–934.

10. *Transforming Our World: The 2030 Agenda for Sustainable Development*. New York: United Nations; 2015.

11. *World Health Statistics 2021*. Geneva: World Health Organization; 2021.

12. *Saving Lives, Spending Less: The Case for Investing in Noncommunicable Diseases*. Geneva: World Health Organization; 2021.

13. Beaglehole R, Bonita R, Horton R, et al. Priority actions for the non-communicable disease crisis. *Lancet*. 2011;377:1438–1447.

14. DiMeglio LA, Evans-Molina C, Oram RA. Type 1 diabetes. *Lancet*. 2018;391:2449–2462.

15. *IDF Diabetes Atlas*. 9th ed. Brussels: International Diabetes Federation; 2019.

16. *Pocketbook for Management of Diabetes in Childhood and Adolescence in Under-Resourced Countries*. 2nd ed. Brussels: International Diabetes Federation; 2017.

17. Nolan CJ, Damm P, Prentki M. Type 2 diabetes across generations: from pathophysiology to prevention and management. *Lancet*. 2011;378:169–181.

18. Zimmet P, Alberti KGMM, Shaw J. Global and societal implications of the diabetes epidemic. *Nature*. 2001;414:782–787.

19. NCD Risk Factor Collaboration (NCD-RisC). Worldwide trends in diabetes since 1980: a pooled analysis of 751 population-based studies with 4.4 million participants. *Lancet*. 2016;387:1513–1530.

20. IDF Clinical Guidelines Task Force. *Global Guideline for Type 2 Diabetes*. Brussels: International Diabetes Federation; 2012.

21. *Use of Glycated Haemoglobin (HbA1c) in the Diagnosis of Diabetes Mellitus: Abbreviated Report of a WHO Consultation*. Geneva: World Health Organization; 2011.

22. Tabák AG, Herder C, Rathmann W, Brunner EJ, Kivimäki M. Prediabetes: a high-risk state for diabetes development. *Lancet*. 2012;379:2279–2290.

23. McIntyre HD, Catalano P, Zhang C, Desoye G, Mathiesen ER, Damm P. Gestational diabetes mellitus. *Nat Rev Dis Primers*. 2019;5:47.

24. Chan JCN, Lim LL, Wareham NJ, et al. The Lancet Commission on diabetes: using data to transform diabetes care and patient lives. *Lancet*. 2020;396:2019–2082.

25. *Global Report on Diabetes*. Geneva: World Health Organization; 2016.

26. Williams R, Karuranga S, Malanda B, et al. Global and regional estimates and projections of diabetes-related health expenditure: results from the International Diabetes Federation Diabetes Atlas, 9th edition. *Diabetes Res Clin Pract*. 2020;162:108072.

27. Ali M, Siegel K, Chandrasekar E, et al. Diabetes: an update on the pandemic and potential solutions (chapter 12). In: Prabhakaran D, Anand S, Gaziano TA, Mbanya J-C, Wu Y, Nugent R, eds. *Disease Control Priorities: Cardiovascular, Respiratory, and Related Diseases*. 3rd ed. Vol. 5. Washington DC: IBRD/World Bank; 2017:209–234.

28. *IDF Clinical Practice Recommendations for Managing Type 2 Diabetes in Primary Care*. Brussels: International Diabetes Federation; 2017.

29. *Global Surveillance, Prevention and Control of Chronic Respiratory Diseases: A Comprehensive Approach*. Geneva: World Health Organization; 2007.

30. Martinez FD, Vercelli D. Asthma. *Lancet*. 2013;382:1360–1372.

31. Burney P, Perez-Padilla R, Marks G, Wong G, Bateman E, Jarvis D. Chronic lower respiratory tract diseases (chapter 15). In: Prabhakaran D, Anand S, Gaziano TA, Mbanya J-C, Wu Y, Nugent R, eds. *Disease Control Priorities: Cardiovascular, Respiratory, and Related Diseases*. 3rd ed. Vol. 5. Washington DC: IBRD/World Bank; 2017:263–286.

32. *The Global Asthma Report 2018*. Auckland New Zealand: Global Asthma Network; 2018.

33. Boulet LP, Boulay ME. Asthma-related comorbidities. *Expert Rev Respir Med*. 2011;5:377–393.

34. Rabe KF, Adachi M, Lai CK, et al. Worldwide severity and control of asthma in children and adults: the global asthma insights and reality surveys. *J Allergy Clin Immunol*. 2004;114:40–47.

35. Decramer M, Janssens W, Miravitlles M. Chronic obstructive pulmonary disease. *Lancet*. 2012;179:1341–1351.

36. Taylor JD. COPD and the response of the lung to tobacco smoke exposure. *Pulm Pharmacol Ther*. 2010;23:376–383.

37. Decramer M, Janssens W. Chronic obstructive pulmonary disease and comorbidities. *Lancet Respir Med*. 2013;1:73–83.

38. *Prevention and Control of Noncommunicable Diseases: Guidelines for Primary Health Care in Low-Resource Settings*. Geneva: World Health Organization; 2012.

39. Leung CC, Yu ITS, Chen W. Silicosis. *Lancet*. 2012;379:2008–2018.

40. Verbeek J, Ivanov I. Essential occupational safety and health interventions for low- and middle-income countries: an overview of the evidence. *Saf Health Work*. 2013;4:77–83.

41. *IARC Monographs on the Evaluation of Carcinogenic Risks to Humans: Review of Human Carcinogens. Tobacco.* Vol. 100E. Lyon France: International Agency for Research on Cancer; 2012:43–211.

42. Benowitz NL. Nicotine addiction. *N Engl J Med.* 2010;362:2295–2303.

43. Walley SC, Jenssen BP. Electronic nicotine delivery systems. *Pediatrics.* 2015;136:1018–1026.

44. *How Tobacco Smoke Causes Disease: The Biology and Behavioral Basis for Smoking-Attributable Disease: A Report of the Surgeon General.* Atlanta GA: Centers for Disease Control and Prevention; 2010.

45. *The Health Consequences of Smoking: 50 Years of Progress: A Report of the Surgeon General.* Atlanta GA: Centers for Disease Control and Prevention; 2014.

46. *WHO Framework Convention on Tobacco Control.* Geneva: World Health Organization; 2005.

47. Glynn T, Seffrin JR, Brawley OW, Grey N, Ross H. The globalization of tobacco use: 21 challenges for the 21st century. *CA Cancer J Clin.* 2010;60:50–61.

48. Shibuya K, Ciecierski C, Guindon E, Bettcher DW, Evans DB, Murray CJL. WHO Framework Convention on Tobacco Control: development of an evidence based global public health treaty. *BMJ.* 2003;327:154–157.

49. Roemer R, Taylor A, Lariviere J. Origins of the WHO Framework Convention on Tobacco Control. *Am J Public Health.* 2005;95:936–938.

50. *WHO Report on the Global Tobacco Epidemic, 2021.* Geneva: World Health Organization; 2021.

51. GBD 2019 Tobacco Collaborators. Spatial, temporal, and demographic patterns in prevalence of smoking tobacco use and attributable disease burden in 204 countries and territories, 1990–2019: a systematic analysis from the Global Burden of Disease Study 2019. *Lancet.* 2021;397:2337–2360.

52. *WHO Global Report on Trends in Prevalence of Tobacco Use 2000–2025.* 4th ed. Geneva: World Health Organization; 2021.

53. Beaglehole R, Bonita R, Yach D, Mackay J, Reddy KS. A tobacco-free world: a call to action to phase out the sale of tobacco products by 2040. *Lancet.* 2015;385:1011–1018.

54. Ramakrishnan K, Scheid DC. Diagnosis and management of acute pyelonephritis in adults. *Am Fam Physician.* 2005;71:933–942.

55. Chadban SJ, Atkins RC. Glomerulonephritis. *Lancet.* 2005;365:1797–1806.

56. Lameire NH, Bagga A, Cruz D, et al. Acute kidney injury: an increasing global concern. *Lancet.* 2013;382:170–179.

57. Ronco R, Bellomo R, Kellum JA. Acute kidney injury. *Lancet.* 2019;394:1949–1964.

58. Kalantar-Zadeh K, Jafar TH, Nitsch D, Neuen BL, Perkovic V. Chronic kidney disease. *Lancet.* 2021;398:786–802.

59. Murtagh FE, Addington-Hall J, Higginson IJ. The prevalence of symptoms in end-stage renal disease: a systematic review. *Adv Chronic Kidney Dis.* 2007;14:82–99.

60. Bello AK, Alrukhaimi M, Ashuntantang GE, et al. Complications of chronic kidney disease: current state, knowledge gaps, and strategy for action. *Kidney Int Suppl.* 2017;7:122–129.

61. GBD Chronic Kidney Disease Collaborators. Global, regional, and national burden of chronic kidney disease, 1990–2017: a systematic analysis for the Global Burden of Disease Study 2017. *Lancet.* 2017;395:709–733.

62. Luyckx VA, Tuttle KR, Garcia-Garcia G, et al. Reducing major risk factors for chronic kidney disease. *Kidney Int Suppl.* 2017;7:71–87.

63. Jha V, Garcia-Garcia G, Iseki K, et al. Chronic kidney disease: global dimension and perspectives. *Lancet.* 2013;382:260–272.

64. Bello AK, Levin A, Lunney M, et al. Status of care for end stage kidney disease in countries and regions worldwide: international cross sectional survey. *BMJ.* 2019;367:l5873.

65. Liyanage T, Ninomiya T, Jha V, et al. Worldwide access to treatment for end-stage kidney disease: a systematic review. *Lancet.* 2015;385:1975–1982.

66. Tsochatzis EA, Bosch J, Burroughs AK. Liver cirrhosis. *Lancet.* 2014;393:1749–1761.

67. Younossi Z, Anstee QM, Marietti M, et al. Global burden of NAFLD and NASH: trends, predictions, risk factors and prevention. *Nat Rev Gastroenterol Hepatol.* 2017;15:11–20.

68. Asrani SK, Devarbhavi H, Eaton J, Kamath PS. Burden of liver diseases in the world. *J Hepatol.* 2019;70:151–171.

69. Steward B, Khanduri P, McCord C, et al. Global disease burden of conditions requiring emergency surgery. *Br J Surg.* 2014;101:e9–e22.

70. Alkire BC, Raykar NP, Shrime MG, et al. Global access to surgical care: a modelling study. *Lancet Glob Health.* 2015;3:e316–e323.

71. Rose J, Weiser TG, Hider P, Wilson L, Gruen RL, Bickler SW. Estimated need for surgery worldwide based on prevalence of diseases: a modelling strategy for the WHO Global Health Estimate. *Lancet Glob Health.* 2015;3:S13–S20.

72. Meara JG, Leather AJM, Hagander L, et al. Global Surgery 2030: evidence and solutions for achieving health, welfare, and economic development. *Lancet.* 2015;386:569–624.

73. Holmer H, Lantz A, Kunjumen T, et al. Global distribution of surgeons, anaesthesiologists, and obstetricians. *Lancet Glob Health.* 2015;3:S9–S11.

74. *Neurological Disorders: Public Health Challenges.* Geneva: World Health Organization; 2006.

75. Vaughan KA, Ramos CL, Buch VP, et al. An estimation of the global volume of surgically treatable epilepsy based on a systematic review and meta-analysis of epilepsy. *J Neurosurg.* 2019;130:1127–1141.

76. Moshé SL, Perucca E, Ryvlin P, Tomson T. Epilepsy: new advances. *Lancet.* 2015;385:884–898.

77. Newton CR, Garcia HH. Epilepsy in poor regions of the world. *Lancet.* 2012;380:1193–1201.

78. *Epilepsy: A Public Health Imperative.* Geneva: World Health Organization; 2019.

79. Saylor D, Steiner TJ. The global burden of headache. *Semin Neurol.* 2018;38:182–190.

80. *The International Classification of Headache Disorders.* 3rd ed. London: International Headache Society; 2017.

81. Woldeamanuel YW, Cowan RP. Migraine affects 1 in 10 people worldwide featuring recent rise: a systematic review and meta-analysis of community-based studies involving 6 million participants. *J Neurol Sci.* 2017;372:307–315.

82. Ashina M, Katsarava Z, Do TP, et al. Migraine: epidemiology and systems of care. *Lancet.* 2021;397:1485–1495.

83. Bloem BR, Okun MS, Klein C. Parkinson's disease. *Lancet.* 2021;397:2284–2303.

84. Dickson DW. Neuropathology of Parkinson disease. *Parkinsonism Relat Disord.* 2018;46(Suppl 1):S30–S33.

85. Espay AJ, Morgante F, Merola A, et al. Levodopa-induced dyskinesia in Parkinson disease: current and evolving concepts. *Ann Neurol.* 2018;84:797–811.

86. Dorsey ER, Bloem BR. The Parkinson pandemic: a call to action. *JAMA Neurol.* 2018;75:9–10.

87. Kister I, Bacon TE, Chamot E, et al. Natural history of multiple sclerosis symptoms. *Int J MS Care.* 2013;15:146–158.

88. Olek MJ. Multiple sclerosis. *Ann Intern Med.* 2021;174:81–96.

89. Tremlett H, Zhao Y, Rieckmann P, Hutchinson M. New perspectives in the natural history of multiple sclerosis. *Neurology.* 2010;74:2004–2015.

90. Walson C, King R, Rechtman L, et al. Rising prevalence of multiple sclerosis worldwide: insights from the Atlas of MS, 3rd edition. *MS J.* 2020;26:1816–1821.

91. Goldberg AD, Allis CD, Bernstein E. Epigenetics: a landscape takes shape. *Cell.* 2007;128:635–638.

92. Mégarbané A, Ravel A, Mircher C, et al. The 50th anniversary of the discovery of trisomy 21: the past, present, and future of research and treatment of Down syndrome. *Genet Med.* 2009;11:611–616.

93. Bondy CA, Turner Syndrome Study Group. Care of girls and women with Turner syndrome: a guideline of the Turner Syndrome Study Group. *J Clin Endocrinol Metab.* 2007;92:10–25.

94. Gusella JF, Lee JM, MacDonald ME. Huntington's disease: nearly four decades of human molecular genetics. *Hum Mol Genet.* 2021;30:R254–R263.

95. Bell SC, Mall MA, Gutierrez H, et al. The future of cystic fibrosis care: a global perspective. *Lancet Respir Med.* 2019;8:65–124.

96. Modell B, Darlison M. Global epidemiology of haemoglobin disorders and derived service indicators. *Bull World Health Organ.* 2008;86:480–487.

97. Muncie HL, Campbell JS. Alpha and beta thalassemia. *Am Fam Physician.* 2009;80:339–344.

98. Ware RE, de Montalembert M, Tshilolo L, Abboud MR. Sickle cell disease. *Lancet.* 2017;390:311–323.

99. Piel FB, Patil AP, Howes RE, et al. Global distribution of the sickle cell gene and geographical confirmation of the malaria hypothesis. *Nat Commun.* 2010;1:104.

100. Mannucci PM, Tuddenham EG. The hemophilias: from royal genes to gene therapy. *N Engl J Med.* 2001;344:1773–1779.

101. Luzzatto L, Nannelli C, Notaro R. Glucose-6-phosphate dehydrogenase deficiency. *Hematol Oncol Clin North Am.* 2016;30:373–393.

102. Hartvigsen J, Hancock MJ, Kongsted A, et al. What low back pain is and why we need to pay attention. *Lancet.* 2018;391:2356–2367.

103. Foster NE, Anema JR, Cherkin D, et al. Prevention and treatment of low back pain: evidence, challenges, and promising directions. *Lancet.* 2018;391:2368–2383.

104. Palazzo C, Nguyen C, Lefevre-Colau MM, Rannou F, Poiraudeau S. Risk factors and burden of osteoarthritis. *Ann Phys Rehabil Med.* 2016;59:134–138.

105. Hunter DJ, Bierma-Zeinstra S. Osteoarthritis. *Lancet.* 2019;393:1745–1759.

106. Tracy A, Buckley CD, Raza K. Pre-symptomatic autoimmunity in rheumatoid arthritis: when does the disease start? *Sem Immunopathol.* 2017;39:423–435.

107. Whitacre CC. Sex differences in autoimmune disease. *Nature Immunol.* 2001;2:777–780.

108. McInnes IB, Schett G. Pathogenetic insights from the treatment of rheumatoid arthritis. *Lancet.* 2017;389:2328–2337.

109. La MCV, Ghetu MV, Bieniek M. Systemic lupus erythematosus: primary care approach to diagnosis and management. *Am Fam Physician.* 2016;94:284–294.

110. Rees F, Doherty M, Grainge MJ, Lanyon P, Zhang W. The worldwide incidence and prevalence of systematic lupus erythematosus: a systematic review of epidemiological studies. *Rheumatol.* 2017;56:1945–1961.

111. Curtis EM, Moon RJ, Harvey NC, Cooper C. The impact of fragility fracture and approaches to osteoporosis risk assessment worldwide. *Bone.* 2017;104:29–38.

112. Dehlin M, Jacobsson L, Roddy E. Global epidemiology of gout: prevalence, incidence, treatment patterns and risk factors. *Nature Rev Rheumatol.* 2020;16:380–390.

113. Burton MJ, Ramke J, Marques AP, et al. The Lancet Global Health Commission on Global Eye Health: vision beyond 2020. *Lancet Glob Health.* 2021;9:e489–e551.

114. *International Statistical Classification of Diseases and Related Health Problems.* 11th ed. (ICD-11). Geneva: World Health Organization; 2020.

115. *World Report on Vision.* Geneva: World Health Organization; 2019.

116. GBD 2019 Blindness and Vision Impairment Collaborators. Trends in prevalence of blindness and distance and near vision impairment over 30 years: an analysis for the Global Burden of Disease Study. *Lancet Glob Health.* 2021;9:e130–e143.

117. GBD 2019 Blindness and Vision Impairment Collaborators. Causes of blindness and vision impairment in 2020 and trends over 30 years, and prevalence of avoidable blindness in relation to VISION 2020: the Right to Sight: an analysis for the Global Burden of Disease Study. *Lancet Glob Health.* 2021;9:e144–e160.

118. Liu YC, Wilkins M, Kim T, Malyugin B, Mehta JS. Cataracts. *Lancet.* 2017;390:600–612.

119. Weinreb RN, Aung T, Medeiros FA. The pathophysiology and treatment of glaucoma: a review. *JAMA.* 2014;311:1901–1911.

120. Mitchell P, Liew G, Gopinath B, Wong TY. Age-related macular degeneration. *Lancet.* 2018;392:1147–1159.

121. *Universal Eye Health: A Global Action Plan 2014–2019.* Geneva: World Health Organization; 2013.

122. Resnikoff S, Lansingh VC, Washburn L, et al. Estimated number of ophthalmologists worldwide (International Council of Ophthalmology update): will we meet the needs? *Br J Ophthalmol.* 2020;104:588–592.

123. *World Report on Hearing.* Geneva: World Health Organization; 2021.

124. GBD 2019 Hearing Loss Collaborators. Hearing loss prevalence and years lived with disability, 1990–2019: findings from the Global Burden of Disease Study 2019. *Lancet.* 2021;397:996–1009.

125. Kros CJ, Steyger PS. Aminoglycoside- and cisplatin-induced ototoxicity: mechanisms and otoprotective strategies. *Cold Spring Harb Perspect Med.* 2019;9:a033548.

126. Basner M, Babisch W, Davis A, et al. Auditory and non-auditory effects of noise on health. *Lancet.* 2014;383:1325–1332.

127. Bisgaard N, Zimmer S, Laureyns M, Growth J. A model for estimating hearing aid coverage worldwide using historical data on hearing aid sales. *Int J Audiol.* 2021. doi:10.1080/14992027.2021.196 2551

128. Bodington E, Saeed SR, Smith MCF, Stocks NG, Morse RP. A narrative review of the logistic and economic feasibility of cochlear implants in lower-income countries. *Cochlear Implants Int.* 2021;22:7–16.

129. *Multi-country Assessment of National Capacity to Provide Hearing Care.* Geneva: World Health Organization; 2013.

130. Avena-Woods C. Overview of atopic dermatitis. *Am J Managed Care.* 2017;23:S115–S123.

131. Parisi R, Symmons DP, Griffiths CE, et al. Global epidemiology of psoriasis: a systematic review of incidence and prevalence. *J Invest Dermatol.* 2013;133:377–385.

132. Zaenglein AL. Acne vulgaris. *New Engl J Med.* 2018;379:1343–1352.

133. Raff AB, Kroshinsky D. Cellulitis. *JAMA.* 2016;316:325–337.

134. Peres MA, Macpherson LMD, Weyant RJ, et al. Oral diseases: a global public health challenge. *Lancet.* 2019;394:249–260.

135. *The Oral Health Atlas.* 2nd ed. Geneva: FDI World Dental Federation; 2015.

136. Frencken JE, Sharma P, Stenhouse L, Green D, Laverty D, Dietrich T. Global epidemiology of dental caries and severe periodontitis: a comprehensive review. *J Clin Periodontol.* 2017;44(Suppl 18):S94–S105.

137. Gallagher JE, Hutchinson L. Analysis of human resources for oral health globally: inequitable distribution. *Int Dental J.* 2018;68:183–189.

138. Watt RG, Daly B, Allison P. Ending the neglect of global oral health: time for radical action. *Lancet.* 2019;394:261–272.

Mental Health Promotion

Depression, anxiety disorders, substance use disorders, and other mental health disorders are among the most frequent causes of disability worldwide. Although effective therapies for many mental health disorders exist, only a small proportion of people who would benefit from them are currently accessing mental healthcare services.

16.1 Mental Health and Global Health

Mental health disorders are a global health priority because they have high prevalence rates worldwide and they cause significant reductions in quality of life.[1] A **disorder** is a functional impairment that may or may not be characterized by measurable structural or physiological changes. Approximately one in five people meets the criteria for a mental health disorder in any one-year period.[2] Many of these individuals will have days of reduced productivity at work and home because of their mental health conditions, and many will experience times when it takes extreme effort to perform routine daily activities.[3] Some people with severe mental health disorders will have extended periods of time when they have great difficulty with self-care, interpersonal relationships, and other life activities.[4] These challenges make mental health disorders one of the leading cause of disability worldwide, accounting for about one-sixth of all years lived with disability (YLDs) generated annually (**Figure 16.1**).[5]

While there is some variation in regional prevalence rates, every part of the world bears a significant burden from mental health disorders.[6] The most frequently diagnosed and disabling mental health conditions include depressive disorders, anxiety disorders, schizophrenia, bipolar disorder, and alcohol and drug use disorders (**Figure 16.2**).[5] Even though these mental health disorders are known to have high prevalence rates, most of these conditions remain poorly understood.[7] Mental health disorders likely arise from a complex set of genetic, biological, psychological, social, developmental, and environmental factors, but few risk factors have been confirmed.[8] Without greater clarity about the causes of mental health disorders, it is difficult to develop effective preventive interventions.[9] Improved scientific knowledge about mental health disorders will be necessary to make progress toward achieving the Sustainable Development Goal (SDG) targets that aim

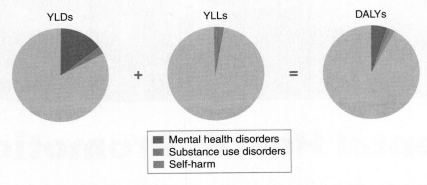

Figure 16.1 Years lived with disability (YLDs), years of life lost (YLLs), and disability-adjusted life years (DALYs) from mental health disorders (including substance abuse and self-harm), as a percentage of the total worldwide burden of disease.

Data from GBD 2019 Diseases and Injuries Collaborators. Global burden of 369 diseases and injuries in 204 countries and territories, 1990–2019: a systematic analysis for the Global Burden of Disease Study 2019. *Lancet.* 2020;396:1204–1222.

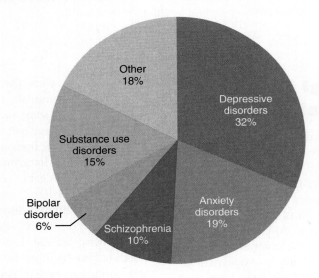

Figure 16.2 Distribution of years lived with disability (YLDs) from various types of mental health and substance use disorders.

Data from GBD 2019 Diseases and Injuries Collaborators. Global burden of 369 diseases and injuries in 204 countries and territories, 1990–2019: a systematic analysis for the Global Burden of Disease Study 2019. *Lancet.* 2020;396:1204–1222.

to "promote mental health and well-being" (SDG 3.4) and "strengthen the prevention and treatment of substance abuse, including narcotic drug abuse and harmful use of alcohol" (SDG 3.5).[10]

Improved global mental health is also necessary for making progress toward realization of universal human rights. Although medications and various types of therapy and support are effective at improving quality of life for people with neuropsychiatric conditions, most people who would benefit from these interventions experience major barriers to accessing mental health diagnoses and effective treatment.[11] In many communities, people with psychiatric disorders are maltreated. They may be imprisoned or involuntarily detained in hospitals for long periods of time without any legal recourse, denied access to hospitalization when it is needed, and subjected to various types of violence and abuse.[12] Poverty and discrimination exacerbate the challenges faced by many people with psychiatric conditions.[1] The global burden from mental health, neurological, and substance use disorders will not be reduced without vigorous international commitments to work together to develop effective new treatments, increase access to specialty care, and reduce the stigma associated with mental health disabilities.[13]

16.2 Depressive Disorders

A **depressive disorder** is characterized by sadness; hopelessness; loss of interest in usual activities; fatigue; poor concentration; and other negative thoughts, feelings, and physical symptoms that interfere with routine daily activities.[14] People with severe depression may not have the energy to get out of bed, eat, go to work, meet with friends, or conduct other routine daily activities. Major depressive disorder is sometimes called unipolar depressive disorder to distinguish it from bipolar disorder. **Unipolar depressive disorder** is characterized by depression without the cycles of mania that occur among people with bipolar disorder.

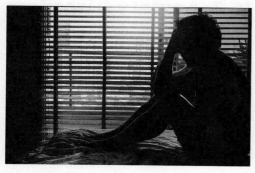

© TZIDO SUN/Shutterstock

Depression is a leading cause of disability globally because it causes significant reductions in productivity at work, home, and school for an estimated 280 million people worldwide each year.[5] About 5% of adults worldwide meet the clinical definition of depression during the course of one year.[15] The American Psychiatric Association guidelines published in the *Diagnostic and Statistical Manual of Mental Disorders* (DSM-5), usually simply called "the DSM," spell out the defining features of dozens of mental health issues, including depression.[16] Children, adolescents, and adults can be clinically diagnosed as having mild, moderate, or severe depression based on criteria in the DSM. However, the diagnosis of depression and other mental health disorders is, in part, dependent on cultural norms and perceptions.[17] Many disorders exist as part of a spectrum where the distinction between what is classified as "normal" and what is classified as a "disorder" is blurry. The variation in the country-specific prevalence rates of depression is partly due to differences in diagnostic criteria (**Figure 16.3**).[5] Countries with a higher prevalence of depression tend to include milder cases of depression in their statistics, while countries with a lower prevalence of depression tend to report only the moderate and severe cases of depression that cause significant impairment.[18]

Most people who experience an episode of acute depression do not develop chronic depression. However, for about one in five people, especially those who were young when they first experienced depression and those with comorbid mental health disorders, depression becomes a persistent depressive disorder.[19] Chronic depression and other long-lasting mental health disorders are associated with a variety of adverse physical health conditions. Chronic pain, fatigue, and other disabling conditions increase the likelihood of depression, and depression can make it difficult to manage chronic noncommunicable diseases that require daily medications and frequent monitoring.[20]

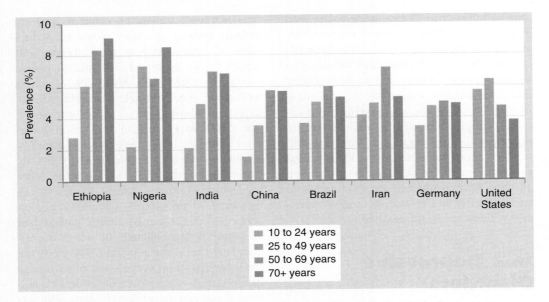

Figure 16.3 Prevalence of depression by age group in selected countries in a typical recent year.

Data from GBD 2019 Diseases and Injuries Collaborators. Global burden of 369 diseases and injuries in 204 countries and territories, 1990–2019: a systematic analysis for the Global Burden of Disease Study 2019. *Lancet.* 2020;396:1204–1222.

In most countries, the prevalence of depression increases with age and is higher among females than males.[5] This may be partly because the prevalence of chronic diseases increases with age and some disabling chronic diseases occur more often among women than men.

Most cases of depression can be successfully treated with low-cost medications and psychotherapy, such as **cognitive behavioral therapy** (CBT), a form of talk therapy in which a therapist helps an individual understand his or her thoughts, feelings, and behaviors and identify actions that can be taken to correct concerns.[21] Both amitriptyline (a tricyclic antidepressant) and fluoxetine (a selective serotonin reuptake inhibitor, or SSRI) are included in the World Health Organization (WHO) list of essential medicines,[22] and several other types of antidepressants are also effective at lessening symptoms among many people experiencing depression.[23]

The barriers to accessing mental health care include perceptions that medication is not needed; structural barriers, such as the financial costs and time constraints associated with seeking health services; and attitudinal barriers, such as the perception that treatment will be ineffective, the belief that the problem will resolve on its own with time, and concerns about stigma.[24] Integrating depression screening, diagnosis, and treatment with care for other health concerns may increase access to treatment for depression.[25]

16.3 Anxiety Disorders

Anxiety disorders are characterized by a disproportionate fear of imminent danger and worry about potential future threats.[26] There are several types of anxiety disorders. **Generalized anxiety disorder** is characterized by persistent excessive worrying about numerous concerns, and it is often accompanied by sleep disturbances, muscle tension, and fatigue.[27] **Panic disorder** is defined by repeated panic attacks that last for several intense minutes and cause a racing heartbeat, shortness of breath, dizziness or weakness, shaking, nausea, and other disturbing symptoms.[28] Social anxiety disorder (previously called social phobia) is characterized by extreme fear of being negatively perceived by others or feeling embarrassed or awkward in social situations.[29] Other anxiety disorders include separation anxiety disorder, agoraphobia (fear of unfamiliar environments and uncontrollable situations that can make it difficult to even leave one's home), and other specific phobias.[16]

Anxiety disorders are diagnosed based on extreme emotional and physical responses to minor threats that cause the individual to be unable to function at work or school or in other environments. Almost everyone feels apprehensive or nervous sometimes and has some level of discomfort in some social situations, and it is appropriate to feel fear in response to specific dangerous situations. Experiencing some anxiety in stressful situations does not mean that an anxiety disorder is present. While 13% of adults have experienced at least one panic attack and about two-thirds of people who have ever had a panic attack have experienced repeated attacks, only about 15% of people who have ever experienced one or more panic attacks meet the criteria for a panic disorder diagnosis.[30]

Even when only cases that meet rigorous clinical diagnostic criteria are counted, the prevalence of anxiety disorders is high after grouping the burden from generalized anxiety disorder, panic disorder, and related conditions.[31] About 4% of adults experience generalized anxiety disorder at some point in their lifetimes, about 2% in a typical year, and about 1% in a typical month.[32] About 2% of all adults meet the clinical criteria for panic disorder at some point in their lifetimes.[30] More than 300 million adults and children are living with an anxiety disorder, making anxiety disorders the most prevalent group of mental health disorders globally and one of the leading causes of disability worldwide.[33] The prevalence of anxiety disorders is higher among females than males, but prevalence rates are similar for younger and older adults (**Figure 16.4**).[5]

Antianxiety medications and CBT can be effective treatments for people who experience anxiety disorders.[8] CBT for panic disorders may include education about the physiology of panic attacks, practice applying relaxation and coping techniques, and interoceptive exposure in which clients increase their heart rates by running or intentionally hyperventilating so they can become accustomed to feeling these sensations in a safe and controlled setting.[34] However, many people with anxiety disorders in countries of all income levels are not aware that therapy could improve their quality of life.[35] This lack of knowledge about treatment options contributes to low rates of healthcare service use for anxiety disorders.

16.4 Schizophrenia

Schizophrenia is a mental health disorder characterized by distorted perceptions of reality.[36] People with schizophrenia and other psychotic disorders may experience delusions and hallucinations. A **delusion** is a false belief that is irrational but seems very real to the person experiencing it. For example, some people with paranoid thinking firmly believe they are being robbed by family members or tracked by the police, even when the reality is that they are not being targeted. Some people with delusions believe they have superpowers, even though others would disagree with that perception. A **hallucination** is a sensory distortion that causes a person to hear, see, feel, smell, or taste something that in reality is not present. For example, a person experiencing auditory hallucinations may hear the voices of people who are not actually nearby. People with schizophrenia may also express disorganized thinking and speech. These "positive" or psychotic symptoms are often accompanied by "negative" or deficit symptoms, such

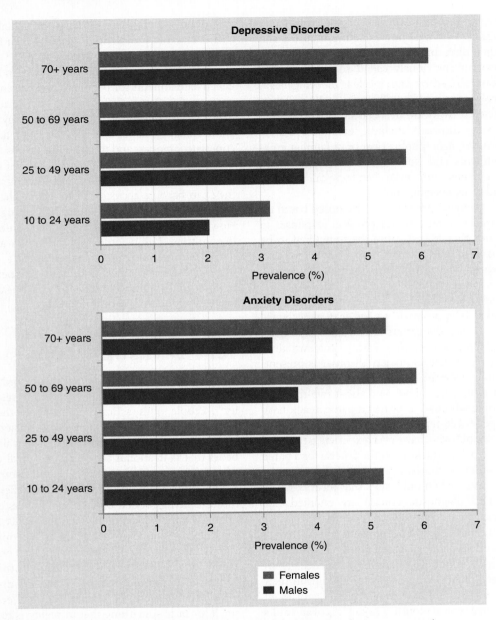

Figure 16.4 Prevalence of depressive disorders and anxiety disorders by age group and sex.

Data from GBD 2019 Diseases and Injuries Collaborators. Global burden of 369 diseases and injuries in 204 countries and territories, 1990–2019: a systematic analysis for the Global Burden of Disease Study 2019. *Lancet.* 2020;396:1204–1222.

as a flat affect and low energy. Additionally, people with schizophrenia may exhibit cognitive issues, such as impaired decision-making and memory.

Approximately 7 per 1,000 people are diagnosed with schizophrenia during their lifetimes.[37] Most initial diagnoses are made during early adulthood, often in the mid-20s.[38]

With medication and other therapies, many people with a schizophrenia diagnosis are able to achieve remission.[39] Antipsychotic medications are often effective in treating most psychotic symptoms. Psychosocial interventions, such as patient therapy, family support groups, and community-based rehabilitation, are also helpful in enabling people with schizophrenia to lead independent lives.[40] However, relapses and chronic disability occur often. Nearly 25 million people worldwide are living with schizophrenia.[5]

One of the major barriers to favorable outcomes for people diagnosed with schizophrenia is limited access to psychiatric services. About two-thirds of people with schizophrenia and related disorders who live in low- and middle-income countries are not receiving specialized mental health care.[41] Another challenge is the stigma associated with the disorder. **Stigma** is a term used to describe negative attitudes about members of a population group. Those negative perceptions often lead to discrimination, social exclusion, and other forms of marginalization. The majority of people with schizophrenia report having experienced rejection, avoidance, and other forms of interpersonal and social stigma.[42] The stigma of mental health disorders can be countered with education, social interactions between members of majority populations and stigmatized populations, and social activism that promotes more inclusive attitudes and behaviors.[43]

16.5 Bipolar Disorder

Bipolar disorder, formerly called manic depression, is characterized by alternating periods of depression and mania or hypomania.[44] Acute mania is characterized by euphoria, sleeplessness, grandiose delusions, racing thoughts, talkativeness, irritability, and impulsive behaviors that last for a week or longer. Hypomania is similar to mania, but the symptoms are milder, last for a shorter duration, and do not require hospitalization. People with bipolar disorder experience dramatic shifts in mood, energy level, appetite and sleep habits, and self-image. These cycles may be relatively rapid or may occur slowly over a period of months.

It is likely that about 1% of adults have bipolar disorder, perhaps about 40 million people worldwide,[5] but it is difficult to ascertain the actual prevalence because diagnosis can be clinically challenging.[45] Many people who meet the clinical definition for bipolar disorder also meet the criteria for anxiety disorders and other concurrent mental health disorders. These complexities may make it difficult for people with bipolar disorder to receive an accurate diagnosis and achieve long-term management of their mental health. Fewer than 10% of people with bipolar disorder are accessing clinical care for the condition.[46]

Antipsychotic medications can alleviate the symptoms of acute mania. Lithium and other pharmaceutical agents can help prevent relapses. These medications are most effective at managing the disorder when their use is combined with psychotherapy.[47] Stigma associated with bipolar disorder may make it difficult for people with the condition to receive an accurate diagnosis; maintain access to high-quality care; continue taking prescribed medication; and feel supported by family, friends, coworkers, and even healthcare providers.[48]

16.6 Drug Use Disorders

Addiction is a cognitive and neurological condition characterized by adverse behaviors related to physical or psychological dependence.[49] While the term is primarily used to refer to dependence on substances, addiction is also used to describe some compulsive behaviors, such as excessive gambling.[50] The American Society of Addiction Medicine has identified the ABCs of addiction as follows[51]:

- The inability to **A**bstain from harmful substances or behaviors
- **B**ehavior control impairment
- **C**raving substances or experiences
- **D**iminished recognition of the problems with individual functioning and interpersonal relationships
- Dysfunctional **E**motional responses

Substance use disorders include misuse of alcohol, caffeine, cannabis, hallucinogens (including phencyclidine, more commonly called PCP), inhalants, opioids, sedatives, hypnotics, anxiolytics, stimulants, tobacco, and other substances.[16]

Cannabis products, such as marijuana, are the most widely used illicit drugs worldwide, but the greatest disability is associated with injectable drugs, such as amphetamines, opioids (including heroin, morphine, and fentanyl), and cocaine.[52] A **person who injects drugs** (PWID), also called an **injecting drug user** (IDU), is an individual who injects illicit drugs for nonmedical use. People who use illicit drugs may face numerous negative health outcomes, including an increased risk of viral hepatitis, HIV infection, and premature mortality. These substances also harm relationships, decrease economic status, and increase the likelihood of participation in criminal activity.[53] There is an additional and growing burden from the nonmedical use of prescription medications.[54]

It can be difficult to measure the level of harm caused by problematic drug use because data about illegal activities are not easily gathered. Even so, it is easy to observe the major adverse effects that substance abuse has on public health in many countries. An estimated 4% of adults worldwide used marijuana in the past year, and more than 1% used injectable drugs (amphetamines, opioids, and/or cocaine).[55] In the United States, about 12% of all people who are 12 years old or older report that they have used an illicit drug in the past year, including about 10% who report marijuana use and 2% who report misuse of

psychotherapeutic drugs (such as antidepressants, antianxiety agents, and stimulants); the rates are higher among people ages 18–25 years, with about 24% reporting illicit drug use, including 22% using marijuana and almost 4% misusing psychotherapeutic medications.[56] About 5% of Americans report misusing prescription pain relievers, 1.8% using cocaine or crack, 1.8% using hallucinogens, and 0.3% using heroin in the past year.[57] The number of overdose deaths in the United States increased from more than 50,000 in 2015 to more than 70,000 in 2017 and more than 90,000 in 2020 as more synthetic opioids were used.[58]

While many countries have attempted to reduce drug addiction problems through substance abuse awareness campaigns, enforcement of drug laws, and imprisonment of drug users, few policies and programs have proven to be effective at reducing the burden from harmful drug use.[53] Opioid antagonist medications like naloxone and naltrexone are used by emergency medical personnel to reverse opioid overdoses, but many people die from overdoses before anyone is able to call for help. From a prevention science perspective, the best interventions are ones that prevent initiation of drug use. Unfortunately, few drug use initiation prevention programs have proven to be highly effective.[59]

16.7 Alcohol Use Disorders

Excessive alcohol use causes cirrhosis and other forms of liver damage; significantly increases the risk of a diversity of cancers, some types of cardiovascular disease, and some other noncommunicable diseases; increases the risk of both unintentional injuries and intentional injuries; and increases the risk of premature death.[60] The types of alcoholic beverages consumed vary by country (**Figure 16.5**),[61] but it is the volume of pure alcohol ingested that

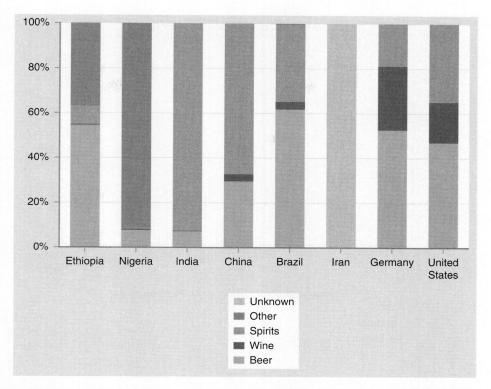

Figure 16.5 Types of alcoholic beverages consumed by liters of pure alcohol in selected countries.

Data from *Global Status Report on Alcohol and Health 2018*. Geneva: World Health Organization; 2018.

predicts the health outcomes, not the particular type of alcoholic beverage consumed.[62] About 9% of adult males worldwide have an alcohol use disorder, including 5% with alcohol dependence, which is characterized by lack of self-control when impaired by alcohol, and 4% who consume large volumes of alcohol but are not dependent on it; about 2% of adult females have an alcohol use disorder, including 1% with alcohol dependence and 1% with other types of harmful use.[61]

The typical male consumes much more alcohol than the typical female and is more likely to practice binge drinking (**Figure 16.6**).[61] In the United States, for example, about 29% of males and 21% of females who are 12 years old or older report binge drinking (five or more drinks within a few hours by males or four or more drinks within a few hours by females)

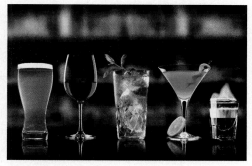

© Petereleven/Shutterstock

in the last month, and about 8% of males and 4% of females report heavy alcohol use (binge drinking on five or more days in the past month).[56] Because males consume more alcohol than females, males have higher rates of cirrhosis, alcohol-related cancers, road traffic injuries, and other adverse health outcomes associated

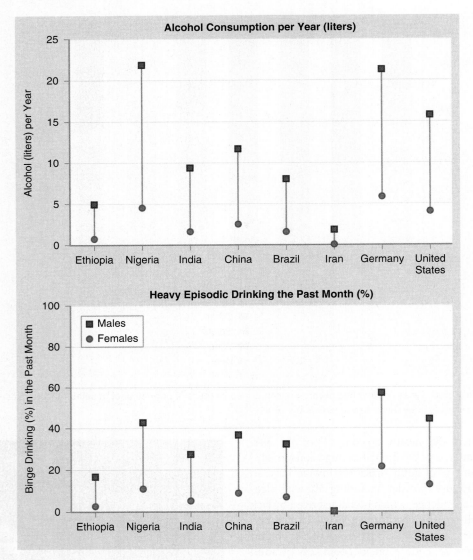

Figure 16.6 Annual alcohol per capita consumption in liters of pure alcohol and prevalence of heavy episodic drinking (binge drinking of 60+ grams of pure alcohol on at least one occasion) in the past month among adults (ages 15+ years) in selected countries, by sex.

Data from *Global Status Report on Alcohol and Health 2018*. Geneva: World Health Organization; 2018.

with the harmful use of alcohol.[60] In many countries, more than 10% of the total disability among young and middle-aged adult men is attributable to alcohol use (**Figure 16.7**).[63]

Several screening tools are available to assist in identifying problematic use of alcohol. The Alcohol Use Disorders Identification Test

(AUDIT), developed by the WHO, includes 10 questions about alcohol consumption and harmful experiences related to drinking.[64] The CAGE questionnaire asks whether adults feel they need to **C**ut down on their drinking, whether others have been **A**nnoyed by or criticized their drinking, whether they feel bad or **G**uilty about their

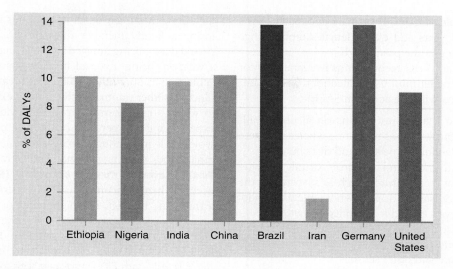

Figure 16.7 Percentage of disability-adjusted life years (DALYs) lost to alcohol consumption among men ages 20–54 years in selected countries.

Data from GBD 2019 Risk Factors Collaborators. Global burden of 87 risk factors in 204 countries and territories, 1990–2019: a systematic analysis for the Global Burden of Disease Study 2019. *Lancet.* 2020;396:1223–1249.

drinking, and whether they have felt the need to consume an **E**ye-opener drink first thing in the morning because of a hangover.[65]

Many males and females begin consuming alcohol and engaging in harmful alcohol consumption practices as adolescents (**Figure 16.8**).[61] For adolescents, the CRAFFT screening tool evaluates harmful use of alcohol and other substances by asking whether the individual has ever ridden in a **C**ar when the driver was under the influence; used alcohol or drugs to **R**elax, feel better, or fit in; used substances when **A**lone; forgotten ("**F**orget") things done when under the influence; been told by **F**amily or **F**riends to cut down on drinking or drug use; or gotten in **T**rouble because of substance use.[66] In the United States, for

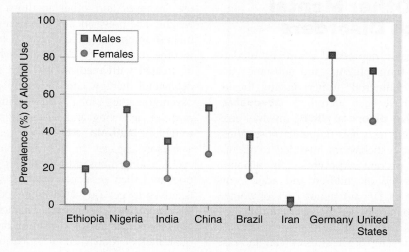

Figure 16.8 Current drinking among adolescents (ages 15–19 years) in selected countries, by sex.

Data from *Global Status Report on Alcohol and Health 2018.* Geneva: World Health Organization; 2018.

example, about 5% of male adolescents ages 12–17 years and 6% of females report binge drinking in the past month.[56]

The WHO recommends five strategies for reducing harmful use of alcohol that are summarized with the acronym SAFER:

- **S**trengthen restrictions on alcohol availability, such as regulating when and where alcohol can be sold and distributed
- **A**dvance and enforce drunk driving countermeasures, such as suspending the licenses of drivers whose blood alcohol levels exceed legal limits
- **F**acilitate access to screening, brief interventions, and treatment in primary health care and other settings
- **E**nforce bans or comprehensive restrictions on alcohol advertising, sponsorship, and promotion (especially marketing to legal minors)
- **R**aise prices on alcohol through taxes and other pricing policies[67]

For people who have alcohol use disorders, community-based detoxification and self-help groups can be effective interventions for reducing harmful drinking behaviors.[68]

16.8 Other Mental Health Disorders

Besides major depressive disorders, anxiety disorders, schizophrenia, and substance use disorders, numerous other mental health disorders have been identified. **Obsessive-compulsive disorder (OCD)** involves anxiety-inducing recurrent thoughts (obsessions) and repetitive behaviors intended to reduce distress or prevent bad events (compulsions). About 2.5–3% of children and adolescents experience OCD,[69] and about 1.5% of women and 1.0% of men experience OCD during their adult years.[70] CBT can effectively treat OCD.[69]

Trauma and other stresses can increase the risk of a mental health disorder. The most frequently occurring types of traumatic events include witnessing a death or a serious injury, losing a family member or friend to unexpected death, being mugged or threatened with a weapon, being involved in a serious motor vehicle collision, and having a life-threatening illness.[71] Other traumas include being exposed to war or other forms of collective violence, experiencing interpersonal or intimate partner violence, living through a natural disaster, and other types of personal and family traumas. **Posttraumatic stress disorder (PTSD)** occurs when someone who has experienced a traumatic incident has nightmares or other types of distressing recollections of the event and exhibits physiological signs of hyperarousal, such as hypervigilance and insomnia.[72] People with PTSD typically seek to avoid reminders of the traumatic event. Trauma-focused CBT, eye movement desensitization and reprocessing therapy, and other types of CBT can be effective at reducing symptoms.[73]

Individuals with feeding and eating disorders exhibit unhealthy eating behaviors. The word **anorexia** means a lack of appetite. **Anorexia nervosa** is an eating disorder in which a person has a distorted body image and feels overweight even when emaciated. A person with anorexia nervosa may follow a very restricted diet, exercise excessively, and use laxatives and other methods of losing weight. The prevalence of anorexia nervosa is highest among adolescent females from high-income countries.[74] Anorexia nervosa can be treated with medication (such as SSRIs), behavioral therapy, family therapy, and other psychotherapies along with nutritional support for achieving and sustaining a healthy weight.[75] **Bulimia nervosa** occurs when a person engages in frequent binge–purge cycles, eating thousands of calories at one sitting, and then inducing vomiting and using laxatives to get rid of the ingested calories. **Binge-eating disorder** is characterized by repeated incidents of consumption of large quantities of food without subsequent purging. In high- and upper-middle-income countries, about 1% of people experience bulimia nervosa during their lifetimes, and about 2% experience binge-eating disorder.[76] CBT can be effective for treating bulimia nervosa and binge-eating disorder.[77]

A variety of other mental health issues are described in the DSM-5, including dissociative disorders; somatic disorders; sleep–wake disorders such as insomnia and narcolepsy; sexual dysfunctions; a variety of disruptive, impulse-control, and conduct (DIC) disorders; and personality disorders.[16] The DSM is mostly designed for the U.S. population. Constructs like stress and depression, which are well understood in the U.S. population, may be framed differently in other cultures, such as being described as "thinking too much."[78] Clinical guidelines in other countries may use alternative diagnostic criteria that incorporate their own cultural concepts of distress.[79]

16.9 Suicide

Suicide is the intentional act of ending one's own life. Thinking about suicide is not uncommon. Each year about 2% of adults have thoughts about committing suicide (suicidal ideation), about 0.7% think about how they would commit suicide (suicidal planning), and about 0.4% make a suicide attempt (**Figure 16.9**).[80] The rates of suicidal ideating, planning, and attempting are similar in countries across the income spectrum. Most people who report having suicidal thoughts do not attempt suicide, and most suicide attempts do not result in death. Globally, there are about 20 suicide attempts and other potentially fatal acts of self-harm for every one reported suicide death.[81] However, it is important for all people who are thinking about suicide to understand the thoughts, feelings, and behaviors that led to suicidal ideation. Trained mental health workers are best able to assist with this process.

As awareness of suicide warning signs and effective prevention strategies has increased, the mortality rate from self-harm

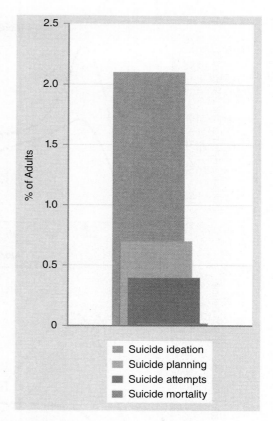

Figure 16.9 Percentage of adults reporting suicidal ideation, planning, and attempts in a one-year period.

Data from Borges G, Nock MK, Haro Abad JM, et al. Twelve month prevalence of and risk factors for suicide attempts in the WHO World Mental Health Surveys. *J Clin Psychiatry.* 2010;71:1617–1628.

has decreased in most world regions.[82] However, suicide continues to be a significant cause of preventable mortality. Globally, the proportion of deaths from self-harm is highest among younger adults, but the rate of death from self-harm is highest among older adults (**Figure 16.10**).[5] Young adults have a high proportionate mortality rate from suicide because the overall mortality rate in this age group is low. With few young adults dying from chronic diseases and other conditions each year, suicide stands out as a relatively frequent cause of mortality. By contrast, older adults have a high overall mortality rate, with many members of this age

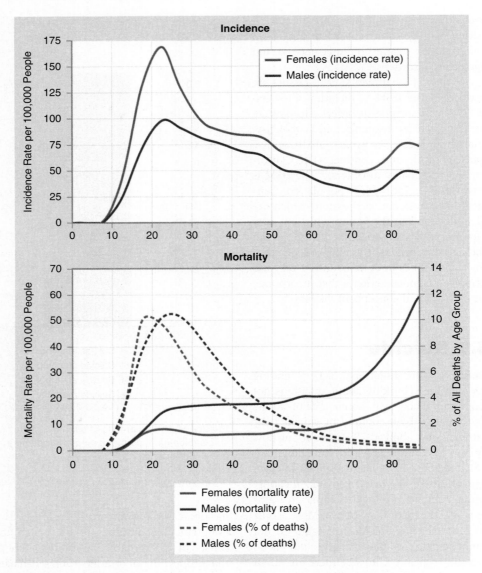

Figure 16.10 Incidence rate per 100,000 people, mortality rate per 100,000 people, and percentage of deaths from self-harm, by sex.

Data from GBD 2019 Diseases and Injuries Collaborators. Global burden of 369 diseases and injuries in 204 countries and territories, 1990–2019: a systematic analysis for the Global Burden of Disease Study 2019. *Lancet.* 2020;396:1204–1222.

cohort dying each year from cardiovascular diseases, cancers, and other chronic conditions. Because the overall death rate is high, deaths from self-harm are a small percentage of all deaths of older adults, even in countries where the suicide rate is highest among the oldest people. The suicide rate varies significantly between countries, even within the same world region, but the general pattern of higher suicide mortality rates per 100,000 in older adulthood is observed in most countries (**Figure 16.11**).[5]

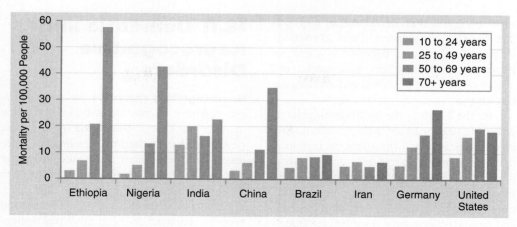

Figure 16.11 Mortality rate from self-harm per 100,000 people by age group in selected countries.

Data from GBD 2019 Diseases and Injuries Collaborators. Global burden of 369 diseases and injuries in 204 countries and territories, 1990–2019: a systematic analysis for the Global Burden of Disease Study 2019. *Lancet.* 2020;396:1204–1222.

Suicides are preventable, and numerous interventions from the individual to the societal level can help reduce the suicide rate. The WHO's "LIVE LIFE" approach calls for four key interventions:

- Limit access to firearms, pesticides, other poisons, and other means of suicide
- Interact with the media to improve responsible reporting of suicide and remove harmful content
- Foster social and emotional skills among adolescents
- Early identification, assessment, and management of suicidal behaviors at all ages[83]

Access to clinical mental health care is critical for people who are thinking or talking about ending their lives or are expressing hopelessness and ambivalence about living or dying. Community-based social support services, including crisis hotlines, can be lifesaving for people who have survived wars and disasters, been displaced from their home communities or imprisoned, encountered systemic discrimination, been abused or bullied, suffered from chronic pain, or experienced other forms of trauma and social disconnection.[84]

Many types of mental health disorders are associated with an increased risk of suicide, including schizophrenia, depressive disorders, bipolar disorder, some types of anxiety disorders, and substance use disorders.[80] However, most people with mental health disorders do not engage in self-harm, and suicide is not the leading cause of the increased risk of premature death among people with mental health disorders.[85] Instead, psychiatric disorders lead to reduced use of preventive health services (such as vaccination and cancer screening), poorer management of other chronic health conditions (such as hypertension and diabetes), and the adoption of unhealthy behaviors (such as tobacco use and physical inactivity), and those risk factors increase the risk of premature mortality.[86] Access to comprehensive health services, not just access to emergency psychiatric care, is required to reduce the rate of preventable mortality among people with mental health disorders and others who may be contemplating suicide.

16.10 Autism and Neurodevelopmental Disorders

Mental health disorders are often grouped with developmental disorders and neurological disorders under a broader umbrella of neuropsychiatric disorders. **Neurodevelopmental disorders** are neurological and developmental disorders that present in childhood. Early intervention for neurodevelopmental disorders is helpful for improving behavior, school achievement, and quality of life among children and enabling the best long-term outcomes as they age.[87]

In the DSM-5, the neurodevelopmental disorder category includes intellectual disabilities, communication disorders, autism spectrum disorder, attention-deficit/hyperactivity disorder (ADHD), specific learning disorders, motor disorders, and other early-onset conditions.[16] The most prevalent childhood mental and neurodevelopmental disorders are anxiety disorders, ADHD, conduct disorder, autism, and intellectual disabilities.[88] The prevalence of anxiety disorders is estimated to increase from about 2% among 5- to 9-year-olds to 4% among 10- to 14-year-olds and 5% among 15- to 19-year-olds.[5] CBT can successfully treat anxiety disorders in children and adolescents.[89] About 3% of schoolchildren have ADHD,[5] and about half of those young people will continue to have ADHD in adulthood.[90] Medications can be effective for managing the symptoms of ADHD.[91] About 3% of schoolchildren have conduct disorder, with the rate twice as high among boys than among girls, and family therapy and medications can help manage symptoms.[92]

Autism is a lifelong neurodevelopmental disorder that begins in early childhood and causes mild to severe challenges with social communication and other functions.[93] About 1 in 130 people worldwide may have an autism spectrum disorder, and this rate appears to be roughly consistent across regions when the same diagnostic criteria are applied.[94] There is uncertainty about whether the prevalence of autism has increased over the past few decades or whether changing definitions have added additional cases to the "spectrum" that is covered by autism spectrum disorders; the causes of autism remain poorly understood.[95] Early interventions can improve cognitive and language skills as well as behavior among children with autism spectrum disorders.[96]

16.11 Dementia and Neurocognitive Disorders

Neurocognitive disorders are neurological and cognitive disorders that typically develop in older adulthood. **Dementia** is a chronic syndrome characterized by memory loss, confusion, and other signs of impaired cognitive function. Over time, people with dementia often develop speech and communication difficulties, disorientation to time and place, and mood and behavior changes.[97] As the symptoms of dementia become worse, adults with the condition may be unable to live independently. **Alzheimer's disease** is the most prevalent form of dementia, accounting for about two-thirds of diagnosed dementia cases.[98] Dementia may also be caused by blocked blood vessels and strokes (vascular dementia), the buildup of alpha-synuclein proteins in the brain (Lewy body dementia), and other pathological processes.[99]

About 5–7% of adults aged 60 years and older have a form of dementia; the prevalence of dementia increases dramatically with age, increasing from less than 1% at age 60 years to more than 10% by age 80 years and more than 25% by age 90 years.[100] Nearly 50 million people worldwide had dementia in 2015, and the prevalence is expected to increase to at least 75 million by 2030 and more than 130 million by 2050 as the world population grows and ages.[98] About 10 million people develop dementia each year. Many people with dementia remain undiagnosed. Among those who have been diagnosed as having dementia, many are not receiving care or are receiving inadequate health care and social support.[101] Families provide most of the care for people with dementia, and they often experience physical, emotional, and financial stress.[102] Dementia awareness campaigns can reduce stigma, increase social inclusion, and protect the dignity and human rights of people with dementia; healthcare, psychological, and social support services for people with dementia and their families, including caregiver education and respite services for caregivers, can support quality of life as the dementia progresses.[98]

Not all neurocognitive disorders are related to aging. Some are the result of injuries. **Traumatic brain injury (TBI)** is short- or long-term damage arising from a concussion or other form of intracranial injury sustained during a traffic collision, fall, violent encounter, sporting event, or other cause of head trauma.[103] Severe and moderate TBI can cause death or permanent cognitive impairment. Even mild TBI may cause several months of cognitive deficits. A variety of rehabilitation strategies can improve memory, cognition, social communication, emotional regulation, and other functions after a TBI.[104]

16.12 Mental Health Care

Most mental health disorders are treatable (**Figure 16.12**). Medications can relieve symptoms and prevent relapses, therapy can help people with mental health disorders understand and change their thoughts and behaviors, and social rehabilitation that focuses on practical skills can help people with psychiatric conditions return to typical activities. A variety of professionals are equipped to offer mental health care. A **psychiatrist** is a physician with advanced training in mental health care who is licensed to prescribe medications. A **psychologist** has advanced training in counseling and is licensed to offer a variety of types of individual and group therapy. Nurses, social workers, and other healthcare and social service professionals may also be trained and licensed to offer mental health care.

Psychiatric hospitals, mental health clinics, the psychiatric departments of general hospitals, and other medical facilities may offer medications, CBT, psychotherapy (talk therapy), and other medical treatments for mental health disorders as well as behavioral health services that use holistic approaches to change behaviors related to substance abuse, eating disorders, and other behaviors that adversely affect overall well-being. Primary

Level of Prevention	Primordial Prevention	Primary Prevention	Secondary Prevention	Tertiary Prevention
Goal	Prevent risk factors for mental health disorders	Mitigate risk factors in people without mental health disorders	Detect mild mental health disorders	Manage moderate and severe mental health disorders
Examples of interventions	■ Practice a healthy lifestyle, such as getting regular exercise and adequate sleep ■ Support healthy social environments ■ Combat the stigma associated with mental health disorders ■ Avoid harmful substances	■ Manage stress ■ Manage physical health problems ■ Cultivate healthy relationships	■ Screen for depression	■ Engage in cognitive behavioral therapy and other types of counseling ■ Take medications to manage psychosis, depression, anxiety, and other conditions

Figure 16.12 Examples of interventions for mental health.

care providers and community service organizations, including religious organizations, may also provide services for individuals and families seeking assistance with mental and behavioral health.[105]

Many people who would benefit from mental and behavioral health services do not have access to specialty care. Considerably fewer than half of adults with severe mental health disorders receive any mental healthcare services, and an even lower proportion of people with mild or moderate mental health disorders receive medical care.[106] Access is especially limited in lower-income countries. There are far fewer psychiatrists, psychiatric nurses, psychologists, and other mental healthcare workers per capita in low-income countries than in high-income countries (**Figure 16.13**).[107] High-income countries have about 30 times more inpatient psychiatric hospital beds per capita, 20 times more inpatient admissions per 100,000 population, and more than 60 times higher outpatient treatment visits per capita than low-income countries.[107] The prevalence of mental health disorders is similar across countries and cultures, so the need for psychiatric care is similar across countries. The very low rates of treatment in lower-income countries are evidence that millions of people with severe mental health disorders are not receiving necessary medical care.

Even when mental health services are available, they may be underused. Many people do not know that medical or behavioral care can help them manage their symptoms and improve their quality of life, so they do not seek clinical help. Fear of the stigma of being diagnosed with a mental illness prevents some people from seeking treatment. Additionally, the risk factors for mental health disorders include living in poverty, experiencing a conflict or disaster, and having a severe physical disease, so the populations that have the greatest need for mental health services often have the least ability to access them.[108]

The majority of the funding allocated to mental health care is spent on long-term inpatient care rather than on more cost-effective interventions like community-based treatment.[109] The public health actions for improving mental health care include educating the public about mental health disorders, providing mental health treatment as part of primary health care, and involving communities and families in caring for people with psychiatric conditions.[110] When social groups, employers, and public service providers (including the healthcare, education, and justice systems) are prepared to support people with mental health disorders, most people with psychiatric conditions are able to actively engage in social events, participate in the economy, and be protected from discrimination and violence.[111]

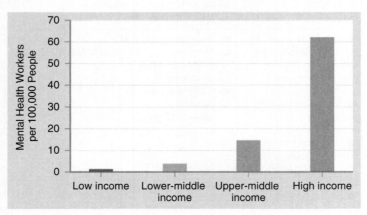

Figure 16.13 Mental health workers per 100,000 people by country income level (including psychiatrists, psychiatric nurses, psychologists, mental health social workers, and other paid mental health workers).

Data from *Mental Health Atlas 2020*. Geneva: World Health Organization; 2021.

Interventions that support healthy behaviors, stress management, self-efficacy, resilience, and other dimensions of holistic well-being can increase the psychosocial health of all people.[112] For example, all adolescents can benefit from interventions that help them develop emotional regulation and interpersonal skills and reduce risk behaviors.[113] A shift toward preventing mental health disorders rather than treating them after they occur would require major investments in research and a willingness to overhaul the entire healthcare system.[114] However, there is already evidence that mental health promotion across the life span would be valuable for supporting individual physical, mental, and social health and achieving population-level goals for health equity.[1]

References

1. Patel V, Saxena S, Lund C, et al. The Lancet Commission on global mental health and sustainable development. *Lancet.* 2018;392:1553–1598.

2. Steel Z, Marnane C, Iranpour C, et al. The global prevalence of common mental disorders: a systematic review and meta-analysis 1980–2013. *Int J Epidemiol.* 2014;43:476–493.

3. Bruffaerts R, Vilagut G, Demyttenaere K, et al. Role of common mental and physical disorders in partial disability around the world. *Br J Psychitar.* 2012;200:454–461.

4. Sánchez J, Rosenthal DA, Chan F, Brooks J, Bezyak JL. Relationships between World Health Organization International Classification of Functioning, Disability and Health constructs and participation in adults with severe mental illness. *Rehabil Res Policy Educ.* 2016;30:286–304.

5. GBD 2019 Diseases and Injuries Collaborators. Global burden of 369 diseases and injuries in 204 countries and territories, 1990–2019: a systematic analysis for the Global Burden of Disease Study 2019. *Lancet.* 2020;396:1204–1222.

6. *Depression and Other Common Mental Disorders: Global Health Estimates.* Geneva: World Health Organization; 2017.

7. Patel V, Chisholm, Parikh R, et al. Global priorities for addressing the burden of mental, neurological, and substance use disorders (chapter 1). In: Patel V, Chisholm D, Dua T, Laxminarayan R, Medina-Mora ME, eds. *Disease Control Priorities: Mental, Neurological, and Substance Use Disorders.* 3rd ed. Vol. 4. Washington DC: IBRD/World Bank; 2015:1–28.

8. Hyman S, Collins PY, Parikh R, Patel V. Adult mental disorders (chapter 4). In: Patel V, Chisholm D, Dua T, Laxminarayan R, Medina-Mora ME, eds. *Disease Control Priorities: Mental, Neurological, and Substance Use Disorders.* 3rd ed. Vol. 4. Washington DC: IBRD/World Bank; 2015:67–86.

9. Collins PY, Patel V, Joestl SS, March D, Insel TR, Daar AS. Grand challenges in global mental health. *Nature.* 2011;475:27–30.

10. *Transforming Our World: The 2030 Agenda for Sustainable Development.* New York: United Nations; 2015.

11. Whiteford HA, Ferrari AJ, Degenhardt L, Feigin V, Vos T. Global burden of mental, neurological, and substance use disorders: an analysis from the Global Burden of Disease Study 2010 (chapter 2). In: Patel V, Chisholm D, Dua T, Laxminarayan R, Medina-Mora ME, eds. *Disease Control Priorities: Mental, Neurological, and Substance Use Disorders.* 3rd ed. Vol. 4. Washington DC: IBRD/World Bank; 2015:29–40.

12. *Guidance on Community Mental Health Services: Promoting Person-Centered and Rights-Based Approaches.* Geneva: World Health Organization; 2021.

13. Becker AE, Kleinman A. Mental health and the global agenda. *New Engl J Med.* 2013;369:66–73.

14. Malhi GS, Mann JJ. Depression. *Lancet.* 2018;392: 2299–2312.

15. Ferrari AJ, Somerville AJ, Baxter AJ, et al. Global variation in the prevalence and incidence of major depressive disorder: a systematic review of the epidemiological literature. *Psychol Med.* 2013;43:471–481.

16. *Diagnostic and Statistical Manual of Mental Disorders (DSM-5).* 5th ed. Arlington VA: American Psychiatric Association Publishing; 2013.

17. Kessler RC, Bromet EJ. The epidemiology of depression across cultures. *Annu Rev Public Health.* 2013;34:119–138.

18. Simon GE, Goldberg DP, Von Korff M, Ustün TB. Understanding cross-national differences in depression prevalence. *Psychol Med.* 2002;32:585–594.

19. Hölzel L, Härter M, Reese C, Kriston L. Risk factors for chronic depression: a systematic review. *J Affect Disord.* 2011;129:1–13.

20. Lotfaliany M, Bowe SJ, Kowal P, Orellana L, Berk M, Mohebbi M. Depression and chronic diseases: co-occurrence and communality of risk factors. *J Affect Dis.* 2018;241:461–468.

21. Patel V, Simon G, Chowdhary N, Kaaya S, Araya R. Packages of care for depression in low- and middle-income countries. *PLoS Med.* 2009;6:e1000159.

22. *World Health Organization Model List of Essential Medicines, 22nd list.* Geneva: World Health Organization; 2021.

23. Ramsberg J, Asseburg C, Henrisksson M. Effectiveness and cost-effectiveness of antidepressants in primary care: a multiple treatment comparison meta-analysis and cost-effectiveness model. *PLoS One.* 2012;7:e42003.

24. Andrade LH, Alonso J, Mneimneh Z, et al. Barriers to mental health treatment: results from the WHO World Mental Health (WMH) surveys. *Psychol Med.* 2014;44:1303–1317.

25. *mhGAP Operations Manual.* Geneva: World Health Organization; 2018.

26. Penninx BWJH, Pine DS, Holmes EA, Reif A. Anxiety disorder. *Lancet.* 2021;397:914–927.

27. Stein MB, Sareen J. Generalized anxiety disorder. *N Engl J Med.* 2015;373:2059–2068.

28. Nardi AE, Balon R. The 40th anniversary of panic disorder. *J Clin Pharmacol.* 2020;40:105–108.

29. Leichsenring F, Leweke F. Social anxiety disorder. *N Engl J Med.* 2017;376:2255–2264.

30. De Jonge P, Roest AM, Lim CCW, et al. Cross-national epidemiology of panic disorder and panic attacks in the World Mental Health Surveys. *Depress Anxiety.* 2016;33:1155–1177.

31. Hovenkamp-Hermelink JHM, Jeronimus BF, Myroniuk S, Riese H, Schoevers RA. Predictors of persistence of anxiety disorders across the lifespan: a systematic review. *Lancet Psychiatr.* 2021;8:428–443.

32. Ruscio AM, Hallion LS, Lim CCW, et al. Cross-sectional comparison of the epidemiology of DSM-5 generalized anxiety disorder across the globe. *JAMA Psychiatr.* 2017;74:465–475.

33. COVID-19 Mental Disorders Collaborators. Global prevalence and burden of depressive and anxiety disorders in 204 countries and territories in 2020 due to the COVID-19 pandemic. *Lancet.* 2021;398:1700–1712.

34. Pompoli A, Furukawa TA, Efthimiou O, Imai H, Tajika A, Salanti G. Dismantling cognitive-behaviour therapy for panic disorder: a systematic review and component network meta-analysis. *Psychol Med.* 2018;48:1945–1953.

35. Alonso J, Liu Z, Evans-Lacko S, et al. Treatment gap for anxiety disorders is global: results of the World Mental Health Surveys in 21 countries. *Depress Anxiety.* 2018;35:195–208.

36. Tandon R, Gaebel W, Barch DM, et al. Definition and description of schizophrenia in the DSM-5. *Schizophr Res.* 2013;150:3–10.

37. McGrath J, Saha S, Chant D, Welham J. Schizophrenia: a concise overview of incidence, prevalence, and mortality. *Epidemiol Rev.* 2008;30:67–76.

38. Rajji TK, Ismail Z, Mulsant BH. Age at onset and cognition in schizophrenia: meta-analysis. *Br J Psychiatry.* 2009;195:286–293.

39. AlAqeel B, Margolese HC. Remission in schizophrenia: critical and systematic review. *Harv Rev Psychiatry.* 2012;20:281–297.

40. De Jesus MJ, Razzouk D, Thara R, Eaton J, Thornicroft G. Packages of care for schizophrenia in low- and middle-income countries. *PLoS Med.* 2009;6:e1000165.

41. Lora A, Kohn R, Levav I, McBain R, Morris J, Saxena S. Service availability and utilization and treatment gap for schizophrenic disorders: a survey in 50 low- and middle-income countries. *Bull World Health Organ.* 2012;90:47–54B.

42. Gerlinger G, Hauser M, De Hert M, Lacluyse K, Wampers M, Correll CU. Personal stigma in schizophrenia spectrum disorders: a systematic review of prevalence rates, correlates, impact and interventions. *World Psychiatry.* 2013;12:155–164.

43. Corrigan PW, Morris SB, Michaels PJ, Rafacz JD, Rüsch N. Challenging the public stigma of mental illness: a meta-analysis of outcome studies. *Psychiatr Serv.* 2012;63:963–973.

44. McIntyre RS, Berk M, Brietzke E, et al. Bipolar disorders. *Lancet.* 2020;396:1841–1856.

45. Merikangas KR, Jin R, He JP, et al. Prevalence and correlates of bipolar spectrum disorder in the World Mental Health Survey initiative. *Arch Gen Psychiatry.* 2011;68:241–251.

46. Jaeschke K, Hanna F, Ali S, Chowdhary N, Dua T, Charlson F. Global estimates of service coverage for severe mental disorders: findings from the WHO Mental Health Atlas 2017. *Glob Ment Health.* 2021;8:e27.

47. Geddes JR, Miklowitz DJ. Treatment of bipolar disorder. *Lancet.* 2013;381:1672–1682.

48. Hawke LD, Parikh SV, Michalak EE. Stigma and bipolar disorder: a review of the literature. *J Affect Disord.* 2013;150:181–191.

49. O'Brien C. Addiction and dependence in DSM-V. *Addiction.* 2011;106:866–867.

50. Alavi SS, Ferdosi M, Jannatifard F, Eslami M, Alaghemandan H, Setare M. Behavioral addiction versus substance addiction: correspondence of psychiatric and psychological views. *Int J Prev Med.* 2012;3:290–294.

51. *Public Policy Statement: Definition of Addiction.* Chevy Chase MD: American Society of Addiction Medicine; 2011.

52. Degenhardt L, Hall W. Extent of illicit drug use and dependence, and their contribution to the global burden of disease. *Lancet.* 2012;379:55–70.

53. Degenhardt L, Stockings E, Strang J, Hall WD. Illicit drug dependence (chapter 6). In: Patel V, Chisholm D, Dua T, Laxminarayan R, Medina-Mora ME, eds. *Disease Control Priorities: Mental, Neurological, and Substance Use Disorders.* 3rd ed. Vol. 4. Washington DC: IBRD/World Bank; 2015:109–126.

54. *World Drug Report 2016.* Vienna: United Nations Office on Drugs and Crime (UNODC); 2016.

55. Peacock A, Leung J, Larney S, et al. Global statistics on alcohol, tobacco and illicit drug use: 2017 status report. *Addiction.* 2018;113:1905–1926.

56. *Health, United States, 2019.* Hyattsville MD: National Center for Health Statistics; 2021.

57. *Facing Addition in America: The Surgeon General's Report on Alcohol, Drugs, and Health.* Washington DC: U.S. Department of Health & Human Services; 2016.

58. Ahmad FB, Rossen LM, Sutton P. *Provisional Drug Overdose Death Counts.* Hyattsville MD: National Center for Health Statistics; 2021.

59. Werb D, Bluthenthal RN, Kolla G, et al. Preventing injection drug use for initiation: state of the evidence and opportunities for the future. *J Urban Health.* 2018;95:91–98.

60. Medina-Mora M, Monteiro M, Room R, Rehm J, Jernigan D, Sanchez-Moreno D. Alcohol use and alcohol use disorders (chapter 7). In: Patel V, Chisholm D, Dua T, Laxminarayan R, Medina-Mora ME, eds. *Disease Control Priorities: Mental, Neurological, and Substance Use Disorders.* 3rd ed. Vol. 4. Washington DC: IBRD/World Bank; 2015:127–144.

61. *Global Status Report on Alcohol and Health 2018.* Geneva: World Health Organization; 2018.

62. Rehm J, Mathers C, Popova S, Thavorncharoensap M, Teerawattananon Y, Patra J. Global burden of disease and injury and economic cost attributable to alcohol use and alcohol use disorders. *Lancet.* 2009;373:2223–2233.

63. GBD 2019 Risk Factors Collaborators. Global burden of 87 risk factors in 204 countries and territories, 1990–2019: a systematic analysis for the Global Burden of Disease Study 2019. *Lancet.* 2020;396:1223–1249.

64. Saunders JB, Aasland OG, Babor TF, de la Fuente JR, Grant M. Development of the Alcohol Use Disorders Identification Test (AUDIT): WHO collaborative project on early detection of persons with harmful alcohol consumption – II. *Addiction.* 1993;88:791–804.

65. Dhalla S, Kopec JA. The CAGE questionnaire for alcohol misuse: a review of reliability and validity studies. *Clin Invest Med.* 2007;30:33–41.

66. Knight JR, Shrier LA, Bravender TD, Farrell M, Vander Bilt J, Shaffer HJ. A new brief screen for adolescent substance abuse. *Arch Pediatr Adolesc Med.* 1999;153:591–596.

67. *The SAFER Technical Package: Five Areas of Intervention at National and Subnational Levels.* Geneva: World Health Organization; 2019.

68. Benegal V, Chand PK, Obot IS. Packages of care for alcohol use disorders in low- and middle-income countries. *PLoS Med.* 2009;6:e100170.

69. Soomro GM. Obsessive compulsive disorder. *BMJ Clin Evid.* 2012;2012:1004.

70. Fawcett EJ, Power H, Fawcett JM. Women are at greater risk of OCD than men: a meta-analytic review of OCD prevalence worldwide. *J Clin Psychiatr.* 2020;81:19r13085.

71. Benjet C, Bromet E, Karam EG, et al. The epidemiology of traumatic event exposure worldwide: results from the World Mental Health Survey Consortium. *Psychol Med.* 2016;46:327–343.

72. Yehuda R. Post-traumatic stress disorder. *N Engl J Med.* 2002;346:108–114.

73. Bisson JI, Roberts NP, Andrew M, et al. Psychological therapies for chronic post-traumatic stress disorder (PTSD) in adults. *Cochrane Database Syst Rev.* 2013;2013:CD003388.

74. Smink FRE, van Hoeken D, Hoek HW. Epidemiology of eating disorders: incidence, prevalence and mortality rates. *Cu,r Psychiatry Rep.* 2012;14:406–414.

75. Murray SB, Quintana DS, Loeb KL, Griffiths S, Le Grange D. Treatment outcomes for anorexia nervosa: a systematic review and meta-analysis of randomized controlled trials. *Psychol Med.* 2019;49:535–544.

76. Kessler RC, Berglund PA, Chiu WT, et al. The prevalence and correlates of binge eating disorder in the WHO World Mental Health surveys. *Biol Psychiatry.* 2013;73:904–914.

77. Hilbert A, Petroff D, Herpertz S, et al. Meta-analysis of the efficacy of psychological and medical treatments for binge-eating disorder. *J Consult Clin Psychol.* 2019;87:91–105.

78. Lewis-Fernández R, Kirmayer LJ. Cultural concepts of distress and psychiatric disorders: understanding symptom experience and expression in context. *Transcultural Psychiatr.* 2019;56:786–803.

79. Kohrt BA, Rasmussen A, Kaiser BN, et al. Cultural concepts of distress and psychiatric disorders: literature review and research recommendations for global mental health epidemiology. *Int J Epidemiol.* 2014;43:365–406.

80. Borges G, Nock MK, Haro Abad JM, et al. Twelve month prevalence of and risk factors for suicide attempts in the WHO World Mental Health surveys. *J Clin Psychiatry.* 2010;71:1617–1628.

81. Vijayakumar L, Phillips MR, Silverman MM, Gunnell D, Carli V. Suicide (chapter 9). In: Patel V, Chisholm D, Dua T, Laxminarayan R, Medina-Mora ME, eds. *Disease Control Priorities: Mental, Neurological, and Substance Use Disorders.* 3rd ed. Vol. 4. Washington DC: IBRD/World Bank; 2015:163–182.

82. Alicandro G, Malvezzi M, Gallus S, La Vecchia C, Negri E, Bertuccio P. Worldwide trends in suicide mortality from 1990 to 2015 with a focus on the global recession time frame. *Int J Public Health*. 2019;64:785–795.

83. *Live Life: An Implementation Guide for Suicide Prevention in Countries*. Geneva: World Health Organization; 2021.

84. *Preventing Suicide: A Global Imperative*. Geneva: World Health Organization; 2014.

85. Charlson FJ, Baxter AJ, Dua T, Degenhardt L, Whiteford HA, Vos T. Excess mortality from mental, neurological, and substance use disorders in the Global Burden of Disease Study 2010 (chapter 3). In: Patel V, Chisholm D, Dua T, Laxminarayan R, Medina-Mora ME, eds. *Disease Control Priorities: Mental, Neurological, and Substance Use Disorders*. 3rd ed. Vol. 4. Washington DC: IBRD/World Bank; 2015:41–66.

86. Walker ER, McGee RE, Druss BG. Mortality in mental disorders and global disease burden implications: A systematic review and meta-analysis. *JAMA Psychiatry*. 2015;72:334–341.

87. Kieling C, Baker-Henningham H, Belfer M, et al. Child and adolescent mental health worldwide: evidence for action. *Lancet*. 2011;378:1515–1525.

88. Scott JG, Rahman A, Mihalopoulos C, Erskine HE, Roberts J. Childhood mental and developmental disorders (chapter 8). In: Patel V, Chisholm D, Dua T, Laxminarayan R, Medina-Mora ME, eds. *Disease Control Priorities: Mental, Neurological, and Substance Use Disorders*. 3rd ed. Vol. 4. Washington DC: IBRD/World Bank; 2015:145–162.

89. James AC, Reardon T, Soler A, James G, Creswell C. Cognitive behavioural therapy for anxiety disorders in children and adolescents. *Cochrane Database Syst Rev*. 2020;11:CD013162.

90. Caye A, Spadini AV, Karam RG, et al. Predictors of persistence of ADHD into adulthood: a systematic review of the literature and meta-analysis. *Eur Child Adolesc Psychiatry*. 2016;25:1151–1159.

91. Thapar A, Cooper M. Attention deficit hyperactivity disorder. *Lancet*. 2016;387:1240–1250.

92. Fairchild G, Hawes DL, Frick PJ, et al. *Conduct disorder. Nat Rev Dis Primers*. 2019;5:43.

93. Constantino JN, Charman T. Diagnosis of autism spectrum disorder: reconciling the syndrome, its diverse origins, and variation in expression. *Lancet Neurol*. 2016;15:279–291.

94. Baxter AJ, Brugha TS, Erskine HE, Scheurer RW, Vos T, Scott JG. The epidemiology and global burden of autism spectrum disorders. *Psychol Med*. 2015;45:601–613.

95. Hodges H, Fealko C, Soares N. Autism spectrum disorder: definition, epidemiology, causes, and clinical evaluation. *Transl Pediatr*. 2020;9(Suppl 1):S55–S65.

96. Warren Z, McPheeters ML, Sathe N, Foss-Feig JH, Glasser A, Veenstra-Vanderweele J. A systematic review of early intensive intervention for autism spectrum disorders. *Pediatrics*. 2011;127:e1303–e1311.

97. *Dementia: A Public Health Priority*. Geneva: World Health Organization; 2012.

98. *Global Action Plan on the Public Health Response to Dementia 2017–2025*. Geneva: World Health Organization; 2017.

99. *World Alzheimer Report 2021*. London: Alzheimer's Disease International; 2021.

100. Prince M, Bryce R, Albanese E, Wimo A, Ribeiro W, Ferri CP. The global prevalence of dementia: a systematic review and metaanalysis. *Alzheimer's Dement*. 2013;9:65–75.

101. *Global Status Report on the Public Health Response to Dementia*. Geneva: World Health Organization; 2021.

102. *Toward a Dementia Inclusive Society*. Geneva: World Health Organization; 2021.

103. Maas AIR, Menon DK, Adelson PD, et al. Traumatic brain injury: integrated approaches to improve prevention, clinical care, and research. *Lancet Neurol*. 2017;16:987–1048.

104. Cicerone KD, Goldin Y, Ganci K, et al. Evidence-based cognitive rehabilitation: systematic review of the literature from 2009 through 2014. *Arch Phys Med Rehabil*. 2019;100:1515–1533.

105. Shidhaye R, Lund C, Chishold D. Health care platform interventions (chapter 11). In: Patel V, Chisholm D, Dua T, Laxminarayan R, Medina-Mora ME, eds. *Disease Control Priorities: Mental, Neurological, and Substance Use Disorders*. 3rd ed. Vol. 4. Washington DC: IBRD/World Bank; 2015:201–218.

106. Wang PS, Aguilar-Gaxiola S, Alonsa J, et al. Use of mental health services for anxiety, mood, and substance disorders in 17 countries in the WHO World Mental Health Surveys. *Lancet*. 2007;370:841–850.

107. *Mental Health Atlas 2020*. Geneva: World Health Organization; 2021.

108. *Comprehensive Mental Health Action Plan 2013–2030*. Geneva: World Health Organization; 2021.

109. Levin C, Chisholm D. Cost-effectiveness and affordability of interventions, policies, and platforms for the prevention and treatment of mental, neurological, and substance use disorders (chapter 12). In: Patel V, Chisholm D, Dua T, Laxminarayan R, Medina-Mora ME, eds. *Disease Control Priorities: Mental, Neurological, and Substance Use Disorders*. 3rd ed. Vol. 4. Washington DC: IBRD/World Bank; 2015:219–236.

110. Petersen I, Evans-Lacko S, Semrau M, et al. Population and community platform interventions (chapter 10). In: Patel V, Chisholm D, Dua T, Laxminarayan R, Medina-Mora ME, eds. *Disease

Control Priorities: Mental, Neurological, and Substance Use Disorders. 3rd ed. Vol. 4. Washington DC: IBRD/World Bank; 2015:183–200.

111. Herrman H, Saxena S, Moddie R, eds. *Promoting Mental Health: Concepts, Emerging Evidence, Practice: Summary Report.* Geneva: World Health Organization; 2004.

112. Min JA, Lee CU, Lee C. Mental health promotion and illness prevention: a challenge for psychiatrists. *Psychiatry Investig.* 2013;10:307–316.

113. Skeen S, Laurenzi CA, Gordon SL, et al. Adolescent mental health promotion components and behavior risk reduction: a meta-analysis. *Pediatrics.* 2019;144:e20183488.

114. Wainberg ML, Scorza P, Shultz JM, et al. Challenges and opportunities in global mental health: a research-to-practice perspective. *Curr Psychiatry Rep.* 2017;19:28.

CHAPTER 17

Injury Prevention

Road traffic injuries, falls, drowning, burns, self-harm, interpersonal violence, armed conflict, and other causes of unintentional and intentional injuries are significant contributors to disability and death across the life span, especially for men. Most injuries can be prevented with educational, environmental, and policy interventions tailored to populations at risk of specific types of injuries.

17.1 Injuries and Global Health

An **injury** is physical damage to the body inflicted by an external force.[1] An injury may take the form of trauma to the brain or spinal cord, a fracture of a bone, a strain or sprain of a joint, a deep gash that tears through the skin, damage to internal organs, or another type of wound. Mild injuries may cause a few days or weeks of pain and activity limitations. Moderate and severe trauma may cause long-term disability or death. About 1 in 13 deaths worldwide each year is due to an injury.[2] Nonfatal injuries can cause permanent disability, such as cognitive impairment from head trauma, paralysis from spinal trauma, limb amputations from crush wounds, joint contractures from burns, and severe mobility limitations from poorly healed fractures and joint injuries.

Injuries are divided into two main categories—unintentional and intentional—and both types of injuries can be averted.

An **unintentional injury** is an unplanned injury that happens very quickly, like the injuries that occur when someone is involved in a motor vehicle collision, falls off a ladder, slips on ice, spills a pot of hot water, or cuts a finger while chopping vegetables. An **accident** is an unfortunate event that happens by chance. Most unintentional injuries are not inescapable accidents that happen simply because of bad luck. Unintentional injuries can be prevented with safety measures such as the use of safety belts and child car seats in motor vehicles, helmets for cyclists, designated drivers who have not consumed alcohol, safety harnesses when working at dangerous heights, flame-resistant clothing, smoke detectors, fencing around bodies of water, swimming lessons, protective eyewear, and hundreds of other preventive safety measures that can be implemented by individuals, households, workplaces, and communities.[3] An **intentional injury** is a purposefully inflicted physical trauma. Psychosocial interventions can reduce both self-directed violence and violent behaviors that are directed at others.[4]

Injury prevention interventions must be tailored to the types of injuries most likely to affect targeted populations. Males have higher rates of unintentional and intentional injury incidence and mortality than females (**Figure 17.1**).[2] The higher rates in males are attributed to males being more likely than females to spend time on the road, work in hazardous occupations, participate in dangerous recreational activities, use alcohol, and be involved in fighting and armed conflict.[5] For males, the overall rate of new injuries is highest in early adulthood and late adulthood; for females, the injury incidence rate is steady across most age groups prior to increasing in old age (**Figure 17.2**).[2] While the overall death rate from injuries is highest among older adults, the proportionate mortality from injuries—that is, the percentage of deaths within an age group or other population that are attributable to injuries rather than to other causes—is greatest among adolescents and young adults.[2] These health statistics point toward a need for more injury prevention interventions targeted toward males, young adults, and the oldest adults.

People residing in lower-income areas have an increased risk of injuries that are associated with living, working, and attending school in unsafe environments.[6] Exposure to poisons, fire, extreme weather, and physical trauma occurs more often in places where there is limited access to safe waste disposal, food must be prepared over a fire, residential structures are not built to withstand earthquakes and other natural disasters, and enforcement of occupational and

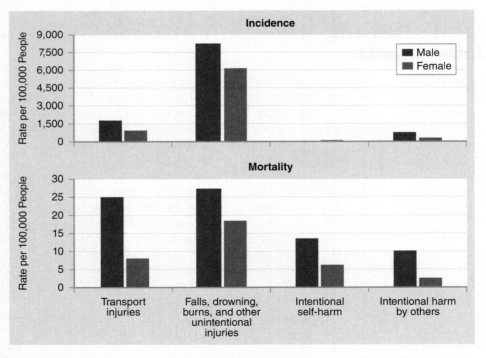

Figure 17.1 Incidence and mortality rates per 100,000 people for major types of injuries, by sex.

Data from GBD 2019 Diseases and Injuries Collaborators. Global burden of 369 diseases and injuries in 204 countries and territories, 1990–2019: a systematic analysis for the Global Burden of Disease Study 2019. *Lancet.* 2020;396:1204–1222.

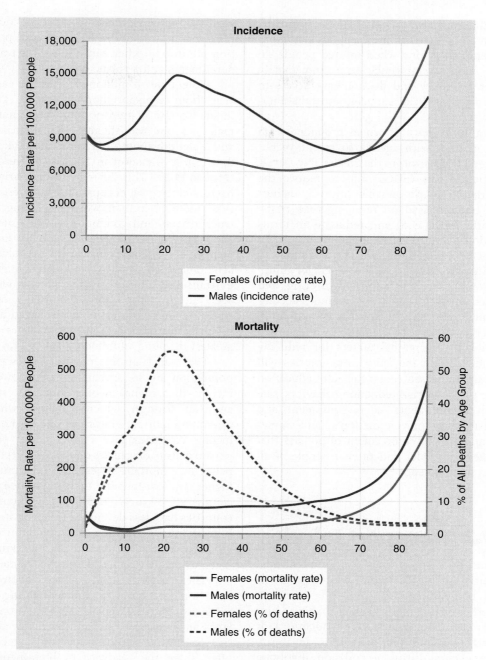

Figure 17.2 Injury incidence rate (new cases) per 100,000 people, injury mortality rate per 100,000 people, and percentage of total deaths from injuries, by sex and age.

Data from GBD 2019 Diseases and Injuries Collaborators. Global burden of 369 diseases and injuries in 204 countries and territories, 1990–2019: a systematic analysis for the Global Burden of Disease Study 2019. *Lancet*. 2020;396:1204–1222.

road safety laws is minimal. The impairment caused by injuries may also be more severe and lasting when injured people do not receive emergency care immediately after an injury and do not have access to advanced medical, surgical, and rehabilitation services.

Injuries have grown in prominence on the global health agenda in recent years.[7] Several targets within the Sustainable Development Goals (SDGs) aim to reduce the burden from preventable injuries, including ones focused on reducing road traffic injuries (SDG 3.6) and reducing all forms of violence (SDG 16.1), including homicide; armed conflict; and physical, psychological, and sexual violence.[8] The "3 Es" of injury prevention are education, engineering, and enforcement. (These are sometimes accompanied by additional Es, such as economics, emergency services, evaluation, and equity.[9]) Achieving the global targets for reducing incidence and mortality from injuries will require increased access to health education that promotes risk-reduction behaviors; safe built environments, safety equipment, and other injury prevention tools; and implementation and enforcement of policies that make roads safer and protect people of all ages from violence.[10]

17.2 Transport Injuries

Transportation injuries are unintentional injuries that occur while people or goods are being conveyed from one place to another via a motor vehicle, ship, train, aircraft, or other carrier. A road injury, or **road traffic injury** (RTI), is an injury that occurs during a collision involving at least one moving motor vehicle.[11] The drivers and passengers of trucks, vans, cars, motorcycles, and other motor vehicles involved in collisions may sustain RTIs and so may bicyclists and pedestrians who are struck by moving vehicles or debris. Most transport injuries are RTIs, but a small portion are due to other causes, such as train derailments and airplane crashes.

More than 1 million people die each year from transportation injuries.[12] The incidence rate of transport injuries among males is about twice the rate among females, and males are about three times more likely to die from transport injuries than females (**Figure 17.3**).[2] This differential likely arises from a variety of occupational differences (like more men than women working as truck drivers and commuting to job sites) and behavioral differences (such as men being more likely to engage in risk-taking activities).[13] The rate of deaths attributable to transport injuries rises gradually with age, but the proportionate mortality rate (the percentage of deaths in a selected age group that are due to transport injuries) is greatest in young adulthood (**Figure 17.4**).[2]

The road transport mortality rates per population are somewhat higher in lower-income than higher-income countries, and an even stronger pattern emerges when examining mortality rates per vehicle. Low-income countries have a much lower per-person density of vehicles on the road, yet the per-vehicle mortality rates tend to be much higher in low-income than high-income countries (**Figure 17.5**).[14] Low-income countries have less developed transportation infrastructure than high-income countries, with fewer paved roads and road markings (such as painted centerlines and edgelines), few safety barriers to divert vehicles away from roadside hazards, limited lighting of roads at night, less signage, few motorcycle lanes and bicycle paths, and few sidewalks and crosswalks.[14] Pedestrians and vehicles often share the roadway. In high-income countries, most vehicle collisions involve two motor vehicles striking one another; in lower-income countries, the victims of a collision are more often motorcyclists or pedestrians who are struck by a car or truck

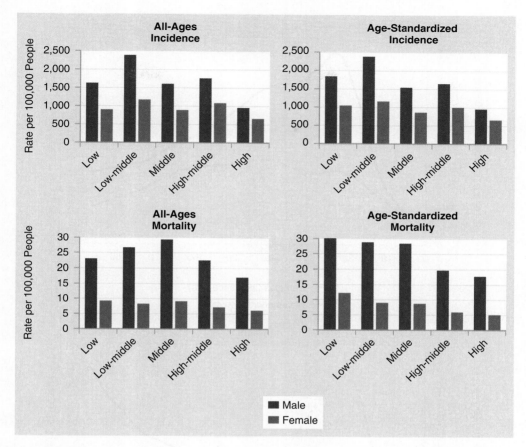

Figure 17.3 All-ages and age-standardized transport injury incidence and mortality rates per 100,000 people, by sex and country sociodemographic group.

Data from GBD 2019 Diseases and Injuries Collaborators. Global burden of 369 diseases and injuries in 204 countries and territories, 1990–2019: a systematic analysis for the Global Burden of Disease Study 2019. *Lancet.* 2020;396:1204–1222.

(**Figure 17.6**).[14] The difference in mortality rates by country income level is exacerbated by people in low- and middle-income countries having less access to emergency medical and surgical care.

The global road mortality rate remained at about 18 per 100,000 people per year from 2000 through 2015, but the mortality rate per 100,000 vehicles decreased from about 135 per 100,000 vehicles to about 65 per 100,000 vehicles.[14] The SDGs aimed to halve the number of RTIs and the annual rate of RTI mortality between 2016 and 2020.[8] That target was not achieved, but

a follow-up plan approved by the United Nations (UN) aims to achieve that 50% reduction between 2021 and 2030.[15]

Transportation laws can help make roads safer and reduce the risk of road injuries.[14] Speed limits can be lowered and enforced, such as limiting urban speed limits to 30 kilometers per hour (20 miles per hour) for local streets that are not highways.[16] Motorcycle helmets can be mandated for drivers and passengers. Seat belts can be required for all car drivers and passengers.[17] The use of child car seats or other restraints for infants and small children can

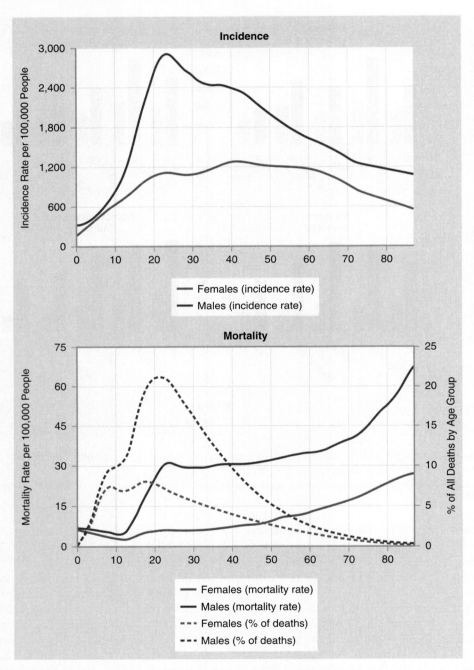

Figure 17.4 Incidence rate per 100,000 people, mortality rate per 100,000 people, and percentage of deaths from transport injuries, by sex and age.

Data from GBD 2019 Diseases and Injuries Collaborators. Global burden of 369 diseases and injuries in 204 countries and territories, 1990–2019: a systematic analysis for the Global Burden of Disease Study 2019. *Lancet.* 2020;396:1204–1222.

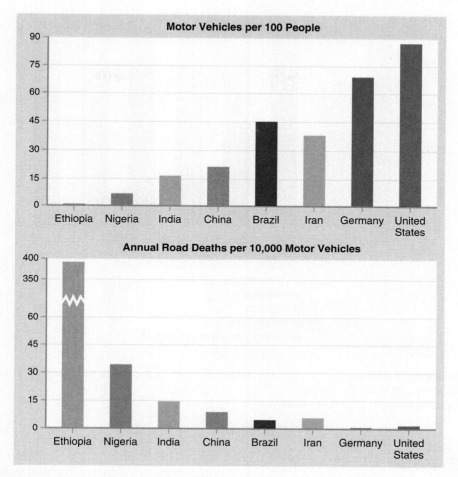

Figure 17.5 Motor vehicles per 100 people and annual rate of road deaths per 10,000 motor vehicles in selected countries.

Data from *Global Status Report on Road Safety 2018*. Geneva: World Health Organization; 2018.

be mandated, and children can be restricted from sitting in the front seats of vehicles. The legal blood alcohol limit can be reduced to 0.05 g/dL or less, with a zero-tolerance policy for any alcohol use among young and inexperienced drivers and commercial drivers who are operating heavy trucks. Restrictions can be set for driving under the influence of any substances that might cause impairment, including prescription medications. Distracted driving can be limited by banning texting and other mobile phone activities while driving. Additionally,

governments can mandate vehicle safety standards, build safer roads with good markings and signage, provide sidewalks and bike lanes to keep pedestrians and cyclists away from car and truck traffic, and promote enforcement of safety laws. These preventive interventions can be very cost effective.[18] Since even the most robust transportation safety policies will not prevent all collisions, governments can also reduce RTI mortality rates by increasing access to post-crash first aid, pre-hospital emergency medical care, in-hospital trauma care, and rehabilitation.[15]

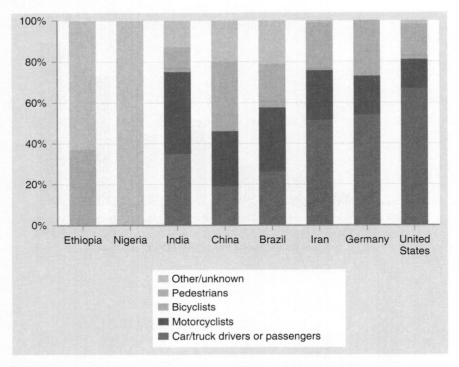

Figure 17.6 Estimated distribution of road injury fatalities (vehicle occupants, motorcyclists, bicyclists, and pedestrians) in selected countries.

Data from *Global Status Report on Road Safety 2018*. Geneva: World Health Organization; 2018.

17.3 Falls

A **fall** is an event that causes a person to land on the ground or floor. Some falls start from a great height, such as falls from ladders, scaffolding, or the tops of buildings; some falls involve only a short distance, such as falls from a bed or chair or a standing position. Most falls do not result in injuries, but some cause mild injuries such as bruises and some cause concussions, spinal cord injuries, fractures, sprains, or other types of moderate or severe trauma.

People of all ages can slip, trip, stumble, and fall, but the rate of fall injuries, the rate of fall-related mortality, and the percentage of deaths due to falls are highest among the oldest adults (**Figure 17.7**).[2] Falls among children, adolescents, and adults up to about 65 years of

age are rarely fatal, but falls among older adults frequently start a trajectory that leads to death.[19] Older adults who fall may sustain soft-tissue damage as well as fractures of hips and other bones.[20] Hip fractures may require surgery to stabilize the pelvis followed by weeks or months of confinement to a bed, and that extended time

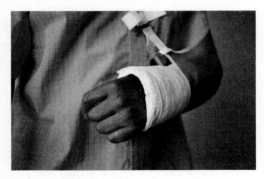

© Sirtravelalot/Shutterstock

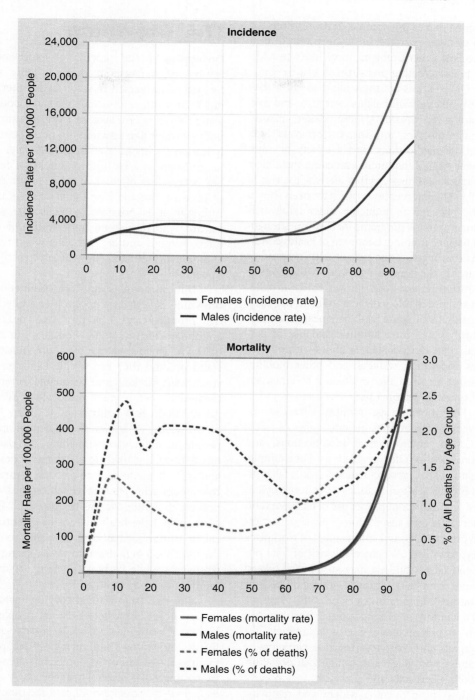

Figure 17.7 Incidence rate per 100,000 people, mortality rate per 100,000 people, and percentage of deaths from fall-related injuries, by sex and age.

Data from GBD 2019 Diseases and Injuries Collaborators. Global burden of 369 diseases and injuries in 204 countries and territories, 1990–2019; a systematic analysis for the Global Burden of Disease Study 2019. *Lancet.* 2020;396:1204–1222.

reclining makes pneumonia, bedsores (infected skin wounds), strokes due to deep vein thromboses, and other problems more likely in addition to exacerbating preexisting frailty.[21]

Older adults are most likely to fall if they have problems with balance, strength, and gait. Neurological disorders, low vision, cardiovascular diseases, arthritis, osteoporosis, side effects of medications, and a variety of other adverse health conditions can cause instability, weakness, and missteps that increase the risk of a fall.[22] The interventions that have been shown to be effective in reducing older adult falls include exercise programs focused on strength and balance training; treatment of health conditions that increase the risk of falls; removal of hazards in the home, such as throw rugs, unstable furniture, and loose power cords; installation and use of safety devices in the home, such as handrails by stairs, grab bars near toilets and bathtubs, and good lighting; and use of personal safety devices such as shoes with nonslip soles and canes, walkers, and other mobility aids that are used after evaluation by an expert and training in proper use.[23]

For younger age groups, strategies for preventing fall injuries include a mix of safety education, environmental modifications, and enforcement of safety regulations. For example, adults may have an occupational risk of fall injuries if they work in factories or at construction sites. Training about proper use of harnesses and other safety gear, installation of physical barriers that prevent falls, and enforcement of workplace safety laws can all reduce the risk of fatal on-the-job falls. Children may sustain fall-related injuries from being dropped, rolling off beds or furniture, climbing on trees or cliffs, tumbling out a window, or playing sports.[3] Teaching children to use protective sports equipment like kneepads and wrist guards when participating in athletic activities with a high risk of falling, installing bed rails and pin locks that prevent windows from opening widely, and removing playground equipment that does not meet current safety standards are ways to reduce risks of fall injuries among young people.

17.4 Drowning

Drowning is the process of experiencing respiratory impairment due to being submerged or immersed in water or another liquid.[24] Drowning can occur in a large body of water like an ocean, lake, or river; in a smaller body of water like a swimming pool, pond, or irrigation ditch; and even in a small water container, such as a bathtub or bucket. Drowning occurs less often than many other types of injuries, but the case fatality rate is high. Although it is possible to resuscitate some victims who have been underwater for only a few minutes and are still alive when rescue attempts are initiated, drowning often results in death.[25]

The mortality rate from unintentional drowning is highest among older adults, but the proportionate mortality rate peaks in childhood (**Figure 17.8**).[2] Toddlers can easily drown in shallow water if they trip and cannot stand up, and they can topple headfirst into small wash buckets and be unable to remove themselves before they suffocate.[26] Alcohol consumption is a contributor to many cases of drowning in adults since alcohol makes people more likely to swim alone or in dangerous settings, less likely to use flotation devices, and more likely to capsize a boat.[27] Untrained bystanders who attempt water rescues often become drowning victims themselves.[28] Older adults may have health issues like neurological or cardiovascular disorders that increase the likelihood of falling into water, losing consciousness while bathing, or being unable to safely exit a body of water.[29]

The risk factors for drowning include a lack of physical barriers between people and bodies of water, lack of close supervision of infants and young children, lack of safe places to cross rivers and other bodies of water, poor swimming skills, alcohol use when near water, lack of safety measures for boats and other vessels, floods from extreme weather, and lack of training in safe rescue and resuscitation.[30] Key actions to reduce the risk of drowning include

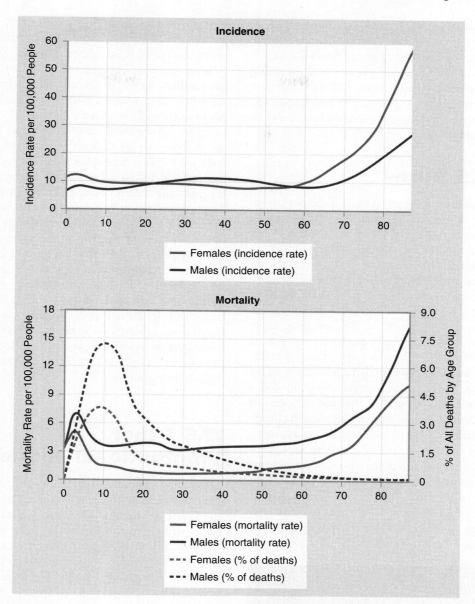

Figure 17.8 Incidence rate per 100,000 people, mortality rate per 100,000 people, and percentage of deaths from drowning, by sex and age.

Data from GBD 2019 Diseases and Injuries Collaborators. Global burden of 369 diseases and injuries in 204 countries and territories, 1990–2019: a systematic analysis for the Global Burden of Disease Study 2019. *Lancet.* 2020;396:1204–1222.

installing barriers to limit access to danger-ous waters, such as covering drinking-water barrels and fencing swimming pools; offering swimming and water safety lessons; enforcing boating and ferry regulations, such as limits to the numbers of passengers per vessel and mandates to have personal flotation devices onboard for all passengers; and preparing people to survive floods by initiating early-warning systems and discouraging unsafe behaviors like driving across flooded streets.[31] The global mortality rate from drowning decreased by more than half over the past 30 years as these types of preventive interventions were implemented in more countries and communities.[32]

17.5 Burns

A **burn** is an injury to skin or deeper tissues that is caused by contact with fire, boiling water, or other very hot substances. Burns may also be caused by radiation, electricity, friction, extreme cold, and some types of chemicals. Burns are classified into three levels of severity. First-degree burns cause redness and pain but do not blister. Second-degree burns penetrate through some layers of skin and often cause painful blisters. Third-degree burns extend through all the layers of skin, causing extensive and possibly fatal damage. Burns that are severe, cover a sizable proportion of the body's surface area, or are on the face or hands or other critical areas often require lengthy hospitalizations.[33] Initial care focuses on managing fluid loss and preventing infection. Skin grafts, amputations, and other advanced wound care techniques may be necessary to prevent death, disability, and disfigurement. Later, contractures (tightened skin that restricts the movement of a joint) and other types of scars may need to be surgically corrected.

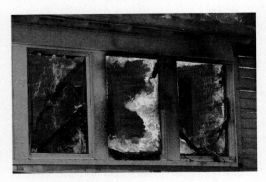

© Elizabeth Castaneda/EyeEm/Getty Images.

The incidence of burn injuries and the percentage of deaths that are attributable to burns peak in early adulthood (**Figure 17.9**).[2] In lower-income countries, many women and the toddlers they care for suffer from burns sustained when cooking over open fires, and house fires are often caused by kerosene lamps or stoves tipping over. Lamps and stoves that are designed to be difficult to tip over can reduce the risk of fires and scalds.[34] In higher-income and urban areas, effective strategies for reducing burns include smoke alarms, devices that limit the temperature of hot water in the home, making children's sleepwear out of fire-resistant fabrics, wiring indoor electrical systems properly, installing sprinklers in buildings, making child-resistant cigarette lighters, and making fireworks safer.[34] After burns occur, access to emergency and specialty care can help prevent disability and mortality. Advanced burn care is rarely available in lower-income countries, so the case fatality rates in those areas are much higher than in high-income countries.[35]

17.6 Other Unintentional Injuries

In addition to transportation injuries, falls, drowning, and burns, unintentional injuries are caused by many other events, including being struck by thrown or falling objects, crushed or jammed between objects, cut by glass or other sharp objects, mangled by a tool or machine, accidentally shot by a firearm, wounded by an exploding or rupturing pressurized device, bit by a dog or other animal, envenomated by a snake, inadvertently poisoned by exposure to toxic substances such as pesticides or carbon monoxide, asphyxiated by aspirated food, or harmed by medical treatments.[36] Injuries may also be caused by exposure to forces of nature, such as extreme heat or cold, an earthquake, a volcanic eruption, an avalanche, a landslide, or a flood.

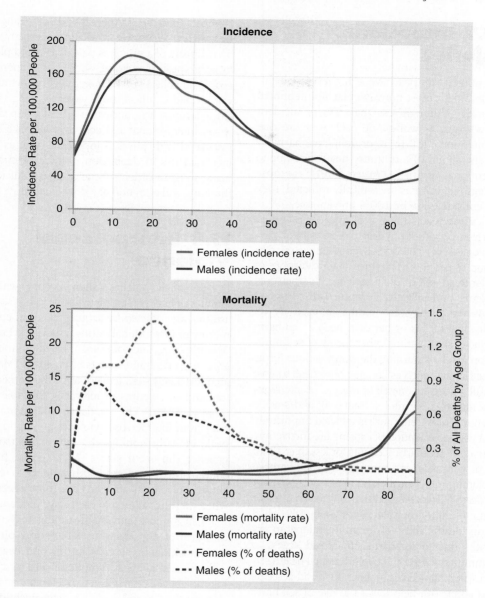

Figure 17.9 Mortality rate per 100,000 people and percentage of deaths from fire, heat, and hot substances, by sex and age.

Data from GBD 2019 Diseases and Injuries Collaborators. Global burden of 369 diseases and injuries in 204 countries and territories, 1990–2019: a systematic analysis for the Global Burden of Disease Study 2019. *Lancet.* 2020;396:1204–1222.

Occupational, environmental, and behavioral prevention strategies must be tailored to site-specific and population-specific risks. For example, poisonings at work can be reduced with restricted use of dangerous substances and mandated use of personal protective equipment, and poisonings at home can be reduced by storing cleaning products and other chemicals in places that cannot be accessed by small children.[37]

17.7 Intentional Injuries

Intentional injuries have a higher case fatality rate than most nonvehicular unintentional injuries. Although less than 7% of incident (new) injuries worldwide each year are due to intentional self-harm or deliberate harm by others, about 29% of injury deaths are due to intentional injuries (**Figure 17.10**).[2] Because intentional injuries are willfully inflicted, they are considered to be 100% preventable.

Violence is the use of force or power to threaten or inflict physical, sexual, and/or psychological harm on oneself, another person, or a group of people.[38] The three main categories of violence are self-directed violence, interpersonal violence, and collective violence. **Self-directed violence** is physical trauma inflicted by an individual on his or her own body.[39] Self-harm includes skin cutting, other forms of self-mutilation (such as burning the skin), various forms of self-injury (such as banging one's head against a wall, punching oneself or objects, or intentionally ingesting harmful substances), and suicide attempts. Most self-injury is inflicted impulsively and with no intention of causing life-threatening damage.[40] Self-harm accounts for less than 1% of all new injuries, and most types of self-harm—including most suicide attempts—do not result in death.[41] However, self-harm remains a major cause of injury mortality, with about 18% of all injury deaths and 60% of all intentional injury deaths due to self-harm.[2] Increased access to community-based and clinical mental health services, including crisis hotlines, for all adolescents and adults can help lower the rate of self-harm injuries and deaths; policies and practices that make it more difficult to access poisons, firearms, and other tools used for self-harm can also reduce the suicide rate.[42]

About 90% of intentional injuries are due to harm deliberately imposed by others.[2] **Interpersonal violence** occurs when one person threatens to harm or actually harms another individual through power and control.[43] Interpersonal violence may be inflicted by a family member, intimate partner, friend, or stranger. **Collective violence** is violence perpetrated by members of a group as part of a shared plan to accomplish a political, social, or economic goal. The collective violence category includes war, armed conflicts, mob violence, gang violence, terrorist acts, and other acts of group violence. Interpersonal and collective violence are associated with physical injuries as well as an increased risk of depression, anxiety, posttraumatic stress disorder, substance abuse, suicidal thinking, and adoption of risky behaviors.[44]

17.8 Interpersonal Violence

Interpersonal violence often occurs within families or between intimate partners, but some assaults are inflicted by acquaintances in community or institutional settings, such as schools or workplaces, and some are inflicted by strangers engaging in random acts of violence.[38] Males are more likely than females to be the perpetrators and the victims of interpersonal violence (**Figure 17.11**).[2] The incidence and mortality rates from interpersonal violence among males peak in early adulthood,[2] but interpersonal violence can occur across the life span, from child maltreatment and youth violence to elder abuse. Prevention activities are most effective when they are tailored to each stage of life.

Child abuse and maltreatment may take the form of physical abuse (including physical punishments, such as hitting and beating a child), sexual abuse, emotional and psychological abuse, or neglect.[45] A global partnership aiming to end violence against children identified seven key strategies for protecting children that can be summarized by the acronym INSPIRE[46]:

- **I**mplementing and enforcing laws that ban corporal punishment of children and criminalize sexual abuse and exploitation
- **N**orms and values changing to create a culture of equity and community involvement in child protection

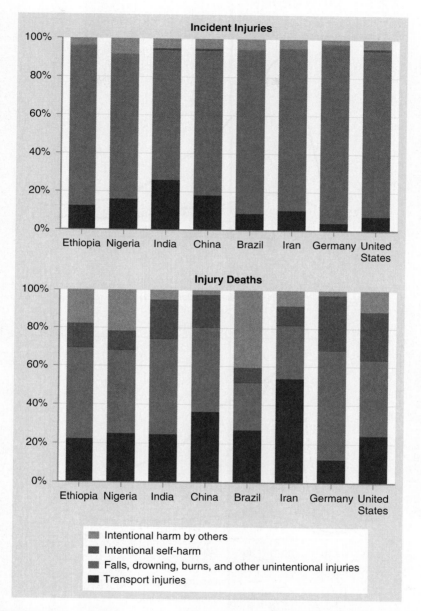

Figure 17.10 Distribution of injury mortality by cause and intentionality in selected countries.

Data from GBD 2019 Diseases and Injuries Collaborators. Global burden of 369 diseases and injuries in 204 countries and territories, 1990–2019: a systematic analysis for the Global Burden of Disease Study 2019. *Lancet*. 2020;396:1204–1222.

- Safe environments being created
- Parent and caregiver support being provided, including parenting education and home visits by nurses

- Income and economic security strengthening to reduce the stresses of poverty on families
- Response and support services being launched and maintained for treating

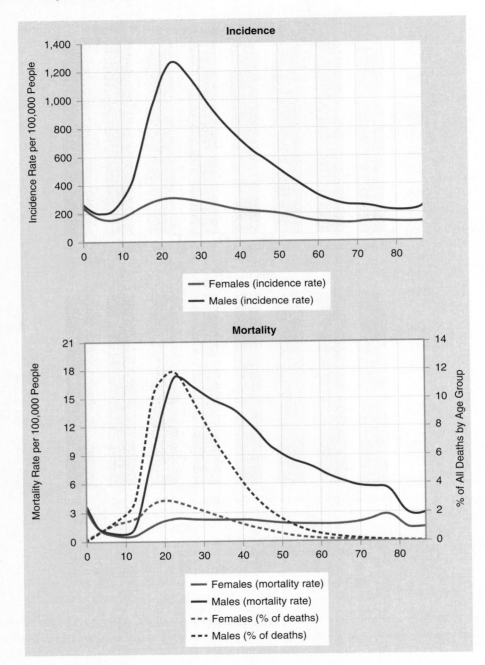

Figure 17.11 Incidence rate per 100,000 people, mortality rate per 100,000 people, and percentage of deaths from interpersonal violence, by sex and age.

Data from GBD 2019 Diseases and Injuries Collaborators. Global burden of 369 diseases and injuries in 204 countries and territories, 1990–2019: a systematic analysis for the Global Burden of Disease Study 2019. *Lancet.* 2020;396:1204–1222.

injuries, investigating and addressing possible cases of abuse, and providing social welfare services to families with vulnerable children

- Education and life skills training being implemented to enhance children's ability to recognize and report abuse and neglect

The SDGs aim to end all forms of violence against children, including physical punishment and psychological aggression by caregivers, by 2030 (SDG 16.2).[8] This is unlikely to be achieved given the UN estimate that about half of all children experienced at least one type of violence in 2020.[47]

Youth violence often involves interpersonal conflict between an adolescent or young adult aggressor and another person of a similar age.[48] The risk factors for involvement in youth violence include being male, being a school dropout or delinquent, performing poorly in school, lacking social connectedness, using alcohol and drugs, living in a low-income household, and having a history of child abuse and exposure to violence.[49] The key strategies to reduce youth violence include anger management and conflict resolution training, school-based bullying prevention programs, counseling for young people already involved in violence, and community-based strategies that reduce poverty and crime.[49] Reducing the harmful use of alcohol and restricting access to guns, knives, and other weapons are also helpful for reducing injuries from violence among young people.[4]

Most abuse of older adults with cognitive or physical impairments (and adults of other ages who have disabilities) is inflicted by a family member or caregiver. Physical abuse may include assaults, the use of physical restraints or unnecessary medications to control the individual, malnutrition and dehydration due to withholding food and water, poor attention to hygiene and cleanliness, untreated medical conditions, and isolation.[38] Other forms of elder abuse include emotional and psychological abuse, neglect, sexual abuse, and financial abuse, such

as withdrawing the adult's money from banks, changing wills, or confiscating property.[50] Up to one in six adults aged 60 years and older may experience elder abuse each year.[51] Strategies for preventing elder abuse and neglect include caregiver support, professional standards for residential care facilities, information campaigns for the public and care professionals, and the availability of adult protective services.[38]

17.9 Gender-Based Violence

Gender-based violence (GBV) is physical, emotional, and/or sexual abuse inflicted on an individual because of that individual's gender. GBV usually involves victimization of women and girls, who may have little power over their own bodies because of gender norms that give men authority over them and because they tend to be smaller and physically weaker than men. Transgender individuals also have a high likelihood of experiencing GBV.[52]

Violence against females may occur at any stage of their lives.[53] Pregnancies with female fetuses may be terminated by sex-selective abortions. Infant daughters may be killed by families with a cultural preference for sons. Young girls may be subjected to female genital cutting (FGC), also called female genital mutilation (FGM), which is the partial or complete removal of the external female genitalia of an infant or child. Women who had this procedure

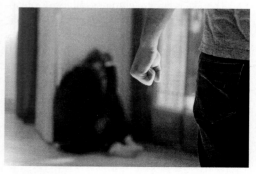

© Sdecoret/Shutterstock

when they were children have significantly increased risks of urinary tract and reproductive tract infections, menstrual problems, sexual dysfunction, and obstetric complications.[54] FGC is still practiced among some populations in parts of Africa and the Middle East as well as among people in other countries with heritage from those regions.[55] Older girls may be forced into early marriages or into pornography, prostitution, and trafficking. Adolescents and adult women may be subjected to dating, courtship, and marriage violence, including coerced sex and rape, and they may experience sexual harassment, forced pregnancies, trafficking, and acts of violence like "honor killings" and acid throwing.[56] The health consequences of GBV may include psychological trauma, serious injuries (including injuries to fetuses when pregnant women are attacked), infections with HIV and other pathogens, and death.

Intimate partner violence (IPV) is physical or sexual violence perpetrated by a current or former spouse or partner, such as being slapped, hit, kicked, choked, or beaten; threatened with a weapon or injured by one; or forced to have sexual intercourse or perform other sexual acts. Most acts of IPV involve men engaging in GBV by abusing women.[57] About 27% of ever-partnered women have experienced IPV during their lifetimes, and about 6% have experienced nonpartner sexual violence; in total, 30% of women aged 15 years or older have experienced some form of IPV or nonpartner sexual violence.[58]

The SDGs aim to "eliminate all forms of violence against all women and girls in the public and private spheres" (SDG 5.2).[8] Ending intimate partner and sexual violence will require social and cultural shifts in thinking about gender equity and healthy relationships as well as individual behavior changes.[44] For example, many women continue to believe that a man has good reason to beat his wife if she does not complete the housework, disobeys her husband, or is unfaithful or if the husband suspects infidelity, and many women believe it is not acceptable for a woman to refuse sex with her husband even if she does not want to have sex, her partner is

drunk or mistreating her, or she is sick.[59] If violence against women is considered to be acceptable in any of these circumstances, GBV will continue. Sustained reductions in GBV will not happen until women and men agree that these types of violence are never acceptable.

The UN uses the acronym RESPECT to describe its framework for preventing violence against women and girls[60]:

- **R**elationship skills strengthened
- **E**mpowerment of women economically and socially
- **S**ervices ensured for survivors of violence, including legal, health, and social services
- **P**overty reduced
- **E**nvironments made safe
- **C**hild and adolescent abuse prevented
- **T**ransformed attitudes, beliefs, and norms about gender, privilege, and subordination

The most effective interventions to reduce GBV engage diverse stakeholders in activities that promote healthy attitudes and behaviors among children and adults of all sexes and genders.[61]

17.10 Conflict and War

A **complex humanitarian emergency** occurs when civil conflict or war causes mass migration of civilian populations, food insecurity, and long-term public health concerns.[62] Natural disasters usually create an immediate period of acute need but quickly transition into recovery mode. By contrast, complex emergencies may remain in an acute phase for years or even decades. Because natural disasters are generally seen as apolitical events, the governments of affected countries typically welcome external aid for survivors. Responses to complex humanitarian emergencies are much more complicated because military commanders and faction leaders engaged in armed conflicts are often disinclined to allow outsiders to assess and assist vulnerable populations.[63]

In addition to an increase in injuries caused by collective violence against combatants and noncombatants, numerous public health challenges arise during complex emergencies. The breakdown of water and sanitation systems and public health services may lead to frequent outbreaks of diarrhea and other infectious diseases. Vaccine-preventable diseases such as measles and meningitis may resurge when routine childhood vaccination programs are interrupted. Respiratory infections like pneumonia and tuberculosis may become more prevalent due to inadequate shelter. Other infectious disease concerns include the intensification of malaria in endemic areas, outbreaks of viral hepatitis, and an increased incidence of sexually transmitted infections, which may be spread through gender-based violence and then remain untreated because of lack of access to health care.[64]

International humanitarian laws are supposed to protect civilians and combatants,[65] but these rules are not always enforced.[66] Rape and sexual violence have been used as military tactics in many conflicts.[67] Reproductive health services (including family planning and obstetric care), emergency medical care, and psychiatric services tend to be severely inadequate during conflicts. Malnutrition is also a major concern during war and civil conflicts.[68] Food production tends to decrease as farms are abandoned, and it is more difficult to import affordable food during times of instability. Food supply chains that enable food products to be processed, transported, stored, and sold are often interrupted by conflict and uncertainty. Large numbers of people may be migrating and in need of a daily supply of nutrients. The combination of too few calories, vitamins, and minerals plus lack of care for other diseases often leads to severe undernutrition.

Two of the most prominent organizations involved in providing health services and other types of assistance during times of war are the Red Cross and Médecins Sans Frontières (MSF). Both groups have been awarded the Nobel Peace Prize (the Red Cross in 1917, 1944, and 1963 and MSF in 1999); both are headquartered in Geneva, Switzerland; both provide direct services to people affected by war and other armed conflicts; and both value impartiality and neutrality. However, their approaches are distinct.

The International Committee of the **Red Cross (ICRC)** is a private humanitarian organization officially sanctioned by the Geneva Convention and international law to provide specific humanitarian services during times of war.[69] The ICRC works with more than 185 national Red Cross and Red Crescent societies and the International Federation of Red Cross and Red Crescent Societies to provide humanitarian aid to both civilian and military victims of conflicts. National Red Cross and Red Crescent societies are autonomous from the ICRC, and they provide a variety of services that meet needs in their communities, such as maintaining blood banks, providing first aid training, and offering assistance to residents who have been affected by natural disasters. National societies also contribute funding and personnel to support ICRC responses.

The ICRC is guided by the principles of humanity, impartiality, neutrality, independence, voluntary service, unity, and universality.[70] The ICRC and its affiliates attempt to avoid actions that could appear to take sides with any partisan or political group.[71] ICRC representatives visit prisoners of war to verify that they are being treated humanely and in accordance with the Geneva Conventions; search for missing persons; transmit messages between separated family members; reunify displaced families; monitor compliance with international laws that pertain to armed conflict; and provide basic services to civilians, such as food, water, and medical assistance.[72] The ICRC is funded through governmental support, contributions from national Red Cross and Red Crescent societies, and private donations.

Médecins Sans Frontières (MSF), more often called **Doctors Without Borders** in the United States, is a private humanitarian organization that advocates for human rights and provides medical care to people harmed by violence. Funds that support MSF's work are raised through its main office and more than 20 national offices in other countries.

MSF staff and volunteers care for the victims of violence no matter what their political affiliations are, often setting up clinics in places that are so unstable that other organizations refuse to deploy resources to them.[73] Independence, impartiality, and neutrality are core principles of MSF, and these are seen as a call to bear witness to violations of human rights rather than remaining silent.[74] Impartiality means that all governmental agencies and other entities are equally open to criticism from MSF when they engage in or allow injustices.[75] MSF does not accept donations from groups that do not meet the organization's ethical standards. Only a tiny fraction of MSF's budget comes from governmental funding, and the organization does not accept funds from pharmaceutical, biotechnology, mineral extraction, tobacco, or arms manufacturing companies.[76]

In post-conflict areas, a diversity of local, national, and international organizations typically helps with reconstruction by responding to urgent needs, assisting with long-term recovery, and working to prevent future crises. Political and economic systems need to be rebuilt, and educational and social services need to be restored after a civil conflict or war. Post-conflict areas also need to repair health systems (because of lost infrastructure and personnel, among other issues),[77] expand access to physical rehabilitation and mental healthcare services, and mitigate environmental health concerns.

Contaminated environments often take longer to renovate than hospitals and clinics.[78] For example, **landmines** are buried explosive devices, and they and other unexploded ordnance buried during wartime remain hazards to workers, children, and communities long after a conflict is over.[79] This means, among many other problems, that large tracts of potential farmland are unable to be cultivated because of the risk of encountering a mine while clearing a field. Most people who sustain landmine injuries are civilians. Children may have elevated risk of injuries because they do not know how to recognize

explosive devices and may pick them up and even play with them. Landmines and other explosive remnants of war remain a concern in many parts of the world, killing thousands of civilians each year and seriously injuring thousands of others.[80] The direct costs to injured individuals and their families can be very high when they must pay for surgery, a lengthy hospitalization, and a lifetime of assistive devices for people who survive with lost limbs, burn contractures, blindness, and other permanent disabilities. A **prosthetic** is an artificial body part, such as a substitute leg or arm that might be used after a limb is lost in a landmine explosion. Even a low-tech prosthetic can be expensive, and children with amputated limbs need to be refitted with new devices as they grow.[81]

Access to basic health care is considered to be a fundamental human right, but wars and civil conflicts often restrict access to health services and the foundational tools for health.[82] Police violence, terrorism, and other forms of collective violence also impair health equity. International organizations play important roles in advocating for human rights; providing medical care during and after times of conflict, war, and other forms of violence; and supporting physical, mental, and social health and well-being.[83] In post-conflict areas, multisectoral interventions can facilitate the transition back to peace by strengthening social connections and improving public health.[84]

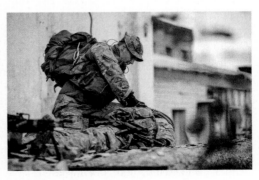

© PRESSLAB/Shutterstock

17.11 Bioterrorism

Bioterrorism is the deliberate release of pathogens, chemicals, or other agents that can cause illness and possibly death of people, animals, or plants. Chemical and biological warfare are not modern inventions.[85] During the Tartar siege of Kaffa, a city on the Crimean Peninsula, in the 14th century, the bodies of plague victims were catapulted over city walls to spark an epidemic. During the French and Indian War in the 1760s, the British army sent smallpox-infected blankets to Native Americans who supported the French. During World War I, several European nations used biological agents against the livestock of enemies. What is new is that there are now more tools available for creating and spreading bioterror agents and the scale on which such acts can occur is much larger.[86]

In the United States, potential bioterror agents are classified into three groups (**Figure 17.12**).[87] Category A represents high-priority agents that pose a significant risk because they can be easily transmitted from one person to another or have high mortality rates. Category A agents include anthrax; botulism; plague; smallpox; tularemia; and viral hemorrhagic fevers like the Ebola, Lassa, and Marburg viruses. Category B agents are moderately easy to spread but usually cause relatively few deaths. Examples of Category B agents include food safety threats (such as *E. coli* O157:H7, *Salmonella*, and *Shigella*), ricin toxin (from the plant *Ricinus communis*, also known as castor bean or castor oil plants), viral encephalitis infections, and water supply threats (such as cholera and cryptosporidiosis). Category C agents are emerging infectious diseases like hantaviruses that are potential bioterror threats. Chemical agents may also pose a

Category	Agents
Category A	■ Anthrax (*Bacillus anthracis*) ■ Botulism (*Clostridium botulinum* toxin) ■ Plague (*Yersinia pestis*) ■ Smallpox (variola major) ■ Tularemia (*Francisella tularensis*) ■ Viral hemorrhagic fevers (such as Ebola, Marburg, Lassa, and Machupo viruses)
Category B	■ Brucellosis (*Brucella* species) ■ Glanders (*Burkholderia mallei*) ■ Melioidosis (*Burkholderia pseudomallei*) ■ Psittacosis (*Chlamydia psittaci*) ■ Q fever (*Coxiella burnetii*) ■ Toxins (such as ricin, *Staphylococcus* enterotoxin, and the epsilon toxin of *Clostridium perfringens*) ■ Typhus fever (*Rickettsia prowazekii*) ■ Food- and waterborne diseases (such as *Cryptosporidium parvum*, *Escherichia coli* O157:H7, hepatitis A virus, *Salmonella*, *Shigella*, and *Vibrio cholerae*) ■ Mosquito-borne encephalitis viruses
Category C	■ Emerging infectious diseases, such as hantavirus, Nipah virus, and drug-resistant pathogens

Figure 17.12 U.S. classifications of potential bioterrorism agents.

Data from Rotz LD, Khan AS, Lillibridge SR, Ostroff SM, Hughes JM. Public health assessment of potential biological terrorism agents. *Emerg Infect Dis.* 2002;8:225–230.

threat (**Figure 17.13**).[88] Biological agents typically cause infections, while chemical agents cause poisoning and other types of injuries. Terrorist attacks could also involve radiological or nuclear agents, explosions, and other types of injury-causing devices.

Potential bioweapons are considered to be greater threats if they are easy to produce and store, have high stability in the environment, can be formulated as an aerosol, can be easily dispersed in large quantities, are highly infectious, have a short or very predictable incubation period, cause most exposed individuals to become ill, are highly lethal, are contagious between individuals through droplet nuclei spread, are not able to be prevented with prophylactic countermeasures like vaccines or antibiotics, cannot be treated with antibiotics or other therapeutics, and cannot be detected with current laboratory assays.[89] However, while the goal of some bioterrorists is to kill or seriously injure large numbers of people, the overarching goal is to cause widespread fear, panic, and social disruption. Even an agent that is not able to be mass-produced and easily dispersed can achieve the goal of inducing chaos.

Anthrax is a bacterial infection (*Bacillus anthracis*) that causes skin lesions when naturally acquired but causes respiratory distress, shock, and death when a weaponized version is inhaled. Naturally occurring cases of anthrax are diagnosed every year in people who work with sheep and livestock because anthrax spores (dormant bacteria) can survive in the soil and some other environments for years. These cases are usually cutaneous (skin) infections. In the laboratory, anthrax can be made into a fine powder that causes inhalation anthrax when breathed in. While most cases of cutaneous anthrax can be cured with antibiotics, there is a high case fatality rate associated with inhalation anthrax.[90] When anthrax was used in a postal bioterrorism attack in the United States in 2001, 22 cases of anthrax were diagnosed and 5 of the 11 people who contracted inhalation anthrax died.[91] Although the number of cases

Category	Examples
Nerve agents	Tabun, sarin, soman, GF, VX
Blood agents	Hydrogen cyanide, cyanogen chloride
Blister agents	Lewisite, nitrogen and sulfur mustards, phosgene oxime
Heavy metals	Arsenic, lead, mercury
Volatile toxins	Benzene, chloroform, trihalomethanes
Pulmonary agents	Phosgene, chlorine, vinyl chloride
Incapacitating agents	BZ
Explosive nitro compounds and oxidizers	Ammonium nitrate combined with fuel oil
Flammable industrial gases and liquids	Gasoline, propane
Poisonous industrial gases, liquids, and solids	Cyanides, nitriles
Corrosive industrial acids and bases	Nitric acid, sulfuric acid
Other agents	Pesticides, dioxins, furans, polychlorinated biphenyls

Figure 17.13 Possible chemical weapons.

Biological and chemical terrorism: strategic plan for preparedness and response. Recommendations of the CDC Strategic Planning Workgroup. *MMWR Recomm Rep.* 2000;49(RR-1):1–14. Reference to specific commercial products, manufacturers, companies, or trademarks does not constitute its endorsement or recommendation by the U.S. Government, Department of Health and Human Services, or Centers for Disease Control and Prevention.

in that bioterror attack was small, people living hundreds of miles from the affected post offices reported experiencing distress related to the event.[92] The attack was also expensive. Decontamination of post offices and office buildings cost more than $300 million dollars.[93]

The best defense against a bioterrorism attack is early detection so that an outbreak can be contained and exposed or at-risk people can receive post-exposure prophylaxis or immunization if available. Detection and response operations are most effective when emergency managers can rely on a strong laboratory network, trained public health departments that are prepared to implement response activities, the cooperation of healthcare providers and emergency responders, and an adequate stockpile of essential vaccines and medications.[87] Effective communication is also critical for keeping the public informed of developments after a chemical, biological, radiological, or nuclear (CBRN) attack and encouraging appropriate personal responses.[94]

At present, many countries do not have the capacity to detect and respond to CBRN threats. The Global Health Security (GHS) Index examines each country's ability to prevent emergence or release of pathogens, detect and report an event, and rapidly respond to an event as well as considering the robustness of each country's health system, its compliance with international norms, and its risk environment and vulnerability to biological threats.[95] Even before the coronavirus pandemic strained public health systems, most countries had GHS Index scores indicating a lack of preparedness to prevent biosecurity threats, respond rapidly to emergencies, link public health and security responses, communicate risk, and deploy medical countermeasures. The pandemic strengthened prevention and response capacity in some countries, but it also revealed how many countries remain highly vulnerable to infectious disease threats.[95]

Responses to acts of terrorism should not infringe on the civil, political, economic, social, and cultural rights of people in affected communities.[96] However, there are situations in which individual rights must be balanced with the public good. For example, freedom of movement for people with highly contagious infections may be temporarily limited during an outbreak so that the health rights of other people can be protected. A **nonderogable right** is a human right that is irrevocable in all circumstances, such as freedom from slavery and torture. A derogable right is one that may be temporarily suspended under special circumstances.[97] If any human rights are derogated during or immediately after a critical incident, the new rules must not be discriminatory, and full rights should be restored as soon as possible.[98] Upholding human rights helps to restore public health and trust after a CBRN attack or another act of collective violence, and promoting human rights might help avert the conditions that can foment future acts of war and terrorism.[99]

References

1. Haddon W Jr. Energy damage and the ten countermeasure strategies. *Human Factors.* 1973;15:355–366.
2. GBD 2019 Diseases and Injuries Collaborators. Global burden of 369 diseases and injuries in 204 countries and territories, 1990–2019: a systematic analysis for the Global Burden of Disease Study 2019. *Lancet.* 2020;396:1204–1222.
3. *World Report on Child Injury Prevention.* Geneva: World Health Organization/UNICEF; 2008.
4. *Violence Prevention: The Evidence.* Geneva: World Health Organization; 2010.

5. Courtenay WH. Behavioral factors associated with disease, injury, and death among men: evidence and implications for prevention. *J Men's Stud.* 2000;9: 81–142.

6. Laflamme L, Burrows S, Hasselberg M. *Socioeconomic Differences in Injury Risks: A Review of Findings and a Discussion of Potential Countermeasures.* Copenhagen: WHO-EURO; 2009.

7. Mock C, Smith KR, Kobusingye O, et al. Injury prevention and environmental health: key messages from the volume (chapter 1). In: Mock CN, Nugent R, Kobusingye O, Smith KR, eds. *Disease Control Priorities: Injury Prevention and Environmental Health.* 3rd ed. Vol. 7. Washington DC: IBRD/World Bank; 2017:1–24.

8. *Transforming Our World: The 2030 Agenda for Sustainable Development.* New York: United Nations; 2015.

9. Giles A, Bauer MEE, Jull J. Equity as the fourth 'E' in the '3 Es' approach to injury prevention. *Inj Prev.* 2020;26:82–84.

10. Mock C, Quansah R, Krishnan R, Arreola-Risa C, Rivara F. Strengthening the prevention and care of injuries worldwide. *Lancet.* 2004;363:2172–2179.

11. Sharma BR. Road traffic injuries: a major global public health crisis. *Public Health.* 2008;122:1399–1406.

12. GBD 2015 Mortality and Causes of Death Collaborators. Global, regional, and national life expectancy, all-cause mortality, and cause-specific mortality for 249 causes of death, 1980–2015: a systematic analysis for the Global Burden of Disease Study 2015. *Lancet.* 2016;388:1459–1544.

13. Ameratunga S, Hijar M, Norton R. Road-traffic injuries: confronting disparities to address a global-health problem. *Lancet.* 2006;367:1533–1540.

14. *Global Status Report on Road Safety 2018.* Geneva: World Health Organization; 2018.

15. *Global Plan: Decade of Action for Road Safety 2021–2030.* Geneva: World Health Organization; 2021.

16. *Managing Speed.* Geneva: World Health Organization; 2017.

17. Vecino-Ortiz AI, Jafri A, Hyder AA. Effective interventions for unintentional injuries: a systematic review and mortality impact assessment among the poorest billion. *Lancet Glob Health.* 2018;6:e523–e534.

18. Bachani A, Peden M, Gururaj G, Norton R, Hyder A. Road traffic injuries (chapter 3). In: Mock CN, Nugent R, Kobusingye O, Smith KR, eds. *Disease Control Priorities: Injury Prevention and Environmental Health.* 3rd ed. Vol. 7. Washington DC: IBRD/World Bank; 2017:35–54.

19. Kannus P, Sievänen H, Palvanen M, Järvinen T, Parkkari J. Prevention of falls and consequent injuries in elderly people. *Lancet.* 2005;366:1885–1893.

20. James SL, Lucchesi LR, Bisignano C, et al. The global burden of falls: global, regional and national estimates of morbidity and mortality from the Global Burden of Disease Study 2017. *Inj Prev.* 2020;26(Suppl 1):i3–i11.

21. Beaupre LA, Jones CA, Saunders LD, Johnston DWC, Buckingham J, Majumdar SR. Best practices for elderly hip fracture patients: a systematic overview of the evidence. *J Gen Intern Med.* 2005;20:1019–1025.

22. Ambrose AF, Paul G, Hausdorff JM. Risk factors for falls among older adults: a review of the literature. *Maturitas.* 2013;75:51–61.

23. Gillespie LD, Robertson MC, Gillespie WJ, et al. Interventions for preventing falls in older people living in the community. *Cochrane Database Syst Rev.* 2012;(9):CD007146.

24. van Beeck EF, Branche CM, Szpilman D, Modell JH, Bierens JJLM. A new definition of drowning: towards documentation and prevention of a global public health problem. *Bull World Health Organ.* 2005;83:853–856.

25. Szpilman D, Bierens JJLM, Handley AJ, Orlowski JP. Drowning. *N Engl J Med.* 2012;366:2102–2110.

26. Jumbelic MI, Chambliss M. Accidental toddler drowning in 5-gallon buckets. *JAMA.* 1990;263: 1952–1953.

27. Hingson R, Howland J. Alcohol and non-traffic unintended injuries. *Addiction.* 1993;88:877–883.

28. Barcala-Furelos R, Graham D, Abelairas-Gómez C, Rodríguez-Núñes A. Lay-rescuers in drowning incidents: a scoping review. *Am J Emerg Med.* 2021;44:38–44.

29. Lin CY, Wang YF, Lu TH, Kawach I. Unintentional drowning mortality, by age and body of water: an analysis of 60 countries. *Inj Prev.* 2015;21:e43–e50.

30. *Global Report on Drowning: Preventing a Leading Killer.* Geneva: World Health Organization; 2014.

31. *Preventing Drowning: An Implementation Guide.* Geneva: World Health Organization; 2017.

32. Franklin RC, Peden AE, Hamilton EB, et al. The burden of unintentional drowning: global, regional and national estimates of mortality from the Global Burden of Disease 2017 Study. *Inj Prev.* 2020;26(Suppl 1):i83–i95.

33. Orgill DP. Excision and skin grafting of thermal burns. *N Engl J Med.* 2009;360:893–901.

34. *Burn Prevention: Success Stories and Lessons Learned.* Geneva: World Health Organization; 2011.

35. Tevlin R, Dillon L, Clover AJP. Education in burns: lessons from the past and objectives for the future. *Burns.* 2017;43:1141–1148.

36. *International Statistical Classification of Diseases and Related Health Problems.* 11th ed. (ICD-11). Geneva: World Health Organization; 2020.

37. Prüss-Ustün A, Wolf J, Corvalán C, Bos R, Neira M. *Preventing Disease Through Healthy Environments: A Global Assessment of the Burden of Disease from Environmental Risks.* Geneva: World Health Organization; 2016.

38. Krug EG, Dahlberg LL, Mercy JA, Zwi AB, Lozano R. *World Report on Violence and Health*. Geneva: World Health Organization; 2002.

39. Rutherford A, Zwi AB, Grove NJ, Butchart A. Violence: a glossary. *J Epidemiol Community Health*. 2007;61:676–680.

40. Nock MK. Self-injury. *Annu Rev Clin Psychol*. 2010;6:339–363.

41. Vijayakumar L, Phillips MR, Silverman MM, Gunnell D, Carli V. Suicide (chapter 9). In: Patel V, Chisholm D, Dua T, Laxminarayan R, Medina-Mora ME, eds. *Disease Control Priorities: Mental, Neurological, and Substance Use Disorders*. 3rd ed. Vol. 4. Washington DC: IBRD/World Bank; 2015:163–182.

42. *Preventing Suicide: A Global Imperative*. Geneva: World Health Organization; 2014.

43. Waters H, Hyder A, Rajkotia Y, Basu S, Rehwinkel JA, Butchart A. *The Economic Dimensions of Interpersonal Violence*. Geneva: World Health Organization; 2004.

44. *Global Status Report on Violence Prevention 2014*. Geneva: World Health Organization; 2014.

45. *Preventing Child Maltreatment: A Guide to Taking Action and Generating Evidence*. Geneva: World Health Organization/International Society for Prevention of Child Abuse and Neglect; 2006.

46. *INSPIRE: Seven Strategies for Ending Violence Against Children*. Geneva: World Health Organization; 2016.

47. *Global Status Report on Preventing Violence Against Children 2020*. Geneva: World Health Organization; 2020.

48. *Hidden in Plain Sight: A Statistical Analysis of Violence Against Children*. New York: UNICEF; 2014.

49. *Preventing Youth Violence: An Overview of the Evidence*. Geneva: World Health Organization; 2015.

50. Pillemer K, Burnes D, Riffin C, Lachs MS. Elder abuse: global situation, risk factors, and prevention strategies. *Gerontologist*. 2016;56(Suppl 2):S194–S205.

51. Yon Y, Mikton CR, Gassoumis ZD, Wilber KH. Elder abuse prevalence in community settings: a systematic review and meta-analysis. *Lancet Glob Health*. 2017;5:e147–e156.

52. Reisner SL, Poteat T, Keatley J, et al. Global health burden and needs of transgender populations: a review. *Lancet*. 2016;388:422–436.

53. Watts C, Zimmerman C. Violence against women: global scope and magnitude. *Lancet*. 2002;359: 1232–1237.

54. *Care of Girls & Women Living with Female Genital Mutilation: A Clinical Handbook*. Geneva: World Health Organization; 2018.

55. *Female Genital Mutilation/Cutting: A Statistical Overview and Exploration of the Dynamics of Change*. New York: UNICEF; 2013.

56. *Global Plan of Action to Strengthen the Role of the Health System Within a National Multisectoral Response to Address Interpersonal Violence, in Particular Against Women and Girls, and Against Children*. Geneva: World Health Organization; 2016.

57. Reed E, Raj A, Miler E, Silverman JG. Losing the "gender" in gender-based violence: the missteps of research on dating and intimate partner violence. *Violence Against Women*. 2010;16:348–354.

58. *Violence Against Women Prevalence Estimates 2018: Global, Regional and National Prevalence Estimates for Intimate Partner Violence Against Women and Global and Regional Prevalence Estimates for Non-Partner Sexual Violence Against Women*. Geneva: World Health Organization; 2021.

59. García-Moreno C, Jansen HAFM, Ellsberg M, Heise L, Watts C. *WHO Multi-Country Study on Women's Health and Domestic Violence Against Women: Initial Results on Prevalence, Health Outcomes and Women's Responses*. Geneva: World Health Organization; 2005.

60. *RESPECT Women: Preventing Violence Against Women*. Geneva: World Health Organization; 2020.

61. Ellsburg M, Arango DJ, Morton M, et al. Prevention of violence against women and girls: what does the evidence say? *Lancet*. 2015;385:1555–1566.

62. Salama P, Spiegel P, Talley L, Waldman R. Lessons learned from complex emergencies over past decade. *Lancet*. 2004;364:1801–1813.

63. Spiegel PB. Differences in world responses to natural disasters and complex emergencies. *JAMA*. 2005;293:1915–1918.

64. Toole MJ, Waldman RJ. The public health aspects of complex emergencies and refugee situations. *Annu Rev Public Health*. 1997;18:283–312.

65. Melzer N. *International Humanitarian Law: A Comprehensive Introduction*. Geneva: ICRC; 2016.

66. Kalshoven F, Zegveld L. *Constraints on the Waging of War*. 4th ed. Cambridge UK: Cambridge University Press; 2011.

67. Kivlahan C, Ewigman N. Rape as a weapon of war in modern conflicts. *BMJ*. 2010;340:c3270.

68. Young H, Borrel A, Holland D, Salama P. Public nutrition in complex emergencies. *Lancet*. 2004; 364:1899–1909.

69. Sandoz Y. *The International Committee of the Red Cross as Guardian of International Humanitarian Law*. Geneva: ICRC; 1998.

70. *The Fundamental Principles of the Red Cross and Red Crescent*. Geneva: ICRC; 2016.

71. Minear L. The theory and practice of neutrality: some thoughts on the tensions. *Int Rev Red Cross*. 1999;833:63–71.

72. *Discover the ICRC*. Geneva: ICRC; 2018.

73. *Hope in Hell: Inside the World of Doctors Without Borders*. 3rd rev. ed. Richmond Hill ON: Firefly Books; 2010.

74. Leebaw B. The politics of impartial activism: humanitarianism and human rights. *Perspect Politics*. 2007;5:223–239.

75. Redfield P. A less modest witness: collective advocacy and motivated truth in a medical humanitarian movement. *Am Ethnologist.* 2006;33:3–26.

76. *International Financial Report 2020.* Geneva: Médecins Sans Frontières; 2021.

77. Kruk ME, Freedman LP, Anglin GA, Waldman RJ. Rebuilding health systems to improve health and promote statebuilding in post-conflict countries: a theoretical framework and research agenda. *Soc Sci Med.* 2010;70:89–97.

78. Brown VJ. BattleScars: Global conflicts and environmental health. *Environ Health Perspect.* 2004;112: A994–A1003.

79. *Landmines, Explosive Remnants of War and IED Safety Handbook.* 3rd ed. New York: United Nations Mine Action Service; 2015.

80. *Landmine Monitor 2020.* Geneva: International Campaign to Ban Landmines; 2020.

81. *Assistance to Victims of Landmines and Explosive Remnants of War: Guidance on Child-Focused Victim Assistance.* New York: UNICEF; 2014.

82. *Protecting Health Care: Key Recommendation.* Geneva: ICRC; 2016.

83. Barnett M. Humanitarianism transformed. *Persp Politics.* 2005;3:723–740.

84. MacQueen G, Santa-Barbara J. Peace building through health initiatives. *BMJ.* 2000;321:293–296.

85. Noah DL, Huebner KD, Darling RG, Waeckerle JF. The history and threat of biological warfare and terrorism. *Emerg Med Clin N Am.* 2002;20:255–271.

86. Beeching NJ, Dance DAB, Miller ARO, Spencer RC. Biological warfare and bioterrorism. *BMJ.* 2002; 324:336–339.

87. Rotz LD, Khan AS, Lillibridge SR, Ostroff SM, Hughes JM. Public health assessment of potential biological terrorism agents. *Emerg Infect Dis.* 2002;8:225–230.

88. Biological and chemical terrorism: strategic plan for preparedness and response. Recommendations of the CDC Strategic Planning Workgroup. *MMWR Recomm Rep.* 2000;49(RR-1):1–14.

89. Cieslak TC, Kortepeter MG, Wojtyk RJ, Jansen HJ, Reyes RA, Smith JO. Beyond the dirty dozen: a proposed methodology for assessing future bioweapon threats. *Mil Med.* 2018;183:e59–e65.

90. Inglesby TV, O'Toole T, Henderson DA, et al. Anthrax as a biological weapon, 2002: updated recommendations for management. *JAMA.* 2002; 287:2236–2252.

91. Jernigan DB, Raghunathan PL, Bell BP, et al. Investigation of bioterrorism-related anthrax, United States, 2001: epidemiologic findings. *Emerg Infect Dis.* 2002;8:1019–1028.

92. Dougall AL, Hayward MC, Baum A. Media exposure to bioterrorism: stress and the anthrax attacks. *Psychiatry.* 2005;68:28–42.

93. Schmitt K, Zacchia NA. Total decontamination cost of the anthrax letter attacks. *Biosecur Bioterror.* 2012;10:98–107.

94. Wray RJ, Becker SM, Henderson N, et al. Communicating with the public about emerging health threats: lessons from the pre-event message development project. *Am J Public Health.* 2008;98:2214–2222.

95. *Global Health Security Index 2021.* Washington DC: Nuclear Threat Initiative; 2021.

96. Annas GJ. Bioterrorism, public health, and civil liberties. *N Engl J Med.* 2002;346:1337–1342.

97. Gostin LO. When terrorism threatens health: how far are limitations on human rights justified? *J Law Med Ethics.* 2003;31:524–528.

98. Thompson AK, Faith K, Gibson JL, Upshur REG. Pandemic influenza preparedness: an ethical framework to guide decision-making. *BMC Med Ethics.* 2006;7:12.

99. Sidel VW, Levy BS. War, terrorism, and public health. *J Law Med Ethics.* 2003;31:516–523.

CHAPTER 18

Promoting Neonatal, Infant, Child, and Adolescent Health

Survival rates for newborns, infants, and young children have improved significantly in recent decades, but the rates in low-income countries continue to lag behind international targets. Expanding access to clinical care, community health and nutrition services, early childhood development interventions, and school health and safety programs will help children thrive as they grow.

18.1 Global Child Health

Childhood can be divided into several developmental stages (**Figure 18.1**):

- The neonatal period is the first four weeks after a live birth. The early neonatal period is typically described as the first 7 days (one week) of life and the late neonatal period as the remaining three weeks of the 28 days.
- An **infant** is a baby of any age between birth and the first birthday. The post-neonatal infancy period encompasses the time between one month after birth and the first birthday.
- An **under-5 child** is a child of any age between birth and the fifth birthday. The post-infancy period of early childhood includes the toddler stage (the time between about the first and third birthdays) and the preschool years (approximately the time between the third and fifth birthdays).

- Middle childhood extends from about age 5 through ages 10 to 12. These are typically the years for primary education.
- Adolescence, or late childhood, includes the preteen and teenage years, which are typically the years for secondary education.

One of the greatest success stories in global health is the steady reduction in child mortality that has been achieved in recent decades. The number of children dying each year has decreased in all age groups even as the number of babies born each year has increased (**Figure 18.2**).[1]

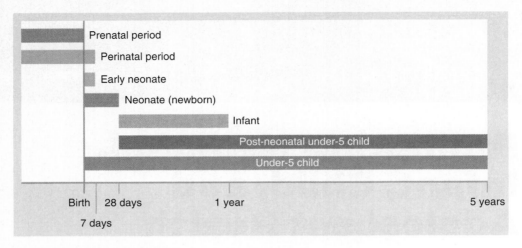

Figure 18.1 Age groups in early childhood.

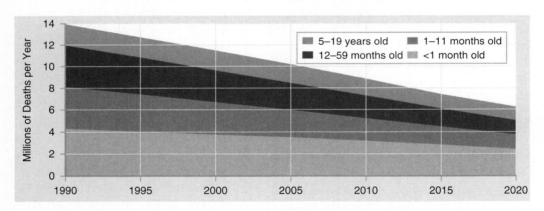

Figure 18.2 Number of deaths per year among infants, children, and adolescents worldwide, 1990–2020.

Data from GBD 2019 Demographics Collaborators. Global age-sex-specific fertility, mortality, healthy life expectancy (HALE), and population estimates in 204 countries and territories, 1950–2019: a comprehensive demographic analysis for the Global Burden of Disease Study 2019. *Lancet.* 2020;396:1160–1203.

The underlying cause of most deaths in early and middle childhood is poverty.[2] Most child mortality occurs in lower-income countries, where limited access to medical care for neonatal health issues, preventable and treatable child infections like diarrhea and pneumonia, and undernutrition continues to cause millions of deaths each year. Most children who die in low-income countries would not have become ill if they had lived in high-income countries. If they had become ill in a high-income rather than a low-income country, most of these children would have survived their illnesses and not died from them. Numerous low-cost interventions are effective at improving infant and child survival, but interventions focused on specific health problems work best when they are accompanied by socioeconomic development initiatives that aim to end the cycle of poverty that makes children born into extreme poverty so much more likely to die than children who happen to be born into wealthier families.

The Millennium Development Goals (MDGs) sought to significantly improve survival among children less than five years old through a mix of poverty reduction and health-specific strategies. The **under-5 mortality** **rate** (U5MR) is the number of infants and children who die before their fifth birthdays per 1,000 live births. The MDGs aimed to reduce the U5MR by two-thirds between 1990 and 2015 (MDG 4), to a rate of less than 30 deaths per 1,000 live births.[3] Although this target was not achieved, the number of under-5 child deaths per year dropped by more than half during those 25 years, from about 12 million deaths in 1990 to less than 6 million under-5 child deaths worldwide in 2015.[4] Reductions in the U5MR occurred in most countries, including in most of the lowest-income countries as well as in high-income countries that already had very low child mortality rates (**Figure 18.3**).

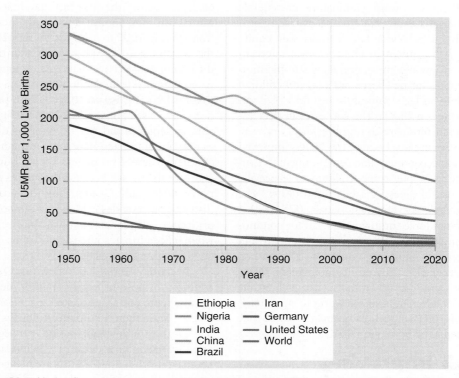

Figure 18.3 Under-5 mortality rate per 1,000 live births, 1950–2020, worldwide and in selected countries.

Data from United Nations Department of Economic and Social Affairs. *World Population Prospects: The 2019 Revision*. New York: United Nations; 2019.

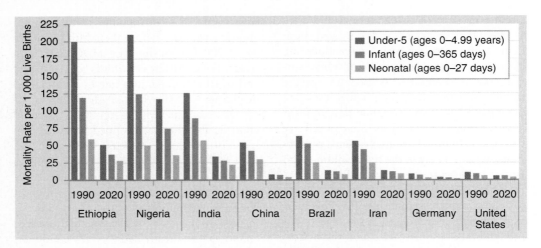

Figure 18.4 Neonatal, infant, and under-5 mortality rates per 1,000 live births in selected countries.

Data from *Levels & Trends in Child Mortality: Report 2020 Estimates Developed by the UN Inter-agency Group for Child Mortality Estimation*. New York: UNICEF; 2020.

Progress toward eliminating preventable child deaths in any country is a gain for global health, but achieving health equity will require greater investment in child survival interventions in low-income countries where the mortality rates for newborns, infants, and children continue to lag significantly behind global targets (**Figure 18.4**).[5] The successes in decreasing child mortality during the MDG era were achieved, in part, because the MDGs improved the socioeconomic and environmental conditions that put some children at especially high risk of illness, disability, and death.[6] The Sustainable Development Goals (SDGs) that will be in force through 2030 call for continuous improvements in poverty reduction and in access to nutrition, education, clean water, sanitation, electricity, adult employment, safety, peace, and the other tools that will enable more children around the world to enjoy long, healthy, productive lives no matter where they happen to be born and raised.[7]

18.2 Improving Neonatal Survival

Neonatal mortality accounts for an increasing percentage of pediatric deaths. The percentage of deaths before the fifth birthday that occur during the first month after birth increased from 35% in 1990 to nearly 50% in 2020, and the percentage of deaths between birth and the end of adolescence that occur among neonates increased from about 30% to 40% across those 30 years (**Figure 18.5**).[8] These proportions increased because the mortality rate among neonates did not decrease as quickly as the mortality rates among older infants and children. There is no preferred distribution of child deaths by age because the goal is to end preventable child deaths, but the changing distribution provides evidence to support prioritization of neonatal survival interventions when allocating resources to various global child health initiatives.

Every day, nearly 7,000 newborns die.[9] In addition to those nearly 2.5 million neonatal deaths, there are an estimated 2 million stillbirths.[9] More than 40% of all stillbirths occur during the intrapartum period between the onset of labor and delivery.[10] While not all neonatal deaths and stillbirths are preventable, up to 3 million of the nearly 4.5 million losses annually could be prevented with improved access to quality obstetric and neonatal care.[9] Until recently, global health reports typically

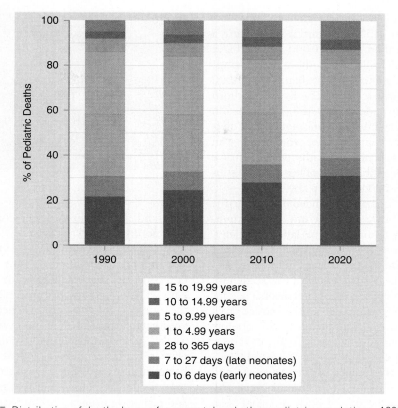

Figure 18.5 Distribution of deaths by age for neonatal and other pediatric populations, 1990–2020.

Data from GBD 2019 Diseases and Injuries Collaborators. Global burden of 369 diseases and injuries in 204 countries and territories, 1990–2019: a systematic analysis for the Global Burden of Disease Study 2019. *Lancet.* 2020;396:1204–1222.

did not include stillbirths in their calculations of lost lives. Including late-in-pregnancy fetal losses with neonatal mortality is a more accurate way to track pregnancy outcomes.[11] In lower-income countries where resuscitation equipment is not consistently available at the places where women give birth, currently high death rates among newborns might be artificially low because they do not include late-term stillbirths in the calculations.[12] (In some high-income countries, intensive resuscitation measures sometimes add newborns with a very low likelihood of survival to the count of live births. Neonatal survival metrics may look slightly less favorable when clinicians are aggressive about attempting to resuscitate very low birthweight neonates

who would be considered stillbirths in places where advanced technologies are not available, but the newborn survival rate in high-income countries is very high even after adding in those early neonatal deaths.)

The **neonatal mortality rate** (NMR) is the number of deaths of babies within 28 days after birth per 1,000 live births. The global NMR decreased from about 35 per 1,000 live births in 1990 to less than 20 per 1,000 live births by 2015,[4] but the rate in many low-income countries remains much higher than the global average. The SDGs aim to "end preventable deaths of newborns" via a target of "all countries aiming to reduce neonatal mortality to at least as low as 12 per 1000 live births" (SDG 3.2) rather than merely aiming to drop the global NMR to less than 12 per 1,000 live births.[7] Achieving a rate of less than 12 per 1,000 live births in all countries will require the global average to drop to significantly less than 12 per 1,000 by 2030 (**Figure 18.6**).[4] The Every Newborn Action Plan endorsed by the World Health Assembly extends this ambitious goal, aiming for every country in the world to have an NMR of less than 10 deaths per 1,000 live births and a stillbirth rate of less than 10 stillbirths per 1,000 total births by 2035.[13]

About 75% of all neonatal deaths are due to preterm birth, asphyxia and other complications and traumas during labor and delivery, and neonatal sepsis and other infections, and an additional 10% are due to congenital birth defects (**Figure 18.7**).[8] (The epidemiological burden from nonfatal neonatal conditions is tiny compared to the burden from neonatal mortality, but the major contributors are nutritional deficiencies (37%), infections (17%), and congenital birth defects (11%).[8]) Because so many neonatal deaths are related to preterm birth and birth traumas, the risk of dying on the day of birth is higher than the cumulative risk of dying across several

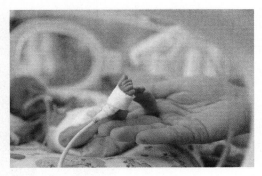

© Kristina Bessolova/Shutterstock

thousand days of life in later childhood or early adulthood.

Interventions on the day of birth are critically important for improving the percentage of pregnancies that result in healthy newborns who will survive into healthy childhood, but the opportunities to improve neonatal survival extend from preconception through the weeks after birth.[14] Immunizing pregnant women with tetanus toxoid protects their babies from tetanus infection. Treating maternal infections (such as malaria and syphilis) and managing maternal health issues (such as diabetes) reduces neonatal mortality.[15] During

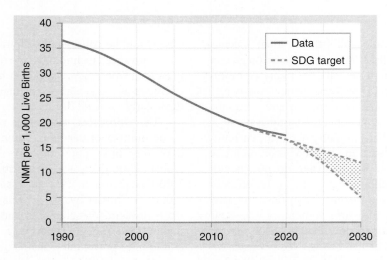

Figure 18.6 Neonatal mortality rate (NMR) per 1,000 live births and the Sustainable Development Goal (SDG) target for 2030.

Data from *Levels & Trends in Child Mortality: Report 2020 Estimates Developed by the UN Inter-agency Group for Child Mortality Estimation.* New York: UNICEF; 2020.

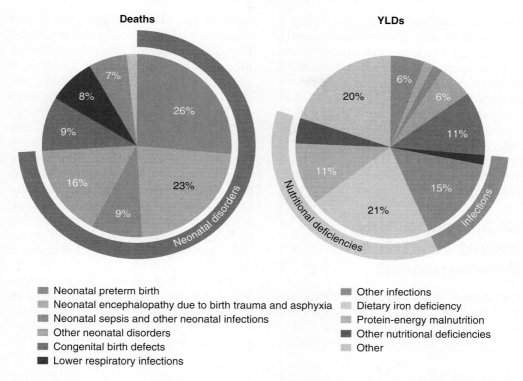

Figure 18.7 Causes of death and years lived with disability (YLDs) during the **neonatal period (ages birth through 27 days)**.

Data from GBD 2019 Diseases and Injuries Collaborators. Global burden of 369 diseases and injuries in 204 countries and territories, 1990–2019: a systematic analysis for the Global Burden of Disease Study 2019. *Lancet.* 2020;396:1204–1222.

the intrapartum period, women and their babies can be saved with actions like giving corticosteroids to women who go into preterm labor in order to prepare the lungs of fetuses to breathe, having skilled attendants care for women in a clean environment during labor and delivery, and managing complications with cesarean sections and other advanced emergency obstetrical procedures when necessary. After delivery, newborn resuscitation, prevention of hypothermia, and initiation of breastfeeding keep newborns alive. Chlorhexidine to clean the umbilical cord and prevent infections, injectable antibiotics to treat newborn sepsis and pneumonia, and other low-cost medical interventions also save lives.[16] In addition to preventing mortality, many of these

interventions help reduce the risk of neurodevelopmental impairment and other long-term disabilities in surviving babies.[17]

The Every Newborn Action Plan (ENAP) emphasizes four key interactions with the healthcare system that improve newborn health and survival[18]:

- Every pregnant woman has at least four prenatal care contacts.
- Every birth is attended by a skilled birth attendant.
- Every newborn receives routine postnatal care within two days of birth.
- Every small or sick newborn receives inpatient care (including respiratory support if needed).

The biggest barriers to expanding access to neonatal health services are not having enough funding, not having enough trained health workers to provide obstetric and neonatal health services, and not having the resources and leadership to manage the logistics of scaling up delivery of quality care.[19] These barriers can be overcome when citizens and communities call for change, governments choose to prioritize progress on child health, and partners make commitments to provide support and accountability.[20]

18.3 Supporting Infant Health and Development

The **infant mortality rate** (IMR), the number of babies who die before their first birthdays per 1,000 live births, has steadily improved in recent decades (**Figure 18.8**).[5] The total number of infant deaths worldwide decreased from about 8.1 million in 1990 to about 3.7 million in 2020, and the total number of post-neonatal infant deaths decreased from about 3.8 million to 1.3 million over those 30 years.[8] Today, about 67% of all post-neonatal infant deaths are due to pneumonia, diarrheal diseases, malaria, and other infectious diseases (**Figure 18.9**).[8] Most of these infectious diseases are preventable and treatable, so there is reason to hope that continued investment in health systems will enable this steady trend toward reduced infant mortality to continue.

The leading causes of years lived with disability (YLDs) for post-neonatal infants include iron deficiency anemia,

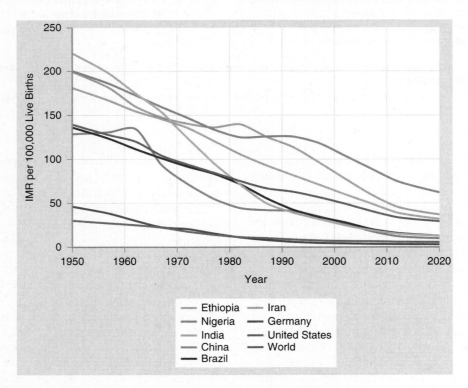

Figure 18.8 Infant mortality rate per 1,000 live births, 1950–2020, worldwide and in selected countries.

Data from United Nations Department of Economic and Social Affairs. *World Population Prospects: The 2019 Revision.* New York: United Nations; 2019.

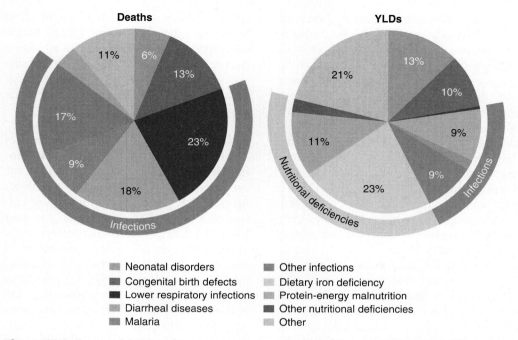

Figure 18.9 Causes of death and years lived with disability (YLDs) during **post-neonatal infancy (ages 1–11 months)**.

Data from GBD 2019 Diseases and Injuries Collaborators. Global burden of 369 diseases and injuries in 204 countries and territories, 1990–2019: a systematic analysis for the Global Burden of Disease Study 2019. *Lancet.* 2020;396:1204–1222.

protein-energy malnutrition, and other nutritional deficiencies (37%); infections (21%); and neonatal disorders and congenital birth defects (16%).[8] Interventions that provide micronutrient supplements such as iron and folic acid to pregnant and breast-feeding women; support exclusive breast-feeding for the first six months after birth; promote continued breastfeeding as complementary foods are added to the infant diet; and distribute micronutrient supplements such as vitamin A, iodine, iron, and zinc to infants and young children who are under-nourished will help reduce the rates of disability and death among infants.[21]

As infant survival rates improve, more emphasis is being placed on interventions that help babies and children thrive rather than merely keeping them alive.[22] **Early childhood development** (ECD) describes the physical, cognitive, emotional, and

social development that occurs during the approximately 1,000 days from conception through the second birthday.[23] By the end of their first year of life, most babies are able to sit without assistance, crawl, pull themselves into a standing position, grasp objects with their hands, understand many words, speak several words, express emotions like happiness and anxiety, and interact meaningfully with caregivers. Infants may not reach these milestones on time if their mothers lacked calories or micronutrients during critical stages of fetal development, if they were born prematurely or experienced birth traumas, if they experience chronic malnutrition and repeated bouts of infection as babies, or if they are abused or neglected by caregivers.

One of the SDGs aims to "ensure that all girls and boys have access to quality early childhood development, care, and pre-primary education, so that they are ready for primary education" (SDG 4.2).[7] During the first two years after birth, motor skills, cognitive development, language acquisition, and socioemotional development are facilitated by psychosocial stimulation from parents and other caregivers that promotes mental development[24]; nutritious food that allows for health, growth, physical activity, and brain development; and a clean and safe environment that protects children from infectious diseases and violence.[25] Child development then continues through the preschool years as children gain the self-regulation and learning skills necessary for success in a primary school classroom.[26]

Access to health services, nutrition, and social interaction with parents and other caregivers in the first months and years of life is critical for health and for preparing young children for success in school and, later on, for healthy and productive adulthood.[27] Economic evaluations show that a diversity of health and nutritional, economic, educational, social, and environmental interventions for young children and their families yield long-term benefits not only for those individuals but also for their communities and nations.[28] ECD initiatives are most effective when they involve cooperation across the health, education, social service, and economic development sectors.[29]

18.4 Health Interventions in Early Childhood

In the late 20th century, several large-scale multinational initiatives improved the lives of millions of young children around the world.[30] Many of these initiatives supported greater access to **primary health care** (PHC), a community-based approach to health that employs community health workers and focuses as much on prevention as on

cures.[31] PHC is a "horizontal" approach to health care that emphasizes routine access to comprehensive primary care rather than a "vertical" approach that targets selected diseases with specific interventions (like special vaccination days) that are managed outside the public healthcare system.[32]

An international conference on PHC hosted in 1978 by what is now the city of Almaty, Kazakhstan, generated the **Declaration of Alma-Ata**, which called for the expanded use of PHC to achieve "Health for All by 2000" through the reduction of barriers to healthcare access, especially in poor and rural areas.[33] Prioritized interventions under a PHC model include prevention of infectious diseases; provision of essential medications and treatments for infectious diseases, noncommunicable diseases, and injuries; promotion of nutrition; programming for maternal and child health, including immunization and family planning; and coordination of health services with traditional health practitioners.[34]

A hallmark of PHC is regularly scheduled health clinics for children younger than five years old in order to monitor child growth and provide recommended immunizations.[35] The Expanded Program on Immunization (EPI) was started in 1974 by the World Health Organization (WHO) to expand the number and types of vaccines routinely given to children. More than four decades later, EPI (now called the Essential Programme on

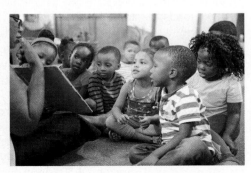

© Monkey Business Images/Shutterstock

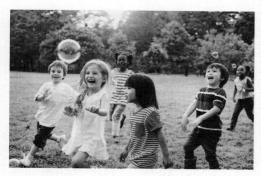

© Rawpixel.com/Shutterstock

Immunization) is still supporting the delivery of essential vaccines to children across the globe.[36] When all children, whether sick or healthy, have frequent interactions with the healthcare system through under-5 health clinics, warning signs for potentially life-threatening conditions in relatively healthy children can be detected early and treated. For example, growth monitoring tracks child weight so that caregivers will know if a child has lost weight or is failing to gain weight. Weight loss or stagnation can be a sign of serious illness, and early detection means that a nutritional intervention can be implemented before a health crisis occurs.

GOBI was an initiative started in the 1980s by UNICEF that focused on increasing child survival by promoting four simple interventions[37]:

- **G**rowth monitoring
- **O**ral rehydration therapy for diarrhea
- **B**reastfeeding
- **I**mmunization

Later, a partnership between UNICEF, the WHO, and the World Bank added three community-focused components to the mix: family planning, food production, and female education—creating a program called GOBI/FFF.[38]

IMCI, the Integrated Management of Childhood Illness, is a package of simple, affordable, and effective home, community, and clinical interventions for major childhood illnesses and undernutrition that was first developed by UNICEF and the WHO in 1995.[39] (The acronym is sometimes expanded to IMNCI, for Integrated Management of Newborn and Childhood Illness.) Integration in IMCI has several layers of meaning.[40] One aspect of integration is an emphasis on the interrelatedness of children's health conditions. A child with malaria is more vulnerable to diarrhea. A child with vitamin A deficiency is more vulnerable to death from measles. Clinicians working under an IMCI framework complete a series of medical assessments on each sick child that allows for diagnosis of underlying conditions in addition to the primary illness. Integration also emphasizes families and communities working together with the staff in various levels of healthcare facilities to care for sick children.

IMCI is intended to improve family and community health practices as well as the case management skills of healthcare staff. To advance this goal, IMCI provides home healthcare guidelines for families with young children and evidence-based decision charts for clinicians to use when assessing children and treating frequently occurring illnesses.[41] For example, the family of a child with diarrhea should know how to prepare oral rehydration therapy correctly and know what symptoms require a sick child to be taken to the local clinic or hospital. The local clinic should support community health education programs, provide care for advanced cases of dehydration, and make referrals for hospital-based treatment if necessary. In places where malaria is endemic, parents should know how to use bednets to prevent mosquito bites and how to recognize fevers and other symptoms of malaria. The local clinic should support those community health education efforts, treat cases of malaria that do occur, and make referrals for advanced treatment when it is needed. **iCCM**, Integrated **C**ommunity **C**ase **M**anagement, is a WHO/UNICEF-led strategy that provides community health workers with algorithms for treating uncomplicated childhood infections in homes.[42] IMCI clinical guidelines, which focus on management of serious childhood diseases at healthcare facilities, are often paired with iCCM guidelines to provide a comprehensive set of clinic- and community-based care recommendations.

Each of these historic international child health programs contributed to significant improvements in global child health metrics. The SDGs aim to further reduce the under-5 child mortality rate to less than 25 deaths per 1,000 live births in all countries by 2030 (SDG 3.2).[7] This will require a decrease in the global U5MR of more than 40% between 2015 and 2030 (**Figure 18.10**).[4] It would be technologically possible to achieve a "grand convergence" of health metrics by the year 2030 by reducing the maternal and child mortality rates in low-income countries to the already-low levels in high-income countries, but this ambitious goal would require doubling funding for maternal and child health.[43]

More than 70% of all deaths in post-infancy early childhood today are due to diarrheal diseases, malaria, pneumonia, and other infectious diseases (**Figure 18.11**).[8] The leading causes of YLDs include iron deficiency anemia and other nutritional deficiencies (26%), infections (18%), neonatal disorders and congenital birth defects (16%), and skin diseases like dermatitis and urticaria (hives) (15%).[8] To ensure that as many children as possible have a healthy start in life, it is important to further improve access to safe drinking water, educate parents about infectious disease prevention and management, support continued breastfeeding and healthy nutrition, increase access to essential medicines and immunizations, and strengthen primary health systems.

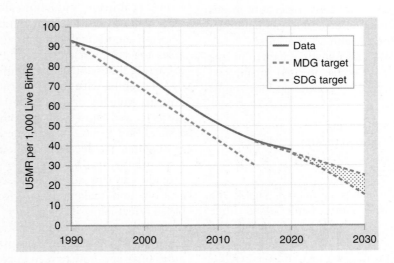

Figure 18.10 Under-5 mortality rate (U5MR) per 1,000 live births and the Sustainable Development Goal (SDG) target for 2030.

Data from *Levels & Trends in Child Mortality: Report 2020 Estimates Developed by the UN Inter-agency Group for Child Mortality Estimation.* New York: UNICEF; 2020.

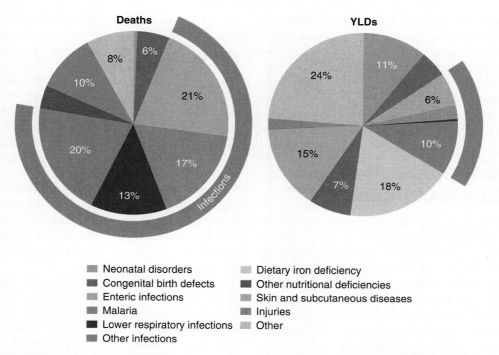

Figure 18.11 Causes of death and years lived with disability (YLDs) during **early childhood (ages one to four years)**.

Data from GBD 2019 Diseases and Injuries Collaborators. Global burden of 369 diseases and injuries in 204 countries and territories, 1990–2019: a systematic analysis for the Global Burden of Disease Study 2019. *Lancet.* 2020;396:1204–1222.

The Partnership for Maternal, Newborn & Child Health (PMNCH), which was launched in 2005 and is hosted by the WHO, brings together more than 1,000 partner groups representing a diversity of sectors.[44] Gavi and other global health partnerships have expanded access to vaccines that protect against measles and other life-threatening infections. UNICEF and other multinational groups have promoted breastfeeding, distributed micronutrients to children, supported agricultural development, and taken other actions to prevent infant and child malnutrition. Ministries of health and collaborating agencies and organizations in low- and middle-income countries have expanded access to tools for preventing and treating pneumonia, diarrhea, malaria,

and other potentially fatal infectious diseases in rural and urban areas within their borders. Each of the funders, channels, and implementers involved in PMNCH and related efforts is playing a role in improving global child health.

Child health is improving because billions of dollars are being invested each year in global child health initiatives.[45] Every Woman Every Child was initiated by the United Nations (UN) in 2010 to accelerate progress on SDG targets related to women, children, and adolescents,[46] and the Global Financing Facility for Every Woman Every Child was started in 2015 by the World Bank and other participants to raise funds for reproductive, maternal, newborn, child, and adolescent health and nutrition interventions. These funds and those from other groups enable partner governments, UN agencies, foundations and other donors, nongovernmental organizations, private sector companies, clinical professional associations, academic institutes, and countless others who are working at the local, national, regional, and global levels to contribute to reducing infant and child mortality and promoting health and well-being in the early years.

18.5 Children with Special Needs

Prevention science seeks to identify opportunities for primary prevention, secondary prevention, and tertiary prevention of health-related issues. Interventions at all three levels can help improve the health and well-being of children with special needs. At the primary prevention level, the goal is to reduce the onset of preventable disabilities. Millions of children have neurodevelopmental disabilities, cerebral palsy, seizure disorders, visual impairment, hearing impairment, and other disabilities related to birth trauma, oxygen deprivation, and other birth complications that could have been prevented if their mothers had access to quality obstetric care before and during delivery and quality neonatal care immediately after birth.[47] Many other children have disabilities that occurred as a result of injuries or untreated infections. Increased access to maternal and child health services could reduce the rate of preventable disability among newborns, infants, and children.

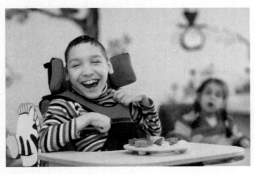

© Olesia Bilkei/Shutterstock

At the secondary prevention level, the goal is to diagnose health issues as early as possible so that interventions can help reduce the duration and severity of disability. For example, babies with cleft palate, which occurs when there is an opening in the roof of the mouth, may suffer from severe malnutrition because they are unable to suck properly. Access to special bottles enables infants with cleft palate to consume breast milk or breast-milk supplements, and the cleft palate can be surgically repaired once babies are several months old and have gained adequate weight. Children who do not have access to nutritional support and surgery may have unnecessarily long durations of disability associated with cleft palate.

At the tertiary prevention level, the goal is for all children with special needs to be able to access the health, educational, and social services they need to reach their full potential. Children with special needs have the healthiest life trajectories when they are able to access various types of physical, occupational, communication, and other therapies early in life.[48] For example, children born with cerebral palsy and other mobility disabilities can develop their motor skills to their highest potential when they have physical therapy and the use of braces, crutches, and walkers from an early age. Unfortunately, many families cannot access (re)habilitation services, and many children with special needs are excluded from educational settings.[49] Those barriers can have negative consequences that persist for a lifetime.[50] Increasing access to (re)habilitation services, assistive devices, and support services for children with special needs and their families is both a public health priority and a human rights issue.[49] Affordable home- and community-based therapies and technologies can help increase function, access, and inclusion for children in places where formal therapy services are not accessible.[51]

18.6 Promoting Health in Middle Childhood

Most of the attention on health in pediatric populations is devoted to under-5 children because the youngest age groups have the highest mortality rates. Although the mortality rate for school-aged children and adolescents is low, health education interventions during these developmental periods can be valuable for keeping older children safe and preparing them for active and healthy adulthood.[52]

Middle childhood is the period between the fifth birthday and early adolescence. The mortality rate is very low, but about 52% of the deaths that do occur are due to enteric infections (such as typhoid and other causes of diarrhea) and other infectious diseases, and about 24% are due to injuries (**Figure 18.12**).[8] The leading nonfatal health losses include iron deficiency anemia and other nutritional deficiencies (21% of YLDs); infectious diseases (16%); skin and subcutaneous diseases such as dermatitis, urticaria (hives), and scabies (14%); and mental health disorders such as anxiety disorder and conduct disorder (10%).[8]

Many health interventions for school-aged children are delivered at primary schools.[53] School health services provide health and hygiene education and support for activities related to infection prevention, nutrition, physical fitness, mental health and well-being, injury prevention and safety awareness, medical and dental care, and healthy relationships, including

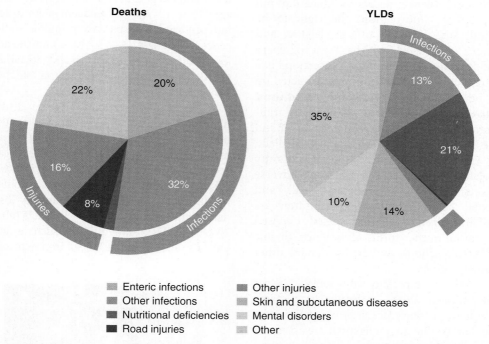

Figure 18.12 Causes of death and years lived with disability (YLDs) during **middle childhood (ages five to nine years)**.

Data from GBD 2019 Diseases and Injuries Collaborators. Global burden of 369 diseases and injuries in 204 countries and territories, 1990–2019: a systematic analysis for the Global Burden of Disease Study 2019. *Lancet.* 2020;396:1204–1222.

bullying prevention.[54] Schools may deliver vaccinations and mass drug administration for intestinal worms in high-risk populations, conduct vision and hearing screenings, monitor growth and nutritional status (such as anemia), provide meals and nutritional supplements, assist students with use of inhalers for asthma and medications for other chronic conditions, and refer students with special needs to other health and social services.

Initiatives to support the rights of children also contribute to protecting their health and enabling them to flourish. In 1989, the General Assembly of the UN adopted the Convention on the Rights of the Child, which declares that the rights of the child include an adequate standard of living; freedom from all forms of exploitation; protection from all forms of violence; access to education and appropriate information; the right to be heard; and the right to rest, leisure, and play.[55] Acknowledging the right of every child in the world to these protections is a start, but this recognition must be acted on to be meaningful.[56] **Adverse childhood experiences (ACEs)** are potentially traumatic events that occur between birth and the 18th birthday, such as abuse, neglect, or exposure to household or community violence. ACEs can have lifelong adverse effects on mental, physical, social, and sexual health.[57] Millions of children are still hungry, neglected or abused, exposed to war and other forms of violence, unable to attend school, and being denied other human rights.

Girls are especially vulnerable to abuse and neglect. When a family has limited resources, girls may face discrimination within the family due to preferential treatment of sons. Daughters may not be allowed to attend school and may be forced into early marriage.[58] In 1995, the UN adopted the Beijing Declaration, which affirms several strategic objectives for promoting the rights of the "girl-child," including eliminating educational discrimination, the exploitation of child laborers, and violence against children. Although some improvements have been achieved, such as increasing school enrollment, significant inequalities between boys and girls remain in many regions of the world. Those inequalities can have significant adverse health effects for girls, young women, and their families.[59]

18.7 Promoting Adolescent Health

Adolescence is a life stage characterized by rapid physical, sexual, neurological, psychological, and social development.[60] Adolescent development may begin at around 10 years of age (especially for girls) and extend until after 19 years of age (especially for boys).[61] Physical maturation begins in early adolescence (about ages 10 to 13 years). Teenagers begin to seek independence from parents in middle adolescence (about ages 14 to 17 years). In late adolescence (about 18 to 20+ years), social and emotional maturation continues as independence is established.[62]

Deaths among adolescents are distributed across injuries (about 30% of all deaths), infectious diseases (about 26% of deaths), and many noncommunicable diseases that each account for only a small share of overall deaths (**Figure 18.13**).[8] The leading causes of nonfatal health loss include depression, anxiety disorders, and other mental health disorders (about 23% of YLDs); skin diseases such as acne vulgaris (about 12% of YLDs); iron deficiency

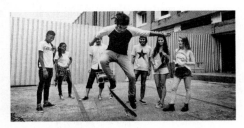

© Rawpixel.com/Shutterstock

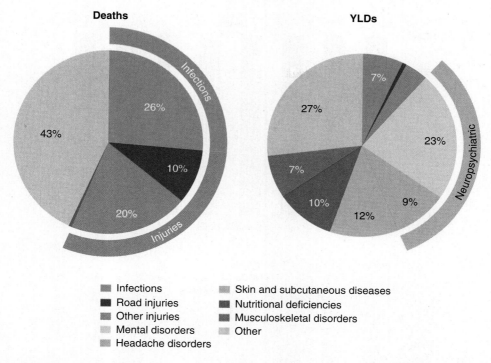

Figure 18.13 Causes of death and years lived with disability (YLDs) during **adolescence (ages 10–19 years)**.

Data from GBD 2019 Diseases and Injuries Collaborators. Global burden of 369 diseases and injuries in 204 countries and territories, 1990–2019: a systematic analysis for the Global Burden of Disease Study 2019. *Lancet*. 2020;396:1204–1222.

anemia and other nutritional deficiencies (about 10% of YLDs); and migraines and other headache disorders (about 9% of YLDs).[8] The causes of YLDs are similar across countries, but infections are the prominent cause of death in lower-income countries while injuries are the dominant cause in higher-income countries (**Figure 18.14**).[8]

The psychosocial risk and protective factors that affect adolescent health can be described using the acronym HEADSSS[63]:

- **H**ome life: parent and family relationships, resources, and communication
- **E**ducation/employment: school performance and involvement in school or work activities that prepare adolescents for responsible adulthood

- **A**ctivities: participation in supervised social activities such as sports, arts, religious, social justice, or community organizations
- **D**rugs: use of alcohol, drugs, or other harmful substances by self, peers, or family members
- **S**exuality: knowledge, attitudes, and behaviors related to sexual activity
- **S**uicide/depression/self-image: stress management, support networks, coping skills, self-esteem, self-acceptance, and other factors related to self-harm and other aspects of mental health
- **S**afety: use of seat belts and other protective gear, skills in nonviolent conflict resolution, exposure to weapons and violence

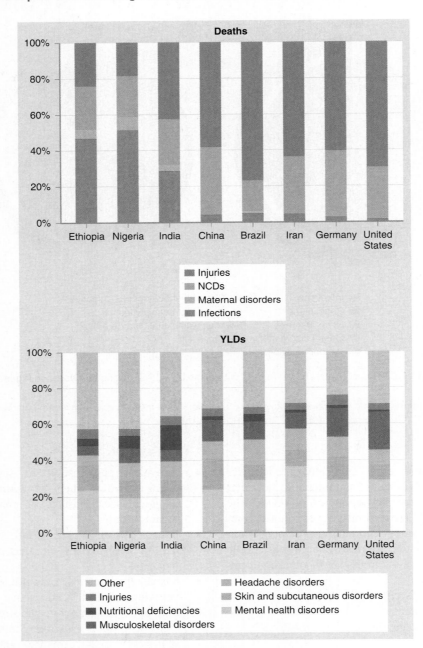

Figure 18.14 Causes of death and years lived with disability (YLDs) among adolescents ages 15–20 years in selected countries.

Data from GBD 2019 Diseases and Injuries Collaborators. Global burden of 369 diseases and injuries in 204 countries and territories, 1990–2019: a systematic analysis for the Global Burden of Disease Study 2019. *Lancet.* 2020;396:1204–1222.

Some versions of this model add an additional "E" for eating or "D" for diet that represents disordered attitudes and practices related to food and weight. A fourth "S" is sometimes added to this model to represent the growing harm associated with excessive social media use that diminishes self-confidence; damages social relationships; and exposes young people to cyberbullying, sexual violence, and other forms of violence.[64]

Adolescent health interventions focus on the immediate needs of youth and on setting the foundation necessary for those young people to become healthy adults.[65] The highest-impact health interventions for adolescents include programs for mental health (including prevention of suicide, alcohol abuse, and drug abuse), injury prevention (including safe driving and prevention of violence), and reproductive health (including access to tools for preventing pregnancy, HIV, and other sexually transmitted infections) as well as interventions that promote nutritious diets, physical activity, tobacco-free living, and other aspects of healthy adult lifestyles.[66] Reducing risky behaviors and adopting protective behaviors has both immediate and long-term benefits for health.[67] Interventions that improve socioenvironmental concerns such as youth unemployment, limited access to advanced education and vocational training, and unhealthy and violent environments also promote improved physical, mental, and social health among adolescents and young adults.[68] Investments in adolescent health generate economic and social returns as well as health benefits.[69]

References

1. GBD 2019 Demographics Collaborators. Global age-sex-specific fertility, mortality, healthy life expectancy (HALE), and population estimates in 204 countries and territories, 1950–2019: a comprehensive demographic analysis for the Global Burden of Disease Study 2019. *Lancet.* 2020;396:1160–1203.
2. *The State of the World's Children 2016: A Fair Chance for Every Child.* New York: UNICEF; 2016.
3. *The Millennium Development Goals Report 2015.* New York: United Nations; 2015.
4. *Levels & Trends in Child Mortality: Report 2020 Estimates Developed by the UN Inter-agency Group for Child Mortality Estimation.* New York: UNICEF; 2020.
5. United Nations Department of Economic and Social Affairs. *World Population Prospects: The 2019 Revision.* New York: United Nations; 2019.
6. *Progress for Children: Beyond Averages: Learning from the MDGs.* New York: UNICEF; 2015.
7. *Transforming Our World: The 2030 Agenda for Sustainable Development.* New York: United Nations; 2015.
8. GBD 2019 Diseases and Injuries Collaborators. Global burden of 369 diseases and injuries in 204 countries and territories, 1990–2019: a systematic analysis for the Global Burden of Disease Study 2019. *Lancet.* 2020;396:1204–1222.
9. *Every Newborn Progress Report 2019.* Geneva: World Health Organization; 2020.
10. *A Neglected Tragedy: The Global Burden of Stillbirths: Report of the UN Inter-agency Group for Child Mortality Estimation.* New York: UNICEF; 2020.
11. Goldenberg RL, McClure EM, Jobe AH, Kamath-Rayne BD, Gravette MG, Rubens CE. Stillbirths and neonatal mortality as outcomes. *Int J Gynaecol Obstet.* 2013;123:252–253.
12. Phillips J, Millum J. Valuing stillbirths. *Bioethics.* 2015;29:413–423.
13. *Every Newborn: An Action Plan to End Preventable Deaths.* Geneva: World Health Organization/UNICEF; 2014.
14. Darmstadt GL, Bhutta ZA, Cousens S, et al. Evidence-based, cost-effective interventions: how many newborn babies can we save? *Lancet.* 2005;365:977–985.
15. Gülmezoglu AM, Althabe F, Souza JP, et al. Interventions to reduce maternal and newborn morbidity and mortality (chapter 7). In: Black RE, Laxminarayan R, Temmerman M, et al., eds. *Disease Control Priorities: Reproductive, Maternal, Newborn, and Child Health.* 3rd ed. Vol. 2. Washington DC: IBRD/World Bank; 2016:115–136.
16. Bhutta ZA, Das JK, Bahl R, et al. Can available interventions end preventable deaths in mothers,

newborn babies, and stillbirths, and at what cost? *Lancet.* 2014;384:347–370.

17. Lawn JE, Blencowe H, Oza S, et al. Every Newborn: progress, priorities, and potential beyond survival. *Lancet.* 2014;384:189–205.

18. *Ending Preventable Newborn Deaths and Stillbirths by 2030: Moving Faster Towards High-Quality Universal Health Coverage in 2020–2025.* Geneva: World Health Organization; 2020.

19. Dickson KE, Simen-Kapeu A, Kinney MV, et al. Health-systems bottlenecks and strategies to accelerate scale-up in countries. *Lancet.* 2014;384:438–454.

20. *Committing to Child Survival: A Promise Renewed. Progress Report 2015.* New York: UNICEF; 2015.

21. *Essential Nutrition Actions: Mainstreaming Nutrition Through the Life-Course.* Geneva: World Health Organization; 2019.

22. Black MM, Walker SP, Fernald LCH, et al. Early childhood development coming of age: science through the life course. *Lancet.* 2017;389:77–90.

23. Britto PR, Lye SJ, Proulx K, et al. Nurturing care: promoting early childhood development. *Lancet.* 2017;389:91–102.

24. Alderman H, Behrman J, Glewwe P, Fernald L, Walker S. Evidence of impact of interventions on growth and development during early and middle childhood (chapter 7). In: Bundy DAP, de Silva N, Horton S, Jamison DT, Patton GC, eds. *Disease Control Priorities: Child and Adolescent Health and Development.* 3rd ed. Vol. 8. Washington DC: IBRD/World Bank; 2017:79–98.

25. Aboud FE, Yousafzai AK. Very early childhood development (chapter 13). In: Black RE, Laxminarayan R, Temmerman M, et al., eds. *Disease Control Priorities: Reproductive, Maternal, Newborn, and Child Health.* 3rd ed. Vol. 2. Washington DC: IBRD/World Bank; 2016:241–262.

26. Anderson LM, Shinn C, Fullilove MT, et al. The effectiveness of early childhood development programs: a systematic review. *Am J Prev Med.* 2003;24(Suppl 3):32–46.

27. *The Global Strategy for Women's, Children's and Adolescents' Health (2016–2030).* New York: Every Woman Every Child; 2015.

28. Denboba AD, Sayre RK, Wodon QT, Elder LK, Rawlings LB, Lombardi J. *Stepping Up Early Childhood Development: Investing in Young Children for High Returns.* Washington DC: World Bank; 2014.

29. Richter LM, Daelmans B, Lombardi J, et al. Investing in the foundation of sustainable development: pathways to scale up for early childhood development. *Lancet.* 2017;389:103–118.

30. Claeson M, Waldman RJ. The evolution of child health programmes in developing countries: from targeting diseases to targeting people. *Bull World Health Organ.* 2000;78:1234–1245.

31. Cueto M. The origins of primary health care and selective primary health care. *Am J Public Health.* 2004;94:1864–1874.

32. Msuya J. *Horizontal and Vertical Delivery of Health Services: What Are the Trade Offs?* Washington DC: World Bank; 2004.

33. Hall JJ, Taylor R. Health for all beyond 2000: the demise of the Alma-Ata Declaration and primary health care in developing countries. *Med J Aust.* 2003;178:17–20.

34. Walley J, Lawn JE, Tinker A, et al. Primary health care: making Alma-Ata a reality. *Lancet.* 2008;372:1001–1007.

35. Rifkin SB, Walt G. Why health improves: defining the issues concerning 'comprehensive primary health care' and 'selective primary health care.' *Soc Sci Med.* 1986;23:559–566.

36. *WHO's Vision and Mission: Immunization and Vaccines 2015–2030.* Geneva: World Health Organization; 2015.

37. Schuftan C. The child survival revolution. *Fam Pract.* 1990;7:329–332.

38. Cash R, Keusch GT, Lamstein J, eds. *Child Health and Survival: The UNICEF GOBI-FFF Program.* London: Croom Helm; 1987.

39. Lambrechts T, Bryce J, Orinda V. Integrated management of childhood illness: a summary of first experiences. *Bull World Health Organ.* 1999;77:582–594.

40. Costello AM, Dalglish SL, Strategic Review Study Team. *Towards a Grant Convergence for Child Survival and Health: A Strategic Review of Options for the Future Building on Lessons Learnt from IMNCI.* Geneva: World Health Organization; 2016.

41. *Child Health in the Community: "Community IMCI" Briefing Package for Facilitators.* Geneva: World Health Organization; 2004.

42. *WHO/UNICEF Joint Statement: Integrated Community Case Management (iCCM).* New York: UNICEF; 2012.

43. Jamison DT, Summers LH, Alleyne G, et al. Global health 2035: a world converging within a generation. *Lancet.* 2013;382:1898–1955.

44. *The Partnership for Maternal, Newborn & Child Health 2021–2025 Strategy.* Geneva: PMNCH; 2020.

45. Dingle A, Schäferhoff M, Borghi J, et al. Estimates of aid for reproductive, maternal, newborn, and child health: findings from application of the Muskoka2 method, 2002–17. *Lancet Glob Health.* 2020;8:e374–e386.

46. *2020 Progress Report on the Every Woman Every Child Global Strategy for Women's, Children's and Adolescents' Health (2016–2030).* Geneva: World Health Organization/UNICEF; 2020.

47. Mwaniki MK, Atieno M, Lawn JE, Newton CRJC. Long-term neurodevelopmental outcomes after intrauterine and neonatal insults: a systematic review. *Lancet.* 2012;379:445–452.

48. *Early Childhood Development and Disability: A Discussion Paper.* Geneva: World Health Organization/UNICEF; 2012.

49. *WHO Global Disability Action Plan 2014–2021: Better Health for All People with Disability.* Geneva: World Health Organization; 2014.

50. Graham N, Schultz L, Mitra S, Mont D. Disability in middle childhood and adolescence (chapter 17). In: Bundy DAP, de Silva N, Horton S, Jamison DT, Patton GC, eds. *Disease Control Priorities: Child and Adolescent Health and Development.* 3rd ed. Vol. 8. Washington DC: IBRD/World Bank; 2017:221–238.

51. *Disabled Village Children: A Guide for Community Health Workers, Rehabilitation Workers, and Families.* Palo Alto CA: Hesperian; 2009.

52. Bundy D, Horton S. Impact of interventions on health and development during childhood and adolescence: a conceptual framework (chapter 6). In: Bundy DAP, de Silva N, Horton S, Jamison DT, Patton GC, eds. *Disease Control Priorities: Child and Adolescent Health and Development.* 3rd ed. Vol. 8. Washington DC: IBRD/World Bank; 2017:72–78.

53. Bundy D, Schultz L, Sarr B, Banham L, Colenso P, Drake L. The school as a platform for addressing health in middle childhood and adolescence (chapter 20). In: Bundy DAP, de Silva N, Horton S, Jamison DT, Patton GC, eds. *Disease Control Priorities: Child and Adolescent Health and Development.* 3rd ed. Vol. 8. Washington DC: IBRD/World Bank; 2017:269–286.

54. *WHO Guidelines on School Health Services.* Geneva: World Health Organization; 2021.

55. *Convention on the Rights of the Child.* New York: United Nations; 1989.

56. Hammarberg T. The UN Convention on the Rights of the Child, and how to make it work. *Human Rights Q.* 1990;12:97–105.

57. Hughes K, Bellis MA, Hardcastle KA, et al. The effect of multiple adverse childhood experiences on health: a systematic review and meta-analysis. *Lancet Public Health.* 2017;2:e356–e366.

58. Ferrant G, Nowacka K, Thim A. *Living Up to Beijing's Vision of Gender Equality: Social Norms and Transformative Change.* Paris: Organisation for Economic Co-operation and Development; 2015.

59. *The Beijing Declaration and Platform for Action Turns 20.* New York: UN Women; 2015.

60. Sawyer SM, Afifi RA, Bearinger LH, et al. Adolescence: a foundation for future health. *Lancet.* 2012;379:1630–1640.

61. *Health for the World's Adolescents: A Second Chance in the Second Decade.* Geneva: World Health Organization; 2014.

62. Curtis AC. Defining adolescence. *J Adolesc Family Health.* 2015;7:2.

63. Goldenring JM, Rosen DS. Getting into adolescent heads: an essential update. *Contemp Pediatr.* 2004;21:64–90.

64. Clark DL, Raphael JL, McGuire AL. HEADS^4: social media screening in adolescent primary care. *Pediatrics.* 2018;141:e20173655.

65. *Global Accelerated Action for the Health of Adolescents (AA-HA!): Guidance to Support Country Implementation.* Geneva: World Health Organization; 2017.

66. Patton GC, Sawyer SM, Santelli JS, et al. Our future: A Lancet commission on adolescent health and wellbeing. *Lancet.* 2016;387:2423–2478.

67. Catalano FR, Fagan AA, Gavin LE, et al. Worldwide application of prevention science in adolescent health. *Lancet.* 2012;379:1653–1664.

68. Viner RM, Ozer EM, Denny S, et al. Adolescence and the social determinants of health. *Lancet.* 2012;379:1641–1652.

69. Sheehan P, Sweeny K, Rasmussen B, et al. Building the foundations for sustainable development: a case for global investment in the capabilities of adolescents. *Lancet.* 2017;390:1792–1806.

CHAPTER 19

Promoting Healthy Adulthood and Aging

Global health seeks to enable as many people as possible to enjoy long, healthy lives. Interventions for young and middle-aged adults seek to establish healthy habits and prevent early death and disability. Interventions for older adults support independence, dignity, and comfort. An aging global population will demand more resources for eldercare.

19.1 Healthy Adulthood

Most of the world's people are adults, and the global population is getting older. The median age of a population is the age of the middle person in the group if everyone is ordered from youngest to oldest. Half of the population is younger than the median age, and half is older than the median age. The global median age increased from about 24 years in 1990 to more than 31 years just 30 years later (**Figure 19.1**).[1] In the typical high-income country, the median age is now older than 40 years; in upper-middle-income countries, the median is over 35 years (**Figure 19.2**).[1] As populations age, more resources need to be allocated to health and social services for older adults.

The Sustainable Development Goals (SDGs) aim to "ensure healthy lives and promote well-being for all at all ages" (SDG 3).[2]

Adulthood is often divided into three developmental stages[3]:

- Early adulthood extends roughly from ages 20 to 39 years, encompassing the typical reproductive years.
- Middle adulthood encompasses the time between about ages 40 and 64 years.
- Late adulthood is the period when adults are about ages 65 years and older.

Many of the health-related interventions with the greatest impact are ones that yield benefits for all age groups, such as ones that improve socioeconomic and environmental conditions for entire communities.[4] For example, clean water prevents diarrheal diseases in people of all ages[5]; clean indoor and outdoor air protects the developing lungs of young children and reduces the risk of cardiovascular and lung disease in older adults[6]; and increased access to

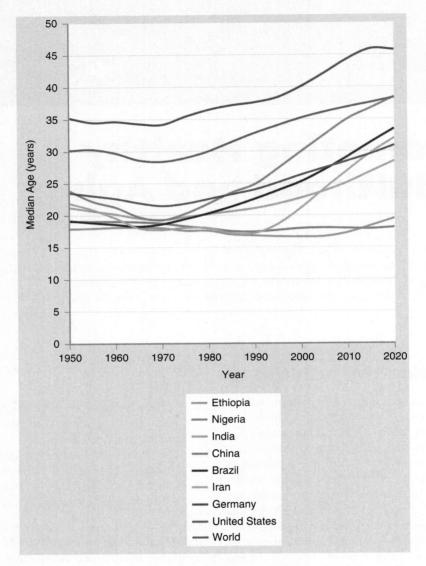

Figure 19.1 Median age of the population, 1950–2020, worldwide and in selected countries.

Data from United Nations Department of Economic and Social Affairs. *World Population Prospects: The 2019 Revision.* New York: United Nations; 2019.

health services benefits young and old alike.[7] However, there are also interventions that are especially relevant for specific age groups.

The overall goal of health promotion among adults is to enable long lives in which physical health, mental health, and social well-being are maintained. For early and middle adulthood, key population health aims

include reducing mortality to as close to zero as possible since any death of a young or middle-aged adult is considered to be premature; decreasing the rates of disease and disability so that as many men and women as possible are leading productive, independent, and pain-free lives; and mitigating risk behaviors and other modifiable exposures that are likely to

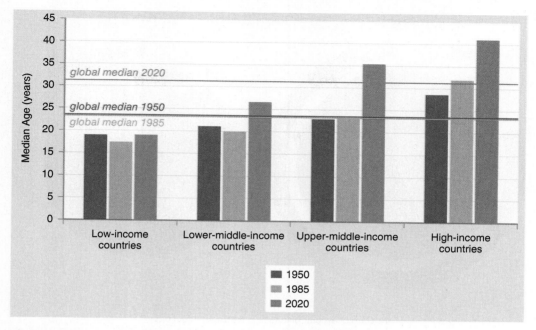

Figure 19.2 Median age of the population today, by country income level.

Data from United Nations Department of Economic and Social Affairs. *World Population Prospects: The 2019 Revision.* New York: United Nations; 2019.

cause disability and premature death later in life. For older adulthood, the aims include preventing premature mortality, minimizing illness and disability, and providing supportive care as needed.

19.2 Promoting Health in Early Adulthood

The mortality rate during early adulthood is low compared to early childhood and late adulthood, but many of the deaths that do occur are ones that could have been prevented. Deaths in early adulthood are distributed across injuries (about 34% of all deaths), infectious diseases (about 24% of deaths), the four major noncommunicable diseases (cardiovascular disease, cancer, chronic respiratory diseases, and diabetes, which together account for about 24% of deaths), and a variety of other noncommunicable

causes (**Figure 19.3**).[8] However, there is considerable variability in the causes of death by country (**Figure 19.4**).[8] Infectious diseases are the most frequent cause of death in most low-income countries but are rare in high-income countries. Mortality reduction interventions for early adult populations must be tailored to the local or national risk profile. Infection control is a leading priority in most low-income countries, and injury prevention is among the top priorities in many middle-income countries.

The overall burden of disease in a population is often calculated in terms of disability-adjusted life years (DALYs) lost, and DALYs are the sum of years lived with disability (YLDs) and years of life lost (YLLs) to premature disability. Global health metrics like YLDs, YLLs, and DALYs may be calculated based on a target survival age in the population as a whole or using target survival ages for each age group rather than the population as a whole. If YLLs

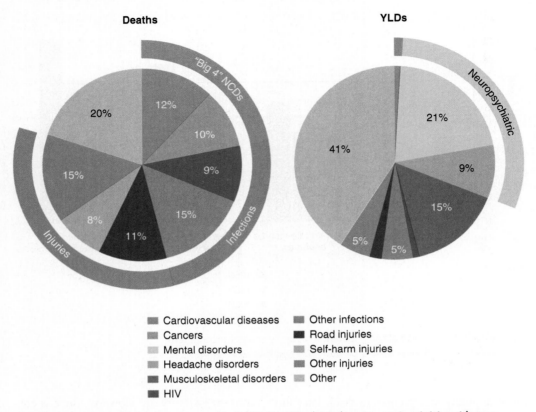

Figure 19.3 Causes of death and years lived with disability (YLDs) during **early adulthood (ages 20–39 years)**.

Data from GBD 2019 Diseases and Injuries Collaborators. Global burden of 369 diseases and injuries in 204 countries and territories, 1990–2019: a systematic analysis for the Global Burden of Disease Study 2019. *Lancet.* 2020;396:1204–1222.

are calculated using a target survival age of 80 years for all age groups, a 90-year-old who dies would not contribute any YLLs to the population total. When age-specific target survival ages are used, target survival for 90-year-olds is based on the expected years of life remaining given that someone has already survived to age 90. This method of calculating YLLs enables even very old adults to still contribute YLLs to the population total. For middle-aged and older adult populations, the number of age-specific YLLs generated each year exceeds the number

of YLDs. By contrast, since there are few deaths in the young adult population, the number of YLDs exceeds the number of YLLs, even though every death of a young adult adds many YLLs to the population total (**Figure 19.5**).[8]

The leading causes of YLDs in early adulthood include depression and other mental health disorders (about 21% of YLDs), low back pain and other musculoskeletal disorders (about 15% of YLDs), migraines and other headache disorders (about 9% of YLDs), and numerous other causes each accounting for a

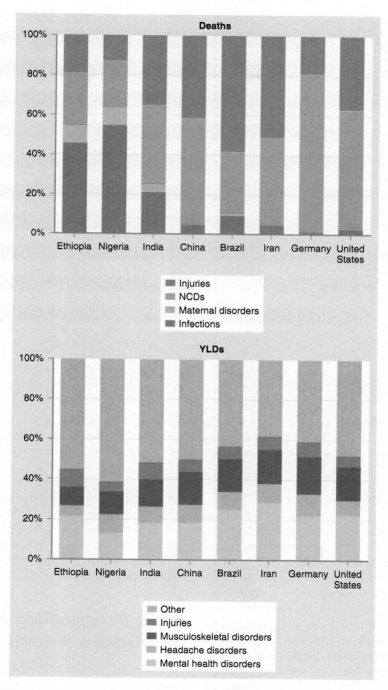

Figure 19.4 Causes of death and years lived with disability (YLDs) during early adulthood (ages 20–39 years) in selected countries.

Data from GBD 2019 Diseases and Injuries Collaborators. Global burden of 369 diseases and injuries in 204 countries and territories, 1990–2019: a systematic analysis for the Global Burden of Disease Study 2019. *Lancet*. 2020;396:1204–1222.

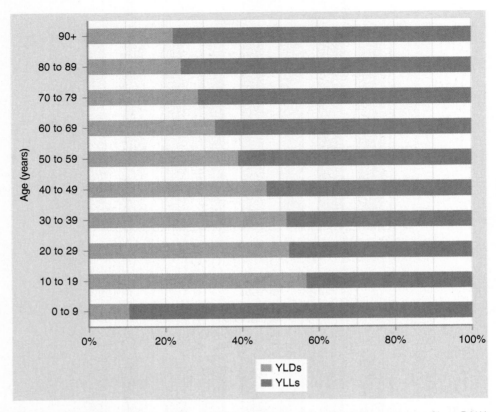

Figure 19.5 Relative proportion of YLDs and YLLs by age group in a typical recent year. Since DALYs are the sum of YLDs and YLLs, each bar represents 100% of the DALYs for the age group.

Data from GBD 2019 Diseases and Injuries Collaborators. Global burden of 369 diseases and injuries in 204 countries and territories, 1990–2019: a systematic analysis for the Global Burden of Disease Study 2019. *Lancet.* 2020;396:1204–1222.

small portion of the total disability.[8] The burden from these major causes of disability is relatively similar across country income levels. Injury prevention and increased access to and utilization of health services, including counseling for mental health conditions and medications for pain management, are important for reducing disability in this age group.

Early adulthood is also an opportune time for young people to establish healthy habits that will increase their likelihood of enjoying a long, healthy life. Key behaviors to establish include avoiding harmful use of alcohol, unsafe sex, harmful drugs, and all tobacco use; maintaining a healthy weight, eating a nutritious diet, and engaging in routine

physical activity; using medications and other approaches if they are necessary to maintain a low blood pressure, healthy blood sugar levels, and low cholesterol levels; and acting to minimize the risks of injury from occupational and recreational exposures.[9]

19.3 Promoting Health in Middle Adulthood

The relative proportion of deaths from infections and injuries shrinks as populations age and the rate of deaths from noncommunicable diseases (NCDs) expands dramatically (**Figure 19.6**).[8] By middle adulthood, most

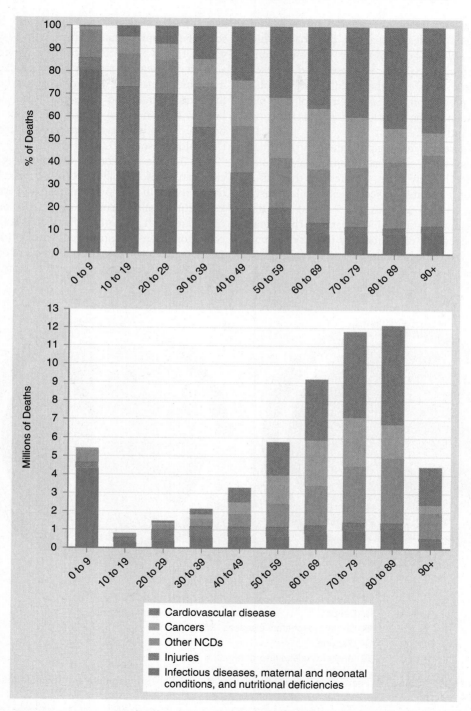

Figure 19.6 Distribution of deaths worldwide by cause and age group in a typical recent year.

Data from GBD 2019 Diseases and Injuries Collaborators. Global burden of 369 diseases and injuries in 204 countries and territories, 1990–2019: a systematic analysis for the Global Burden of Disease Study 2019. *Lancet.* 2020;396:1204–1222.

deaths are attributable to NCDs, including the 64% of deaths that are due to the "big four" NCDs—cardiovascular disease, cancer, chronic respiratory diseases, and diabetes (**Figure 19.7**).[8] For the middle-aged population, prevention and management of the "big four" conditions is the top priority for reducing YLLs and DALYs.

Increases in longevity are only a partial success when those additional years of life are not healthy ones. At present, there is a gap of 10 years between healthy life expectancy (HALE) at birth (63.5 years) and life expectancy at birth (73.5 years).[10] This duration does not vary much by country income level. In countries with low sociodemographic status, there is a 9-year gap between HALE

and life expectancy; in countries with high sociodemographic status, there is a 12-year gap.[10] The typical older adult experiences about a decade of disability prior to death. For many individuals, the years of disability begin in middle adulthood. The population-level burden from nonfatal health conditions can be reduced with interventions targeted toward the major causes of YLDs.

In middle adulthood, the most significant causes of disability are musculoskeletal disorders, including low back pain and arthritis; mental health disorders; and sense organ disorders, such as hearing loss.[8] Some of these conditions can be prevented with worksite safety regulations that reduce the risk of occupational injuries and hearing protection that

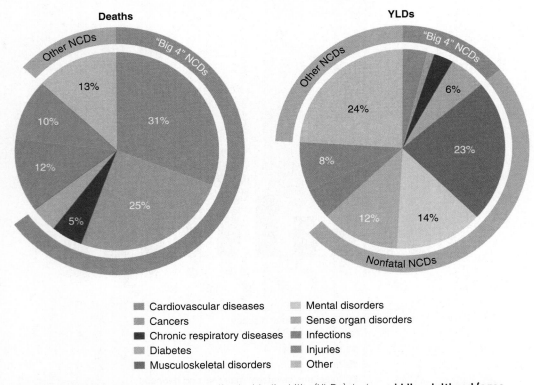

Figure 19.7 Causes of death and years lived with disability (YLDs) during **middle adulthood (ages 40–64 years)**.

Data from GBD 2019 Diseases and Injuries Collaborators. Global burden of 369 diseases and injuries in 204 countries and territories, 1990–2019: a systematic analysis for the Global Burden of Disease Study 2019. *Lancet*. 2020;396:1204–1222.

reduces the noise exposure that can cause hearing loss. Increased access to medical care, medications, mental health counseling, and assistive devices such as hearing aids could significantly reduce the burden of existing disability in this age group.

The number of years an individual adult lives without disability is a function of a lifetime of health-related behaviors in addition to being influenced by personal characteristics like genetics and psychosocial factors.[11] Middle-aged adults can take action to prevent, delay, and treat the health issues that might otherwise become expensive and disabling later in life. The most cost-effective interventions for promoting longevity and postponing age-related disability are ones that enable younger adults—including adults in middle adulthood—to adopt and sustain active lifestyles, seek early diagnosis of health concerns, and manage health problems well.[12]

19.4 The Aging Transition

The **mortality transition** is a health transition characterized by decreases in the rates of death for age groups across the life span. When mortality rates lower, life expectancies increase. The **aging transition** is a health transition characterized by an increase in the percentage of older adults in the population and a decrease in the percentage of children in the population. When both death rates (the mortality transition) and birth rates (the fertility transition) decrease, the number of older adults in a population may grow at a faster rate than the number of children.[13] An aging transition can occur even in places where the number of children is rising as part of overall population growth.

The world population is aging rapidly as more children survive to adulthood and more adults survive to very old age.[14] A substantial increase in the number of older adults and the percentage of older adults in the global population is projected to occur over the coming decades. The number of people worldwide who are 60 years old or older is expected to increase from about 1 billion in 2020 to more than 2 billion by 2050; the number of people who are 80 years old or older did not reach 100 million until after 2005 but is expected to rise to more than 400 million by 2050 (**Figure 19.8**).[1] Globally, the percentage of the total population that is 60 years old or older will more than double between 2000 and 2050, rising from 10% in 2000 to more than 20% by 2050; the percentage of world's people who are aged 80 years or older is expected to rise even faster, from about 1.2% in 2000 to 4.4% in 2050 (**Figure 19.9**).[1]

Cumulative probabilities examine health and survival across the life span, starting at birth. Conditional probabilities examine health and survival based on the "condition" of having already experienced some prior event. For example, a cumulative survival probability might examine the percentage of people who survive from birth to their 85th birthdays. A conditional survival probability might examine the probability of surviving to the 85th birthday given that the person has already survived to the 80th birthday. Surviving to age 80 is the "condition" for the calculation of the additional five years of survival. Even in many lower-income countries, children who survive to their fifth birthdays can now expect to survive to age 70 or older (**Figure 19.10**). The typical 50-year-old in almost every country can now expect to celebrate a 75th birthday, and the typical 70-year-old can expect to celebrate an 80th birthday.[1] As more people survive to middle adulthood and beyond, more people will live to very old age. Countries of all income levels can expect to see increases in the percentage of their residents who are older adults (**Figure 19.11**).[1]

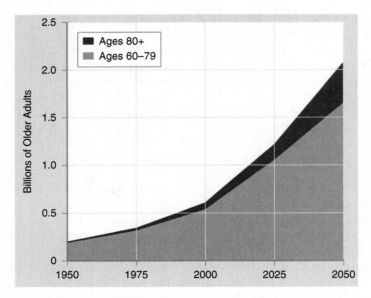

Figure 19.8 Number of people aged 60 years and older worldwide, 1950–2050.

Data from United Nations Department of Economic and Social Affairs. *World Population Prospects: The 2019 Revision*. New York: United Nations; 2019.

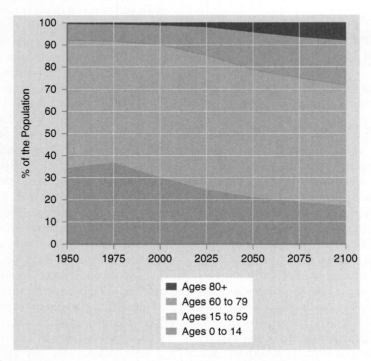

Figure 19.9 Projected distribution of the world's population by age, 1950–2100.

Data from United Nations Department of Economic and Social Affairs. *World Population Prospects: The 2019 Revision*. New York: United Nations; 2019.

	Low - Income Countries	Lower-Middle-Income Countries	Upper-Middle-Income Countries	High-Income Countries	Difference in Years of Life Expectancy Between Low- and High-Income Countries
At least half of **newborns** will live until age . . .	63.5	68.1	75.5	80.9	17.4
At least half of **5-year-old children** will live to age . . .	68.2	71.6	76.6	81.3	13.1
At least half of **15-year-old adolescents** will live to age . . .	69.3	72.3	76.8	81.4	12.1
At least half of **40-year-old adults** will live to age . . .	72.8	74.5	78.2	82.3	9.5
At least half of **60-year-old adults** will live to age . . .	77.1	78.1	80.5	84.4	7.3
At least half of **80-year-old adults** will live to age . . .	85.9	86.8	87.7	89.8	3.9

Figure 19.10 Life expectancy at various ages, by country income levels.

Data from United Nations Department of Economic and Social Affairs. *World Population Prospects: The 2019 Revision*. New York: United Nations; 2019.

19.5 Aging and Global Health

Several social support ratios (also called dependency ratios) calculated from demographic data help social service providers and policymakers understand the current and future needs of the populations they serve.

- The **child support ratio** (also called the child dependency ratio) is a ratio comparing the total number of children (aged 0–14 years) in a population to the number of people aged 15–64 years.
- The **elderly support ratio** (also called the old-age dependency ratio) is a ratio comparing the total number of older adults (aged 65+ years) in a population to the number of people aged 15–64 years.

Populations with relatively few working adults for each older adult have higher aging-related dependency ratios.

- The **total dependency ratio** is a ratio comparing the total number of children (aged 0–14 years) and older adults (aged 65+ years) in a population to the number of people aged 15–64 years.

Similar ratios can also be calculated using different definitions for which age groups define the pediatric and geriatric populations. For example, because many older women and men remain active and economically independent, alternate measurements of the elderly support ratio may include only older adults who are no longer in the formal workforce.

Nearly every country is experiencing a decreasing child support ratio and an increasing elderly support ratio (**Figure 19.12**).[1] In

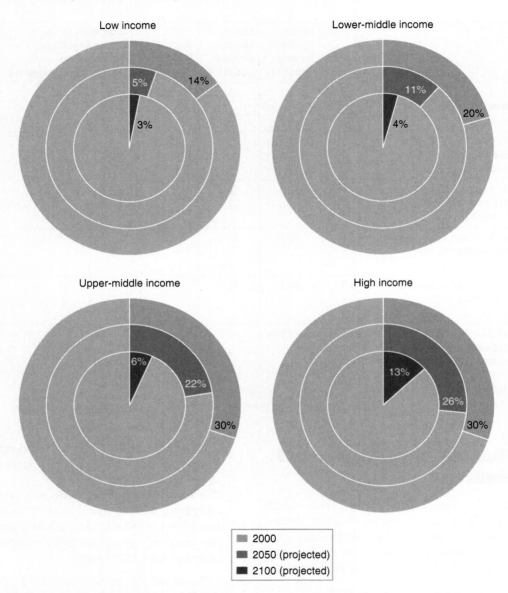

Figure 19.11 Percentage of the population that is aged 65 years or older by country income level, 2000–2100.

Data from United Nations Department of Economic and Social Affairs. *World Population Prospects: The 2019 Revision.* New York: United Nations; 2019.

lower-income countries, the total dependency ratio is currently decreasing because fertility rates are lower than in the past, but that trend will reverse as life expectancies increase. In higher-income countries, the total dependency ratio is rapidly increasing as a result of aging. The trends for these ratios across time point toward a future with greater demands for eldercare in countries of all income levels.

Many older people contribute to their families and communities by taking care of their grandchildren, providing mentorship

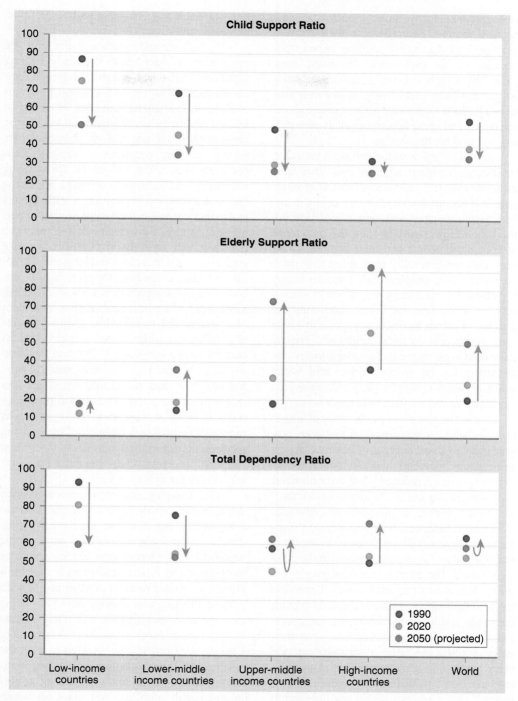

Figure 19.12 Child support ratio, elderly support ratio, and total dependency ratio, by country income level, 1990–2050.

Data from United Nations Department of Economic and Social Affairs. *World Population Prospects: The 2019 Revision*. New York: United Nations; 2019.

and guidance for younger employees, connecting younger generations to their cultural heritage, and sharing the wisdom gained from decades of life experience. However, most older adults will eventually encounter challenges that limit their ability to live independently.[15] These limitations impose demands on the families of aging adults as well as on social support and health systems.

In most of the world, eldercare is provided by spouses, children, siblings, and other family members, and institutionalization of older people is uncommon. Living with family members when assistance with activities of daily living becomes necessary is often the preference of both older people and their families. However, decreasing fertility rates mean that there are fewer young people to care for older family members. The increasing proportion of women who work outside the home also limits the number of people available to provide in-home care. The families of older adults who require daily assistance may incur financial losses due to paying for caregiving services and losing wages as family caregivers drop out of the paid workforce or reduce their paid work hours.

Just as the economic productivity of households is reduced when women and men take time away from other types of labor to care for aging family members, the economic productivity of nations is reduced when large numbers of caregivers step out of the formal workforce.[16] In industrializing middle-income countries where retirement accounts and pension plans are not the norm, aging is expected to become a major social and economic concern in the coming decades. The migration of rural young people to cities means that adult children often live far from their aging parents and cannot provide daily care, and few families have the resources to hire caregivers or nursing assistants.[17] For many older adults, age-based discrimination and other forms of ageism contribute to financial insecurity, social isolation, and reduced health status.[18] Older adults who do not have family support and are no longer able to work—or are no longer able to secure paid employment even

if they are able to work—may end up destitute, homeless, and hungry.

In high-income countries, the growing proportion of older adults is already creating significant challenges for aging adults and their communities. The national pension programs of many industrialized countries, especially in Europe, might be on the pathway to collapse because there are not enough young workers paying into the programs to support retirees adequately.[19] The retirement age is being increased, and retirement benefits are being cut. The increasing proportion of older adults is also burdening healthcare systems because so many adverse health conditions become more prevalent with age. Aging populations create greater demand for acute- and long-term medical care (such as the need for cardiological procedures and management of comorbid NCDs), some types of surgical care (such as treatment of cataracts and stabilization of hip fractures after falls), and rehabilitation services (such as care for stroke survivors).[12] Demand for adult day care, assisted living services, nursing care, hospice care, and community-based services that support the physical needs and psychosocial well-being of older adults also increases as more older adults seek assistance from housing services, transportation networks, nutritional support programs, civic organizations, and other community resources.[20]

The emerging challenges associated with aging can be considered welcome ones because they are the result of the excellent progress that has been made on enabling more people worldwide to live longer lives, but few countries are prepared to finance and provide care for a rapidly increasing number of older people with chronic illnesses and disabilities.[21] Prioritizing care for older populations will likely require budget cuts in other areas, such as education. Creative solutions will be required to meet the resource needs of expanding older adult populations, including the strain that managing age-related health problems will place on health systems, while also maintaining other services that are deemed to be essential. Each nation and each community will need to tailor its responses to aging based on economic realities, cultural considerations, and local preferences. Policymakers will be best equipped to make these important decisions when they can draw on the lessons learned by others from across the globe.

19.6 Supporting Health in Older Adulthood

Nearly 90% of all deaths among older adults are attributable to NCDs, with more than 70% of deaths in a typical recent year due to the "big four" NCDs—cardiovascular disease, cancer, chronic respiratory diseases, and diabetes.[8]

However, these four conditions cause only about 25% of nonfatal health losses. Musculoskeletal disorders (such as back pain and osteoarthritis) and sense disorders (including age-related hearing and vision loss) are major causes of disability along with mental health disorders such as depression and neurological disorders such as Alzheimer's disease and other dementias (**Figure 19.13**).[8] These and other aging-related conditions may cause difficulties with physical movement, sensory perception, energy, balance, cognition (such as memory and orientation), and emotional regulation.[20]

Health promotion and disease prevention initiatives throughout the life span are allowing adults in countries across the income spectrum to live to older ages and enjoy more healthy,

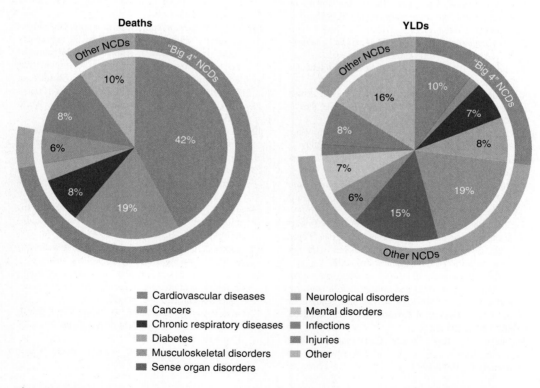

Figure 19.13 Causes of death and years lived with disability (YLDs) among **older adults (ages 65+ years)** in a typical (nonpandemic) year.

Data from GBD 2019 Diseases and Injuries Collaborators. Global burden of 369 diseases and injuries in 204 countries and territories, 1990–2019: a systematic analysis for the Global Burden of Disease Study 2019. *Lancet*. 2020;396:1204–1222.

independent years.[22] However, many older adults eventually require several years of assistance with routine activities of daily living. The quality of life of older adults can be improved with tools that support autonomy, mobility, and social connections. These include affordable preventive and therapeutic healthcare services, including medications for managing chronic health problems and controlling pain; safe, comfortable, and accessible home and community environments; and strong family and social support.[11]

As more assistance with activities of daily living becomes required, the goals for individual care shift from supporting independence toward enabling dignity and comfort for older adults as they experience the final stage of the life course.[23] A good death is one in which the dying individual is not merely avoiding suffering but is encircled by social, spiritual, and other types of support during the final weeks of life.[24]

References

1. United Nations Department of Economic and Social Affairs. *World Population Prospects: The 2019 Revision.* New York: United Nations; 2019.
2. *Transforming Our World: The 2030 Agenda for Sustainable Development.* New York: United Nations; 2015.
3. Levinson DJ. A conception of adult development. *Am Psychol.* 1986;41:3–13.
4. Frieden TR. A framework for public health action: the health impact pyramid. *Am J Public Health.* 2010;100:590–595.
5. Prüss-Üstün A, Bos R, Gore F, Bartram J. *Safe Water, Better Health: Costs, Benefits and Sustainability of Interventions to Protect and Promote Health.* Geneva: World Health Organization; 2008.
6. *Burden of Disease from the Joint Effects of Household and Ambient Air Pollution for 2012.* Geneva: World Health Organization; 2014.
7. *Closing the Gap in a Generation: Health Equity Through Action on the Social Determinants of Health: Final Report of the Commission on Social Determinants of Health.* Geneva: World Health Organization; 2008.
8. GBD 2019 Diseases and Injuries Collaborators. Global burden of 369 diseases and injuries in 204 countries and territories, 1990–2019: a systematic analysis for the Global Burden of Disease Study 2019. *Lancet.* 2020;396:1204–1222.
9. GBD 2019 Risk Factors Collaborators. Global burden of 87 risk factors in 204 countries and territories, 1990–2019: a systematic analysis for the Global Burden of Disease Study 2019. *Lancet.* 2020;396:1223–1249.
10. GBD 2019 Demographics Collaborators. Global age-sex-specific fertility, mortality, healthy life expectancy (HALE), and population estimates in 204 countries and territories, 1950–2019: a comprehensive demographic analysis for the Global Burden of Disease Study 2019. *Lancet.* 2020;396:1160–1203.
11. *Active Ageing: A Policy Framework.* Geneva: World Health Organization; 2002.
12. Prince MJ, Wu F, Guo Y, et al. The burden of disease in older people and implications for health policy and practice. *Lancet.* 2015;385:549–562.
13. Lee R. The demographic transition: three centuries of fundamental change. *J Econ Persp.* 2003;14:167–190.
14. Lutz W, Sanderson W, Scherbov S. The coming acceleration of global population ageing. *Nature.* 2008;451:716–719.
15. Steptoe A, Deaton A, Stone AA. Subjective wellbeing, health, and ageing. *Lancet.* 2015;385:640–648.
16. Bloom DE, Chatterji S, Kowal P, et al. Macroeconomic implications of population ageing and selected policy responses. *Lancet.* 2015;385:649–657.
17. Silverstein M, Giarrusso R. Aging and family life: a decade review. *J Marriage Fam.* 2010;72:1039–1058.
18. *Global Report on Ageism.* Geneva: World Health Organization; 2021.

19. Foster L, Walker A. Active and successful aging: a European policy perspective. *Gerontologist*. 2015; 55:83–90.

20. *Decade of Healthy Ageing: Baseline Report*. Geneva: World Health Organization; 2020.

21. *Multisectoral Action for a Life Course Approach to Healthy Ageing: Draft Global Strategy and Plan of Action on Ageing and Health: Report by the Secretariat (A69/17)*. Geneva: World Health Assembly; 2016.

22. Mathers CD, Stevens GA, Boerma T, White RA, Tobias MI. Causes of international increases in older age life expectancy. *Lancet*. 2015;385:540–548.

23. *WHO Global Strategy on People-Centered and Integrated Health Services: Interim Report*. Geneva: World Health Organization; 2015.

24. Emanuel EJ, Emanuel LL. The promise of a good death. *Lancet*. 1998;351(Suppl 2):S21–S29.

CHAPTER 20

Interprofessionalism in Global Health

Education about the core theories and practices of global health is complemented by course-work in the natural and social sciences, development of interprofessional and intercultural skills, and applied experiential learning and other self-reflective activities. Everyone can contribute to making the world a healthier home for current and future generations.

20.1 Core Knowledge in Global Health

All global health professionals are expected to be knowledgeable about key principles and practices in global health, including the history and values of the field, the connections between globalization and health transitions, the sociocultural determinants of health, environmental and planetary health, human rights and health, the financing and delivery of medical services, the agencies and organizations that fund and implement public health interventions, the global burden of disease, and health promotion across the life span (**Figure 20.1**).[1] These learning objectives are most often achieved through formal coursework in global health and related fields. The teams that design, implement, and evaluate global health projects and programs typically include experts from a variety of disciplinary and professional backgrounds, and a shared set of foundational knowledge and values enables those groups to work together more effectively.[2]

20.2 Multidisciplinary Learning in Global Health

One of the foundational premises of the Sustainable Development Goals (SDGs) is that economic development, environmental sustainability, and improved health are intertwined. Progress on socioeconomic goals, such as ending poverty (SDG 1), improving the quality of education (SDG 4), reducing gender inequalities (SDG 5), expanding employment opportunities (SDG 8), and fostering peace (SDG 16), and progress on environmental goals, such as ensuring access to clean water

#	Learning Objective
1	Describe the history, values, and functions of global health.
2	Explain how travel, trade, and other aspects of globalization contribute to health, disease, and health disparities.
3	Summarize the social, economic, cultural, and political contributors to individual and population health.
4	Examine the connections between human health and environmental health, including considerations of water, sanitation, air quality, urbanization, and ecosystem health.
5	Discuss the relationship between human rights and global health.
6	Compare the financing and delivery of medical care in countries with different types of health systems and different income levels.
7	Evaluate the roles, responsibilities, and relationships of the agencies and organizations involved in financing and implementing public health interventions locally and internationally.
8	Compare the burden of disease, disability, and death from infectious diseases, nutritional deficiencies, maternal and perinatal conditions, noncommunicable diseases, mental health disorders, and injuries in countries with different income levels.
9	Identify evidence-based, cost-effective, sustainable interventions for promoting health and preventing illness across the life span from the prenatal period through older adulthood.
10	Apply an interdisciplinary or interprofessional lens to the evaluation of policies and interventions that seek to solve major population health concerns and achieve health equity.

Figure 20.1 Recommended global health student learning objectives from the Consortium of Universities for Global Health.

Jacobsen KH, Hay MC, Manske JM, Waggett CE. Curricular models and learning objectives for undergraduate minors in global health. *Ann Global Health*. 2020;86:102.

and sanitation (SDG 6), increasing access to affordable clean energy (SDG 7), promoting sustainability (SDG 12), and protecting the environment (SDG 13), will ultimately lead to improved health (SDG 3) and nutrition (SDG 2) across the life span for current and future generations.[3] Just as the SDGs highlight the many different domains that contribute to human flourishing, global health education benefits from intentional engagement with diverse academic disciplines.

Multidisciplinary, interdisciplinary, and transdisciplinary models may be applied to global health education and scholarship (**Figure 20.2**).[4] "Multi-" is a prefix that means more than one, and **multidisciplinary** approaches draw on several traditional areas of academic study to understand complex issues. "Inter-" means between or among, and **interdisciplinary** approaches integrate two or more academic disciplines. "Trans-" means across or beyond, and **transdisciplinary** approaches move beyond traditional disciplinary boundaries to create new ways of thinking and practicing. At the baccalaureate (undergraduate) level, most curricula take a multidisciplinary approach to exploring the theories and frameworks that a variety of distinct academic fields apply to global health. Advanced levels of education may move toward interdisciplinary and transdisciplinary approaches.

The **liberal arts** encompass the humanities, social sciences, and natural sciences. A

Multidisciplinary   Interdisciplinary   Transdisciplinary

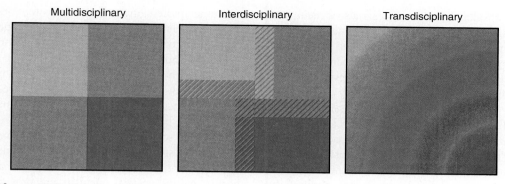

Figure 20.2 Multidisciplinary, interdisciplinary, and transdisciplinary.

liberal arts education is a good foundation for understanding the social–cultural–behavioral and biological–environmental contributors to health and disease. The Council on Education for Public Health, which accredits public health degree programs, recommends that future public health professionals gain familiarity with statistics, environmental science, biology, psychology, sociology, political science, and economics (**Figure 20.3**).[5] All of these public health knowledge areas are also relevant to global health practice, and they highlight the value of completing coursework across a variety of disciplines. (The general education requirements of most colleges and universities in the United States provide broad exposure to the liberal arts that complements focused studies in a particular major or concentration area. Universities in other countries may have more focused curricula.) Students

Profession and Science of Public Health	**Factors Related to Human Health**
Explain public health history, philosophy, and values.	Explain the effects of environmental factors on a population's health.
Identify the core functions and essential services of public health.	Explain the biological and genetic factors that affect a population's health.
Explain the role of quantitative and qualitative methods and sciences in describing and assessing a population's health.	Explain the behavioral and psychological factors that affect a population's health.
List major causes and trends of morbidity and mortality in populations.	Explain the social, political, and economic determinants of health and how they contribute to population health and health inequities.
Discuss the science of prevention in population health.	Explain how globalization affects the global burden of disease.
Explain the critical importance of evidence in advancing public health knowledge.	Explain an ecological perspective on the connections among human health, animal health, and ecosystem health.

Figure 20.3 Foundational public health knowledge identified by the Council on Education for Public Health.

Data from *Accreditation Criteria: Schools of Public Health and Public Health Programs.* Silver Spring MD: Council on Education for Public Health; 2016.

with global health interests also benefit from courses that explore international and global themes. For example, **medical anthropology** studies diverse cultural perspectives on health, disease, illness, sickness, medicine, and healing.

There is no particular checklist of courses that must be taken to be on track for a global health career. An undergraduate major in global health is not a prerequisite for entering the global health workforce, and a master's degree in global health is not required for advancement in the field even though specialized education can be helpful. Studies within a particular major or during advanced professional training can be supplemented with electives that fill gaps in knowledge and enhance skills in the selected area of global health practice in which the learner intends to work.

20.3 Interprofessional Skills for Global Health Practice

Many types of professionals are involved in delivering health-related services to individuals and communities: physicians, surgeons, nurses, dentists, psychologists, therapists, emergency medical technicians, and clinicians with expertise in other practice areas as well as public health workers, social workers, emergency management professionals, program administrators, project managers, and many others. These practitioners and their colleagues may work in or near their home communities to improve access to quality medical, psychological, and other health-related services, or they may work in distant locations to support the goals of global public health partnerships. Another set of global health professionals works on the financing, management, and administration of global health policies and plans. These specialists apply their expertise in public policy, business, law, urban planning, community development, communication,

and other professional practice areas to work at government agencies, foundations and other nonprofit organizations, for-profit corporations, and other groups.

Global health also overlaps with many types of work that are not specifically focused on the financing and delivery of clinical and population health interventions. Scientists working at scales from the molecular level to the ecosystem level and beyond are making discoveries that will inform future global health activities. Social scientists are providing insights about human and organizational behaviors and social systems. Engineers are inventing new tools to support global and ecosystem health. Work advancing any of the SDGs can be considered to promote global health equity. By this standard, anyone working in education, social work, economic development, international relations, security, other sociopolitical fields, technology, agriculture, energy, transportation, sanitation, other environmental resource sectors, or nearly any other area might be contributing to global health.[6]

Interprofessionalism is the ability to work with and communicate well with colleagues in different clinical and nonclinical practice areas who are seeking to achieve a shared goal. Being proficient in any academic discipline or professional practice area requires a mix of knowledge, skills, and abilities (KSAs) specific to the selected area of study and practice. Being a skilled global health professional also requires aptitudes in areas such as collaboration, partnering, and communication; professionalism and ethics; program planning, management, and evaluation; sociocultural and political awareness; and strategic analysis.[7] Global health professionals must be prepared to "translate" the jargon and philosophical underpinnings of their own fields into language that coworkers with different professional vocabularies will understand.[8]

Successful careers are built on both technical aptitudes and **soft skills**, the personal, social, emotional, and communication skills that enable people to productively contribute to and lead work teams and other collaborative activities. Soft skills that are valued across work sectors include communication, courtesy, flexibility, integrity, positive attitude, professionalism, responsibility, social skills, teamwork, and work ethic.[9] Global health workplaces also value compassion, empathy, and a sense of solidarity with other human beings, whether those people live next door or on the other side of the planet.[10]

20.4 Intercultural Communication and Global Health Practice

Communication describes the verbal (spoken), written, and other ways that people share information, ideas, and feelings. Interpersonal communication is the exchange of information between two or more people using words, gestures, body language, and other means. Organizational communication is the formal and informal dissemination of information among members of a business or other group. Mass communication is the distribution of information to large audiences through media such as newspapers, radio, television, and the Internet. Visual communication uses images, maps, graphs, charts, and other visual elements to convey information. **Health communication** describes the communication strategies and methods that are used to promote individual and population health. Health communication includes interpersonal communication, such as communication between clinical care providers and their patients, and health awareness campaigns that use visual and other tools to communicate with large numbers of people. **Intercultural communication** describes communication across different cultures or social groups.

Global health is an international, interdisciplinary, and interprofessional field that requires effective intercultural communication among collaborators and stakeholders in the natural and social sciences, applied health disciplines (such as medicine, nursing, and public health), and other professional fields (such as business, education, engineering, and social work) who come from diverse cultural and language backgrounds. Being proficient in multiple languages is useful (though not required) for individuals who want to work with and perhaps eventually lead global health partnerships, but communication is about much more than language skills.

Cultural competence describes the integration of cultural knowledge, awareness, and skills into professional practice.[11] Cultural competency encompasses awareness of one's own cultural rules and biases, knowledge about other cultures, skills in verbal and nonverbal communication, and characteristics like empathy, curiosity, and openness that enable effective communication.[12] Some cultural scholars prefer to use the term **cultural humility** to describe the lifelong process of becoming self-aware about one's own cultural assumptions and beliefs, understanding and respecting other cultures, and improving one's ability to participate in inclusive and equitable partnerships.[13] Experiencing different cultural worldviews can help individuals develop greater intercultural sensitivity, but only if they genuinely seek to understand and appreciate alternative ways of thinking, believing, and communicating.[14]

20.5 Experiential Learning in Global Health

After foundational knowledge in global health has been acquired, skills and abilities can be developed through applied learning experiences. In global health, the typical options for gaining experience include internships, study abroad (including international clinical electives), service-learning courses, and volunteering with diverse local populations or in international settings.[15] Fellowships and other early career development programs may provide additional opportunities for structured learning experiences.

The best experiential learning opportunities in global health are ones that are beneficial for the learner, the host organization, and the host community.[16] This requires mutual respect and assurances that none of the parties will be exploited, undermined, or harmed.[17] For example, mutual respect means that volunteers should not engage in practices that are beyond the scope of their training. A student without hands-on medical training and clinical certification at home should not provide clinical care in a foreign country. A student without supervised counseling experience and licensure at home should not provide mental health care in another country. Even experienced clinicians should provide services in another country only if they are properly credentialed to do so in the host country.

Voluntourism, or volunteer tourism, is travel for the purpose of volunteering, and it usually combines vacation with international service.[18] Voluntourism is often criticized for exacerbating power imbalances and privilege disparities.[19] Short-term volunteer experiences offer little time to build meaningful relationships with local partners but ample time for even well-intentioned guests to disrupt, offend, and harm the host community.[20] Some visitors post social media content that portrays the visiting team as heroes and violates the dignity of hosts.[21] Some international visitors who provide medical services undermine confidence in local practitioners, and some visiting students eager to log procedures displace local trainees who are working hard to complete their own educational requirements.[22] Engaging in self-reflection before, during, and after an intercultural experience improves learning and helps reduce harm to the host community.[23]

20.6 Professional Development in Global Health

The diversity of professional pathways within global health and adjacent to it means that there are many educational and training tracks that lead to a fulfilling and successful global health career. Professionals who work in global health must remain current within their own primary areas of specialization as well as staying up to date on emerging trends and methods within global health. **Continuing education** (CE) is the completion of approved learning activities in order to maintain a professional licensure or credential. In some professional fields, licensing and credentialing agencies mandate the type and frequency of CE activities that are required. Practitioners in medicine, nursing, and several other fields often can fulfill at least some of their CE requirements with activities related to global health. Global health professionals whose primary fields do not require licenses or certifications to be attained and renewed on a regular basis must set their own learning goals and establish individualized plans for meeting them.

Professional development is an ongoing and intentional process of establishing short- and long-term professional goals; identifying and completing activities that enable systematic progress toward achieving those goals; and routinely evaluating performance, competencies, and growth. Examples of professional development activities include reading reports from global health agencies and organizations, reading research publications, attending lectures and webinars, participating in workshops and conferences, conducting research, becoming an active member of academic and professional organizations, taking formal coursework, earning advanced degrees, and participating in fellowships or other formal training programs. **Mentorship** is a formal or informal relationship in which an experienced mentor offers professional development advice and guidance to a less experienced mentee. Most individuals benefit from having multiple mentors at every stage of their careers who can provide timely advice about how to handle complex situations and long-term guidance about the process of self-reflection, goal setting, and planning for professional success.

20.7 Global Health Matters

As global health has matured as a field of study, research, and application, several activities have emerged as important global health functions, including protecting the world from dangerous infectious diseases, saving the lives of infants and children, and promoting global security and economic growth by finding cost-efficient solutions for expensive health issues.[24] Global health interventions could make unparalleled improvements in the lives of billions of people during the 21st century by promoting health, preventing disease and disability, improving health standards, reducing health disparities, overcoming the health and human security problems associated with extreme poverty, and bringing together people from around the world as equals to solve shared challenges.

A diverse set of health conditions can be considered to fall under the umbrella of global health, including HIV, tuberculosis, and antimicrobial resistance; diarrheal diseases, pneumonia, influenza, and vaccine-preventable infections; malaria, other vector-borne diseases, neglected tropical diseases, and emerging infectious diseases; reproductive and sexual health; undernutrition, overnutrition, and food safety; cardiovascular diseases, cancer, diabetes, chronic respiratory diseases, and other noncommunicable diseases; mental health and substance use disorders; and injuries. Opportunities to improve the health status of individuals, communities, and the world exist throughout the life span, from the prenatal period through older adulthood. Some of these interventions are health specific, but many are not. Improvements in economics, education, employment opportunities, equity, and governance yield benefits for population health. Improvements in access to clean drinking water, toilets, clean energy, unpolluted air, safe jobs, and planned cities and the adoption of sustainable practices enable healthier human living and a healthier planet.

Health and human rights are inextricably linked, and populations are healthier when everyone has access to the tools for health. Medical and public health interventions are financed by a diversity of governmental and charitable groups as well as the individuals who receive services. Local and global health interventions are implemented by people working for governmental and intergovernmental agencies, nonprofit organizations, and for-profit corporations who apply their expertise to solving complex challenges. Health metrics are a tool for evaluating population health needs, selecting cost-effective health interventions, and tracking progress toward achieving goals. While the health profiles of low-income and high-income populations can look quite different when comparing countries or comparing subpopulations within the same country, there are also many shared socioeconomic, environmental, and health concerns.[25] International trade and other globalization processes have exacerbated climate change and increased the risk of pandemics while also creating opportunities to work together to solve shared concerns and enhance security.

Global health matters, and careers and volunteer work that contribute to global health can be very meaningful. A variety of health and health-related interventions are effective in preventing adverse health outcomes and promoting transitions toward improved population health, and a wide range of educational and professional pathways can lead to a career in global health. Everyone can participate in making communities worldwide healthier places for current and future generations.

References

1. Jacobsen KH, Hay MC, Manske JM, Waggett CE. Curricular models and learning objectives for undergraduate minors in global health. *Ann Global Health.* 2020;86:102.

2. Jacobsen KH, Waggett CE. Global health education for the post-pandemic years: parity, people, planet, priorities, and practices. *Glob Health Res Policy.* 2022;7:1.

3. *Transforming Our World: The 2030 Agenda for Sustainable Development.* New York: United Nations; 2015.

4. Choi BCK, Pak AW. Multidisciplinarity, interdisciplinarity and transdisciplinarity in health research, services, education and policy: 1. Definitions, objectives, and evidence of effectiveness. *Clin Invest Med.* 2006;29:351–364.

5. *Accreditation Criteria: Schools of Public Health and Public Health Programs.* Silver Spring MD: Council on Education for Public Health; 2016.

6. Hughes BB, Kuhn R, Peterson CM, Rothman DS, Solórzano JR. *Improving Global Health: Forecasting the Next 50 Years: Patterns of Potential Human Progress.* Vol. 3. Denver CO: Pardee Center for International Futures; 2011.

7. Jogerst K, Callender B, Adams V, et al. Identifying interprofessional global health competencies for 21st-century health professionals. *Ann Global Health.* 2015;81:239–247.

8. Cornwall A. Buzzwords and fuzzwords: deconstructing development discourse. *Dev Pract.* 2007;17:471–484.

9. Robles MM. Executive perceptions of the top 10 soft skills needed in today's workplace. *Bus Commun Q.* 2012;75:453–465.

10. Benatar SR, Daar AS, Singer PA. Global health ethics: the rationale for mutual caring. *Int Affairs.* 2003;79:107–138.

11. Napier AD, Ancarno C, Butler B, et al. Culture and health. *Lancet.* 2014;384:1607–1639.

12. *Intercultural Knowledge and Competence VALUE Rubric.* Washington DC: Association of American Colleges and Universities; 2009.

13. Foronda C, Baptiste DL, Reinholdt MM, Ousman K. Cultural humility: a concept analysis. *J Transcult Nurs.* 2016;27:210–217.

14. Hammer MR, Bennett MJ, Wiseman R. Measuring intercultural sensitivity: the Intercultural Development Inventory. *Int J Intercult Rel.* 2003;27:421–443.

15. Arya AN, Evert J, eds. *Global Health Experiential Education: From Theory to Practice.* New York: Routledge; 2018.

16. Stone GS, Olson KR. The ethics of medical volunteerism. *Med Clin North Am.* 2016;100:237–246.

17. Melby MK, Loh LC, Evert J, Prater C, Lin H, Khan OA. Beyond medical "missions" to impact-drive short-term experiences in global health (STEGHs): ethical principles to optimize community benefit and learner experience. *Acad Med.* 2016;91:633–638.

18. Lasker JN. *Hoping to Help: The Promises and Pitfalls of Global Health Volunteering.* Ithaca NY: Cornell University Press; 2016.

19. Banki S, Schonell R. Voluntourism and the contract corrective. *Third World Q.* 2018;39:1475–1490.

20. Shah S, Lin HC, Loh LC. A comprehensive framework to optimize short-term experiences in global health (STEGH). *Global Health.* 2017;15:27.

21. *How to Communicate the World: A Social Media Guide for Volunteers and Travelers.* Oslo: SAIH; 2017.

22. Loh LC, Cherniak W, Dreifuss BA, Dacso MM, Lin HC, Evert J. Short term global health experiences and local partnership models: a framework. *Global Health.* 2015;11:50.

23. Ventres WB. Facilitating critical self-exploration by global health students. *AMA J Ethics.* 2019; 29:E749–E758.

24. *Global Health and the Future Role of the United States.* Washington DC: National Academies Press; 2017.

25. Frenk J, Gómez-Dantés O, Moon S. From sovereignty to solidarity: a renewed concept of global health for an era of complex interdependence. *Lancet.* 2014;383:94–97.

Glossary

A

abortion the termination or loss of a pregnancy

abstinence the practice of refraining from sexual intercourse and other types of genital contact

abstract a one-paragraph summary of the objectives, methods, results, and implications of a scientific investigation

accident an unfortunate event that happens by chance

acculturation the complex process of adopting the practices, traditions, values, and identity of a new community after migrating

action plan the steps that will be taken to achieve strategic goals and implement approved policies

activated health education model a theoretical framework that describes behavior change as a three-step process: an experiential phase, an awareness phase, and a responsibility phase

active immunity protection against infectious diseases that occurs when the body's immune system produces antibodies against a specific infectious agent

active surveillance the process of public health officials contacting healthcare providers to ask about how often they are diagnosing prioritized diseases

active TB the symptomatic, contagious form of tuberculosis; also called *TB disease*

activities of daily living (ADLs) the routine daily self-care functions that are required for health and survival, such as dressing, eating, ambulating, using the toilet, and taking care of personal hygiene

acute a description of a health condition that has a rapid onset and typically resolves within a few days or weeks

acute respiratory infection an infection of the respiratory tract characterized by rapid onset of symptoms and a relatively short duration of illness

addiction a cognitive and neurological condition characterized by adverse behaviors related to physical or psychological dependence

adolescence a life stage characterized by rapid physical, sexual, neurological, psychological, and social development

adverse childhood experiences (ACEs) potentially traumatic events that occur between birth and the 18th birthday, such as abuse, neglect, or exposure to household or community violence

adverse event a negative outcome that may be the result of a medication, vaccination, or other medical exposure or may be a coincidental occurrence that is not directly related to the exposure

adverse reaction a negative side effect of a medication, vaccination, medical device, or other medical exposure

advocacy the process of increasing awareness of a selected cause in order to influence policies related to that issue

Aedes mosquito a genus of mosquito that has black and white stripes on its body and legs, thrives in urban areas, and can be an aggressive day biter

agent a pathogen or a chemical or physical cause of disease or injury

age standardization the generation of comparable statistics for populations with different age structures

aging transition a health transition characterized by an increase in the percentage of older adults in the population and a decrease in the percentage of children in the population

AIDS the acquired immunodeficiency syndrome that occurs as a result of the destruction of immune system cells by the HIV virus

airborne transmission infection acquired when a susceptible individual breathes in pathogens that have become aerosolized and are suspended as small droplet nuclei in the air

allele a version of a gene

allergy an immune dysfunction in which the body is hypersensitive to foreign substances that are usually not harmful

Alzheimer's disease the most prevalent form of dementia

ambient air pollution the presence of harmful chemicals or other substances in the air outside buildings at concentrations above the thresholds established for human safety; also called *outdoor air pollution*

amino acids organic compounds that contain carbon, hydrogen, oxygen, and nitrogen and are the base units for proteins

anemia a deficiency of red blood cells or hemoglobin that causes fatigue

aneurysm a bulge in a blood vessel that can cause the vessel to rupture

angina chest pain or tightness caused by the heart muscle not getting an adequate supply of oxygen

angiogenesis the formation of new blood vessels that nourish a new cancerous tumor

angioplasty a procedure that physically opens and unclogs a blocked artery

***Anopheles* mosquito** the vector that transmits malaria-causing parasites to humans

anorexia a lack of appetite

anorexia nervosa an eating disorder characterized by a person having a distorted body image and feeling overweight even when emaciated

antenatal care routine preventive healthcare consultations during pregnancy that allow clinicians to identify and ameliorate potential health problems in a woman or fetus; also called *prenatal care*

anthrax a bacterial infection that causes skin lesions when naturally acquired but causes respiratory distress, shock, and death when a weaponized version is inhaled

anthropometry the measurement of the human body

anthroponosis an infectious disease that usually occurs only in humans

antibody a protein produced by the human body in response to the presence of antigens

antigen a substance that originates outside the body and triggers an immune response once inside the body

antigenic drift a minor genetic mutation of an influenza virus that causes a small change in the virus's surface antigens

antigenic shift a major change in the genome of an influenza virus that occurs when the genetic material from two very different types of influenza A viruses recombine to form a new strain

antimicrobial resistance a situation in which a pathogen that used to be susceptible to a therapeutic agent mutates in a way that makes that medication ineffective

antiretroviral a medication for a retroviral infection that suppresses the viral count and slows the progression of symptoms

antiretroviral therapy (ART) combinations of three or more different types of medication that are taken together to combat HIV; also called *HAART*

aortic aneurysm a bulge in the aorta that can rupture and cause a rapid death from internal bleeding

apnea long pauses in breathing, especially during sleep

apoptosis a process of programmed cell death

appropriate technology affordable and environmentally sustainable technology that can be locally operated and maintained

arbovirus an arthropod-borne virus

arrhythmia an abnormal heartbeat that is too fast, too slow, or irregularly paced

arsenicosis chronic arsenic poisoning from being exposed to contaminated water over a long period of time

artemisinin-based combination therapy (ACT) malaria treatment that combines at least two different antimalarial drugs, one of which is an artemisinin-based drug

arthropod an insect or an arachnid

ascariasis an intestinal helminth infection in which long worms dwell in the small intestine

assisted reproductive technologies fertility treatments that handle eggs or embryos

assistive device a tool that helps with the performance of a task

association a statistical relationship between two variables

asthma a chronic but reversible inflammation of the airways that causes episodes of wheezing (especially when exhaling), coughing, chest tightness, and shortness of breath

asylum seeker an involuntary migrant who asks for protection from a host country after arriving in that country rather than waiting for a refugee application to be processed prior to traveling

asymptomatic not symptomatic

atherosclerosis the thickening and hardening of the walls of the arteries that carry oxygen-rich blood from the heart to the rest of the body

Atlas method an estimation method that improves economic comparisons by reducing the impact of market and exchange rate fluctuations on metrics

atrial fibrillation an arrhythmia in which the atria of the heart quiver fast and irregularly rather than contracting and relaxing at a regular beat

autism a lifelong neurodevelopmental disorder that begins in early childhood and causes challenges with social communication and other functions

autochthonous cases of infectious diseases that are locally acquired rather than imported

autoimmune disorder a condition that occurs when the body has difficulty distinguishing between "self" and "nonself" and begins to attack its own cells

autonomy an ethical principle requiring that only an individual (or his or her legal guardians) is authorized to decide whether to volunteer to participate in a research study

autosomal gene a gene that is not located on the sex chromosome and is therefore not sex linked

B

bacterium a single-celled organism that lacks a true nucleus

BCG (Bacillus Calmette-Guérin) a vaccine that confers some protection against TB disease in children

behavior change the process of an individual intentionally adopting and maintaining healthier behaviors

behavioral risk factor a behavior that can be adopted, stopped, or changed in order to reduce the risk of disease

benchmark a standard or point of reference for comparison

beneficence the ethical imperative for a research study to maximize possible benefits

benign prostatic hyperplasia an enlargement of the prostate gland that may cause difficulty with urination and with sexual performance

benign tumor a noncancerous growth that will not spread to another part of the body

beriberi thiamine deficiency that causes heart failure, weakness, and confusion

bilateral aid money given from the government of a higher-income country to the government of a lower-income country to support development activities

Bill & Melinda Gates Foundation the largest private foundation in the world

binge-eating disorder an eating disorder characterized by repeated incidents of consumption of large quantities of food without subsequent purging

bioavailability the proportion of a consumed nutrient that is able to be absorbed and used by the body

biodiversity the presence of a wide variety of plant and animal species within a particular ecosystem

biomass fuel from organic materials like wood, vegetation, or animal waste

biopsy the examination of tissue removed from a living body in order to test for the presence or absence of disease

biostatistics the science of analyzing health data and interpreting the results so that they can be applied to solving public health problems

bioterrorism the deliberate release of pathogens, chemicals, or other agents that can cause illness and possibly death of people, animals, or plants

bipolar disorder a depressive disorder characterized by alternating periods of depression and mania or hypomania

birth asphyxia a birth complication that occurs when a newborn fails to take a first breath immediately after delivery and is therefore deprived of oxygen

birth rate the annual number of births per 1,000 people (or other units) in a population over a one-year period

birth spacing waiting until at least two years after the birth of one child before conceiving the next child

blindness having no light perception or having vision that even with corrective lenses is no better than 20/400 in the best eye

body mass index (BMI) a measure of body composition calculated by taking weight in kilograms and dividing it by the square of the height in meters

Bradford Hill criteria a set of conditions that provide support for the existence of a causal relationship between an exposure and an outcome

brain drain the migration of healthcare professionals trained in low- and middle-income countries to higher-paying jobs in high-income countries

breast cancer the most frequently diagnosed cancer among women

bronchitis inflammation of the bronchi that is characterized by a productive cough, narrowing of the airways, and excess mucus production

built environment structures built by humans for human use

bulimia nervosa an eating disorder characterized by frequent binge–purge cycles

burden of disease the adverse impact of a particular health condition (or group of conditions) on a population

burn an injury to skin or deeper tissues that is caused by contact with fire, boiling water, or other very hot substances

Buruli ulcer a mycobacterial infection that causes painless lesions that can become so deep that they extend from the skin to the underlying tendons and bones of the arms or legs

bypass surgery a surgical procedure that uses a healthy blood vessel from another part of the body to restore blood flow to the heart muscle by bypassing the damaged area

C

calcium a mineral used by the body for strengthening bones

calorie the amount of energy required to raise the temperature of one gram of water by one degree Celsius

cancer a disease that occurs when abnormal cells in the body begin to reproduce uncontrollably

cancer transition a health transition characterized by a shift from many cancers being associated with chronic infections to few cancers being caused by untreated chronic infections

candidiasis an overgrowth of the fungus *Candida*

carbohydrate a chain of sugars

carcinogen a substance that can cause genetic mutations that lead to cancer

carcinoma a cancer that forms in epithelial tissues that line the inside or outside of the body

cardiac arrest the abrupt stopping of the heartbeat

cardiomyopathy a disease of the heart muscles that causes the heart to enlarge and become weaker

cardiovascular disease a disorder of the heart or blood vessels

caries holes (cavities) in the teeth that are created by demineralization and decay

carrier a person with a persistent contagious infection who does not have symptoms of the disease but can pass the infectious agent on to others

carrying capacity the maximum human population the Earth can sustain

case definition a list of the inclusion and exclusion criteria that must be met in order for an individual to be classified as having a particular disease or disability

case detection rate the proportion of people with a disease who are diagnosed as having that disease and, if the condition is a notifiable disease, have that case reported to government health agencies

case fatality rate the proportion of people with a particular disease who die as a result of that condition

cataract a clouding of the lens of an eye that makes vision fuzzy

catastrophe a large-scale critical incident that overwhelms the local response networks and requires extensive outside assistance

causal factor an exposure that has been scientifically tested and shown to occur before the disease outcome and to contribute directly to its occurrence

causation a relationship in which an exposure directly causes an outcome

CD4 a glycoprotein found on the surface of some types of immune system cells

census the collection of demographic data about every individual in a population

Centers for Disease Control and Prevention (CDC) the lead health protection agency in the United States

CEPI a public–private partnership that coordinates development of new vaccines that protect against emerging infectious diseases and ensures that those products are available to everyone

cerebral malaria a neurological complication of *Plasmodium* infection that is characterized by seizures and coma

cerebral palsy a neuromuscular disorder that is associated with birth trauma and is characterized by permanent difficulties with movement, balance, and posture

cesarean section the surgical delivery of a neonate through an incision in the mother's abdomen and uterus

cestode a tapeworm consisting of a mouthpiece and numerous flat segments

Chagas disease a trypanosome infection that can cause chronic heart and intestinal damage

chemotherapy the treatment of disease using chemical substances

chikungunya an arbovirus that can cause long-term disability from joint pain

child labor a violation of child rights that occurs when a child has an excessive workload, unsafe work conditions, or extreme work intensity

child sponsorship a charitable donation model in which a donor selects a child to sponsor and then receives regular updates about that child in exchange for continued monthly contributions to the host organization

child support ratio a ratio comparing the total number of children (aged 0–14 years) in a population to the number of people aged 15–64 years

chlamydia an infection with *Chlamydia trachomatis*, obligate intracellular bacteria that can cause chronic urogenital or eye infections

cholera an infection with *Vibrio cholerae* bacteria, which causes severe watery diarrhea

cholesterol a waxy lipid (fat) that is a major component of the plaque that causes atherosclerosis

chronic a description of a health condition that develops slowly and may worsen over months or years

chronic kidney disease a progressive loss of kidney function characterized by a reduced glomerular filtration rate and increased urinary albumin levels

chronic obstructive pulmonary disease (COPD) a chronic, progressive respiratory disease that limits airflow and causes shortness of breath and productive coughing

chronic respiratory diseases long-term noncommunicable diseases of the airway, bronchi, and lungs

circumcision the surgical removal of the foreskin of the penis

cirrhosis irreversible scarring of the liver that impedes the flow of blood through the liver and prevents the liver from functioning well

cisgender a gender identity that aligns with the sex assigned to an individual at birth

civil rights liberties that are granted by governments

climate change a long-term shift in weather patterns and average temperatures

clinical trial a research study that experimentally tests the safety and efficacy of a health intervention

Codex Alimentarius a compilation of international food standards that provide specific guidelines for keeping food products safe

cognitive behavioral therapy a form of talk therapy in which a therapist helps an individual understand his or her thoughts, feelings, and behaviors and identify actions that can be taken to correct concerns

co-insurance a percentage of the costs of healthcare services that an insured patient must pay for out of pocket

collective violence a form of violence perpetrated by members of a group as part of a shared plan to accomplish a political, social, or economic goal

colostrum the protein-rich breast milk produced in the first days after giving birth

communication the verbal, written, and other ways that people share information, ideas, and feelings

community development a process through which community members identify their own development priorities and take action to achieve them

community-led total sanitation public health programs that encourage toilet use in places where residents are accustomed to open defecation and have not yet adopted new sanitation behaviors

complementary foods soft, semisolid, or solid foods introduced into an infant's diet while continuing to breastfeed the child

complementary proteins foods that individually lack some types of essential amino acids but provide all the essential amino acids when consumed together

complete protein a protein that contains all nine essential amino acids

complex humanitarian emergency a situation that occurs when civil conflict or war causes mass migration of civilian populations, food insecurity, and long-term public health concerns

condom a thin sheath that is used as a physical barrier during sexual contact

contact tracing the process of identifying the contacts of infected individuals so that they can be tested, monitored, and possibly quarantined

continued feeding the process of encouraging individuals with diarrhea to eat the same foods that they usually consume

continuing education the completion of approved learning activities in order to maintain a professional licensure or credential

contraception the intentional prevention of pregnancy

contraindication a condition that makes it unsafe for an individual to receive a particular vaccine, medication, device, procedure, or other medical intervention

control the process of using public health interventions to reduce the incidence or prevalence of an adverse health condition to a substantially lower level within a community or a larger geopolitical area

copay a fixed fee that is paid out of pocket by an insured patient when receiving routine medical services

coronary artery disease a condition that occurs when atherosclerosis of the arteries that provide blood to the heart reduces blood flow to the heart muscle; also called *ischemic heart disease*

corporate social responsibility the positive social and environmental actions a company voluntarily supports

corruption politically powerful people abusing their positions for personal gain

cost-effectiveness analysis an economic analysis that compares the health gains from an intervention to the financial costs of that intervention

counterfeit an illegal product that is marketed deceptively

COVID-19 the disease caused by the SARS-CoV-2 virus

crisis a small-scale incident that can easily be managed with local resources

crude statistic a raw or unadjusted statistical measure

cue to action an internal or external stimulus that prompts an individual to implement a recommended health behavior

***Culex* mosquito** a genus of mosquito that deposits rafts of 100 or more eggs on water rather than laying eggs singly

cultural competence the integration of cultural knowledge, awareness, and skills into professional practice

cultural humility the lifelong process of becoming self-aware about one's own cultural assumptions and beliefs, understanding and respecting other cultures, and improving one's ability to participate in inclusive and equitable partnerships

culture a way of living, believing, behaving, communicating, and understanding the world that is shared by members of a social unit

cycle of transmission a description of how an infectious agent passes between different species

cysticercosis the disease caused by *Taenia solium* tapeworms forming cysts in muscle tissue or other parts of the body

D

DALY an abbreviation for a *disability-adjusted life year*

data raw or unprocessed facts, figures, symbols, or signs

data science an interdisciplinary field that uses statistics, machine learning, and other computational tools to generate information and knowledge from various types of data

DDT a persistent organic compound that used to be widely used as an agricultural pesticide

death rate the number of all-cause or cause-specific deaths per 1,000 people (or other units) in a population during a stated period of time; also called the *mortality rate*

Declaration of Alma-Ata an influential document released in 1978 that called for the expanded use of primary health care to achieve "Health for All by 2000"

deductible the amount that an insured person must spend out of pocket on medical care each year (in addition to premiums) before the insurance company begins paying for health services

DEET a chemical that is an effective insect repellent but does not kill mosquitoes

default rate the proportion of people who are diagnosed with an infectious disease and begin treatment but do not complete the full course of treatment

definitive host the animal host in which a parasite reaches sexual maturity and reproduces

dehydration the excessive loss of water from the body

deliverable a product, service, or other result of a project that fulfills the terms of a contract or other agreement

delusion a false belief that is irrational but seems very real to the person experiencing it

dementia a chronic syndrome characterized by memory loss, confusion, and other signs of impaired cognitive function

demographic transition a health transition characterized by changes in population size and composition that accompany a shift toward lower birth and death rates

demography the study of the size and composition of human populations

dengue a mosquito-borne viral infection that is sometimes called breakbone fever because it can cause severe joint and muscle pain

depressive disorder a mental health disorder characterized by sadness; hopelessness; loss of interest in usual activities; fatigue; poor concentration; and other negative thoughts, feelings, and physical symptoms that interfere with routine daily activities

determinants of health biological, behavioral, social, environmental, political, and other factors that influence the health status of individuals and populations

development a long-term process of improving the socioeconomic and environmental conditions that are associated with suboptimal population health status

development assistance for health external funding designated for health activities in low- or middle-income countries

diabetes a metabolic disorder characterized by an impairment in the production of or response to insulin

diagnostic accuracy the proportion of people who receive a test whose results are true positives or true negatives

dialysis the process of using a machine to filter the blood

diarrhea loose or liquid feces and an increased frequency of defecation

diastolic blood pressure the pressure in the blood vessels when the heart is at rest in between beats

diffusion of innovations model a theoretical framework that describes a process of behavior change in communities that unfolds as new ideas and actions are adopted by community members

diphtheria a vaccine-preventable membranous inflammation of the airway caused by a toxin produced by *Corynebacterium*

diplomacy the process of negotiating agreements between countries, resolving disputes without conflict, and navigating other aspects of international relations

direct transmission infection acquired when an infected person transfers a pathogen to a susceptible person by touching that person or breathing directly into that person's face

disability an activity limitation or participation restriction that is related to an impairment

disability-adjusted life year (DALY) a burden of disease metric that is quantified as the sum of years of life lost (YLLs) to premature death and years lived with disability (YLDs) in a population

disaster a critical incident in which the need for assistance exceeds local capacity

discrimination actions taken against an individual because of that person's membership in a sociocultural group

disease the presence of signs or symptoms of poor health

disorder a functional impairment that may or may not be characterized by measurable structural or physiological changes

distal cause a social, environmental, or other factor that is not an immediate cause but contributes to the causal pathway for an adverse event

distributive justice the ethical principle that needed resources in a population should be fairly allocated

Doctors Without Borders the name used in the United States for the international humanitarian organization Médecins Sans Frontières (MSF)

dominant gene an allele that will be phenotypically expressed if it is inherited from one or both parents

DOTS an acronym for directly observed therapy, short-course

dracunculiasis a painful condition in which a long filarial helminth takes weeks to slowly emerge from its human host; also called *guinea worm disease*

drowning the process of experiencing respiratory impairment due to being submerged or immersed in water or another liquid

dysentery bloody diarrhea

E

early breastfeeding initiating breastfeeding within the first hour after giving birth

early childhood development the physical, cognitive, emotional, and social development that occurs during the approximately 1,000 days from conception through the second birthday

Ebola virus disease a viral hemorrhagic fever caused by a filovirus that is transmitted through the body fluids of infected individuals

echinococcosis the disease caused when humans become the accidental host for a cyst-inducing tapeworm that usually matures in dogs

ecological fallacy the incorrect assumption that individuals follow the trends observed in population-level data

ecological footprint a measure of how much burden human consumption places on the biosphere

ecology the relationships of living things to one another and the environments in which they live

ecosystem all the living things that share a particular environment

ecosystem services the benefits humans receive from various ecosystems

ecotoxicology the study of the impact of toxic exposures on populations, communities, and ecosystems

ectoparasite a parasite that lives on the exterior surface of its host's body

ectopic pregnancy a fertilized egg implanted in a fallopian tube or another location outside the uterus

edema fluid retention in extracellular spaces that causes swelling of the tissues in the arms, legs, and face

edentulism the loss of most or all of one's teeth

effectiveness a measure of the success of an intervention under real-world conditions

efficacy a measure of the success of an intervention under ideal, laboratory-controlled conditions

efficiency an evaluation of the cost effectiveness of an intervention that is based on both its effectiveness and resource considerations

elderly support ratio a ratio comparing the total number of older adults (aged 65+ years) in a population to the number of people aged 15–64 years

elephantiasis chronic lymphedema that causes the skin of an affected limb to thicken and develop a coarse texture

elimination the process of removing all risk of new infection in a defined geopolitical area

emergency a critical incident that stresses local humanitarian resources but can still be managed locally

emergency management the process of overseeing all the resources and responsibilities related to emergencies and disasters, including prevention, preparedness, response, and recovery

emergency obstetric and newborn care (EmONC) a core set of actions that can save the lives of women and neonates during the perinatal period

Emergency Support Functions (ESFs) critical service areas that require immediate attention after a critical incident

emerging infectious disease an infectious disease caused by a pathogen that has not previously caused severe disease in humans or is affecting human populations in new ways

emphysema a disease that occurs when the alveoli (the tiny air sacs in the lungs) lose elasticity and become distended or destroyed

encephalitis an acute inflammation of the brain

endemic an adverse health condition that is always present in a human population

endometriosis a condition in which some of the tissue that lines the uterus is located on the ovaries or in other parts of the abdominal cavity

endoparasite a parasite that lives inside the body of its host

endowment a large donation made to a nonprofit organization so that the funds can be invested and the interest from the investments can be used to support the operation of the charity

enrichment the process of adding nutrients lost during handling, processing, or storage back to food products

enteric infection an infection of the intestinal tract

environment the surroundings in which humans and other organisms live

environmental health the study of the connections between human health and environmental exposures, such as poor water quality, air pollution, and hazardous waste

enzootic an adverse health condition that is always present in an animal population

epidemic an event characterized by an adverse health condition occurring more often than usual in a human population and causing more than a few sporadic occurrences of disease

epidemiologic transition a health transition characterized by a shift from infectious diseases to chronic noncommunicable diseases being the primary cause of deaths and disability in a population

epidemiology the study of the distribution and determinants of health and disease in human populations

epigenetics the differential expression of genetic code through activation or inactivation of genes

epilepsy a chronic seizure disorder characterized by episodes of excessive and abnormal electrical activity in the brain

epizootic an outbreak in an animal population

eradication the process of eliminating an infectious disease globally

essential amino acid an amino acid that cannot be produced by the human body and must be acquired from food

essential medicine a drug that has been identified as a high priority for a country's health system to have in stock at all times because it is a cost-effective treatment for a frequently occurring health issue

estimate a calculation of the likely value of an indicator, metric, or other variable in a population

ethics the principles that guide appropriate conduct in specific situations

ethnicity a social grouping based on many dimensions of cultural heritage, nationality, language, religion, tribal affiliation, and other factors

etiology the cause of a disease or another adverse condition

evaluation an assessment of how well a project, program, or policy has met its goals

exclusive breastfeeding breast milk is the only substance a baby consumes

Expanded Program on Immunization (EPI) a program established by the World Health Organization in 1974 to ensure universal child access to critical vaccines

expatriate a person who is temporarily living in another country and intends to return to his or her home country

exposure a personal characteristic, behavior, environmental encounter, or intervention that might change the likelihood of developing a health condition

extinction the process of destroying all laboratory specimens of an eradicated pathogen so that there is no possibility of the pathogen reentering the human population

extreme poverty surviving on less income than an international poverty line, typically set at an income of less than $1 or $2 per person per day

F

faith-based organization a nongovernmental organization sponsored by a religious or religiously affiliated entity

falciparum malaria an infection with the species of *Plasmodium* that is most likely to cause life-threatening disease

fall an event that causes a person to land on the ground or floor

family planning a process by which adults make informed decisions about how many children they want to have, how many years apart they want those pregnancies to be, and the actions they will take to achieve these goals

famine very low food security in a large proportion of a population

FAO the Food and Agriculture Organization, the specialized agency of the United Nations that serves as its lead agency for improving nutrition and agricultural productivity

fat a lipid of animal origin that is solid at room temperature

fat-soluble vitamin a vitamin that is able to be stored in body tissues

fecal-oral transmission the acquisition of an infectious agent by eating or drinking products contaminated with fecal matter from animals or humans

fertility a woman's total number of births, including live births and stillbirths

fertility transition a health transition characterized by a reduction in the number of children born to the typical woman

fiber a nondigestible complex carbohydrate found in unprocessed plant-based foods

fibroids benign tumors in the uterus that can cause heavy bleeding and pelvic pain

financing the provision of money for an activity and the management of that investment

fluoride a mineral that is essential for the development of strong teeth

folate a B vitamin that is critical for fetal development

folic acid a synthetic form of folate

fomite an inanimate object or surface that has been contaminated with infectious agents

food intoxication illness caused when ingested bacteria produce toxins in the body

food security members of a household or community reliably having access to enough food to be healthy, active, and productive

food system the entire process of growing or producing food, processing and packaging food, distributing and selling food (which may require transportation and storage), and preparing and consuming food

forecast the most likely estimate of future trends based on past data

foreign direct investment a business investment made by a corporation or an individual in another country

foreign policy the strategies and approaches a country uses to engage with other nations while protecting its own interests

fortification the process of adding micronutrients not naturally present in a food's ingredients to a food product

foundation a charitable trust that gives grants to other nonprofit organizations

Framework Convention on Climate Change (FCCC) an international environmental treaty that seeks to reduce greenhouse gas emissions

Framework Convention on Tobacco Control (FCTC) a global health treaty negotiated under the auspices of the World Health Organization that aims to significantly reduce the global prevalence of tobacco use

functional literacy the ability to understand written words well enough to complete routine daily tasks

fungus a spore-producing organism, such as mold or yeast

G

gastroenteritis infection-induced inflammation of the inner lining of the stomach and/or intestines that causes diarrhea, nausea, vomiting, cramps, and fever

Gavi a public–private partnership that works with lower-income countries to identify vaccine priorities and then procure and distribute the vaccines

gender social, cultural, and psychological aspects of expressing maleness or femaleness

gender-based violence physical, emotional, and sexual abuse inflicted on an individual because of that individual's gender

gender identity an individual's sense of maleness or femaleness

gender roles how a cultural group expects men and women to behave based on their genders

generalized anxiety disorder an anxiety disorder characterized by persistent excessive worrying about numerous concerns

generic drug a medication with the same active ingredient as a brand-name drug

genetics the study of genes, genetic variation, and heredity

genotype the set of alleles a person inherits for a particular gene

gestational diabetes elevated blood sugar that is first diagnosed during pregnancy and typically resolves after delivery

gingivitis an inflammation of the gums associated with poor oral hygiene and the presence of bacterial plaques

giardiasis a protozoal disease that can cause persistent diarrhea

Gini coefficient a measure of the inequality in the distribution of incomes within a particular country

glaucoma elevated pressure within the eyeball that causes loss of peripheral vision

Global Burden of Disease (GBD) a massive collaborative effort to quantify the epidemiologic profiles of every country in the world

Global Charter for the Public's Health an international agreement that identifies protection, prevention, and promotion as core public health services and governance, advocacy, capacity, and information as core public health functions

Global Fund a public–private partnership founded in 2002 to support infectious disease control initiatives in low- and middle-income countries

global health a field of academic study, research, and applied practice that seeks to improve population health worldwide

global health security public health interventions implemented by governmental and military personnel in collaboration with other stakeholders in order to protect populations from threats to health and safety

globalization the process of countries around the world becoming more integrated and interdependent across economic, political, cultural, and other domains

global warming a gradual increase in the temperature of Earth's atmosphere

goal a desired future outcome

GOBI an initiative started in the 1980s by UNICEF that focused on increasing child survival by promoting growth monitoring, oral rehydration therapy for diarrhea, breastfeeding, and immunization

goiter a swollen neck caused by an enlarged thyroid gland

gonorrhea a sexually transmitted infection caused by *Neisseria gonorrhoeae* bacteria

gout a painful swelling of a joint, usually the joint at the base of the big toe, due to elevated levels of uric acid in the blood

governance the processes and structures that enable governments to set policies, provide services, and protect human rights

grant a gift of money that does not have to be repaid

gravidity a woman's total number of pregnancies, including miscarriages, abortions, stillbirths, and live births

greenhouse gas a gas in the atmosphere that traps heat and causes surface temperatures to increase

gross domestic product (GDP) the total amount of goods and services produced in one country by domestic- and foreign-owned companies

gross national income (GNI) the total income from the selling of goods and services produced in one country, including consumer spending, government spending, investments, and exports

gross national product (GNP) the total amount of goods and services produced by one country's companies in that country and by companies owned by that country's companies but operating in other countries

guinea worm disease a painful condition in which a long filarial helminth takes weeks to slowly emerge from its human host; also called *dracunculiasis*

H

HAART highly active antiretroviral therapy; combinations of three or more different types of drugs that are taken together to combat HIV; also called *ART*

habilitation the process of learning, maintaining, or improving functional abilities in order to maximize independence and quality of life

hallucination a sensory distortion that causes a person to hear, see, feel, smell, or taste something that in reality is not present

Hansen's disease a chronic mycobacterium infection that can cause nerve damage that leads to amputations; also called *leprosy*

health a state of complete physical, mental, and social well-being and not merely the absence of disease or infirmity

health behavior an individual's intentional or unintentional action that either enhances or impairs health

health belief model a theoretical framework that describes individual health behavior change as a function of personal perceptions of the severity of the disease, susceptibility to the disease, the likely benefits from adopting healthier behaviors, the barriers to action, cues to action, and the self-efficacy to enact change

healthcare-associated infection an infection that is contracted while receiving care in a hospital, nursing or rehabilitation center, or other medical facility; also called a *nosocomial infection*

health communication the communication strategies and methods that are used to promote individual and population health

health diplomacy the use of health projects as part of meeting foreign policy goals

health disparity an avoidable difference in health status between population groups

health equity a status achieved when everyone has an equal opportunity to be as healthy as possible

health information system the technology used to collect, store, analyze, and disseminate health-related data and information

health literacy the ability to access, understand, and apply health information

health promotion an applied social science that encourages individuals and communities to take steps to improve their own health

health system the people, facilities, products, resources, and organizational structures that deliver health services to a population

health transition a shift in the health status of a population that usually occurs in conjunction with socioeconomic development

healthy life expectancy the average number of additional years an individual of a particular age in a population can expect to live without disability

heart failure a chronic condition in which the heart is not able to pump enough blood to meet the body's need for oxygen

helminth a multicellular parasitic worm

hemoglobin a molecule made from iron that holds the oxygen inside red blood cells

hemorrhagic stroke a stroke that occurs when a blood vessel ruptures and causes bleeding in the brain

hepatitis inflammation of the liver

hepatitis A a vaccine-preventable picornavirus infection that is spread through contaminated food and water and can cause acute liver inflammation

hepatitis B a vaccine-preventable hepadnavirus infection that is spread through blood and other body fluids and can cause chronic liver disease

hepatitis C a chronic flavivirus infection that is now transmitted primarily through injecting drug use

hepatitis E a waterborne hepevirus infection that can cause acute liver failure and death in pregnant women

herd immunity a theory that says that when a high proportion of a population is immune to a specific infectious disease, the entire community is protected

herpes a viral infection that can cause painful ulcers, such as genital ulcers or cold sores

Hib a bacterial infection caused by *Haemophilus influenzae* type b

highly pathogenic avian influenza a strain of influenza that causes serious disease and high case fatality rates among infected birds

high-risk screening secondary prevention recommendations that apply to people who are known to have an elevated risk of a particular disease

hookworm an intestinal worm that latches onto the walls of the human intestine

horizontal program a program that strengthens an existing health system so that it can deliver additional health services

hospice care services that provide end-of-life comfort care for people with end-stage illnesses and support for their families

host a human who is susceptible to an infection or another type of disease or injury

household air pollution the presence of harmful chemicals or other substances in the air inside or near buildings at concentrations above the thresholds established for human safety; also called *indoor air pollution*

Human Development Index (HDI) an estimate of national development calculated from data on income, education, and life expectancy at birth

human immunodeficiency virus (HIV) a retrovirus that destroys specialized blood cells that are needed by the immune system to fight infection

human papillomavirus (HPV) a virus associated with the majority of cases of cervical dysplasia

human rights entitlements that are due to every person simply because that person is human

human security freedom from fear and want

hydatid disease the formation of large cysts in the human liver and lungs due to infection with *Echinococcus* tapeworm larvae

hydrocele lymphedema of the scrotum

hygiene the practice of maintaining cleanliness in order to prevent disease

hyperemesis gravidarum relentless nausea and vomiting during pregnancy that causes severe dehydration and significant weight loss

hypertension high blood pressure, typically defined as having a systolic blood pressure of 140 mm Hg or higher or a diastolic blood pressure of 90 mm Hg or higher

hypoxia an inadequate supply of oxygen in body tissues

I

iCCM Integrated Community Case Management; a WHO/UNICEF-led strategy that provides community health workers with algorithms for treating uncomplicated childhood infections in homes

illness a person's perception of his or her own experience of having an adverse health condition

IMCI Integrated Management of Childhood Illness; a package of simple, affordable, and effective home, community, and clinical interventions for major childhood illnesses and undernutrition that was first developed by UNICEF and the WHO in 1995

immigrant a person who has settled in a new country and intends to stay there permanently

immunization the process of a person's immune system developing immunity against a particular infection after receipt of a vaccine

impairment a difference or limitation in an anatomical structure, mental or sensory function, or physiological function that constrains the capacity of an individual to do a task or action

implementation science the scientific study of how to increase uptake of evidence-based practices and policies

inactivated vaccine a vaccine that contains a killed bacterium or an inactive virus that has been rendered harmless by heat, chemicals, or radiation

incidence the number of new cases of a disease in a population during a specified period of time

incidence rate the number of new cases of a disease occurring in a population during a specified time period divided by the total number of people who were at risk of the disease during that period

Incident Command System (ICS) an organizational structure used in the United States to provide a clear chain of command for people who respond to a critical event

income the amount of take-home pay earned by household members in a week, year, or other time period

incubation period the time between exposure to a pathogen and onset of symptoms

indicator a variable used to measure performance, achievement, or change

Indigenous population a group that has maintained unique cultural traditions (and often also languages) for many generations after the colonization or domination of their traditional homeland by another group

indirect transmission infection acquired when an infected person transfers a pathogen to a surface or other item that is subsequently touched (or otherwise encountered) by a susceptible host

indoor air pollution the presence of harmful chemicals or other substances in the air inside or near buildings at concentrations above the thresholds established for human safety; also called *household air pollution*

indoor residual spraying (IRS) the application of long-lasting insecticides to walls and other surfaces where mosquitoes might rest

induced abortion a chemically or surgically terminated pregnancy

industrial hygiene the process of assessing and mitigating workplace hazards

inequality a remediable difference in health status or access to health services between population groups

inequity a health inequality that is considered to be unfair and unjust

infant a baby of any age between birth and the first birthday

infant mortality rate the number of babies who die before their first birthday per 1,000 live births

infection an infectious agent reproducing inside a person

infectivity the capacity of an infectious agent to cause infection when a susceptible host is exposed to the agent

infertility the inability to achieve a pregnancy when sexually active and not using contraception or the inability to maintain a pregnancy through to a live birth

inflammation an immune system response that causes white blood cells to release chemicals that increase blood flow to local tissues

influenza a highly contagious respiratory infection caused by an orthomyxovirus

influenza-like illness a status assigned to people with an acute illness who have fever and a cough but have not tested positive for influenza or another pathogen that causes similar symptoms

information data that have been processed and presented in a format usable for understanding a situation and making decisions

informed consent an individual's voluntary decision to participate in a research study after reviewing essential information about the project

injecting drug user an individual who injects illicit drugs for nonmedical use; also called a *person who injects drugs*

injury physical damage to the body inflicted by an external force

insecticide-treated net (ITN) a mesh sheet dipped in insecticides and then hung over a bed so that it provides a barrier between sleeping humans and mosquitoes while also killing any mosquitoes that land on it

in situ tumor a noninvasive precancerous group of abnormal cells

instrumental activities of daily living (IADLs) the functions required for independent living, such as shopping, housekeeping, managing personal finances, preparing foods, and navigating transportation

insulin a hormone produced by the pancreas that helps the body to maintain a relatively constant level of glucose in the bloodstream so that cells have a relatively consistent supply of energy

insurance a risk management strategy that protects purchasers against major financial losses

intentional injury purposefully inflicted physical trauma

intercultural communication communication across different cultures or social groups

interdisciplinary an approach to education and scholarship that integrates two or more academic disciplines

Intergovernmental Panel on Climate Change (IPCC) a scientific board that reviews and synthesizes scientific data about climate and weather under the auspices of the United Nations

intermediate host an animal host in which an immature parasite develops but does not reach sexual maturity

intermittent preventive treatment (IPT) the routine distribution of anti-infective medications to vulnerable people so that they maintain therapeutic drug levels in their blood during times of high risk for disease

internally displaced person (IDP) a person who fled his or her home community because of civil war, famine, natural disaster, or another crisis but did not cross into another country

International Code of Marketing of Breast-milk Substitutes an international agreement that bans problematic marketing of infant formula

international cooperation financial assistance, technical support, capacity building, and other actions implemented by a donor country in a recipient partner country as part of a foreign policy strategy

international health efforts to alleviate poverty-related health conditions in lower-income areas

International Health Regulations (IHR) a global health security agreement among all United Nations members that mandates reporting of outbreaks of infectious diseases of potential international concern

International Monetary Fund (IMF) a multilateral organization that provides a structure for international monetary policy and

makes loans to countries of any income level that would otherwise not be able to make payments on their other international loans

international NGO a large nongovernmental organization with a diverse portfolio of projects that are implemented in numerous countries

interpersonal violence a form of violence that occurs when one person threatens to harm or actually harms another individual through power and control

interprofessionalism the ability to work and communicate well with colleagues in different practice areas who are seeking to achieve a shared goal

intersectionality the overlapping identities and experiences related to socioeconomic status, gender, sexuality, race, (dis)ability, and other characteristics that align with social privilege or systemic discrimination

intervention a strategic action intended to improve individual and/or population health status

intimate partner violence physical or sexual violence by a current or former spouse or partner

intrauterine device (IUD) a small T-shaped copper or plastic object that is placed in the womb to act as a contraceptive

in vitro fertilization a type of assisted reproductive technology in which a woman's eggs are extracted from her ovaries, fertilized with sperm in a laboratory setting, and then the resulting embryos are transferred to the uterus

iodine an element that is critical for regulating metabolism

iodine deficiency disorders thyroid disorders and intellectual disabilities caused by a lack of dietary iodine

iron a mineral the body uses to make red blood cells

iron deficiency anemia low red blood cell counts resulting from inadequate iron intake

ischemia reduced blood supply

ischemic heart disease a condition that occurs when atherosclerosis of the arteries that provide blood to the heart reduces blood flow to the heart muscle; also called *coronary artery disease*

ischemic stroke a stroke that occurs when a blocked blood vessel cuts off blood flow to a portion of the brain

isolation the physical separation of people who have a contagious infection from people who are susceptible to the infection

J

jaundice a yellowing of the skin and sclera (the whites of the eyes) due to the buildup of bilirubin levels in the blood

K

kidney failure an acute or chronic condition in which the kidneys are not functioning well enough for health

kwashiorkor a form of severe acute undernutrition that is caused by chronic dietary protein deficiency and characterized by very low weight-for-height accompanied by pitting edema

L

landmine a buried explosive device

latent period the time between exposure to a pathogen and onset of contagious disease

latent TB infection (LTBI) a state of having tuberculosis bacteria reproducing within the body without feeling sick or being contagious

laws rules that define enforceable standards of behavior

leishmaniasis a sandfly-transmitted protozoal disease that can cause disfigurement and death

leprosy a chronic mycobacterium infection that can cause nerve damage that leads to amputations; more formally known as *Hansen's disease*

leukemia a blood cancer that begins in the bone marrow, which produces the body's blood

leukocyte a white blood cell

liberal arts the humanities, social sciences, and natural sciences

life expectancy the average number of additional years of life an individual of a particular age can be expected to survive based on population mortality patterns

life expectancy at birth the average number of years a newborn in a population can be expected to survive based on population mortality patterns at the time of birth

lifestyle diseases noncommunicable diseases that are associated with health-related behaviors such as unhealthy diets, sedentariness, tobacco use, and heavy alcohol consumption

lipid a fatty acid, which is a carbohydrate chain with other chemical groups at the ends of the chain

literacy the ability to read and write and apply those communication skills

live attenuated vaccine a vaccine that contains a pathogen that has been intentionally weakened

LMIC an abbreviation for low- or middle-income country

loan borrowed money that must be repaid with interest

logistics the process of coordinating complex operations, especially the movement of supplies and equipment

long-lasting insecticidal net (LLIN) a bednet that has been impregnated with a pesticide that remains effective for two years or longer before requiring retreatment

low birthweight a birthweight less than 5.5 pounds (2,500 grams)

lower respiratory infection an acute infection of the bronchi, bronchioles, or lungs

low vision not being able to see better than 20/60 in the best eye even when using corrective lenses

lung cancer the most frequent cause of cancer death worldwide

lupus an autoimmune disorder that causes a butterfly rash on the face and swollen joints and adversely affects numerous other body systems

lymphatic filariasis a mosquito-borne helminth infection that can block lymph nodes and cause fluid buildup in affected legs and other body parts

lymphedema the swelling of body parts due to retained lymph fluid in the tissues

lymphocyte a type of white blood cell that attacks viruses, bacteria, and other pathogens

lymphoma an immune system cancer that affects white blood cells and lymph nodes

M

M&E monitoring and evaluation, the systematic collection of information about an ongoing intervention and the determination of whether the intervention achieved its objectives

macronutrient a nutrient such as a carbohydrate, protein, fat, or oil that is required to be consumed in relatively large quantities because it provides energy

macular degeneration loss of central vision that occurs when a portion of the retina deteriorates

malaria a mosquito-borne parasitic infection with *Plasmodium* protozoa that can cause cyclic fevers, anemia, neurological complications, and death

malarial anemia the destruction of so many red blood cells by malaria-causing parasites that the body cannot adequately transport oxygen through the bloodstream

malignant tumor a cancerous growth that can spread to other parts of the body

malnutrition deficiencies, excesses, or imbalances in the intake and processing of energy and nutrients

mammogram an X-ray of a breast

marasmus a form of severe acute undernutrition that is caused by prolonged calorie deprivation and characterized by very low weight-for-height without edema

mass drug administration the distribution of preventive chemotherapy to large population groups at regular time intervals as part of strategies for preventing and controlling infectious diseases

maternal and child health an area of public health practice that focuses on the health of mothers, infants, and children

maternal mortality the death of a woman from a pregnancy-related cause during pregnancy, childbirth, or the six weeks after delivery

maternal mortality ratio (MMR) the number of women who die of pregnancy-related causes per 100,000 live births

MDR-TB a multidrug-resistant tuberculosis strain that does not respond to two of the standard antibiotic therapies, rifampicin and isoniazid

measles a very contagious vaccine-preventable viral infection that infects immune system cells and causes several months of immunosuppression

Médecins Sans Frontières (MSF) a private humanitarian organization that advocates for human rights and provides medical care to people harmed by violence

Medicaid a federal program in the United States that provides funding to states to support state-sponsored health coverage for very low-income citizens

medical anthropology the study of diverse cultural perspectives on health, disease, illness, sickness, medicine, and healing

Medicare the federal health funding system in the United States that provides coverage for people aged 65 years and older as well as some younger people with serious permanent disabilities

medicine the practice of preventing, diagnosing, and treating health problems in individuals and families

megacity a metropolitan area with 10 million or more inhabitants

melanoma cancer that originates in melanin-producing skin cells

menarche the first menstrual period

meningitis an inflammation of the meninges, the membranes that cover the brain and spinal cord

meningococcus infection with the bacterium *Neisseria meningitidis*

menopause the cessation of menstruation

menstruation the shedding of the lining of the uterus (the endometrium) that occurs approximately monthly for most nonpregnant women of childbearing age

mentorship a formal or informal relationship in which an experienced mentor offers professional development advice and guidance to a less experienced mentee

metabolism the rate at which a person's body uses energy

metastasis a secondary cancerous tumor that is located at a different site in the body than the primary tumor

metric a composite indicator derived from two or more other measures

miasma foul-smelling gases produced by poorly managed waste that were thought to cause disease prior to the discovery of pathogenic microorganisms

microcephaly an abnormally small head that is a sign of aberrant brain development

micronutrient a nutrient that the body requires in small amounts, such as a vitamin or mineral

mid-upper arm circumference (MUAC) a measure of arm-circumference-for-age that is used as an indicator of wasting in a child

migraine a recurrent severe headache that is often accompanied by nausea, vomiting, and sensitivity to light and sound

migrant a person who has moved across an international border and is residing in a new country

Millennium Development Goals (MDGs) a set of eight goals endorsed by the United Nations and hundreds of partners that aimed to significantly reduce global poverty between 2000 and 2015

mineral an inorganic chemical element

ministry of health a term used in many countries to describe the lead governmental health agency

miscarriage the spontaneous loss of a pregnancy prior to the fetal age of viability

mitigation the process of implementing preemptive measures to protect people and property from hazards

model a set of equations that define relationships among many variables

modifiable risk factor a risk factor that can be avoided or mitigated

monitoring ongoing assessment of a project or program to track progress toward achieving predefined targets

monogenic disorder a genetic disorder that results from a child inheriting a single disease-causing gene from one or both parents

morals the beliefs and customs that shape how a society defines what is right and wrong

morbidity the presence of nonfatal illness or disease

mortality death

mortality rate the number of all-cause or cause-specific deaths per 1,000 people (or other units) in a population during a stated period of time; also called the *death rate*

mortality transition a health transition characterized by decreases in the rates of death for age groups across the life span

mother-to-child transmission the transmission of a pathogen from an infected pregnant woman to her offspring during pregnancy, delivery, or breastfeeding; also called *vertical transmission*

MRSA methicillin-resistant *Staphylococcus aureus*

MSM a classification that emphasizes sexual behavior rather than sexual identity by encompassing all men who have sex with men

multicausality a causal pathway in which many different risk factors contribute to an adverse event occurring

multidisciplinary an approach to education and scholarship that draws on several traditional areas of academic study

multilateral aid funding for development activities that is pooled from many donor countries

multiple sclerosis a chronic, progressive disease that causes inflammatory demyelination of the sheaths of nerve cells in the central nervous system

multisectoral an approach to policies and partnerships that involves representatives and resources from governments, businesses, and nonprofit groups

mumps a vaccine-preventable viral infection that causes the parotid salivary glands in the cheeks to swell

mutation a permanent change in the sequence of bases that make up DNA that occurs after birth in response to exposure to radiation, chemicals, pollutants, or other substances

mycetoma a chronic granulomatous inflammatory disease of the subcutaneous tissue of the foot

myocardial infarction the death of a portion of the heart muscle due to lack of oxygen that occurs when a coronary blood vessel becomes mostly or fully occluded

N

National Incident Management System (NIMS) an emergency response framework in the United States that specifies how governmental agencies and nongovernmental organizations work together to respond to disasters

National Institutes of Health (NIH) the lead health research agency within the U.S. Department of Health and Human Services

natural environment aspects of the biological and physical world that are not created by humans

natural history of disease the typical timeline from initial infection with a pathogen to either recovery or death for progression of an adverse health condition from onset to resolution if treatment is not received

negative predictive value the proportion of people who test negative for a disease who truly do not have the disease

neglected tropical diseases (NTDs) infectious diseases that primarily occur in the poorest regions of the world and have not historically been a priority for global policymakers, funding agencies, or pharmaceutical companies

nematode a cylindrically shaped roundworm

neonatal mortality rate the number of deaths of babies within 28 days after birth per 1,000 live births

neonate a newborn within his or her first 28 days (four weeks) after birth

neoplasm a word for a tumor that is derived from root words meaning "new formation"

neurocognitive disorders neurological and cognitive disorders that typically develop in older adulthood

neurocysticercosis the disease caused by *Taenia solium* tapeworms invading the human nervous system and causing seizures

neurodevelopmental disorders neurological and development disorders that present in childhood

niacin a B vitamin that is necessary for skin health and digestive and nervous system function

noncommunicable disease (NCD) an adverse health condition that is not contagious

nonderogable right a human right that is irrevocable in all circumstances

nongovernmental organization a nonprofit organization that is privately managed and receives at least some of its funding from private sources

nonmaleficence the ethical imperative for a research study to do no harm

nonmodifiable risk factor a risk factor for a disease that cannot be changed through health interventions

nonprofit organization a mission-driven group that reinvests surplus revenue in the organization rather than distributing extra income to owners or shareholders

norovirus the most frequent cause of severe diarrhea among adults

nosocomial infection an infection that is contracted while receiving care in a hospital, nursing or rehabilitation center, or other medical facility; also called a *healthcare-associated infection*

nutrition the consumption of foods that allow the body to survive, grow, heal, and be healthy and the processing of those nutrients within the body

nutrition transition a health transition characterized by a shift from having undernutrition and nutrient deficiencies as the most prevalent nutritional concerns in a population to having overweight and obesity as the dominant nutritional disorders

obesity a body mass index (BMI) of 30 or greater

obesity transition the typical progression of which demographic groups develop obesity as the nutrition transition occurs

obsessive-compulsive disorder a mental health disorder characterized by anxiety-inducing recurrent thoughts and repetitive behaviors intended to reduce distress or prevent bad events

obstetric fistula a hole between the rectum or bladder and the vagina that is caused by obstructed labor and constantly leaks urine or feces

obstetric transition a health transition characterized by a shift from a high maternal mortality ratio to a very low rate

obstructed labor an obstetric complication that occurs when the unborn baby is wedged so tightly into the birth canal that blood flow to surrounding tissues is cut off and the tissues start to die

occupational health an applied public health field focused on primary prevention of injuries and other work-related health problems

OECD (Organisation for Economic Co-operation and Development) an intergovernmental organization that represents about three dozen of the world's richest countries

official development assistance money given by the government of a high-income country to the government of a low-income country to support socioeconomic development

OIE the Office International des Epizooties, an intergovernmental group that helps to control the spread of zoonotic infectious diseases and to promote food safety

oil a lipid of plant origin that is a liquid at room temperature

onchocerciasis a fly-borne helminth infection that can cause blindness

One Health a concept that emphasizes the interconnectedness of human health, animal health, and ecological health

open defecation free a community status that is earned when all members are consistently using designated toilet facilities

opportunistic infection an infection that occurs when the body's immune system is weakened enough to give a pathogen an opportunity to invade

oral contraceptives pills that prevent ovulation when taken as prescribed so no eggs are released from the ovaries and a pregnancy cannot occur

oral rehydration salts (ORS) a mixture of sugar, salt, and other chemicals that restores the balance of electrolytes in the blood when they are mixed with clean drinking water and consumed to replace lost fluids

oral rehydration therapy (ORT) drinking enough water to prevent or treat the dehydration caused by diarrhea

osteoarthritis a degenerative disease that slowly causes loss of cartilage in the joints, causing pain, stiffness, and disability

osteomalacia vitamin D deficiency in adults

osteoporosis a loss of bone density that significantly increases the risk of fractures of the hip, vertebrae, and other bones in older adults

Ottawa Charter an international agreement that identifies healthy public policies, supportive environments, strong communities, skilled personnel, and expanded access to preventive health services as core health promotion actions

outbreak an event characterized by at least several people becoming ill from a disease that is not usually present in a population

outdoor air pollution the presence of harmful chemicals or other substances in the air outside buildings at concentrations above the thresholds established for human safety; also called *ambient air pollution*

out-of-pocket payments cash disbursements made by patients and their families in order to receive health services

overdiagnosis the detection of cancers or other conditions that would have gone away on their own or caused no symptoms during the diagnosed individual's lifetime

overnutrition a form of malnutrition caused by excessive intake of calories and nutrients

overpopulation a situation that occurs when a population becomes so large that the amount of food and other environmental resources available is insufficient to support all members of the population

overtreatment the unnecessary provision of therapy for a condition that is unlikely to cause health problems during the diagnosed individual's lifetime and the therapy has harmful side effects

overweight a body mass index (BMI) of 25 to 29.9

oxytocin a hormone that strengthens uterine contractions during labor and delivery and then helps control postpartum bleeding

P

palliative care clinical interventions that improve the quality of life of people with serious chronic illnesses by managing pain, reducing emotional distress, and providing other types of support to patients and their families

pandemic a worldwide epidemic

panic disorder an anxiety disorder characterized by repeated panic attacks that last for several intense minutes and cause a racing heartbeat, shortness of breath, and other disturbing symptoms

parasite an organism that survives by living in or on a host organism

parasitemia the presence of parasites in the blood

parenteral infection an infection that enters the body through a route other than the digestive tract

parity a woman's total number of live births

Parkinson's disease a chronic, progressive neurodegenerative disorder characterized by motor symptoms such as slowed movement, rigidity or stiffness in an arm or leg or other body part, and tremors when a limb is resting

particulate matter substances that are small enough to remain suspended in the air for long periods of time and travel deep into the lungs

partner notification the process of a patient diagnosed with an STI communicating with his or her sexual partners (or a public health official communicating with the partners of the diagnosed individual) about their need to be tested

passive immunity temporary protection against infectious diseases that is conferred by antibodies produced by another human or an animal

passive surveillance the compilation of mandatory reports of notifiable disease diagnoses from medical laboratories

pasteurization a process of heating foods to kill the bacteria that might be present

patent the exclusive legal right for one company to sell a new product for several years before other companies are allowed to produce and sell the product

pathogen a bacterium, virus, or other microorganism that can cause disease

pathogenicity the capacity of an infectious agent to cause disease in an infected host

peer review the process of a scientific manuscript being evaluated by experts who scrutinize the methodology and the reasonableness of the results prior to a report being published

pellagra niacin deficiency that is characterized by dermatitis, dementia, and diarrhea

pelvic inflammatory disease an infection in the female reproductive system that can cause pain and lead to scarring and infertility

PEPFAR the U.S. President's Emergency Plan for AIDS Relief, which provides financing for increasing access to antiretroviral therapy and other HIV prevention and treatment services in low- and middle-income countries

percentage a ratio expressed in units of "per 100"

perinatal mortality stillbirths and deaths within the first seven days (one week) after a live birth

perinatal period the time period that extends from about 22 weeks of gestation through seven days after a live birth

periodontitis chronic inflammation of the gums due to infection

peripheral artery disease narrowed blood vessels in the extremities that impair blood circulation and can cause severe leg pain and cramping when walking

persistent organic pollutant an organic compound that does not degrade easily

personal protective equipment gowns, gloves, face masks, eye protection, and other barriers that prevent infection

person who injects drugs an individual who injects illicit drugs for nonmedical use; also called an *injecting drug user*

pertussis a vaccine-preventable bacterial infection that causes whooping cough

PHEIC a public health emergency of international concern, a declaration that can be made under the 2005 International Health Regulations when an infectious disease outbreak is causing serious illness, is likely to spread to other countries, and requires a coordinated global response

phenotype the way a particular set of alleles is expressed in physical appearance, the way a person develops or functions physiologically, or disease status

physical inactivity the failure to regularly engage in exercise of moderate or vigorous intensity

placenta the organ that lines the uterus during pregnancy and provides oxygen and nutrients to a fetus during fetal development

placental abruption a pregnancy complication in which the placenta separates from the uterine wall prior to delivery

placenta previa a pregnancy complication in which the placenta covers part or all of the cervix and causes bleeding

planetary health a concept that emphasizes the dependence of human health on the Earth and seeks to understand the damage that human actions impose on ecosystem health

Plasmodium the genus of protozoans that cause malaria

pneumococcus infection with the bacterium *Streptococcus pneumoniae*

pneumoconiosis a restrictive lung disease caused by exposure to various types of occupational hazards

pneumonia an infection-induced inflammation that causes the air sacs of the lung to fill with fluid

policy a set of principles and procedures established by governments or other groups to guide decision-making and resource allocation

polio a vaccine-preventable viral infection that can attack the spinal cord and cause permanent paralysis

pooled risk the assumption that if many low-risk people and a few high-risk people pay premiums to an insurance system over many years, there will be a pot of money that can be used to pay for major expenses when they occur

population a group of individuals, communities, nations, or other entities

population-based screening secondary prevention recommendations that apply to large demographic groups

population health the health outcomes and determinants of health in groups of humans at the community, regional, national, and/or worldwide level

population planning the practice of promoting a population growth rate that aligns with a country's demographic goals

population pyramid a graphic that displays the number of females and males by age group in a population

positive predictive value the proportion of people who test positive for a disease who truly have the disease

post-exposure prophylaxis (PEP) the process of taking medications after exposure to a pathogen in order to reduce the likelihood of contracting an infection

postpartum hemorrhage severe bleeding within several hours after giving birth

posttraumatic stress disorder (PTSD) a mental health disorder that occurs when someone who has experienced a traumatic incident has nightmares or other types of distressing recollections of the event and exhibits physiological signs of hyperarousal

power the authority to control or influence the actions of others

precaution a condition that might make a vaccine ineffective at producing immunity or might increase the likelihood of an adverse reaction in a particular individual

prediabetes elevated blood glucose levels that are below the threshold for a type 2 diabetes diagnosis

preeclampsia a combination of worsening hypertension in the final months of pregnancy along with the presence of protein in the urine that can progress to seizures and death

pre-exposure prophylaxis (PrEP) the process of taking medications prior to a likely exposure to a pathogen in order to reduce the likelihood of contracting an infection

prejudice a perception about an individual based solely on preconceived notions about a sociocultural group to which that person belongs

premature mortality any death before a selected target survival age

premium a monthly fee paid for health insurance

prenatal care routine preventive healthcare consultations during pregnancy that allow clinicians to identify and ameliorate potential health problems in a woman or fetus; also called *antenatal care*

preterm birth the delivery of a baby before the 37th week of pregnancy

prevalence the percentage of members of a population who have a given trait at a particular time

prevention science the process of determining which preventive health interventions are effective at improving health status, how successful those interventions are in various populations, and how readily they can be scaled up for widespread implementation

preventive chemotherapy the use of a safe medicine as part of a public health strategy to prevent and control an infectious disease

primary health care a community-based approach to health that employs community health workers and focuses as much on prevention as on cures

primary infertility infertility in someone who has never achieved a live birth

primary prevention protective actions that help keep an adverse health event from ever occurring

primordial prevention the general lifestyle habits and environmental conditions that prevent risk factors for adverse health events from developing

professional development an ongoing and intentional process of establishing short- and long-term professional goals; identifying and completing activities that enable systematic progress toward achieving those goals; and routinely evaluating performance, competencies, and growth

program a portfolio of related projects that together achieve part of an action plan

project a series of coordinated tasks that are completed within a limited time period in order to achieve a specific target

project management the process of initiating, planning, executing, monitoring, and closing out projects

projection the future outcomes that can be anticipated if various interventions are implemented or other events occur

proportion a ratio in which the numerator is a subset of the denominator

proportionate mortality rate the percentage of all people who die in a population whose death is the result of a particular cause

prosthetic an artificial body part

protein a chain of amino acids

protozoan a single-celled organism that has animal-like characteristics

proximal cause the most immediate cause of an adverse event

psychiatrist a physician with advanced training in mental health care

psychologist a mental health professional with advanced training in counseling

public health the actions taken at the population level to promote health and prevent illnesses, injuries, and early deaths

public policy the process by which laws, regulations, policies, and government-sponsored programs are developed, implemented, enforced, funded, administered, and evaluated

public–private partnership (PPP) a long-term collaboration in which the costs, risks, and benefits are shared by governmental and nongovernmental entities

purchasing power parity (PPP) an estimation method that improves economic comparisons by adjusting metrics based on how many goods, services, and other products can be purchased in various populations with a fixed amount of money

Q

qualitative research a research approach that uses in-depth interviews, focus group discussions, participant–observation, and other unstructured or semistructured methods to explore attitudes and perceptions, identify themes and patterns, and formulate new theories

quality-adjusted life year (QALY) a metric used in health economics to represent the additional duration of life and quality of life conferred to populations by successful public health interventions

quantitative research a research approach that uses structured, hypothesis-driven approaches to gather data that can be statistically analyzed

quarantine the restriction of freedom of movement of healthy contacts of people with an infectious disease as part of a strategy to contain the spread of a contagious disease

R

rabies a lethal zoonotic virus infection transmitted through the bites of infected mammals

race superficial categories that group individuals based primarily on physical attributes like skin color

radiation therapy the use of high-energy ionizing radiation to damage the DNA of cancer cells, which causes the cells to stop dividing or die

rapid diagnostic test a test that can quickly detect the presence of a pathogen or markers for a pathogen in blood or another body fluid

rate a ratio in which the numerator and denominator have different units

ratio a comparison of two numbers

rational model a theoretical framework that considers behavior change to be a function of knowledge, attitudes, and practices

ready-to-use therapeutic foods (RUTF) premade food products that are high in energy and protein and are often made from a peanut base

recessive gene an allele that must be inherited from both parents in order to be phenotypically expressed

Red Cross (ICRC) a private humanitarian organization officially sanctioned by the Geneva Convention and international law to provide specific humanitarian services during times of war

refugee a person who has been forced to move across an international border because of security concerns like war, civil conflict, political strife, or persecution based on race, tribe, religion, political affiliation, or membership in some other group

rehabilitation the process of restoring lost function to the greatest extent possible in order to maximize independence and quality of life

relative poverty living on less than the nationally defined poverty line

relative survival rate a comparison of the likelihood of survival to selected time points after diagnosis of an adverse health condition with survival rates for people of the same age who do not have the condition

relief aid that meets the immediate needs of people who might otherwise not have access to water, food, shelter, emergency medical care, and other urgent necessities

remittances funds transferred by international workers to family members in their home communities

renewable energy energy derived from a source like wind or solar power that is not depleted when it is used

replacement population a demographic pattern in which the average woman gives birth to two children

reproductive health issues related to fertility and infertility, pregnancy and childbirth, contraception, the prevention and treatment of sexually transmitted infections, and other aspects of gynecological and urological health

reproductive rights the freedom of women and their partners to decide how many children they want without interference from governments or other organizations

research the process of systematically investigating a topic in order to discover new insights about the world

reservoir the environmental home for an infectious agent

resilience the ability to resist, survive, adapt to, and recover from adverse events

respect for persons a research principle that emphasizes autonomy, informed consent, voluntariness, and protection of potentially vulnerable individuals

respiratory syncytial virus (RSV) a frequent cause of severe pneumonia among neonates and other young infants

rheumatic heart disease an inflammatory condition that causes irreversible damage to the heart and heart valves as a result of an untreated infection with group A *Streptococcus*

rheumatoid arthritis an autoimmune disorder characterized by chronic inflammation that damages the cartilage and bones in many joints

rickets vitamin D deficiency in children, whose bones are still growing

Rift Valley fever a zoonotic arboviral infection that can cause outbreaks of pregnancy loss in livestock herds

rinderpest an eradicated zoonotic disease that decimated cattle herds

risk factor an exposure that increases the likelihood of experiencing a particular health outcome

risk transition a health transition characterized by a shift from exposures like undernutrition, unsafe water, and indoor air pollution that increase the risk of childhood infectious diseases causing most preventable morbidity and mortality in a population to exposures like obesity, physical inactivity, and tobacco use that increase the risk of chronic diseases being the most prominent risk factors

road traffic injury an injury that occurs during a collision involving at least one moving motor vehicle

rotavirus the most frequent cause of severe diarrhea among infants and young children

rubella a vaccine-preventable viral infection that can cause miscarriage and birth defects when contracted early in pregnancy

rurality the degree to which a particular location is rural

S

saccharides the molecular units that form carbohydrates

safe drinking water an adequate supply of affordable clean drinking water in or near the home

SAFE strategy a trachoma control plan that combines surgery, antibiotics, facial cleanliness, and environmental improvements

sanitation the safe disposal of human excreta (feces)

sarcoma a cancer that arises from connective tissues like bones or muscles

SARS severe acute respiratory syndrome caused by the SARS-CoV virus

saturated fatty acid a fatty acid with only single bonds between its carbon atoms

scabies an intensely itchy condition that occurs when mites burrow into skin and lay eggs

scheme an operationalized plan that spells out the desired outcomes and completion timelines for an action plan

schistosomiasis a blood fluke disease that can increase the risk of bladder cancer among people with chronic infection

schizophrenia a mental health disorder characterized by distorted perceptions of reality

screening a type of secondary prevention in which all members of a well-defined group of people are encouraged to be tested for a disease based on evidence that members of the population are at risk for the disease and early intervention improves health outcomes

scurvy vitamin C deficiency that is characterized by bleeding gums and loose teeth

secondary infertility the inability to have additional offspring when attempting to conceive after giving birth

secondary prevention the detection of health problems in asymptomatic individuals at an early stage when the conditions have not yet caused significant damage to the body and can be treated more easily

sedentariness sitting for long durations each day

selection a biological term that describes the preferential survival and reproduction of advantaged organisms

self-directed violence physical trauma inflicted by an individual on his or her own body, such as cutting and suicide attempts

self-efficacy an individual's confidence in his or her ability to successfully achieve a performance goal

Sendai Framework a global agreement that aims to significantly reduce the number of deaths and the magnitude of destruction caused by natural disasters

sensitivity the proportion of people who truly have a disease who test positive for the disease

sentinel surveillance the continuous collection and analysis of high-quality data from a limited number of clinics or hospitals

sepsis widespread inflammation in the body that is triggered by the chemicals released by the body's immune system in response to an infection

severe acute malnutrition a state of extreme undernutrition that is present when a child has a weight-for-height z-score below $z = -3$

sex the biological classification of people as male or female based on genetics and reproductive anatomy

sexual health the enjoyment of safe, voluntary, and nonviolent sexual experiences

sexually transmitted infection an infection spread through sexual intercourse or other types of sexual contact

sexual orientation an individual's sexual attraction, identity, and behavior

sickle cell disease a genetic disorder that causes some red blood cells to become misshapen in a way that can cause painful blockages in small blood vessels

sickness the ways in which a person with a physical or mental health condition relates to and is regarded by his or her community

sign an objective indicator of disease that can be clinically observed, such as a rash, cough, fever, or elevated blood pressure

skilled birth attendant an obstetrician or gynecologist, another type of physician, a midwife, a nurse, or another licensed clinician who is proficient in recognizing and treating potential complications of women and newborns during and after labor and delivery

smallpox an eradicated viral disease that caused blisters to form over the body and could cause death or permanent disability

social cognitive theory a theoretical framework stipulating that behavior change is about both inner motivation and environmental realities because behavior is a function of personal factors, behaviors, and environmental conditions

social determinants of health the personal factors and community conditions that enable or hinder access to health

social ecological model a theoretical framework that considers individual health and health behaviors to be a function of the social environment, which includes intrapersonal (individual), interpersonal, institutional (organizational), community, and public policy dimensions

social justice the principle that moving toward greater equality in the distribution of income and wealth, opportunities for education and employment, access to health and security, and involvement in civic and political activities is valuable for human flourishing

social marketing the use of advertising strategies to change behaviors in targeted populations

social media electronic communication tools that allow users to generate and share content

Sociodemographic Index (SDI) an estimate of national development calculated from data on income per capita, the average number of years of education, and fertility rates

socioeconomic status (SES) an individual's standing in a society based on individual and household income, education, gender, occupation, ethnicity and race, and other characteristics; also called *socioeconomic position*

soft skills the personal, social, emotional, and communication skills that enable people to successfully contribute to and lead work teams and other collaborative activities

soil-transmitted helminth a nematode infection contracted by contact with soil that contains feces contaminated with worm eggs or larvae

specificity the proportion of people who are truly free of a disease who test negative for it

spontaneous abortion the miscarriage of a pregnancy prior to the fetal age of viability

stages of change model a theoretical framework that describes individual behavior change as a multistage process from precontemplation to contemplation, preparation for action, action, and maintenance; also called the *transtheoretical model*

stakeholder a person who has an interest in the success or failure of a group and can influence or be affected by that group's decisions or actions

standard of health targets that governments set for improving the health of the populations they govern

statistic a measured characteristic of a sample population

steatosis fatty liver disease caused by the accumulation of lipids in the liver

sterilization the use of medical or surgical procedures to intentionally make it difficult or impossible for a person to reproduce

stigma negative attitudes about members of a population group that often lead to discrimination, social exclusion, and other forms of marginalization

stillbirth the death of a fetus late in pregnancy but prior to delivery

Stop TB Partnership an international network that coordinates the efforts of hundreds of organizations working on tuberculosis control

strategy a big-picture plan for how to achieve a major goal

strep throat a Group A *Streptococcus* infection of the pharynx that if left untreated can lead to complications such as rheumatic fever

stroke the death of cells in the brain due to lack of oxygen

strongyloidiasis a threadworm infection that is usually soil transmitted but has the capacity to reproduce entirely within a human host

stunting a condition in which a child has low height-for-age

suicide the intentional act of ending one's own life

supplementation the process of delivering micronutrients through a pill, tablet, capsule, or other nonfood substance

supply chain management the process of coordinating all steps from selecting and procuring products through transporting, storing, and delivering them

surgery an operation to confirm whether a disease is present or to remove a tumor or repair a part of the body

surveillance the process of continually monitoring health events in a population so that emerging public health threats can be detected and appropriate control measures can be implemented quickly

survival analysis statistical evaluation of the distribution of the durations of time that individuals in a population experience from an initial time point (such as birth) until some well-defined event (such as death)

sustainability a concept that emphasizes the need to provide for current human needs without compromising the ability of future generations to meet their needs

Sustainable Development Goals (SDGs) a set of 17 goals endorsed by the member nations of the United Nations at the end of 2015 that aim, by 2030, to end poverty, protect the planet, and promote prosperity and peace

symptom a subjective indication of illness that is experienced by an individual but cannot be observed by others

syndemic two or more diseases clustering within a population in part due to social and structural conditions and the interaction between the diseases making the health outcomes worse

syndrome a collection of signs and symptoms that occur together

syndromic surveillance the process of tracking potential outbreaks or other disease events based on reports of symptoms and other types of data rather than relying solely on counts of laboratory-confirmed diagnoses

syphilis a sexually transmitted infection with *Treponema pallidum* that can cause chronic cardiovascular and nervous system impairments

systems thinking the process of identifying the underlying causes of complex problems so that sustainable solutions can be developed and implemented

systolic blood pressure the pressure in blood vessels when the heart beats

T

taeniasis having tapeworms that cycle between pigs or cattle and humans living in human intestines

target a specific, measurable objective that contributes to achieving a desired future outcome

TB disease the symptomatic, contagious form of tuberculosis; also called *active TB*

T cells lymphocytes that form in the bone marrow, then mature in the thymus

teratogen a substance that can cause birth defects

tertiary prevention interventions that reduce impairment, minimize pain and suffering, and restore function in people with symptomatic health problems

tetanus a sustained muscle contraction that is often caused by a neurotoxin from the bacterium *Clostridium tetani*

thalassemia a genetic disorder characterized by impaired production of hemoglobin, the molecules in red blood cells that carry oxygen

theory of planned behavior a theoretical framework that builds on the theory of reasoned action by emphasizing that follow-through on implementing plans for a healthier lifestyle is dependent on the individual's perceived self-efficacy and control over the change

theory of reasoned action a theoretical framework positing that follow-through on implementing plans for a healthier lifestyle is dependent on the individual's belief that the outcome of the change will be worth the effort and his or her confidence that others will support the change

thiamine a B vitamin that is necessary for nerve, muscle, and heart function

total dependency ratio a ratio comparing the total number of children (aged 0–14 years) and older adults (aged 65+ years) in a population to the number of people aged 15–64 years

total fertility rate the average number of children a woman gives birth to during her childbearing years

toxicology the study of the harmful effects that chemicals and other environmental hazards can have on living things

trachoma a bacterial eye infection that can lead to blindness in people who do not practice good facial hygiene

traditional birth attendant a lay midwife who has been trained through an apprenticeship rather than a formal educational program

trafficking the crime of arranging for a person to relocate with the intention of forcing that migrant into sex work, debt bondage, slavery, or other types of forced labor

transdisciplinary an approach to education and scholarship that moves beyond traditional disciplinary boundaries to create new ways of thinking and practicing

trans fat a liquid oil that has been transformed into a semisolid fat through hydrogenation

transgender a gender identity that does not match the sex assigned at birth

transient ischemic attack a mini stroke in which a temporary blockage of an artery causes stroke-like symptoms that quickly resolve

transmissibility the ease with which an infectious agent is passed from an infected host to another individual

transtheoretical model a theoretical framework that describes individual behavior change as a multistage process from precontemplation to contemplation, preparation for action, action, and maintenance; also called the *stages of change model*

traumatic brain injury (TBI) short- or long-term damage arising from a concussion or other form of intracranial injury

trematode a fluke that typically has a complex life cycle involving two different animal hosts

trichomoniasis a protozoal sexually transmitted infection caused by *Trichomonas vaginalis*

trichuriasis an intestinal whipworm infestation that can cause colitis

TRIPS Agreement an international agreement negotiated through the World Trade Organization that protects patents, copyrights, registered trademarks, and industrial designs across international boundaries

trypanosomiasis African sleeping sickness, an often fatal infection transmitted by tsetse flies

tuberculosis (TB) the disease caused by infection with *Mycobacterium tuberculosis* bacteria

tumor an abnormal growth of a body tissue

type 1 diabetes a form of diabetes in which the body does not produce enough insulin

type 2 diabetes a form of diabetes in which the body stops responding appropriately to insulin even when the hormone is still being produced by the body

U

UNAIDS the Joint United Nations Programme on HIV/AIDS, an entity co-sponsored by 10 UN system agencies to advance HIV/AIDS prevention and control

under-5 child a child of any age between birth and the fifth birthday

under-5 mortality rate the number of children who die before their fifth birthdays per 1,000 live births

underemployment a situation in which a person is involuntarily working part-time rather than full-time or is a low-wage worker whose earnings are below the local poverty level even after working long hours

undernutrition malnutrition resulting from deficiencies in the amount of food or types of nutrients eaten or from poor absorption of the nutrients that have been consumed

underweight a condition in which a child has low weight-for-age

UNDP the United Nations Development Programme, the UN program focused on poverty reduction

unemployment the inability of a person who is not working for pay to secure a paid position despite actively seeking a paid job

UNEP the United Nations Environment Programme, the UN program that promotes healthy ecosystems and sustainable use of natural resources

UNFPA the United Nations Population Fund (formerly the UN Fund for Population Activities), the UN program that supports reproductive health programs

UNICEF the United Nations Children's Fund (formerly the UN International Children's Emergency Fund), the UN program that advocates for children's rights and provides humanitarian assistance for children

unintentional injury an unplanned injury that happens very quickly

unipolar depressive disorder a depressive disorder characterized by depression without cycles of mania

United Nations the world's largest intergovernmental organization

Universal Declaration of Human Rights an international agreement unanimously adopted by the member states of the UN in 1948 that spells out more than two dozen civil, political, economic, social, and cultural human rights

universal health coverage (UHC) a population-level status achieved when everyone in a country has access to high-quality health services and is protected from major health-associated financial shocks

universal precautions the use of barriers like gloves to prevent contact with blood or body fluids

unsaturated fatty acid a fatty acid that contains at least one double bond in the carbon chain

upper respiratory infection an acute infection of the nose, sinuses, pharynx, larynx, or trachea

urbanicity the degree to which a particular location is urban

urbanization a shift toward more people living in cities and fewer people living in rural areas

USAID the U.S. Agency for International Development, which is the lead international cooperation agency in the United States

V

vaccination the intentional delivery of a substance into the body in order to stimulate development of immunity against a particular disease

vaccine hesitancy the decision to delay receiving recommended vaccines or to refuse offered vaccines

values general principles that define what is good or evil and what is meaningful

vector an organism (usually a nonvertebrate, such as an insect) that transmits a pathogen to another organism

vector-borne infection an infection caused by a pathogen that is transmitted to humans via an arthropod

vector control interventions that reduce the size and density of arthropod populations

ventricular tachycardia an arrhythmia that occurs when the ventricles of the heart begin contracting extremely rapidly

vertical program a program that delivers disease-specific clinical services that are not fully integrated into the health system

vertical transmission the transmission of a pathogen from an infected pregnant woman to her offspring during pregnancy, delivery, or breastfeeding; also called *mother-to-child transmission*

VIA visual inspection with acetic acid, an inexpensive method for detecting signs of cervical cancer

violence the use of force or power to threaten or inflict physical, sexual, and psychological harm on oneself, another person, or a group of people

virion an assembled virus with nucleic acid and an outer protein coating

virulence the ability of an infectious agent to cause severe disease or death in a host

virus a nucleic acid (DNA or RNA) encased in a protein shell

vital statistics population-level quantifications of births, deaths, and other life events

vitamin a micronutrient organic compound that cannot by synthesized by the body

vitamin A a fat-soluble vitamin critical for vision

vitamin A deficiency a vitamin deficiency that causes visual impairment

vitamin C a vitamin essential for collagen formation and iron absorption

vitamin D a vitamin that is necessary for bone health because it assists the body with calcium absorption

voluntary counseling and testing a process of being tested for HIV or another infection and receiving counseling about risk reduction, treatment referrals, and communication strategies

voluntourism volunteer tourism, travel for the purpose of volunteering

W

WASH program an intervention that combines improved access to water and sanitation systems with hygiene promotion

wasting a condition in which a child has low weight-for-height

water-soluble vitamin a vitamin that is easily dissolved in the body but is not able to be stored in body tissues

wealth the accumulated worth of a household's resources

West Nile virus an arbovirus that has become endemic to the United States and can cause encephalitis

World Bank a multilateral investment bank that makes loans to developing countries

World Food Programme the UN program that aims to eliminate hunger and malnutrition associated with natural disasters and armed conflict

World Health Organization a specialized agency of the United Nations that serves as its primary health agency

World Organisation for Animal Health (OIE) an intergovernmental group that helps to control the spread of zoonotic infectious diseases and to promote food safety

World Trade Organization (WTO) a UN-related organization that negotiates and enforces trade agreements among United Nations member nations

X

XDR-TB an extensively drug-resistant tuberculosis strain that does not respond to rifampicin, isoniazid, fluoroquinolones, and at least one second-line injectable TB medication

xerophthalmia a severe dryness of the eye

Y

yaws an endemic treponematosis that causes disfiguring skin lesions and has been targeted for eradication

years lived with disability (YLDs) a burden of disease metric used to quantify the population-level reductions in health status attributable to nonfatal conditions

years of life lost (YLLs) a burden of disease metric used to quantify population-level reductions in health status due to premature mortality

yellow fever a vaccine-preventable arbovirus infection that causes the skin and eyes of infected people to become yellow due to jaundice

YLD an abbreviation for a year *lived* with *disability*

YLL an abbreviation for a year of *life lost*

Z

Zika virus an arbovirus infection that is usually asymptomatic but has been linked to an increased risk of microcephaly in babies born to women who contract the virus during the pregnancy

zinc a mineral that is important for immune function and wound healing

zoonosis an infectious disease that usually occurs in animals and only occasionally infects humans

z-score a statistical indicator of how many standard deviations away from the population mean an individual's measure is

Index

Note: Page numbers followed by "*f*" indicate figures

A

ABCs of addiction, 463–464
abortion, 308
abstinence, sexual, 308
abstract, 46
Abt Associates, 170
academic sector, 171
acceptable, feasible, affordable, sustainable, and safe (AFASS), 193
accident, 481
acculturation, 68
ACE inhibitors. *See* angiotensin-converting enzyme (ACE) inhibitors
ACEs. *See* adverse childhood experiences (ACEs)
Acinetobacter baumannii, 228
acne vulgaris, 451
ACT. *See* artemisinin-based combination therapy (ACT)
Actinomycetes, 278
action, 2*f*
action plan, 156
activated health education model, 371
active immunity, 235
active surveillance, 128
active TB, 197
activities of daily living (ADLs), 114, 115*f*
acute, 224
acute flaccid paralysis, 287
acute liver failure, 243
acute lymphoblastic leukemia (ALL), 414
acute mania, 463
acute myelogenous leukemia (AML), 414
acute respiratory infection (ARI), 224–228, 225*f*
addiction, 463
ADHD. *See* attention-deficit/hyperactivity disorder (ADHD)

ADLs. *See* activities of daily living (ADLs)
adolescence, 507, 522–525
adulthood
    early adulthood, 531–534
    middle adulthood, 534–537, 535–536*f*
    older adulthood, 543–544
adverse childhood experiences (ACEs), 522
adverse event, 237
adverse reaction, 237
advocacy, 158
Aedes mosquitoes, 265, 266*f*, 269
AEDs. *See* automated external defibrillators (AEDs)
Aeromonas, 218
AFASS. *See* acceptable, feasible, affordable, sustainable, and safe (AFASS)
African eye worm, 271
African Programme for Onchocerciasis Control, 271
afterbirth. *See* placenta
age-based discrimination, 542
Agency for Healthcare Research and Quality (AHRQ), 168
Agency for Toxic Substances and Disease Registry (ATSDR), 168
2030 Agenda for Sustainable Development, 30
agent, 179
age standardization, 38, 38*f*
aging and global health, 539–543
aging transition, 12*f*, 537–539, 538*f*, 539*f*, 540*f*
Agreement on Trade-Related Aspects of Intellectual Property Rights. *See* TRIPS Agreement
AHRQ. *See* Agency for Healthcare Research and Quality (AHRQ)
AIDS, 182. *See also* HIV/AIDS

airborne pathogens, 230
airborne transmission, 229
air pollution, 75, 100, 380
    burden of disease to, 86*f*
alcohol use disorders, 464–468, 465–467*f*
Alcohol Use Disorders Identification Test (AUDIT), 466
ALL. *See* acute lymphoblastic leukemia (ALL)
allele, 444
allergy, 445
alveoli, 225
Alzheimer's disease, 472
ambient air pollution, 85
American sleeping sickness. *See* Chagas disease
amino acids, 333–334
amitriptyline, 460
AML. *See* acute myelogenous leukemia (AML)
amoebas, 256
Ancylostoma duodenale, 274
anemia, 347, 518
aneurysm, 379
angina, 375
angiogenesis, 393
angioplasty, 378
angiotensin-converting enzyme (ACE) inhibitors, 382, 437
angiotensin II receptor blockers (ARBs), 382, 437
Anopheles mosquitoes, 257
anorexia, 468
anorexia nervosa, 468
antenatal care, 311
anthrax, 502
anthropometry, 337
anthroponosis, 233
antibody, 235
antigen, 233
antigenic drift, 233
antigenic shift, 233

antimicrobial resistance (AMR), 205–207
antiretroviral medications (ARVs), 113, 182, 193*f*
antiretroviral therapy (ART), 182–184
　HIV treatment, 190, 191*f*
anxiety disorders, 460–461, 462*f*
aortic aneurysm, 385–386
apicomplexans, 256
apnea, 240
apoptosis, 393
appendicitis, 440
appropriate technology, 168
arbovirus, 267, 268*f*
ARBs. *See* angiotensin II receptor blockers (ARBs)
ARI. *See* acute respiratory infection (ARI)
arrhythmia, 386
arsenicosis, 122
ART. *See* antiretroviral therapy (ART); assisted reproductive technologies (ART)
artemisinin-based combination therapy (ACT), 258
arthropod, 266
ARVs. *See* antiretroviral medications (ARVs)
ascariasis, 273
Ascaris lumbricoides, 273, 273*f*
asphyxia, 512
assisted reproductive technologies (ART), 322
assistive devices, 116
association, 10
asthma, 430
asylum, 68–69, 69*f*
atherosclerosis, 375, 377
Atlas method, 48
atrial fibrillation, 386
ATSDR. *See* Agency for Toxic Substances and Disease Registry (ATSDR)
attention-deficit/hyperactivity disorder (ADHD), 472
AUDIT. *See* Alcohol Use Disorders Identification Test (AUDIT)
autism, 472
autochthonous, 260
autoimmune disorder, 445
automated external defibrillators (AEDs), 386
autonomy, 111
autosomal gene, 444

B

Bacillus anthracis, 502
Bacillus Calmette-Guérin (BCG) vaccine, 203
bacterium, 180–181
Barrett's esophagus, 413
basic emergency obstetric and newborn care (BEmONC), 315
basic human needs, access to, 121–122
BCG vaccine. *See* Bacillus Calmette-Guérin (BCG) vaccine
behavioral risk factor, 11
behavior change, 371
Beijing Conference, 298, 522
BEmONC. *See* basic emergency obstetric and newborn care (BEmONC)
benchmark, 31
beneficence, 111
benign prostatic hyperplasia (BPH), 324, 410
benign tumor, 393
beriberi, 350
Bhopal incident, India, 91
bilateral aid, 163
bilharzia. *See* schistosomiasis
Bill & Melinda Gates Foundation, 27, 149
binge-eating disorder, 468
bioavailability, 346
biodiversity, 99
biomass, 84, 86
biopsy, 403
biostatistics, 36
bioterrorism, 501–503
　chemical weapons, 502*f*
　classifications of, 501*f*
bipolar disorder, 463
birth asphyxia, 320
birth control pills, 308
birth rate, 34
birth spacing, 306, 308
bladder cancer, 415
blindness, 447
blood cancer, 414
blood flukes, 257
blood, path of, 225*f*
blood poisoning, 245
blood pressure, 382
BMI. *See* body mass index (BMI)
body mass index (BMI), 351–352, 352*f*

BPH. *See* benign prostatic hyperplasia (BPH)
Bradford Hill criteria, 10, 10*f*
brain drain, 120
breast cancer, 398, 407–409, 407*f*
　interventions for, 408*f*
breastfeeding, 335–337, 336*f*
bronchitis, 431
budgeting, 173
built environment, 75
bulimia nervosa, 468
burden of disease metrics, 41–43, 42*f*
burns, 492, 493*f*
Buruli ulcer, 277
bypass surgery, 378

C

calcium, 348
calorie, 332
Campylobacter jejuni, 218
CA-MRSA. *See* community-acquired MRSA (CA-MRSA)
cancer, 391–416
　biology, 392–394, 394*f*
　breast cancer, 407–409
　care by country income level, 404, 404*f*
　cervical cancer, 409–410
　with chronic infections, 400*f*
　colorectal cancer, 413–414
　epidemiology, 394–398
　esophageal cancer, 413–414
　and global health, 391–392
　liver cancer, 412–413
　lung cancer, 406–407
　mortality rate, 395*f*, 396*f*, 397*f*, 398*f*
　other cancers, 414–416
　patients, 405*f*
　prevention, 398–400
　prostate cancer, 410–411
　screening, 401–402, 401*f*
　screening tests, 403*f*
　signs and symptoms, 393
　stomach cancer, 413–414
　treatment, 402–406
cancer transition, 399
candidiasis, 181
cannabis, 464
carbohydrate, 333
carcinogens, 90
carcinoma, 393
cardiac arrest, 386
cardiac rehabilitation, 379

cardiomyopathy, 386
cardiovascular disease (CVD),
    361–387
  burden of disease from, 369*f*
  epidemiologic transition, 363–365
  epidemiology, 365–367
  and global health, 361–363
  health behavior change, 371–373
  hypertension, 381–384
  interventions for, 370*f*
  ischemic heart disease, 375–379
  mortality rate, 362*f*, 363*f*, 367, 368*f*
  other diseases, 384–387
  physical inactivity and
      sedentariness, 373–375
  prevention, 367–371
caries, dental, 451
carrier, 221
carrying capacity, 98
case definition, 40
case detection rate (CDR), 199
case fatality rate (CFR), 38
cataract, 447
catastrophe, 124
Catholic Relief Services, 151
causal factor, 10
causation, 10
CBRN attack. *See* chemical,
    biological, radiological, or
    nuclear (CBRN) attack
CBT. *See* cognitive behavioral
    therapy (CBT)
CD4 cells, 182
  count, 182, 183*f*
CDR. *See* case detection rate (CDR)
CE. *See* continuing education (CE)
CEA. *See* cost-effectiveness analysis
    (CEA)
cellulitis, 451
CEmONC. *See* comprehensive
    emergency obstetric and
    newborn care (CEmONC)
census, 34
Centers for Disease Control and
    Prevention (CDC), 27, 28*f*,
    167, 253
Centers for Medicare & Medicaid
    Services, 168
CEPI. *See* Coalition for Epidemic
    Preparedness Innovations
    (CEPI)
cerebral malaria, 258
cerebral palsy (CP), 320, 520
cervical cancer, 398, 409–410
  interventions for, 409*f*

cesarean section, 315, 316*f*
cestode, 257
CFR. *See* case fatality rate (CFR)
Chagas disease, 274–275
Charity Navigator, 152
chemical, biological, radiological, or
    nuclear (CBRN) attack, 503
chemical hazards, 91
Chemonics International, Inc., 170
chemotherapy, 403
Chernobyl incident, 91
chikungunya, 267
child growth, 337–341, 338*f*
Child Growth Standards, 337, 339*f*
child health, 507–510
  adolescence, 522–525
  children with special needs, 520
  early childhood, 516–520
  infant health and development,
      514–516
  middle childhood, 521–522
  neonatal survival, 510–514
childhood vaccinations, 239*f*
  recommended doses of, 241*f*,
      242*f*
child labor, 91
children with special needs, 520
child sponsorship, 151
child support ratio, 539, 541*f*
chlamydia, 195
Chlamydia pneumoniae, 228
Chlamydia trachomatis, 195, 277
Chlamydophila psittaci, 228
chlorhexidine, 513
cholera, 218–219
cholesterol, 377
chromoblastomycosis, 279
chronic condition, 224
chronic kidney disease (CKD),
    436–437, 438–439*f*
chronic obstructive pulmonary
    disease (COPD), 76, 431, 432*f*
chronic respiratory diseases (CRDs),
    429–432
cigarette smoking. *See* tobacco
    smoking
ciliates, 256
circulating vaccine-derived
    poliovirus (cVDPV), 288
circumcision, 194
cirrhosis, 437
cisgender, 325
civil rights, 108
CKD. *See* chronic kidney disease
    (CKD)

claudication, 375
climate change, 101
  and human health, 100–103,
      101*f*, 102*f*
clinical trials, 111, 237
Clinton Health Access Initiative, 150
Clonorchis, 257, 257*f*
Clonorchis sinensis, 281
Clostridium botulinum, 221
Clostridium difficile infections, 206
Clostridium tetani, 321
CLTS programs. *See* community-led
    total sanitation (CLTS)
    programs
CMAM. *See* community-based
    management of acute
    malnutrition (CMAM)
Coalition for Epidemic
    Preparedness Innovations
    (CEPI), 150, 166
Coccidioidomycosis, 228
cochlear implants, 450
Codex Alimentarius, 356
cognitive behavioral therapy (CBT),
    460, 461
co-insurance, 143
collective violence, 494
colorectal cancer, 396, 398,
    413–414
  interventions for, 413–414, 414*f*
colostrum, 335
communication, 551
community-acquired MRSA
    (CA-MRSA), 206
community-based management of
    acute malnutrition (CMAM),
    343
community development, 158
community-led total sanitation
    (CLTS) programs, 82
complementary foods, 335, 335*f*
complementary proteins, 334
complete protein, 334
complex humanitarian emergency,
    498
comprehensive emergency obstetric
    and newborn care (CEmONC),
    315
computed tomography (CT), 379
condom, 308
cone-nosed bugs, 274
conflict and war, 498–500
conjugate vaccine, 236
contact tracing, 234
continued feeding, 223

continuing education (CE), 552
contraception, 308–311, 309f, 310f
contraindication, 237
control, 283
Convention on the Rights of Persons with Disabilities, 117
cooperation, international, 159–160
copay, 143
COPD. *See* chronic obstructive pulmonary disease (COPD)
copepods, 286
coronary artery disease, 375
coronavirus, 234–235
  vaccines, 242
corporate sector, 170–171
corporate social responsibility (CSR), 150
corruption, 71, 71f
corticosteroid injections, 513
cost-effectiveness analysis (CEA), 172–173
Council on Education for Public Health, 549, 549f
counterfeit drug, 112
country income level and health, 46–50, 47f, 49f, 50f
COVAX, 166
COVID-19, 3, 44, 99, 163, 235
  deaths, 38–39, 39f
Coxiella burnetii (Q fever), 228
CP. *See* cerebral palsy (CP)
C-reactive protein (CRP), 378
crisis, 124
cross-cultural communication, 169. *See also* intercultural communication
crude statistic, 38
Cryptococcus, 182
cryptosporidiosis, 221
Cryptosporidium, 218, 256
C-section. *See* cesarean section
CSR. *See* corporate social responsibility (CSR)
cue to action, 371
Culex mosquitoes, 268
cultural competence, 551
cultural humility, 551
cultural rights, 108
culture, 65–67
cVDPV. *See* circulating vaccine-derived poliovirus (cVDPV)
cycle of transmission, 266
cysticercosis, 281
cystic fibrosis, 444

D

DAC. *See* Development Assistance Committee (DAC)
DAH. *See* Development assistance for health (DAH)
DAI, 170
DALYs. *See* disability-adjusted life years (DALYs)
data, 44
data science, 44
DBP. *See* diastolic blood pressure (DBP)
DCP project. *See* Disease Control Priorities (DCP) project
DDT (dichloro-diphenyltrichloroethane), 260
deafness, 114. *See also* hearing loss
death rate, 36. *See also* mortality rates
Declaration of Alma-Ata, 516
deductible, 143
DEET (N,N-diethyl-mtoluamide), 262
default rate, 206
definitive host, 256
dehydration, 217
deliverable, 156
delusion, 461
dementia, 472–473
demographic transition, 12f, 299, 299f
demography, 299
dengue, 265–266
dental and oral health, 451–452, 452f
deoxygenated blood, 361
Department of Defense (DOD), 147
Department of Political and Peacebuilding Affairs, 161
depression, 459
depressive disorders, 459–460, 460f
dermatitis, 451
determinants of health, 4. *See also* environmental determinants of health; socioeconomic determinants of health
development, 158
Development Assistance Committee (DAC), 147
development assistance for health (DAH), 146, 148f, 178f
  United States, 146, 148f
  funding channels for, 157f
diabetes (diabetes mellitus), 425–429, 426–429f

diagnostic accuracy, 401
Diagnostic and Statistical Manual of Mental Disorders (DSM-5), 459
dialysis, 437
diarrhea, 217, 508, 519
  causing pathogens, 217–218
  interventions, 221–224, 222f
  mortality, 224f
diastolic blood pressure (DBP), 381
diffusion of innovations model, 372
digestive diseases, 440–442
dilated cardiomyopathy, 386
diphtheria, 239f, 240
diplomacy, 159, 160
direct transmission, 229
directed donations, 168
directly observed therapy, short-course (DOTS), 202
disabilities, 114–117, 114f
disability-adjusted life years (DALYs), 42, 42f, 43f, 62f, 77f, 531, 534f
disaster, 124
discrimination, 66
disease, 197
Disease Control Priorities (DCP) project, 27
Diseases of Workers (book), 89
disorder, 457
distal cause, 8
distributive justice, 111
Doctors Without Borders, 499
DOD. *See* Department of Defense (DOD)
Doha Declaration, 113
dominant gene, 444
donors, 145, 168
DOTS. *See* directly observed therapy, short-course (DOTS)
dracunculiasis, 285–287, 287f
drinking water, 79–84, 110, 121–122
drowning, 490–492, 491f
drug-resistant TB (DR-TB), 205–206
drug susceptibility testing (DST), 206
drug use disorders, 463–464
DSM-5. *See* Diagnostic and Statistical Manual of Mental Disorders (DSM-5)
DST. *See* drug susceptibility testing (DST)
dysentery, 221
dyskinesia, 443

E

early adulthood, 531–534
early breastfeeding, 335
early childhood, 507, 508*f*
   health interventions in, 516–520
early childhood development
   (ECD), 515
earthquake in Haiti, in 2010, 151
Ebola virus disease, 288
ECD. *See* early childhood
   development (ECD)
echinococcosis, 281
Echinococcus granulosus, 281
Echinococcus multilocularis, 281
ecological fallacy, 400
ecological footprint, 98, 99*f*
ecology, 99
Economic and Social Council, 161
economic rights, 108
economics, 56–59
ecosystem health, 99–100
ecosystem services, 99
ecotoxicology, 91
ectoparasite, 279
ectopic pregnancy, 311
eczema, 451
ED. *See* erectile dysfunction (ED)
edema, 342
edentulism, 452
education, 59–61
effectiveness, 172
efficacy, 172
efficiency, 172
EIDs. *See* emerging infectious
   diseases (EIDs)
elderly support ratio, 539, 541*f*
electricity, 85–86, 85*f*
elephantiasis, 269, 270*f*
elimination, 283
emergency, 124
emergency management, 123–126
   disaster types, 123*f*
   stages of, 123*f*
emergency obstetric and newborn
   care (EmONC), 315
Emergency Support Functions
   (ESFs), 125
emerging infectious diseases (EIDs),
   288–290
   risk factors for, 290*f*
EmONC. *See* emergency obstetric
   and newborn care
emotional and psychological abuse,
   497

emphysema, 431
employment, 63–65, 63*f*, 64*f*
ENAP. *See* Every Newborn Action
   Plan (ENAP)
encephalitis, 245
endemic, 128
END Fund, 150
Ending Preventable Maternal
   Mortality initiative, 317
endometriosis, 323
endoparasite, 279
endowment, 149
end-stage renal disease (ESRD), 437
End TB Strategy, 203
energy, 84–88
enrichment, 346
Entamoeba histolytica, 218
enteric infections, 217
enteropathogenic *E. coli* (EPEC),
   220
enterotoxigenic *E. coli* (ETEC), 220
environment, 75
environmental determinants of
   health
   climate change and health,
      100–103
   ecosystem health, 99–100
   energy and air quality, 84–88
   occupational and industrial
      health, 88–92
   and SDGs, 75–79
   sustainability, 96–99
   urbanization, 92–96
   water/sanitation/hygiene, 79–84
environmental health, 75
environmental risk factors, 77*f*
enzootic, 235
EPEC. *See* enteropathogenic *E. coli*
   (EPEC)
EPI. *See* Expanded Program on
   Immunization (EPI)
epidemic, 128
epidemiologic transition, 12*f*,
   363–365
epidemiology, 36, 179
epigenetics, 443
epilepsy, 442
epizootic, 284
equity, 2*f*
eradication, 283–285, 284*f*
erectile dysfunction (ED), 324
Escherichia coli, 181, 218, 219
ESFs. *See* Emergency Support
   Functions (ESFs)
"3 Es" of injury prevention, 484
esophageal cancer, 413–414

ESRD. *See* end-stage renal disease
   (ESRD)
essential amino acid, 334
essential medicines, access to,
   111–114
estimate, 44
ETEC. *See* enterotoxigenic *E. coli*
   (ETEC)
ethics, 108
ethnicity, 66
etiology, 8
eukaryote, 255
evaluation, 172
Every Newborn Action Plan
   (ENAP), 319, 512, 513
Every Woman Every Child (UN),
   519
exclusive breastfeeding, 335
Expanded Program on
   Immunization (EPI), 238,
   516
expatriate, 68
experiential learning, 551–552
exposure, 9
extensively drug-resistant TB
   (XDR-TB), 206
extinction, 285
extreme poverty, 57

F

faith-based organization (FBO),
   168
falciparum malaria, 257
falls, 488–490, 489*f*
family planning, 306–308
famine, 344
FAO, 162. *See* Food and Agriculture
   Organization (FAO)
Fasciola gigantica, 281
Fasciola hepatica, 281
fat, 334
fat-soluble vitamin, 345
FBO. *See* faith-based organization
   (FBO)
FCCC. *See* Framework Convention
   on Climate Change (FCCC)
FCTC. *See* Framework Convention
   on Tobacco Control (FCTC)
FDA. *See* Food and Drug
   Administration (FDA)
FDI. *See* foreign direct investment
   (FDI)
fecal-oral transmission, 222, 287
female genital cutting (FGC), 497
female genital mutilation (FGM),
   497

fertility, 306
 rates, 307, 307*f*
fertility transition, 12*f*, 299–302, 537
FGC. *See* female genital cutting (FGC)
FGM. *See* female genital mutilation (FGM)
FHI (Family Health International), 170
fiber, 333
fibroids, 323
financial abuse, 497
financing, 137
flagellates, 256
fluoride, 348–349
fluoxetine, 460
flying toilet, 81
folate, 350
folic acid, 350
fomite, 222
Food and Agriculture Organization (FAO), 162
Food and Drug Administration (FDA), 168
foodborne infectious diseases, 355
foodborne NTDs, 279–282, 280*f*
food intoxication, 220
food safety, 216, 355–356
food security, 343–345
food supply, 344*f*
food system, 345
forecast, 45
foreign aid expenditures, in United States, 146, 147*f*
foreign direct investment (FDI), 148
foreign policy, 159, 166
fortification, 346
foundations, 149–150
fractional vaccines, 236
Framework Convention on Climate Change (FCCC), 102
Framework Convention on Tobacco Control (FCTC), 434
"5 Fs," 222
functional literacy, 59
funder–channel–implementer pathway, 145*f*
funding sources, 141, 141*f*
fungus, 181

G

GAPPD. *See* Global Action Plan for Pneumonia and Diarrhea (GAPPD)
gastroenteritis, 217

gastroesophageal reflux disease (GERD), 413
Gates Foundation, 27, 149
Gavi. *See* Global Alliance for Vaccines and Immunization (Gavi)
GBV. *See* gender-based violence (GBV)
gender, 61–63, 62*f*
gender-based violence (GBV), 497–498
gender identity, 325
gender roles, 61
generalized anxiety disorder, 460
generic drug, 112
genetic blood disorders, 443–445
genetics, 443
genital prolapse, 324
genotype, 444
geohelminth, 273
GERD. *See* gastroesophageal reflux disease (GERD)
German measles. *See* rubella
gestational diabetes, 427
GFR. *See* glomerular filtration rate (GFR)
GHG. *See* greenhouse gas (GHG)
Giardia, 218, 221, 256, 256*f*
giardiasis, 221
gingivitis, 451
Gini coefficient, 49
"girl-child," rights of, 522
GiveWell, 152
glaucoma, 447
Global Action Plan for Pneumonia and Diarrhea (GAPPD), 223, 230
Global Action Plan for the Prevention and Control of Noncommunicable Diseases, 422
Global Alliance for TB Drug Development, 150
Global Alliance for Vaccines and Immunization (GAVI), 166, 242, 519
Global Burden of Disease (GBD) project, 45
Global Charter for the Public's Health, 134
Global Financing Facility for Every Woman Every Child (2015), 519
Global Fund, 150, 166, 177
global health
 achievements, 17–18

aging and, 539–543
burden of disease metrics, 41–43
cancer and, 391–392
cardiovascular disease and, 361–363
core knowledge in, 547
country income level and, 46–50
defining, 1–3
experiential learning in, 551–552
history and functions of, 15–17
HIV/AIDS, TB, and, 177–179
infectious diseases and, 213–217, 214*f*, 215*f*, 216*f*
and injuries, 481–484
interprofessionalism and, 547–553
malaria and neglected tropical diseases, 253–255
mental health and, 457–459
Millennium Development Goals, 28–30, 29*f*
morbidity and, 40–41, 40*f*
mortality and, 36–39
noncommunicable diseases (NCDs), 419–425
nutrition and, 331–332
PACES of, 1, 2*f*, 3
prioritization strategies, 24–28
reproductive health and, 297–299
sources of health information, 44–46, 45*f*
transitions, 1–18
United Nations (UN), 107, 108*f*
vital statistics, 34–36
global health channels and implementers, 145, 155–157
global health financing, 135–137
 health insurance, 143–144
 health systems, 137–140
 medicine and public health, 133–135
 paying for global health interventions, 145–146
 paying for personal health, 141–142
 personal donations, 150–152
global health implementation
 corporate sector, 170–171
 development banks, 163–165
 global partnerships, 165–166
 international cooperation, 159–160
 local and national governments, 166–168
 measuring impact, 171–173
 nonprofit sector, 168–170
 research and academic sector, 171
 United Nations, 160–163

global health interventions, 157–159

global health security, 22–24

Global Health Security Agenda (GHSA), 24

Global Health Security (GHS) Index, 503

global health statistics, 34–43, 44

Global Hunger Index, 341, 341*f*

globalization
defined, 21
and health, 21–22

Global Nutrition Targets, 339, 340*f*, 383

global partnerships, 165–166

Global Polio Eradication Initiative (GPEI), 288

Global Programme to Eliminate Lymphatic Filariasis (GPELF), 270

global warming, 101–102

Global Yaws Control Programme, 278

glomerular filtration rate (GFR), 436

glomerulonephritis, 436

glucose-6-phosphate dehydrogenase (G6PD) deficiency, 444

GNI. *See* gross national income (GNI)

goal, 29

GOBI, 517

goiter, 348

gonorrhea, 195

gout, 446

governance, 70–72, 71*f*

government
public health activities, 167, 167*f*
spending, on health and education, 140, 140*f*

G6PD deficiency. *See* glucose-6-phosphate dehydrogenase (G6PD) deficiency

GPEI. *See* Global Polio Eradication Initiative (GPEI)

GPELF. *See* Global Programme to Eliminate Lymphatic Filariasis (GPELF)

Grand Challenges in Global Health, 27

grant, 164

gravidity, 306

GreatNonprofits, 152

greenhouse gas (GHG), 101–102

gross domestic product (GDP), 46, 135

gross national income (GNI), 46, 148

gross national product (GNP), 46

GuideStar, 152

guinea worm. *See* dracunculiasis

gynecological health, 323–324

H

HAART. *See* highly active antiretroviral therapy (HAART)

habilitation, 116

HACCP. *See* hazard analysis and critical control point (HACCP)

Haemophilus influenzae type b (Hib), 228, 245
vaccine, 240

HAI. *See* healthcare-associated infection (HAI)

Haiti earthquake, 151, 218

HALE. *See* healthy life expectancy (HALE)

hallucination, 461

handwashing, 206

Hansen's disease. *See* leprosy

hazard analysis and critical control point (HACCP), 356

hazardous exposures, 89–90, 90*f*

HBV. *See* hepatitis B virus (HBV)

HCC. *See* hepatocellular carcinoma (HCC)

HCV. *See* hepatitis C virus (HCV)

HDI. *See* Human Development Index (HDI)

headache disorders, 442

HEADSSS acronym, 523

health. *See also* global health
defined, 3–4
standard of, 107

health behavior, 371

health behavior change, 371–373
"5 As and 5 Rs" model of, 372, 372*f*

health belief model, 371

healthcare-associated infection (HAI), 206

health communication, 551

health diplomacy, 159

health disparity, 15

health equity, 2, 56

"Health for All by 2000," 516

health information, sources of, 44–46

health information system, 44, 139

health insurance, 143–144

health interventions, 157–158

health literacy, 59

health metrics, 41–46, 48–49, 52

health promotion, 134
for adolescents, 522–525
in early adulthood, 531–534
in early childhood, 516–520
in middle adulthood, 534–537, 535–536*f*
in middle childhood, 521–522

Health Resources and Services Administration (HRSA), 168

health services
access to, 110–111, 137*f*
coordination of, 516

health spending, based on country income level, 135, 136*f*, 141*f*

health systems, 137–140
building blocks of, 139

health trajectories, 5*f*

health transitions, 12–15, 12*f*

healthy life expectancy (HALE), 36, 36*f*, 536

healthy pregnancy, 311–313

hearing impairment, 449–451

hearing loss, 449–451, 450*f*. *See also* deafness

heart failure, 387

Helicobacter pylori infection, 413

helminth diseases, 255–257

hemoglobin, 346

hemophilia, 444

hemorrhagic stroke, 379

hepatitis A, 242

hepatitis B, 243

hepatitis B virus (HBV), 412

hepatitis C, 244

hepatitis C virus (HCV), 412

hepatitis E, 244

hepatocellular carcinoma (HCC), 412–413

herd immunity, 237

herpes, 196

HHS. *See* United States, Department of Health and Human Services (HHS)

Hib. *See* Haemophilus influenzae type b (Hib)

highly active antiretroviral therapy (HAART), 184

highly pathogenic avian influenza (HPAI), 233

high-risk screening, 401

Hispanic/Latino, 66

Histoplasma capsulatum, 228
HIV/AIDS, 113, 181–184, 183*f*
  deaths, 186–188*f*
  epidemiology, 184–189
  interventions, 189–195, 190*f*
  new cases of, 186*f*, 189*f*
  people living with, 185, 185*f*
  and tuberculosis, 177–179
H1N1 influenza pandemic (2009), 234
Hodgkin lymphoma, 415
hookworm, 274
horizontal program, 158
hospice care, 404
host, 179
household air pollution, 84
HPAI. *See* highly pathogenic avian influenza (HPAI)
HPV. *See* human papillomavirus (HPV)
HRSA. *See* Health Resources and Services Administration (HRSA)
human African trypanosomiasis (HAT), 275
Human Development Index (HDI), 48
  versus Gini coefficient, 50*f*
  over time, 50*f*
humanitarian response clusters, 125*f*
human needs. *See* basic human needs, access to
human papillomavirus (HPV), 196, 240, 409
human rights
  access to basic human needs, 121–122
  access to essential medicines, 111–114
  access to health services, 110–111
  emergency management, 123–126
  health and, 107–128
  health workforce, 119–121
  International Health Regulations, 126–128
  people with disabilities, 114–117
  prisons, 117–119
human security, 22–24, 23*f*
Hurricane Katrina, 151
hydatid disease, 281
hydrocele, 270
hygiene, 80
hyperemesis gravidarum, 311
hypertension, 381–384, 383*f*, 384*f*

hypertrophic cardiomyopathy, 386
hypothermia, 513
hypoxia, 225

I

IADLs. *See* instrumental activities of daily living (IADLs)
IAEA. *See* International Atomic Energy Agency (IAEA)
IARC. *See* International Agency for Research on Cancer (IARC)
IAVI. *See* International AIDS Vaccine Initiative (IAVI)
IBRD. *See* International Bank for Reconstruction and Development (IBRD)
iCCM (Integrated Community Case Management), 518
ICPD. *See* International Conference on Population and Development (ICPD)
ICRC. *See* International Committee of the Red Cross (ICRC)
ICS. *See* Incident Command System (ICS)
IDA. *See* iron deficiency anemia (IDA)
IDD. *See* iodine deficiency disorders (IDD)
IDP. *See* internally displaced person (IDP)
IDU. *See* injecting drug user (IDU)
IGRA blood test. *See* interferon-gamma release assay (IGRA) blood test
IHD. *See* ischemic heart disease (IHD)
IHR. *See* International Health Regulations (IHR)
ILI. *See* influenza-like illness (ILI)
illness, 65
ILO. *See* International Labour Organization (ILO)
IMCI (Integrated Management of Childhood Illness), 517
IMF. *See* International Monetary Fund (IMF)
immigrant, 68
immunization, 235–238, 512
Immunization Agenda 2030, 242
impairments, 114, 115*f*
implementation science, 6
IMR. *See* infant mortality rate (IMR)
inactivated vaccine, 235
incarceration, 118
incidence, 40
incidence rate, 40, 187

Incident Command System (ICS), 125
income, 56
incubation period, 197
Indian Ocean tsunami, in 2004, 151
indicator, 29
Indigenous population, 67
indirect transmission, 229
indoor air pollution, 84
  DALYs to, 87*f*
indoor residual spraying (IRS), 260
induced abortion, 308
industrial health, 88–92
industrial hygiene, 89
inequality, 56
inequity, 56
infant, 507
infant health and development, 514–516
infantile paralysis. *See* polio
infant mortality rate (IMR), 514, 514*f*
infant nutrition, 335–337
infection, 197
infectious diseases, 177–207, 213–245, 253–290
  big three, 254
  emerging, 288–290
  and global health, 213–217, 214*f*, 215*f*, 216*f*
  mortality, 215*f*, 216*f*
  percentage of deaths in children in 2025, 231*f*
infectivity, 288
infertility, 322–323
inflammation, 378
influenza, 230–234
influenza-like illness (ILI), 234
information, 44
informed consent, 111
INGO. *See* international NGO (INGO)
injecting drug user (IDU), 464
injury prevention, 481–503
  bioterrorism, 501–503
  burns, 492
  conflict and war, 498–500
  drowning, 490–492
  "3 Es," 484
  falls, 488–490
  injuries and global health, 481–484
  intentional injuries, 494
  interpersonal violence, 494–497
  transport injuries, 484–488
  unintentional injuries, 492–493

in-kind donations, 150
insecticide-treated net (ITN), 261, 262f
insect-transmitted infections, 100
in situ tumor, 393
INSPIRE acronym, 494–497
Institute for Health Metrics and Evaluation (IHME), 45
instrumental activities of daily living (IADLs), 115, 115f
insulin, 425
insulin-dependent diabetes. See type 1 diabetes
insurance, 143
Integrated Community Case Management (iCCM), 518
Integrated Management of Childhood Illness (IMCI), 517
intensive resuscitation, 511
intentional injuries, 481, 494, 495f
interagency coordination, 126
intercultural communication, 551
interdisciplinary approach, 548, 549f
interferon-gamma release assay (IGRA) blood test, 198
Intergovernmental Panel on Climate Change (IPCC), 101
intermediate host, 256
intermittent preventive treatment (IPT), 259
internally displaced person (IDP), 69
International Agency for Research on Cancer (IARC), 44
International AIDS Vaccine Initiative (IAVI), 150, 178
International Atomic Energy Agency (IAEA), 161
International Bank for Reconstruction and Development (IBRD), 164
International Centre for Diarrhoeal Disease Research, Bangladesh (ICDDR,B), 150
International Code of Marketing of Breast-milk Substitutes, 336
International Committee of the Red Cross (ICRC), 499
International Conference on Population and Development (ICPD), 297
international cooperation, 159–160, 160f
international health, 16

International Health Regulations (IHR), 126–128
international humanitarian laws, 499
International Labour Organization (ILO), 91
International Monetary Fund (IMF), 164
international NGO (INGO), 168
International Organization for Migration (IOM), 161
International Rescue Committee, 151
interpersonal violence, 494–497
    mortality rate, 495–496f
interprofessionalism, 547–553
    defined, 550
intersectionality, 121
interventions, 5, 6f
intimate partner violence (IPV), 498
intrauterine device (IUD), 308
in vitro fertilization (IVF), 322–323
involuntary migrant, 68–70
iodine deficiency disorders (IDD), 348
IOM. See International Organization for Migration (IOM)
IPCC. See Intergovernmental Panel on Climate Change (IPCC)
IPT. See intermittent preventive treatment (IPT)
IPT in pregnancy (IPTp), 259
IPT of infants (IPTi), 259
IPV. See intimate partner violence
iron deficiency anemia (IDA), 346–348, 514
iron deficiency disorders, 348
ischemia, 375
ischemic heart disease (IHD), 375–379
    CVD deaths due to, 375, 375f
    mortality rates, 381f
    risk factors, 376–377
ischemic stroke, 379
isolation, 234
ITN. See insecticide-treated net (ITN)
IUD. See intrauterine device (IUD)
IVF. See in vitro fertilization (IVF)

J

Japan International Cooperation Agency (JICA), 159
jaundice, 243
Jhpiego, 170
JICA. See Japan International Cooperation Agency (JICA)

"J-shaped" growth pattern, 97, 98f
juvenile-onset diabetes. See type 1 diabetes

KAP. See knowledge, attitudes, and practices (KAP)
kidney failure, 436
kissing bugs, 274
Klebsiella pneumoniae, 228
knowledge, attitudes, and practices (KAP), 371
kwashiorkor, 342

L

landmines, 500
"late, long, few" policy, 306
latent period, 197
latent TB infection (LTBI), 197
laws, 108
LBW. See low birthweight (LBW)
Legionella pneumophila, 228
Legionnaires' disease, 228
Leishmania, 256
leishmaniasis, 276, 276f
lending groups, 145
leprosy, 276–278
leukemia, 414
leukocyte, 181
liberal arts, 548
licensed vaccines, 237
life expectancies, 34
    at birth, 34, 35f
    at various ages, 539f
lifestyle diseases, 421
Lind, James, 89
lipid, 334
literacy, 59, 60f, 61f
live attenuated vaccine, 236
"LIVE LIFE" approach, 471
liver cancer, 412–413
    interventions for, 413f
liver diseases, 437–440, 441f
liver flukes, 257
LLIN. See long-lasting insecticidal net (LLIN)
LMICs. See low- and middle-income countries (LMICs)
loan, 164
local governments, 166–168, 167f
lockjaw. See tetanus
logistics, 158
loiasis, 271
long-lasting insecticidal net (LLIN), 261

low- and middle-income
        countries (LMICs), 46, 47*f*
low birthweight (LBW), 320, 321*f*
lower respiratory infection (LRI), 225
        mortality among children, 232*f*
low vision, 447
LRI. *See* lower respiratory infection
        (LRI)
LTBI. *See* latent TB infection (LTBI)
lung cancer, 396, 398, 406–407,
        406*f*
        interventions for, 407*f*
lung flukes, 257
lupus, 446
lymphatic filariasis (LF), 269–270
lymphedema, 269
lymphoma, 414–415
lymphocyte, 181–182

M

macronutrients, 332–335, 333*f*
macular degeneration, 447
Madura foot. *See* mycetoma
malaria, 257–259, 512, 519
        cases and deaths, 259–260, 265*f*
        epidemiology, 259–260
        history, 253
        interventions, 260–265, 261*f*
malarial anemia, 258
Malaria Vaccine Initiative, 263
malignant tumor, 393
malnutrition, 331
Malthus, Thomas, 97
MAM. *See* moderate acute
        malnutrition (MAM)
mammogram, 408
Mantoux tuberculin skin test (TST),
        198
marasmus, 342
mass drug administration (MDA),
        270, 274
maternal and child health (MCH),
        298
maternal health issues, 512
maternal mortality, 313–317,
        314–315*f*
        interventions for, 317*f*
maternal mortality ratio (MMR),
        316, 318*f*
mathematical model, 45
MCH. *See* maternal and child health
        (MCH)
MDA. *See* mass drug administration
        (MDA)
MDG. *See* Millennium Development
        Goal (MDG)

MDGs. *See* Millennium
        Development Goals (MDGs)
MDR-TB. *See* multidrug-resistant TB
        (MDR-TB)
measles, 238, 239*f*
Médecins Sans Frontières (MSF),
        499
Medicaid, 144
medical anthropology, 550
Medicare, 143
medicine, 133
        versus public health, 135*f*
Medicines for Malaria Venture, 263
MEDLINE, 46
megacity, 96
melanoma, 415, 415*f*
menarche, 323
meningitis, 245
meningitis belt, 245
meningococcus, 245
meningoencephalitis, 245
menopause, 323
men's health, 61–63, 324–325
menstruation, 323
mental health
        alcohol use disorders, 464–468
        anxiety disorders, 460–461
        autism and neurodevelopmental
                disorders, 471–472
        bipolar disorder, 463
        care, 473–474*f*, 473–475
        dementia and neurocognitive
                disorders, 472–473
        depressive disorders, 459–460
        drug use disorders, 463–464
        and global health, 457–459
        other disorders, 468–469
        promotion, 457–475
        schizophrenia, 461–463
        suicide, 469–471
mentorship, 552
men who have sex with men (MSM),
        189, 324
Mercy Corps, 151
MERS. *See* Middle East respiratory
        syndrome (MERS)
metabolism, 348
metastasis, 393
methicillin-resistant *Staphylococcus
        aureus* (MRSA), 206
metric, defined, 41
miasma, 76
microcephaly, 269
micronutrients, 345–346
middle adulthood, 534–537
middle childhood, 521–522

Middle East respiratory syndrome
        (MERS), 235
mid-upper arm circumference
        (MUAC), 337
migraine, 442
migrant health, 67–70
Millennium Development Goals
        (MDGs), 28–30, 29*f*, 82, 83*f*,
        214, 255, 317, 509
mineral deficiencies, 348–349
minerals, 345, 346*f*
Ministry of Health, 167
miscarriage, 308
mitigation, 123
MMR. *See* maternal mortality ratio
        (MMR)
model, statistical, 45
moderate acute malnutrition
        (MAM), 342
modifiable risk factor, 10
monitoring, 172
monitoring and evaluation (M&E),
        172
monogenic disorder, 444
morals, 108
morbidity, 40–41, 40*f*
*Morbidity and Mortality Weekly
        Report* (MMWR), 44
mortality, 36–39, 37*f*
        premature, 41
mortality rates, 12*f*, 36
        cancer, 395*f*, 396*f*, 397*f*, 398*f*
        cardiovascular disease (CVD),
                362*f*, 363*f*, 367, 368*f*
        diabetes (diabetes mellitus), 426*f*
        diarrhea, 224*f*
        drowning, 490, 491*f*
        gender-based violence (GBV),
                497–498
        HIV/AIDS, 186–188*f*, 190
        infant mortality rate (IMR), 514
        injuries, 482–483*f*
        interpersonal violence, 495–496*f*
        ischemic heart disease (IHD),
                381*f*
        measles, 238, 239*f*
        neonatal mortality rate (NMR),
                511
        transport injuries, 485–486*f*
        tuberculosis, 202, 204*f*
        under-5 mortality rate, 509
mortality transition, 12*f*, 537
mother-to-child transmission
        (MTCT), 192
MPI. *See* Multidimensional Poverty
        Index (MPI)

MPOWER acronym, 434
MRSA. *See* methicillin-resistant *Staphylococcus aureus* (MRSA)
MS. *See* multiple sclerosis (MS)
MSF. *See* Médecins Sans Frontières (MSF)
MSM. *See* men who have sex with men (MSM)
MTCT. *See* mother-to-child transmission
MUAC. *See* mid-upper arm circumference (MUAC)
multicausality, 8
Multidimensional Poverty Index (MPI), 59
multidisciplinary learning, 548–550, 548*f*, 549*f*
multidrug-resistant TB (MDR-TB), 205
multilateral aid, 163
multilateral lending groups, 145
multiple sclerosis (MS), 443
multisectoral, 158
mumps, 240
musculoskeletal disorders, 445–446, 446*f*
mutation, 443
mycetoma, 278, 279*f*
Mycobacterium leprae infection, 277
Mycobacterium tuberculosis, 197
Mycobacterium ulcerans infection. *See* buruli ulcer
Mycoplasma pneumoniae, 228
myocardial infarction, 375

N

NAFLD. *See* nonalcoholic fatty liver disease (NAFLD)
National Academies of Sciences, Engineering, and Medicine, 23
national governments, 166–168, 167*f*
national health agency, 167
national health plan, 139, 139*f*
National Health Service (NHS), 138
National Incident Management System (NIMS), 125
National Institutes of Health (NIH), 168
natural environment, 75
natural history of disease, 184
NCDs. *See* noncommunicable diseases (NCDs)
Necator americanus, 274
negative predictive value (NPV), 402
neglected tropical diseases (NTDs), 254, 254*f*, 255

foodborne, 279–282
skin, 278–279
Neisseria gonorrhoeae, 195
Neisseria meningitidis, 245
nematode, 257
neonatal mortality, 317–322, 322*f*, 510–514
neonatal mortality rate (NMR), 511, 511*f*, 512*f*
neonatal period, 507
neonatal sepsis, 512
neonate, 319
neoplasms, 393
neurocognitive disorders, 472–473
neurocysticercosis, 281
neurodevelopmental disorders, 471–472, 520
neurological disorders, 442–443
NGO. *See* nongovernmental organization (NGO)
NHL. *See* non-Hodgkin lymphoma (NHL)
NHS. *See* National Health Service (NHS)
niacin, 350
nicotine, 433
NIH. *See* National Institutes of Health (NIH)
NIMS. *See* National Incident Management System (NIMS)
NMR. *See* neonatal mortality rate (NMR)
N, N-diethyl-mtoluamide (DEET), 262
NNRTIs. *See* non-nucleoside reverse transcriptase inhibitors (NNRTIs)
nonalcoholic fatty liver disease (NAFLD), 440
noncommunicable diseases (NCDs), 15, 364, 364*f*, 365*f*, 419–452. *See also* cancer; cardiovascular disease (CVD)
chronic kidney disease (CKD), 436–437
deaths from, 420*f*, 421*f*, 423*f*, 424*f*
dental and oral health, 451–452
diabetes, 425–429
digestive diseases, 440–442
genetic blood disorders, 443–445
and global health, 419–425
hearing loss, 449–451
liver diseases, 437–440
musculoskeletal disorders, 445–446

neurological disorders, 442–443
skin diseases, 451
tobacco control, 433–436
vision impairment, 446–449
voluntary global targets for, 422*f*
nonderogable right, 503
nongovernmental organization (NGO), 168
non-Hodgkin lymphoma (NHL), 415
non-insulin-dependent diabetes. *See* type 2 diabetes
nonmaleficence, 111
nonmelanoma skin cancer, 396, 451
nonmodifiable risk factor, 10
non-nucleoside reverse transcriptase inhibitors (NNRTIs), 184
nonprofit organization (NPO), 151, 168
norovirus, 217, 218
Norwalk-like virus, 218
nosocomial infection, 206
NPO. *See* nonprofit organization (NPO)
NPV. *See* negative predictive value (NPV)
NRTIs. *See* nucleoside reverse transcriptase inhibitors (NRTIs)
nucleoside reverse transcriptase inhibitors (NRTIs), 184
nutrition, 331–356
breastfeeding and infant, 335–337
child growth, 337–341
food safety, 355–356
food security 343–345
food systems, 343–345
and global health, 331–332
iodine deficiency disorders, 348
iron deficiency anemia, 346–348
macronutrients, 332–335
micronutrients, 345–346
mineral deficiencies, 348–349
overweight and obesity, 350–353
severe acute malnutrition, 341–343
vitamin A deficiency, 349
nutrition transition, 12*f*, 332

OA. *See* osteoarthritis (OA)
obesity, 350–353
among adults, 353*f*
interventions, 353–355
in pediatric population, 353*f*
obesity transition, 352

obsessive-compulsive disorder (OCD), 468
obstetric fistula, 313
obstetric transition, 12*f*, 316
obstructed labor, 313
occupational hazards, 76, 93
occupational health, 88–92
OCD. *See* obsessive-compulsive disorder (OCD)
ODF status. *See* open defecation free (ODF) status
OECD. *See* Organisation for Economic Co-operation and Development (OECD)
Office for Disaster Risk Reduction (UNDRR), 161
Office for the Coordination of Humanitarian Affairs, 161
Office of the United Nations High Commissioner for Refugees (UNHCR), 69
official development assistance (ODA), 146–149
OIE (*Office International des Epizooties*). *See* World Organisation for Animal Health
oil, 334
older adulthood, 543–544
onchocerciasis, 270–271
Onchocerciasis Elimination Program, 271
One Health, 99
open defecation, 80
open defecation free (ODF) status, 82
Ophithorchis felineus, 281
Ophithorchis viverini, 281
opportunistic infections (OIs), 182
OPV. *See* oral polio vaccine (OPV)
oral contraceptives, 308
oral polio vaccine (OPV), 287
oral rehydration salts (ORS), 223
oral rehydration therapy (ORT), 223, 517
Organisation for Economic Co-operation and Development (OECD), 46, 120
Development Assistance Committee (DAC), 147
ORS. *See* oral rehydration salts (ORS)
ORT. *See* oral rehydration therapy (ORT)
osteoarthritis (OA), 445
osteomalacia, 350
osteoporosis, 446

Ottawa Charter, 134
outbreak, 128
outdoor air pollution, 85
DALYs to, 87*f*
out-of-pocket payments, 141
overdiagnosis, 402
overnutrition, 350
overpopulation, 97
overtreatment, 402
overweight, 350–353, 352*f*, 353*f*
oxygenated blood, 361
oxytocin, 314

PACES (populations, action, cooperation, equity, and security), 1–3, 2*f*, 25–27, 25–27*f*
palliative care, 404
pancreatic cancer, 414
pandemic, 128
Pandemic Alert System (WHO), 234
panic disorder, 460
Paragonimus, 257
parasitemia, 258
parasites, 255–257
parenteral infection, 243
parity, 306
Parkinson's disease (PD), 442–443
parrot fever. *See* psittacosis
particulate matter, 84
partner notification, 197
Partnership for Maternal, Newborn & Child Health (PMNCH), 519
passive immunity, 235
passive surveillance, 128
pasteurization, 356
patent, 112
PATH, 150
pathogen, 21
pathogenicity, 288
Patient Protection and Affordable Care Act (ACA) of 2010, 143
PC. *See* preventive chemotherapy (PC)
PCOS. *See* polycystic ovary syndrome (PCOS)
PCP. *See Pneumocystis carinii* pneumonia (PCP)
PD. *See* Parkinson's disease (PD)
pediatric deaths, 510
peer review, 46
pellagra, 350
pelvic inflammatory disease (PID), 195
PEP. *See* post-exposure prophylaxis (PEP)

PEPFAR. *See* President's Emergency Plan for AIDS Relief (PEPFAR)
percentage, 34
perinatal mortality, 319
perinatal period, 315
periodontitis, 451
peripheral artery disease, 375
persistent organic pollutant (POP), 260
personal donations, 150–152
personal health, paying for, 141–142
personal protective equipment (PPE), 234
person who injects drugs (PWID), 464
pertussis, 240
pharmaceutical companies, 150
PHC. *See* primary health care (PHC)
PHEIC. *See* public health emergency of international concern (PHEIC)
phenotype, 444
physical abuse, 497
physical inactivity, 373, 374*f*
PICE (potential injury-creating event) nomenclature, 124*f*
PID. *See* pelvic inflammatory disease (PID)
pit latrine, 81
placenta, 312
placental abruption, 312
placenta previa, 312
planetary health, 100
Plasmodium parasites, 256, 257
life cycle of, 258*f*
PMDD. *See* premenstrual dysphoric disorder (PMDD)
PMI. *See* President's Malaria Initiative (PMI)
PMNCH. *See* Partnership for Maternal, Newborn & Child Health (PMNCH)
PMR. *See* proportionate mortality rate (PMR)
PMS. *See* premenstrual syndrome (PMS)
PMTCT. *See* prevention of MTCT (PMTCT)
pneumococcus, 226
pneumoconiosis, 431
Pneumocystis carinii pneumonia (PCP), 184
pneumonia, 8–11, 225, 508, 519
interventions, 228–230, 229*f*
policy, 158

polio, 240, 287–288
 vaccine, infants receiving, 289*f*
political rights, 108
politics, 70–72
polycystic ovary syndrome (PCOS), 323
pooled risk, 143
POP. *See* persistent organic pollutant (POP)
population-based screening, 401
population planning, 302–306, 305*f*
population pyramid, 300, 304*f*
populations, 2*f*, 300
 defined, 4
 health, 3–4
Population Services International, 150
positive predictive value (PPV), 402
post-exposure prophylaxis (PEP), 193
postpartum hemorrhage, 314
posttraumatic stress disorder (PTSD), 468
Pott, Percivall, 89
poverty, 56–59, 58*f*, 78, 508
power, 70
PPE. *See* personal protective equipment (PPE)
PPP. *See* public–private partnership (PPP); purchasing power parity (PPP)
PPV. *See* positive predictive value (PPV)
praziquantel, 272
precaution, 237
prediabetes, 427
preeclampsia, 312
pre-exposure prophylaxis (PrEP), 193
pregnancy, 311–313
 immunization during, 512
prejudice, 66
premature mortality, 41
premenstrual dysphoric disorder (PMDD), 323
premenstrual syndrome (PMS), 323
premiums, 143
prenatal care. *See* antenatal care
PrEP. *See* pre-exposure prophylaxis (PrEP)
President's Emergency Plan for AIDS Relief (PEPFAR), 178, 194
President's Malaria Initiative (PMI), 178
preterm birth, 319, 320*f*, 512
prevalence, 40
prevention of MTCT (PMTCT), 192
prevention science, 6

preventive care, insurance for, 143, 144
preventive chemotherapy (PC), 270
primary health care (PHC), 516
primary infertility, 322
primary prevention, 6, 7*f*
primordial prevention, 9
prioritization strategies, 24–28
prisons, health in, 117–119, 118*f*, 119*f*
private health insurance, 143
private voluntary organization (PVO), 168
professional development, 552–553
program, 156
PROGRESS acronym, 55, 56*f*
project, 156
projection, 45
project management, 156
proportion, 34
proportionate mortality rate (PMR), 38
prostate cancer, 396, 398, 410–411, 410*f*
 interventions for, 411, 411*f*
prostate-specific antigen (PSA) test, 411
prosthetic, 500
protein, 334
protozoans, 255–257
proximal cause, 8
PSA test. *See* prostate-specific antigen (PSA) test
Pseudomonas aeruginosa, 228
psittacosis, 228
psychiatrist, 473
psychologist, 473
PTSD. *See* post-traumatic stress disorder (PTSD)
public health, 76, 133–135, 134*f*, 172
 medicine *versus*, 135*f*
public health emergency of international concern (PHEIC), 128, 235
public policy, 158
public–private partnership (PPP), 165
pulmonary tuberculosis, 197
purchasing power parity (PPP), 48
purified protein derivative (PPD) test, 198
PVO. *See* private voluntary organization (PVO)
PWID. *See* person who injects drugs (PWID)
pyelonephritis, 436

Q

qualitative research, 171
quality-adjusted life year (QALY), 42
quantitative research, 171
quarantine, 234

R

RA. *See* rheumatoid arthritis (RA)
rabies, 282–283
race, 66
radiation therapy, 403–404
Ramazzini, Bernardino, 89
rapid diagnostic test (RDT), 258, 259*f*
rate, 34
ratio, 34
rational model, 371
RDT. *See* rapid diagnostic test (RDT)
ready-to-use therapeutic foods (RUTF), 343
recessive gene, 444
Red Cross, 499
reduviids, 274
refractive errors, 447
refugee, 68
refugee health, 67–70
rehabilitation, 116
relative poverty, 57
relative survival rate, 393
relief, 157
remittances, 148
renewable energy sources, 87, 87*f*, 88*f*
replacement population, 300
reproductive health, 297, 525
 family planning, 306–308
 fertility transition, 299–302
 and global health, 297–299
 gynecological health, 323–324
 healthy pregnancy, 311–313
 infertility, 322–323
 maternal mortality, 313–317
 men's, 324
 population planning, 302–306
 sexual minority health, 324–325
 stillbirths and neonatal mortality, 317–322
reproductive rights, 297
research, 171
reservoir, 273
resilience, 124
RESPECT acronym, 498
respect for persons, 111
respiratory syncytial virus (RSV), 228
rheumatic heart disease, 385

rheumatoid arthritis (RA), 445
rickets, 350
Rift Valley fever, 269
right to health, 110–111
rinderpest, 284
risk factor, 8–11, 9f
   behavioral, 11
   defined, 9
   modifiable, 10
   nonmodifiable, 10
risk transition, 12f
river blindness. *See* onchocerciasis
road traffic injury (RTI), 484
Roll Back Malaria, 263
rotavirus, 218
RSV. *See* respiratory syncytial virus
   (RSV)
RTI. *See* road traffic injury (RTI)
RTI International, 170
rubella, 240
rurality, 92
RUTF. *See* ready-to-use therapeutic
   foods (RUTF)

S

saccharides, 333
safe drinking water, 79, 79f, 82, 83
SAFER acronym, 468
SAFE strategy, 278
Salmonella, 218
salt, 383, 385f
SAM. *See* severe acute malnutrition
   (SAM)
sanitation, 80, 81f
   access to, 83–84, 84f
sarcoma, 393
Sarcoptes scabiei var. *hominis*, 279
SARS. *See* severe acute respiratory
   syndrome (SARS)
saturated fatty acid, 334
Save the Children, 151
SBA. *See* skilled birth attendant (SBA)
scabies, 279
scheme, 156
Schistosoma, 257
Schistosoma mansoni, 272
schistosomiasis, 272–273
schizophrenia, 461–463
screening
   cancer, 401–402, 401f
   characteristics of programs, 402f
scurvy, 350
SDGs. *See* Sustainable Development
   Goals (SDGs)
SDI. *See* Sociodemographic Index (SDI)
secondary infertility, 322
secondary prevention, 7, 7f

security, 2f
sedentariness, 373
seizure disorders, 442
selection, 206
selective serotonin reuptake
   inhibitor (SSRI), 460
self-directed violence, 494
self-efficacy, 371
Sendai Framework, 126
sensitivity, 401
sentinel surveillance, 127
sepsis, 314
septic tanks, 81
SES. *See* socioeconomic status (SES)
severe acute malnutrition (SAM),
   341–343
severe acute respiratory syndrome
   (SARS), 235
sex, 61
sexual abuse, 494
sexual health, 297
sexually transmitted infection (STI),
   195–197, 196f
sexual minority health, 324–325
sexual orientation, 324
SHAKE package, 383
Shiga toxin-producing *E. coli*
   (STEC), 220
sickle cell disease, 444
sickness, 65
sign, 182
skilled birth attendant (SBA), 312
skin cancers, 415, 415f
skin diseases, 451
skin NTDs, 278–279
sleep, leisure, occupation,
   transportation, and home-
   based (SLOTH) model, 373
SLOTH model. *See* sleep, leisure,
   occupation, transportation, and
   home-based (SLOTH) model
smallpox, 285
smoking. *See* tobacco smoking
snakebite envenoming, 282–283
social cognitive theory, 372
social determinants of health, 55
social ecological model, 372
social isolation, 542
social justice, 56
social marketing, 165
social media, 158
social rights, 108
Sociodemographic Index (SDI), 48
socioeconomic determinants of
   health, 55–72
   economics, 56–59
   education, 59–61

   employment, 63–65
   gender, 61–63
   governance and politics, 70–72, 71f
   health equity and SDGs, 55–56
   migrant and refugee health, 67–70
socioeconomic status (SES), 55
   key components of, 63
sodium, 383, 385f
soft skills, 550
soil-transmitted helminths, 273–274
solar panels, 86
solid fuels, 85
specificity, 401
spending on health services, 135, 136f
spontaneous abortion, 308
sputum smear test, 198
SSRI. *See* selective serotonin
   reuptake inhibitor (SSRI)
stages of change model, 372
stakeholder, 165
standard of health, 107
Staphylococcus, 181, 451
Staphylococcus aureus, 228
statistic, 34
steatosis, 440
sterilization, 308
stigma, 463
stillbirths, 317–322, 319f, 511
stomach cancer, 396, 413–414
Stop TB Partnership, 203
Stop TB Strategy, 203
strategy, 156
strep throat, 225
Streptococcus, 226, 245, 451
stroke, 379–381
   hemorrhagic, 379
   ischemic, 379
Strongyloides stercoralis, 274
strongyloidiasis, 274
stunting, 337
substance use disorders. *See* alcohol
   use disorders; drug use disorders
suicide, 469–471, 469–471f
sulfadoxone/pyrimethamine (SP), 258
supplementation, 346
supply chain management, 170
supporting health in older
   adulthood, 543–544
surgery, 402, 440–442
surveillance, 127, 127f
survival analysis, 34
sustainability, 96–99
Sustainable Development Goals
   (SDGs), 30–34, 31f, 32f, 33f,
   113, 140, 255, 255f, 297, 298f,
   332, 367, 457, 484, 510, 512f,
   529, 547

environmental health and, 75–79
and health equity, 55–56
neonatal mortality rate, 512*f*
SDG 1, 547
SDG 2, 332, 548
SDG 3, 548
SDG 4, 547
SDG 5, 297, 547
SDG 6, 82, 548
SDG 7, 86, 548
SDG 8, 65, 92, 547
SDG 9, 92
SDG 10, 67, 70
SDG 11, 96
SDG 12, 97, 548
SDG 13, 548
SDG 16, 71, 547
targets related to health, 33*f*
under-5 mortality rate, 518*f*
symptom, 182
syndemic, 288
syndrome, 182
syndromic surveillance, 128
syphilis, 196, 512
systems thinking, 6
systolic blood pressure, 381, 385*f*

T

Taenia, 257*f*
taeniasis, 281
target, 29
TBA. *See* traditional birth attendant
(TBA)
TB disease, 197
T cells, 182
teratogens, 90
tertiary prevention, 7, 7*f*
tetanus, 321
Tetra Tech, Inc, 170
TFR. *See* total fertility rate (TFR)
thalassemia, 444
theory of planned behavior, 372
theory of reasoned action, 372
thiamine, 350
TIA. *See* transient ischemic attack
(TIA)
TNM classification system, 393
tobacco control, 433–436, 433*f*
tobacco smoking, 433, 433*f*, 435–436*f*
among adults, 435*f*
by sex, 436*f*
toilets, 80–82
total dependency ratio, 539, 541*f*
total fertility rate (TFR), 299*f*, 300,
302*f*
toxicology, 89
toxoid vaccine, 236

Toxoplasma gondii, 282
trachoma, 277
Trade-Related Aspects of Intellectual
Property Rights (TRIPS)
Agreement, 113
traditional birth attendant (TBA), 313
trafficking, 68
transdisciplinary approach, 548, 549*f*
trans fat, 334
transgender, 325
transient ischemic attack (TIA), 379
transitions, global health, 1–18
transmissibility, 288
transport injuries, 484–488,
485–488*f*
mortality rates, 485–486*f*
transtheoretical model, 372
traumatic brain injury (TBI), 473
trematode, 257
Treponema carateum, 278
Treponema pallidum, 196, 278
Trichomonas vaginalis, 196, 256
trichomoniasis, 196
trichuriasis, 273–274
Trichuris trichiura, 273
TRIPS Agreement, 113
Trypanosoma brucei, 275, 275*f*
Trypanosoma brucei gambiense, 275
Trypanosoma brucei rhodesiense, 275
Trypanosoma cruzi, 256
trypanosomiasis, 274, 275
TST. *See* Mantoux tuberculin skin
test (TST)
tsunami, Indian Ocean (2004), 151
tuberculosis (TB), 177–179, 197–199
epidemiology, 199–202,
200–201*f*
incidence rate, 204*f*
interventions, 202–205, 202*f*
mortality, 202, 204*f*
in prison, 118
skin test, 198*f*
spending on, 205*f*
TB Drug Accelerator program, 178
X-ray of, 198*f*
tumor, 393
type 1 diabetes, 425
type 2 diabetes, 425, 430*f*
typhoid, 217, 221

U

UDHR. *See* Universal Declaration of
Human Rights (UDHR)
UHC. *See* universal health coverage
(UHC)
U5MR. *See* under-5 mortality rate
(U5MR)

UN. *See* United Nations (UN)
UNAIDS. *See* United Nations
Programme on HIV/AIDS
(UNAIDS)
under-5 child, 507
underemployment, 64
under-5 mortality rate (U5MR), 509,
509*f*, 510*f*
undernutrition, 341
underweight, 337
UNDP. *See* United Nations
Development Programme
(UNDP)
unemployment, 64
UN Environment Programme
(UNEP), 161
UNEP. *See* UN Environment
Programme (UNEP)
UNFPA. *See* UN Population Fund
(UNFPA)
UNHCR. *See* Office of the United
Nations High Commissioner
for Refugees (UNHCR)
UNICEF. *See* United Nations
Children's Fund (UNICEF)
unintentional injuries, 481,
492–493
unipolar depressive disorder, 459
United Nations (UN), 160–163,
161*f*
Every Woman Every Child, 519
General Assembly, 160, 161
and global health, 107, 108*f*
Human Settlements Programme,
162
programs and funds, 161, 161*f*
Security Council, 161
specialized agencies, 162, 162*f*
United Nations Children's Fund
(UNICEF), 162, 517–518
United Nations Development
Programme (UNDP), 161
United Nations Programme on
HIV/AIDS (UNAIDS), 163,
177, 185
United States
Centers for Disease Control and
Prevention (CDC), 167, 253
Department of Health and
Human Services (HHS), 167
disease-specific charities, 145
food consumed in, 356*f*
foreign aid expenditures, 146,
147*f*
nonprofit organizations, 151
Patient Protection and Affordable
Care Act (ACA) of 2010, 143

United States Agency for International Development (USAID), 147, 170
Universal Declaration of Human Rights (UDHR), 107–108, 109f, 110
universal health coverage (UHC), 139, 139f, 142f
universal precautions, 194
UNODC. See UN Office on Drugs and Crime (UNODC)
UN Office for the Coordination of Humanitarian Affairs (OCHA), 125
UN Office on Drugs and Crime (UNODC), 161
UN Population Fund (UNFPA), 161
unsaturated fatty acid, 334
upper respiratory infection, 224
urbanicity, 92, 92f, 95f, 96f
  health risks, 93, 94f
urbanization, 92–96, 290
urinary bladder cancers, 415
urticaria, 451
USAID, 159. See United States Agency for International Development (USAID)
U.S. Centers for Disease Control and Prevention (CDC), 17f, 18f
uterine cancer, 410

V

vaccinations, 17, 110, 133, 135, 196–197, 235, 238–242
  available, 241f
vaccine-associated paralytic poliomyelitis (VAPP), 287
vaccine hesitancy, 237
vaccine-preventable infections, 238–242
vaccines, 60
Valley fever. See Coccidioidomycosis
values, 108
VAPP. See vaccine-associated paralytic poliomyelitis (VAPP)
variola major, 285
variola minor, 285
vasectomies, 308
VCT. See voluntary counseling and testing (VCT)
vector, 257
vector-borne disease. See specific disease
vector-borne infection, 266, 267f

vector control, 265
ventilation-improved pit (VIP) latrine, 81
ventricular tachycardia, 386
vertical program, 158
vertical transmission, 192
VIA. See visual inspection with acetic acid (VIA)
Vibrio cholerae, 218
violence, 494
viral hepatitis, 242–244
  types of, 243f
viral infections, 180
virion, 180
virulence, 288
viruses, 179
vision impairment, 446–449, 448f
visual inspection with acetic acid (VIA), 409
vital statistics, 34–36
vitamin A, 349
vitamin A deficiency, 349–350
vitamin C, 350
vitamin D, 350
vitamins, 345, 346f
VMMC. See voluntary male medical circumcision (VMMC)
voluntary counseling and testing (VCT), 192
voluntary male medical circumcision (VMMC), 194
voluntourism, 552

W

WASH program, 82
wasting, 337
water, and nutrition, 334–335
water privatization, 122
water, sanitation, and hygiene (WASH) programs, 82
water scarcity, 122
water service level, 79f
water-soluble vitamin, 345
water sources, 80
  access to, 83–84, 84f
  global percentage of, 83
wealth, 57
Weekly Epidemiological Record, 44
West Nile virus, 268
WFP. See World Food Programme (WFP)
WHA. See World Health Assembly (WHA)
whipworm. See trichuriasis

WHO. See World Health Organization (WHO)
WHO/UNICEF Joint Monitoring Programme for Water Supply and Sanitation, 83–84
whooping cough. See pertussis
wild poliovirus (WPV), 288
women's health, 61–63, 323–324
workforce, health, 119–121
World Bank, 164
World Food Programme (WFP), 162
World Health Assembly, 162, 339, 422, 434
World Health Organization (WHO), 3, 24, 162, 223, 260, 263, 270, 370, 383, 434, 468, 517–518
  Child Growth Standards, 337, 339f
  Expanded Program on Immunization (EPI), 238, 516
World Obesity Federation, 355
World Organisation for Animal Health (OIE), 163
World Trade Organization (WTO), 112
World Vision, 151
WPV. See wild poliovirus (WPV)
WTO. See World Trade Organization (WTO)

X

XDR-TB. See extensively drug-resistant TB (XDR-TB)
xerophthalmia, 349

Y

yaws, 278
years lived with disability (YLDs), 41, 457, 458f, 513f, 514, 515f, 519f, 521f, 523f, 524f, 531, 532f, 533f, 534f, 536f, 543f
years of life lost (YLLs), 41, 531–532, 534f
yellow fever, 267–268
YLDs. See years lived with disability (YLDs)
YLLs. See years of life lost (YLLs)

Z

Zika virus, 269
zinc, 349
zoonosis, 233
z-score, 337–338